EUROPEAN FEDERATION OF NATIONAL ASSOCIATIONS
OF ORTHOPAEDICS AND TRAUMATOLOGY

EUROPEAN INSTRUCTIONAL COURSE LECTURES

VOLUME 5

2001

European Federation of National Associations of Orthopaedics and Traumatology

European Federation of National Associations of Orthopaedics and Traumatology

EUROPEAN INSTRUCTIONAL COURSE LECTURES

VOLUME 5 2001

Edited by:

K.-G. THORNGREN
University Hospital in Lund
Sweden

P. N. SOUCACOS
University of Iaonnina, Iaonnina
Greece

F. HORAN
Editor, Journal of Bone and Joint Surgery
London

J. SCOTT
Associate Editor, Journal of Bone and Joint Surgery
London

Published by
The British Editorial Society of Bone and Joint Surgery
22 Buckingham Street
London

The British Editorial Society of Bone and Joint Surgery

Chairman: David L. HAMBLEN
Editor: Frank HORAN
General Manager: Stephen BISHOP
Production Manager: Fay MILLER
Production Editor: Kate TAYLOR

ISBN: 0-9525921-3-4
ISSN: 1359-2335

The British Editorial Society of Bone and Joint Surgery
22 Buckingham Street
London WC2N 6ET
U.K.
Tel: 44(0)20-7782-0010
Fax: 44(0)20-7782-0995

Printed in U.K.

CONTENTS

Tumours

Primary bone disease

Spine

Upper extremity

Hip

Knee

Foot and ankle

PREFACE

The Instructional Course Lectures (ICL) of the European Federation of National Associations of Orthopaedics and Traumatology (EFORT) constitute a major source of updated information within a wide spectrum of orthopaedics including trauma of the locomotor system. The information contained here will first be presented in early June 2001 at the fifth EFORT Congress in Rhodes, Greece. For the future, the full text will be available and further spread through the present issue of the EFORT Instructional Course Lectures. Together with the previous volumes of EFORT ICL they provide a base for both specialist education and continued postgraduate learning throughout Europe. The lectures would also be useful for this purpose in a wider international perspective.

As Editor of these ICL of 2001 it is a great challenge to fulfil the high goals and ambitions of EFORT on education. This is only possible through the great effort of all the authors of this volume. On behalf of EFORT I want to thank them for all the dedicated work needed to make their specialised knowledge available to their colleagues in this way. The editorial ambition behind this ICL volume has been to highlight actual and important aspects of a wide spectrum of diseases and trauma of the locomotor system with the selection of experts from most parts of Europe. The number of lectures has been expanded to 26 in this volume. The authors have been asked to write a comprehensive current concepts review aimed at both a general and a subspecialist orthopaedic audience. I am grateful for the suggestions made through the EFORT network of national associations and the advice for selection from the Scientific Committee. I am furthermore grateful for the fruitful collaboration with my Co-Editor, Panayotis Soucacos, who is also Chairman of the Organising Committee for the Rhodes Congress and to Frank Horan, the Editor of the British volume of the *Journal of Bone and Joint Surgery*, and his staff who have facilitated this publication.

The high quality of EFORT educational material is only possible through this whole-hearted support of all the membership associations. The combined resources of our Federation provide a strong platform for the present and future spread of existing knowledge and new achievements within the whole field of diseases and trauma of the locomotor system.

Karl-Göran Thorngren

FOREWORD

The fifth EFORT Congress in Rhodes continues the tradition of the Instructional Course Lecture series initiated at the first EFORT Congress held in Paris. The Instructional Course Lectures have become pivotal to the EFORT educational programme, by presenting the latest and most noteworthy developments in orthopaedic surgery and discussing current issues in clinical practice and surgery, as well as landmarks in orthopaedic research.

The fifth volume of the Instructional Course series contains 26 lectures from renowned surgeons representing the entirety of the European orthopaedic family which were selected and edited expertly by Professor Karl-Göran Thorngren. The production of this volume was achieved under the careful eye of the *Journal of Bone and Joint Surgery* and its Editor, Frank Horan. As an integral part of the EFORT Congresses, the Instructional Course Book is distributed free to all congress participants. With the assistance of the authors, Professor Thorngren and Mr Horan, the EFORT Instructional Course Series has become a cornerstone in the continuing educational programme of European orthopaedic surgeons.

Panayotis N. Soucacos
Chairman, Organising Committee
Fifth EFORT Congress

CONTRIBUTORS

Robin Allum
The Consulting Rooms, 9 Beaumont Road, Windsor, Berks SL4 1HY, UK

F. Alvarez
Hospital Sant Rafael, Barcelona, Spain

P. Beaufils
Centre Hospitalier de Versailles, Hôpital André Mignot, 177 rue de Versailles, 78157 Le Chesnay Cedex, France

X. Cassard
Clinique des Cèdres, Toulouse, France

Tore Dalén
Umeå University Hospital, 901 85 Umeå, Sweden

Ioannis N. Gaitanis
Department of Orthopaedic Surgery and Traumatology, University of Crete, School of Health Sciences, University General Hospital, PO Box 1352, Heraklion, 711 10, Crete, Greece

S. Giannini
Istituto Ortopedico Rizzoli, Via G. C. Pupilli 1, 40136 Bologna, Italy

Ph. Gillet
Centre Hospitalier Universitaire, Domaine Universitaire du Sart Tilman - B.35, B-4000 Liège, Belgium

D. Goutallier
Hôpital Henri Mondor, 51 avenue Marchal de Lattre de Tasigny, 94010 Créteil, France

N. P. Haas
Charite Universitätsklinikum Medizinische Fakultät der Humboldt zu Berlin, Augustenburger Platz 1, D- 13353 Berlin, Germany

Alexander G. Hadjipavlou
Department of Orthopaedic Surgery and Traumatology, University of Crete, School of Health Sciences, University General Hospital, PO Box 1352, Heraklion, 711 10, Crete, Greece

P. Hardy
Hôpital Ambroise Paré, Boulogne, France

P. Hoffmeyer
Clinique d'orthopédie et de chirurgie de l'appareil moteur, Hôpital Cantonal, 24 rue Micheli-du-Crest, CH-1211, Genève 14, Switzerland

D. Huten
Groupe Hospitalier Bichat Claude-Bernard, 46 rue Henri Huchard, 75877 Paris, France

Andreas B. Imhoff
Abteilung und Poliklinik für Sportorthopädie, der Technischen Universität München, Connollystrasse 32, 80809 München, Germany

Andrew M. Jackson
107 Harley Street, London W1, UK

M. Kasparek
Orthopädisches Spital Wien-Speising, Speisingerstrasse 109, A-1134 Wien, Austria

K. Knahr
Orthopädisches Spital Wien-Speising, Speisingerstrasse 109, A-1134 Wien, Austria

Manvilius Kocius
Clinic of Traumatology and Orthopaedics, Vilnius University Emergency Hospital, Siltnamiu 29, 2043 Vilnius, Lithuania

R. Krauspe
Heinrich Henine Universität Düsseldorf, Orthopädische Klinik, Postfach 10 10 07, D-40001 Düsseldorf, Germany

Martin Krismer
Universitätsklinik für Orthopädie, Anischstrasse 35, A-6020 Innsbruck, Austria

J. Krugluger
Orthopädisches Spital Wien-Speising, Speisingerstrasse 109, A-1134 Wien, Austria

P. Leguilloux
Henri Mondor Hospital, Créteil, France

Vladimir Martinek
Abteilung und Poliklinik für Sportorthopädie, der Technischen Universität München, Connollystrasse 32, 80809 München, Germany

Werner Müller
Kantonsspital, CH 4101 Bruderholz, Basel, Switzerland

Martyn J. Parker
Peterborough District Hospital, Thorpe Road, Peterborough PE3 6DA, UK

J. M. Postel
Henri Mondor Hospital, Créteil, France

David I. Rowley
Dundee Royal Infirmary, Barrack Road, Dundee DD1 9ND, Scotland

W. Schneider
Orthopädisches Spital Wien-Speising, Speisingerstrasse 109, A-1134 Wien, Austria

Jan Skowroński
Department of Orthopaedics and Trauma, Medical University of Bialystok, 24A Sklodowskiej Curie Street, 15-275 Bialystok, Poland

Michael M. Stephens
The Childrens Hospital, Temple Street, Dublin 1, Ireland

Panayotis P. Symeonides
3 Gregoriou Palama Street, 54622 Thessaloniki, Greece

A. Viladot Jr
Hospital Sant Rafael, Barcelona, Spain

R. Viladot
75 calle Dr Roux, 08017 Barcelona, Spain

Geert H. I. M. Walenkamp
Academisch Ziekenhuis Maastricht, P. Debyelaan 25, Postbus 5800, 6202 AZ Maastricht, The Netherlands

B. Westhoff
Heinrich Henine Universität Düsseldorf, Orthopädische Klinik, Postfach 10 10 07, D-40001 Düsseldorf, Germany

A. Wild
Heinrich Henine Universität Düsseldorf, Orthopädische Klinik, Postfach 10 10 07, D-40001 Düsseldorf, Germany

W. Winkelmann
Klinik und Poliklinik für Allgemeine Orthopädie, Albert Schweitzer Strasse 33, 48129 Münster, Germany

Theodore A. Xenakis
Department of Orthopaedic Surgery, University of Ioannina, School of Medicine, Ioannina 45110, Greece

BLOOD-SAVING PROCEDURES IN ORTHOPAEDIC SURGERY

TORE DALÉN

From Umea University Hospital, Sweden

Interest in reducing the need for allogeneic blood transfusion has increased in recent years mainly because of the fear of transmission of disease. Transfusion of blood is extremely safe, but has several potentially fatal hazards. Blood itself has been of great interest for centuries and the use of blood transfusion is banned by some religions. Orthopaedic surgery is a large consumer of banked blood both in elective and emergency surgery. To be able to avoid allogeneic blood transfusion, the necessity for the requirement of blood has to be understood better and the efficacy of current practices critically evaluated. With proper planning and the use of a number of different procedures, most operations can be completed successfully without the need for transfusion.

HISTORY

Blood is associated with many myths and beliefs. In ancient Greece Galenos thought blood was one of the four liquids constituting the body. This belief is thought to be responsible for the centuries-old custom of blood-letting in order to get rid of 'bad blood'. In literature blood is often used in magical rites, for example in the opera *Faust*.[1] There are also many religious opinions about blood; Jehovah's Witnesses refuse blood transfusions and all food made of animal blood.

In the early 1800s an important contribution was made by the surgeon and obstetrician James Blundell in London, also called the 'father of modern autotransfusion'. He tried to find a way of preventing death from postpartum haemorrhage in young women and developed a method for the collection, temporary storage and reinfusion of the shed blood.[2] Miller[3] and later Duncan[4] independently reported the successful reinfusion of shed blood after amputation of the lower limbs. In the early 1900s the ABO antigen system was discovered and a better explanation was given for the problems of incompatibility at transfusion.[5] During World War I the need for replacement of blood loss was further recognised, and methods were developed for the collection and storage of blood to be available for emergencies. In 1921 preoperative blood collection for subsequent reinfusion at surgery was used in a patient with polycythaemia and a cerebellar meningioma.[6]

Banked blood was used during World War II and the experience gained stimulated the growing number of blood banks after the war. Homologous transfusion was necessary for many operations and regarded as practically free from risk in the first decades after World War II. Major complications such as transfusion reactions and hepatitis occurred so infrequently that they were of little concern.[7] Most reactions were febrile responses which disappeared when the transfusion was stopped. Fatal reactions were extremely rare. Many patients who had reactions to blood transfusions later experienced difficulties in cross-matching blood, but the connection to the former transfusion was not obvious for many years. Initially, the association between transfusion and hepatitis was not recognised, but testing of donor blood for possible contamination or diseases was slowly introduced into transfusion practice. This changed rapidly when acquired immune deficiency syndrome (AIDS) was discovered in the last years of the 1970s, and it was found that it could also be transmitted by blood transfusion. This led to a growing demand for the avoidance of allogeneic transfusions to offset possible problems.

RISKS WITH HOMOLOGOUS BLOOD

Transfusion of homologous bank blood involves a risk of complications. Apart from human error, these can be divided into transfusion reactions, transmission of disease and immunomodulation. Mistransfusions leading to major morbidity or death by human error occur, and are the major cause of complications of transfusion of blood or its components.[8]

Transfusion reactions, which occur in approximately 5% of transfusions in the USA,[9] can be separated into acute intravascular immune haemolytic reactions, delayed extravascular immune haemolysis and febrile reactions.[10] The risk of a non-fatal haemolytic reaction is 1 in 25 000 and for a fatal reaction is less than 1 in a million. Febrile reactions occur in 1 in 100.[11] Blood-group incompatibility can cause an acute intravascular haemolytic reaction, with symptoms such as haemoglobinuria, fever, chills, coagulopathy, chest pain, and circulatory collapse. In a patient under anaesthesia the symptoms can be hypotension or unexpected haemorrhage. Delayed extravascular haemolytic reactions are caused by non-ABO antigen-antibody incompatibility.[10] These reactions present as either fever, malaise, hyperbilirubinaemia or a falling haematocrit. They are difficult to recognise because there is a delay of 3 to 10 days before they occur. A febrile response is the most common reaction to a transfusion and is normally caused by circulating recipient antibodies to donor leukocytes or platetets.[12] Blood can transmit a wide range of diseases, both viral and bacterial, and also rickettsias and parasites. The most common is cytomegalovirus (CMV), since 70% to 80% of donors have CMV antibodies and 1% to 4% may transmit the disease.[13-15] Transmission of hepatitis B (HBV) and C (HCV) has been radically reduced in the last few years (HBV 1/63 000 units of blood, HCV 1/103 000 units).[16] The risk of a hepatitis-infected patient developing cirrhosis within five years is about 25%.[17] The most serious transmittable viruses are human immunodeficiency virus (HIV) and human T-cell lymphotropic virus I and II (HTLV), but these risks have also decreased in recent years (HIV 1/493 000 units, HTLV 1/641 000 units).[17] In France the prevalence of seropositive donations for HIV was 1/588 000 units, for HBV 1/112 000 units and for HCV 1/217 000 units.[18] Infection by transfusion of Creutzfeldt-Jakob disease has been suggested but so far is of only theoretical concern. It is probable that other blood-transmittable agents will be discovered.[19]

Probably the most important reaction is immunomodulation. Homologous blood transfusion has an immunosuppressive effect which is mediated both by cellular and humoral factors and this has been demonstrated in a variety of animal studies.[20-24]

The immunosuppressive effect seen in recipients of a renal allograft in which there is a higher rate of survival of the allograft when homologous blood is transfused, is evidence for this effect in a clinical situation.[25] There have also been effects from different cell populations of leukocytes among patients receiving blood transfusions.[26-29] Storage of blood leads to increased levels of cytokines which can be reduced by early leukodepletion. In orthopaedic surgery allogeneic transfusions account for a higher rate of postoperative infection, mainly urinary infections and pneumonia.[30,31] These raised rates may be one factor responsible for the longer hospitalisation and subsequent increased costs when allogeneic blood is used.[30,32] The rate of recurrence after cancer surgery when allogeneic blood has been transfused is debatable. The negative immunological effects of allogeneic transfusion are probably mainly linked to the amount of leukocytes present in the blood and the use of leukodepleted blood could probably reduce the negative effects of the transfusion.[33] Whether immunomodulation also has an effect on the healing of fractures or the process of loosening of joint prostheses is not known. Fluid overload necessitating the use of a diuretic is also more frequently associated with the use of allogeneic transfusion compared with autologous or no transfusion.[30]

SURGERY AND THE NEED FOR TRANSFUSION

Most operations do not need a blood transfusion, but in extensive surgery in which homeostasis is a problem, such as major cardiothoracic operations, prostate resections and major orthopaedic operations, transfusions are common. Orthopaedic surgery is the specialty requiring the largest number of blood transfusions in Sweden. Total joint arthroplasty is one of the more common orthopaedic surgical procedures and despite refinements in fixation and design leading to increased survival of the prosthesis, the avoidance of transfusion still remains a problem. A total knee replacement (TKR) has an estimated mean blood loss of between 600 and 1500 ml, and patients are often transfused with a mean of two units of blood.[19,34-38] With bilateral TKR the loss is doubled and revision procedures require larger volumes of blood than primary replacements due to the exposure of large areas of soft tissue, cancellous bone, often with more extensive soft-tissue release and violation of the femoral and tibial medullary canals. The amount of blood loss is also dependent on gender, the method of fixation of the prosthesis, the use of a tourniquet, postoperative salvage drains and the extent of the surgical exposure. Total joint replacements are done primarily on older people with smaller margins for blood loss and these operations would be much more dangerous to perform if blood were not available. Recent studies have reported a transfusion rate (autologous and/or allogeneic) of 39% to 57% after joint replacements, with a higher frequency in hip replacements.[30,39]

In a regular orthopaedic ward, without any blood-conservation programme, blood transfusions for joint replacement account for about half of the blood used; the other half is mainly for fractures and spinal and tumour surgery.

INDICATIONS FOR TRANSFUSION

There are operations which cannot be done without blood transfusions, but when to transfuse is debatable. In the past, the trigger point for transfusion was usually a haemoglobin level below 100 g/l or a haematocrit below 30%. In 1988, the NIH (National Institute of Health) in the USA stated that: "..otherwise healthy patients with haemoglobin values of 100 g/l or greater rarely require peroperative transfusion, whereas those with acute anaemia with resulting haemoglobin levels of less than 70 g/l will frequently require red blood cell transfusions".[40] The need for transfusion at levels of haemoglobin above 80 g/l has been discussed and it has been shown that postoperative mortality has not been reduced, even in older orthopaedic patients.[41] Patients who are Jehovah's Witnesses with Hb concentrations of 5 g/dl or less have shown an increased rate of mortality.[42] An important predictor of the requirement of postoperative blood transfusion is the preoperative level of Hb. Patients under the age of 65 years with a level

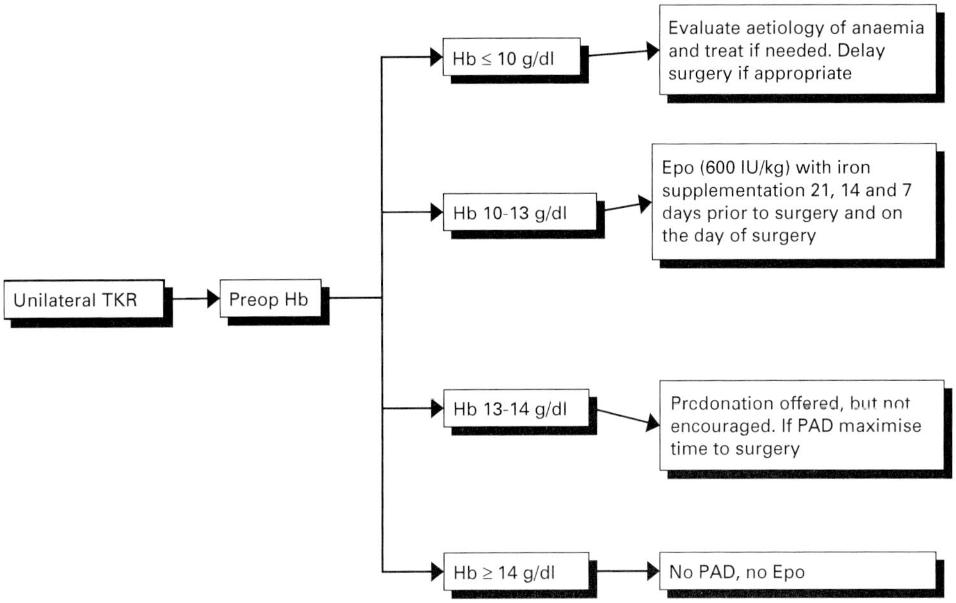

Fig. 1

Diagram of a preoperative algorithm used for TKR at the Insall Scott Kelly Institute for Orthopaedics and Sports Medicine.

between 13 and 15 g/dl have a minimal risk of requiring transfusion after primary joint replacement.[39] The lower the preoperative Hb level, the higher is the transfusion rate.[43]

The postoperative Hb and haematocrit levels are directly proportional to the energy levels of the patients and the ability to exercise and regain strength.[44] The level of the postoperative haematocrit is also correlated with the number of medical complications.[45]

DIFFERENT METHODS FOR REDUCTION OF BLOOD LOSS

Surgical. Preoperative planning for surgery is important. An algorithm to calculate the expected blood loss and to indicate how much can be tolerated in the specific patient should be used.[46] In this way the necessity for the individual planning of different blood-conservation methods becomes apparent (Fig. 1). Planning should also include giving detailed information of the risks, benefits and alternatives to the patient and/or his family on the options for reduction of blood loss. There is also a need for more specific orthopaedic planning including the timing of the surgery, the use of less invasive procedures (arthroscopic *v* open surgery, external fixator *v* open reduction-internal fixation), fixation of implants (cemented *v* uncemented) and also preoperative templating of the implants. Removal of cement with the help of ultrasound causes less bleeding than by the standard techniques.

A thorough preoperative history which includes the personal and family history, bleeding disorders, known anaemia, known cardiac, pulmonary, renal or hepatic disease or any medications which may cause bleeding disturbance, must be taken. A physical examination with emphasis on signs of bleeding disorders and/or hepatomegaly or splenomegaly should also be done. Laboratory tests should include the blood count and clotting studies if an abnormality is suspected. Microsampling techniques should be used for blood tests to reduce the amount of blood lost in the test procedure. Sensors applied to the skin can monitor tissue oxygen levels and other blood gases accurately without drawing blood.

During the operation the positioning of the patient has a role in the amount of bleeding. The surgical field should be positioned above the level of the heart and compression which may cause obstruction of venous reflow should be avoided, for example in spinal surgery. Positioning should aim at promoting venous drainage away from the surgical field. In total hip replacement (THR) the lateral position has been shown to decrease blood loss.[47,48] Careful operation with gentle tissue handling, dissection along anatomical planes and the frequent use of electrocautery is crucial. The least vascular approach should be selected; for example, trochanteric osteotomy should be avoided if possible. Vessels should be controlled before cutting and local haemostatic agents should be used. Checks should be made to ensure that all bleeding has stopped before closure. Interventional radiological procedures may be performed before surgery to minimise blood loss, or after surgery to help stem bleeding. Temporary occlusion of a vessel can be done by a balloon catheter or permanently with coils or pieces of haemostatic agent, which is the most common procedure in trauma and tumour surgery. Most bleeding in joint replacement operations occurs during sawing or milling. A tourniquet should be used in limb surgery and is important if postoperative salvage by drains is planned. If salvage is not planned, the use of drains is controversial and probably in many cases not beneficial.[49]

Anaesthesiological. The method of anaesthesia is important. Regional anaesthesia has been shown to reduce the intraoperative blood loss to less than half of the normal level.[50,51] Parameters under the immediate control of the anaesthetist such as the intravascular pressure, cardiac output and levels of CO_2 can influence intraoperative blood loss. Controlled hypotension has been advocated for reducing blood loss with excellent results.[52] Hypotension can be achieved by a reduction in cardiac output, systemic vascular resistance, or both. Blood flow sufficient to maintain adequate tissue oxygenation and metabolism must be provided. Usually controlled hypotension is achieved by decreasing vascular resistance with only a limited reduction in cardiac output. This is usually accomplished by deepening the level of anaesthesia, the use of spinal/epidural anaesthesia or of rapid-acting antihypertensive medication. Close monitoring together with appropriate patient selection is essential when controlled hypotension is used. Maintaining the body temperature is important, as a general cooling of the body increases the blood loss. In THR this is partly caused by deranged coagulation.[53] Active warming of the patient during operation is shown to reduce the requirements of homologous blood.[54] The use of plasma-volume expanders is common practice in patients who are hypovolaemic or need resuscitation. Aggressive fluid replacement with crystalloid infusion in non-fatal uncontrolled haemorrhage can increase the volume of haemorrhage and mortality. Therefore restoration of blood pressure should not be attempted until definite operative control of the haemorrhage has been obtained.[55] Artificial oxygen carriers such as Hb solutions and perfluorocarbon emulsions are a possible alternative in the future. There are problems and unsolved side-effects with these options but promising clinical results have been obtained.[56]

Pharmacological. Different agents can be utilised either generally or locally. Preoperative anaemia can often be treated with erythropoietin alpha combined with iron supplementation.[57] Erythropoietin is a glycoprotein normally secreted by peritubular cells in the kidney. Secretion is triggered by hypoxaemia but the normal rate of response is reduced by chronic inflammation and uraemia. It is commercially available and will increase the Hb and reticulocyte counts resulting in a decrease in the number of postoperative transfusions.[58] The main disadvantage is its relatively high cost and the optimal dose remains to be established.

Anaemia can also be caused by deficiency of iron, folic acid or vitamin B12, and can be treated with appropriate medication. Certain blood deficiencies can be treated prophylactically with either special fractions of blood or more often nowadays with recombinant factors such as anti-haemophilic factor VIIa, VIII and IX for different haemophilic diseases. Vitamin K is required for the production of certain blood-clotting factors in the liver. Deficiency of vitamin K can be caused by inadequate dietary intake or drug interactions. Anabolic androgenic steroids stimulate the synthesis of cellular protein and can stimulate the production of red blood cells. The preoperative withdrawal of agents affecting thrombocyte aggregation, such as non-steroidal anti-inflammatory drugs, is important. The recently introduced COX-2 inhibitors do not influence thrombocyte aggregation or the bleeding time and medication can continue until operation.[59] A prolonged bleeding time caused by thrombocyte malfunction, usually caused by the intake of analgesics, or different haemophilias, can sometimes be treated with desmopressin,[19] which causes a dose-dependent increase in factor VIII. Large doses can increase the activity of factor VIII and von Willebrand factor in patients with mild to moderate haemophilia A and B or von Willebrand's disease and also in patients with uraemia. This medication may also constrict blood vessels resulting in limited blood loss. Postoperative fibrinolysis with breakdown of blood clots can be drastically reduced or stopped with tranexamic acid.[34] This can significantly reduce the bleeding if given before the start of operation in THR or before tourniquet release in TKR. Aminocaproic acid has also been tried, but is less effective than tranexamic acid. Aprotinin inhibits the haemostatic defect induced by tissue plasminogen activator without significantly inhibiting clot lysis. It also inhibits fibrinolysis. It has been widely used in open-heart surgery, where it has been shown to reduce the total amount of transfusions by 35% to 97%.[60] A significant reduction of blood loss has also been shown in primary hip surgery with the use of high-dose aprotinin therapy.[61] The drawback is that it is a relatively costly drug with the potential to cause hypersensitivity reactions.

The local application of topical haemostatic agents such as pads, powders, pastes, sponges, solutions, meshes and special dressings may be used before and during surgery to control blood loss from open wounds. Thrombin is a commercially available haemostatic agent of bovine origin. Haemostatic agents (Actifoam, Avitene, Gelfoam, Oxycel, Surgicel, Thrombostat) are not a substitute for surgical technique or the use of a haemostatic surgical instrument, but properly used they can in certain cases reduce the bleeding by over 50%. Fibrin glue is a human-derived tissue adhesive that may be used for haemostasis and the sealing of tissues. Local cold compression dressings can also decrease bleeding.[62]

AUTOLOGOUS BLOOD

Autologous blood can be utilised in four different ways. Preoperative donation of blood is a well-known method widely used and well documented.[7,63,64] The blood can be collected and stored for up to six weeks before operation. Patients are often motivated and interested, but there are drawbacks. The main disadvantage with predonation is that it is costly. There is also a demand for a thorough planning of operations beforehand, and there must be an interested blood-bank service. Several reports have also shown that a large number of predonating patients do not receive any blood back. The predonated blood is then discarded. This waste of autologous blood is reported to be around 45%,[30,39] although it has been recommended that all blood should be given back.[45] There are also reports showing a poor erythropoietic response in patients donating autologous blood before operation.[65-67] This can lead to a progressive decrease in Hb and haematocrit and the overall gain of the donation is questionable. Patients who have donated blood may still require allogeneic transfusions, but the need is reduced. The risk for allogeneic transfusion is higher among patients with a low preoperative Hb. In one report 34% of patients donating blood had a preoperative Hb between 10 and 13 g/dl; 28% of these required allogeneic transfusion.[30]

The second way of obtaining autologous blood is by acute preoperative normovolaemic haemodilution. Just before operation 1 to 4 units of blood are collected from the patient and temporarily stored. Crystalloid or colloid solution is used to replace the blood loss. Fewer red blood cells are lost during the procedure because surgical bleeding occurs at a lower hematocrit. When a transfusion is needed the blood collected is readily available.[68] Close monitoring is necessary during operation, combined with the attention of an experienced anaesthesiologist. The final gain in blood and economy is debatable.[69-71.]

The third method is the collection of shed blood intraoperatively. During operation the blood is salvaged with suction, and heparin or citrate is added for anticoagulation. The blood is treated by centrifugation and washed with a saline solution in a so-called 'cell saver' machine[63] or treated by washing and ultrafiltration for haemoconcentration.[72] The advantages of these collecting-and-washing methods are that the product consists mainly of concentrated erythrocytes, and the number of contaminants from the unwashed blood is reduced. The method is also used in the emergency/trauma setting for rapid recovery and immediate reinfusion of warm blood to patients with a wide range of different injuries. The disadvantages are the cost, and when used in orthopaedic surgery there is only a gain of 30% to 60% of lost erythrocytes.[73,74] For peroperative haemorrhage below 1.0 to 1.5 l, the value of using this method is doubtful,[75,76] but it should be considered for operations with larger blood loss such as revision hip surgery, bilateral joint replacement, major spinal surgery or trauma surgery.

The fourth way of using autologous blood is by collecting shed blood after surgery. The blood is collected by drainage and returned to the patient either after centrifugation and washing as described above, or through a filtering technique. The drained blood is filtered in different steps and there are special procedures to reduce the fat content. The first filter removes large debris such as cell fragments, clotted blood, and bone substances and possible bone-cement particles. The last filter has usually the same pore size as regular transfusion filters (40 μm) or smaller. No anticoagulant is needed because the blood is free from fibrinogen. The drained blood has low counts of leukocytes and platelets, especially initially. The blood should not be retransfused later than six to eight hours hours after operation. The filter method is simple and relatively cheap and if salvaged volumes are moderate the method is safe.[49] It is considered particularly effective for knee arthroplasty.

The transfusion of autologous blood is not without risk, despite the obvious advantages. Adverse immunological reactions have been reported such as allergic reactions, febrile non-haemolytic reactions, immune and non-immune haemolysis and coagulopathies.[77-79] Bacterial contamination and fluid overload are also a concern. Most of these reactions are probably due to clerical error in that allogeneic blood is mistakenly given instead of the donated autologous unit. These errors occur in approximately 1 in 24 000 autologous transfusions.[80]

SPECIAL SITUATIONS

Infected patients requiring revision of a joint replacement are not suitable for preoperative donation or reinfusion of autologous blood during or after surgery. They may have anaemia as a result of the infection, and they will also lose more blood than usual in the surgical procedure because of the inflammation and extensive surgery, often done in two stages. In these patients other methods must be used.

Intra- and postoperative blood salvage is contraindicated in tumour surgery because of contaminating tumour cells and the risk of systemic dissemination. With irradiation of salvaged blood with 50 Gy, all cancer cells are eliminated from the blood.[81] These preliminary results mean that autotransfusion could probably also be used in clinical practice during cancer surgery.

In trauma surgery the priority should be to stop the bleeding first before proceeding to definitive reconstruction. Salvage of blood should be done from cavities and surgical sites with the use of a 'cell-saver'. Hypotension should be tolerated until bleeding is under control, and then normovolaemia should be restored. If bleeding persists the patient must return for further surgery and if the circulatory system is not stable or the patient is still bleeding, transfer between hospitals should be avoided. Embolisation or hyperoxic ventilation should be borne in mind. Some patients refuse blood donation because of religious or other reasons. Most of these are Jehovah's Witnesses who refuse all blood transfusions if the bloodstream is disconnected from the body in any way. This means that preoperative donation and acute preoperative normovolaemic haemodilution cannot be used. Peroperative and postoperative salvage of blood can be used if a continuous line with stopcocks is prepared before the salvage starts. Usually all other procedures such as pharmacological and anaesthesiological methods are accepted, but this can vary and in elective surgery must be thoroughly discussed with each patient before operation.

SUMMARY

Blood is an important prerequisite for many major orthopaedic operations. Transfusion of allogeneic blood is associated with a certain risk of transmission of disease, although blood transfusion is an extremely safe procedure. Today the prevention of human error is the most important step in clinical practice. Immunomodulation caused by the transfusion may result in postoperative infections. Reducing blood loss by careful pre- and intraoperative planning is vital and eliminating the need for allogeneic transfusions must be the goal to optimise the outcome. If blood is needed at or after an operation, autologous blood is a natural choice when there is an option. There is an ongoing refinement of salvage techniques of autologous blood. Pharmacological methods to reduce blood loss will probably be further developed and research is currently in progress in regard to blood substitutes which can act as an oxygen carrier.

REFERENCES

1. **Goethe JW von.** Faust: eine Tragödie: I und II. *Teil* 1808-33.
2. **Blundell J.** Experiments on the transfusion of blood by the syringe. *Medicochirurgical Transactions* 1818;9:56-92.
3. **Miller AG.** Case of amputation at hip-joint, in which reinjection of blood was performed, and rapid recovery took place. *Edinb Med J* 1885-86;31:721-2.
4. **Duncan J.** On re-infusion of blood in primary and other amputations. Tr Med-Chir Soc Edinb 1885-86, n.s., v, 42-48. *Br Med J* 1886;I:192.
5. **Landsteiner K.** Uber Agglutinationserscheinungen normalen menschlichen Blutes. *Wien Klin Wochenschr* 1901;14:1132-4.
6. **Grant FC.** Autotransfusion. *Ann Surg* 1921;74:253-4.
7. **Spence RK, Cenaianu AC, Carson J, Del Rossi AJ.** Transfusion and surgery. *Curr Prob Surg* 1993;30:12.
8. **Williamson LM, Lowe S, Love EM, et al.** Serious hazards of transfusion (SHOT) initiative: analysis of the first two annual reports. *BMJ* 1999;319:16-9.
9. **Goodnough LT, Shuck JM.** Risks, options and informed consent for blood transfusion in elective surgery. *Am J Surg* 1990;59:602-7.
10. **Pisciotto PT.** *Transfusion reactions.* In: blood transfusion therapy: a physicians handbook, 3rd ed. Arlington, Va: American Association of Blood Banks, 1989:77-85.
11. **Aubuchon JP, Busch M, Epstein JS, et al.** *Increasing the safety of blood transfusions.* Washington DC: American Red Cross, 1992.
12. **Heddle NM, Klama LN, Griffith L, et al.** A prospective study to identify the risk factors associated with acute reactions to platelet and red cell transfusions. *Transfusion* 1993;33:794-97.
13. **Leikola J.** Transfusion transmitted infectious agents, excluding hepatitis and human immunodeficiency viruses. *Acta Anaesth Scand* 1988;32 Suppl 89:20-5.
14. **Lindholm A.** Safety of blood products in Scandinavia today. *Acta Anaesth Scand* 1988;32 Suppl 89:35-8.
15. **Mollison PL, Engelfreit CP, Contreras M.** *Blood transfusion in clinical medicine.* 8th ed. Oxford: Blackwell Scientific Publictions, 1987.
16. **Schreiber GB, Busch MP, Kleinman SH, Korelitz JJ.** The risk of transfusion-transmitted viral infections. *N Engl J Med* 1996;334:1685-90.
17. **Mattson L.** Chronic non-A, non-B hepatitis, with special reference to the transfusion-associated form. Thesis. Stockholm: Karolinska Institutet, 1989.
18. **Baron JF.** The hemovigilance network: The French experience. In: *Building a Blood System for the 21st Century. Proceedings and Recommendations.* Health Canada, 1997:37-9.
19. **Flordal PA.** Haemostatic mechanism and blood loss in total hip replacement, with special reference to the effects of desmopressin. Thesis. Danderyd: Karolinska Institutet, 1992.
20. **Blumberg N, Heal JM.** Transfusion and recipient immune function. *Arch Pathol Lab Med* 1989;113:246-53.
21. **Bradley JA.** The blood transfusion effect: experimental aspects. *Immunol Lett* 1991;29:127-32.
22. **Perkins HA.** Transfusion-induced immunologic unresponsiveness. *Transfus Med Rev* 1988;2:196-203.
23. **Van Aken WG.** Does perioperative blood transfusion promote tumor growth? *Transfus Med Rev* 1989;III:243-52.
24. **Waymack JP, Yurt RW.** The effect of blood transfusions on immune function v the effect on the inflammatory response to bacterial infections. *J Surg Res* 1990;48:147-53.
25. **Ahmed Z, Terasaki PI.** *Effects of transfusions in clinical transplants 1991.* Terasaki P, ed. Los Angeles: UCLA Tissue Typing Laboratory, 1991:305-12.
26. **Fernandez LA, MacSween JM, You CK, Gorelick M.** Immunologic changes after blood transfusion in patients undergoing vascular surgery. *Am J Surg* 1992;163:263-9.
27. **Gascon P, Zoumbos NC, Young NS.** Immunological abnormalities in patients receiving multiple blood transfusions. *Ann Intern Med* 1984;100:173-7.
28. **Kaplan J, Sarnaik S, Gitlin J, Lusher J.** Diminished helper/suppressor lymphocyte ratios and natural killer activity in recipients of repeated blood transfusions. *Blood* 1984;64:308-10.
29. **Triulzi DJ, Vanek K, Ryan DH, Blumberg N.** A clinical and immunologic study of blood transfusion and postoperative infection in spinal surgery. *Transfusion* 1992;32:517-24.
30. **Bierbaum BE, Callaghan JJ, Galante JO, et al.** An analysis of blood management in patients having a total hip or knee arthroplasty. *J Bone Joint Surg [Am]* 1999;81-A:2-10.
31. **Carson JL, Altman DG, Duff A, et al.** Risk of bacterial infection associated with allogeneic blood transfusion among patients undergoing hip fracture repair. *Transfusion* 1999;39:694-700.
32. **Sonnenberg FA, Gregory P, Yomtovian R, et al.** The cost-effectiveness of autologous transfusion revisited: implications of an increased risk of bacterial infection with allogeneic transfusion. *Transfusion* 1999;39:808-17.
33. **Van de Watering LMG, Hermans J, Houbiers JGA, et al.** Beneficial effects of leukocyte depletion of transfused blood on postoperative complications in patients undergoing cardiac surgery: a randomized clinical trial. *Circulation* 1998;97:562-8.
34. **Benoni G.** Fibrinolysis and blood loss in major arthroplasty: the effect of tranexamic acid. Thesis. Malmö: Lund University, 1997.
35. **Dalén T, Skak S, Thorsen K.** Blood salvage in total hip arthroplasty with Solcotrans postoperative drainage. *Acta Orthop Scand* 1993;64 Suppl 253:70-1.
36. **Kristensen PW, Sorensen LS, Thyregod HC.** Autotransfusion of drainage blood in arthroplasty: a prospective controlled study of 31 operation. *Acta Orthop Scand* 1992;63:377.
37. **Lotke PA, Faralli VJ, Orestein EM, Ecker ML.** Blood loss after total knee replacement: effects of tourniquet release and continuous passive motion. *J Bone Joint Surg [Am]* 1991;73-A:1037-40.
38. **Mylod AG, Franace MP, Muser DE, Parsons JR.** Perioperative blood loss associated with total knee arthroplasty: a comparison of procedures performed with and without cementing. *J Bone Joint Surg [Am]* 1990;72-A:1010.
39. **Hatzidakis AM, Mendlick RM, McKillip T.** Preoperative autologous donation for total joint arthroplasty. *J Bone Joint Surg [Am]* 2000;82-A:89-100.
40. **Office of Medical Applications of Research, National Institutes of Health.** Perioperative red blood cell transfusion. *JAMA* 1988;260:2700-3.
41. **Carson JL, Duff A, Berlin JA, et al.** Perioperative blood transfusion and postoperative mortality. *JAMA* 1998;279:199-205.
42. **Viele MK, Weiskopf RB.** What can we learn about the need for transfusion from patients who refuse blood?: the experience with Jehovah's Witnesses. *Transfusion* 1994;34:396-401.
43. **Cushner FD, Scott WN.** Evolution of blood transfusion management for a busy knee practice. *Orthopedics* 1999;2 Suppl:145-7.

44. Keating ME, Ranawat CS, Baril WC. Assessement of postoperative vigor in patients undergoing elective total joint arthroplasty: a concise patient and caregiver instrument. *Orthopedics* 1999;2:119-28.

45. Lotke PA, Parth P, Garino JP, Cook EF. Predonated autologous blood transfusion after total knee arthroplasty. *Arthroplasty* 1999;14:647-50.

46. Nelson CL, Fontenot HJ, Flahiff C, Stewart J. An algorithm to optimize perioperative blood management in surgery. *Clin Orthop* 1998;357:36-42.

47. Hovelius L, Hussenius A, Thorling J. Posterior versus lateral approach for hip arthroplasty. *Acta Orthop Scand* 1977;48:47-51.

48. Roberts JM, Fu FH, McClain EJ, Ferguson AB Jr. A comparison of the posterolateral and anterolateral approaches to total hip arthroplasty. *Clin Orthop* 1984;187:205-10.

49. Dalén T. Postoperative autotransfusion after total knee arthroplasty. Thesis. Umea University, 1998.

50. Keith I. Anaesthesia and blood loss in total hip replacement. *Anaesthesia* 1977;32:444-50.

51. Modig J. Regional anaesthesia and blood loss. *Acta Anaesth Scand* 1988;32:44-8.

52. Sharrock NE, Salvati EA. Hypotensive epidural anesthesia for total hip arthroplasty: a review. *Acta Orthop Scand* 1996;67:91-107.

53. Schmied H, Kurz A, Sessler DI, Kozek S, Reiter A. Mild hypothermia increases blood loss and transfusion requirements during total hip arthroplasty. *Lancet* 1996;347:289-92.

54. Schmied H, Schiferer A, Sessler DI, Meznik C. The effects of red-cell scavenging, hemodilution and active warming on allogenic blood requirements in patients undergoing hip or knee arthroplasty. *Anesth Analg* 1998;86:387-91.

55. Gross D, Landau EH, Klin B, Krausz MM. Treatment of uncontroflled hemorrhagic shock with hypertonic saline solution. *Surg Gynecol Obstet* 1990;170:529-36.

56. Spahn DR, Van Brempt R, Theilmeier G, et al. Perflubron emulsion delays blood transfusions in orthopedic surgery: European Perflubron Emulsion Study Group. *Anesthesiology* 1999;91:1195-208.

57. Faris PM, Ritter MA. Epoetin alfa: a bloodless approach for the treatment of perioperative anemia. *Clin Orthop* 1998;357:60-7.

58. Faris PM, Ritter MA, Abels RI. The effects of recombinant human erythropoietin on perioperative transfusion requirements in patients having major orthopaedic operations: the erythropoietin study group. *J Bone Joint Surg [Am]* 1996;78-A:62-72.

59. Leese PT, Hubbard RC, Karim A, et al. Effects of celecoxib, a novel cyclooxygenase-2 inhibitor, on platelet function in healthy adults: a randomised, controlled trial. *J Clin Pharmacol* 2000;40:124-32.

60. Davis R, Whittinton R. Aprotinin: a review of its pharmacology and therapeutic efficacy in reducing blood loss associated with cardiac surgery. *Drugs* 1995;49:954-83.

61. Jansens M, Joris J, David JL, Lemaire R, Lamy M. High-dose aprotinin reduces blood loss in patients undergoing total hip replacement surgery. *Anesthesiology* 1994;80:23-9.

62. Levy AS, Marmar E. The role of cold compression dressings in the postoperative treatment of total knee arthroplasty. *Clin Orthop* 1993;297:174-8.

63. Elawad AAR. Autotransfusion in total hip arthroplasty. Thesis. Malmö: Lund University, 1991.

64. Toy PTCY. The use of autologous blood: the National Blood Resource Education Program Expert Panel. *JAMA* 1990;263:414-7.

65. Cohen JA, Brecher ME. Preoperative autologous blood donation: benefit or detriment?: a mathematical analysis. *Transfusion* 1995;35:640-4.

66. Goodnough LT, Brittenhem GM. Limitations of the erythropoietic response to serial phlebotomy: implications for autologous blood donor programs. *J Lab Clin Med* 1990;115:28-35.

67. Kicker TS, Spivak JL. Effect of repeated whole blood donations on serum immunoreactive erythropoietin levels in autologous donors. *JAMA* 1988;260:65-7.

68. Hur S-R, Huizenga BA, Major M. Acute normovolemic hemodilution combined with hypotensive anesthesia and other techniques to avoid homologous transfusion in spinal fusion surgery. *Spine* 1992;17:867-73.

69. Bennet SR. Perioperative autologous blood transfusion in elective total hip prosthesis operations. *Ann R Coll Surg Engl* 1994;76:95-8.

70. Bryson GGGL, Laupacis A, Wells GA. Does acute normovolemic hemodilution reduce perioperative allogeneic transfusion: a meta-analysis. *Anesth Analg* 1998;86:9-15.

71. Oishi CS, D'Lima DD, Morris BA, et al. Hemodilution with other blood reinfusion techniques in total hip arthroplasty. *Clin Orthop* 1997;339:132-9.

72. Bellhouse BJ, Lewis RWH. A high efficiency membrane separator for donor plasmapheresis. *ASAIO Transactions* 1988;34:747-54.

73. Wilson WJ. Intraoperative autologous transfusion in revision total hip arthroplasty. *J Bone Joint Surg [Am]* 1989;71-A:8-14.

74. Woolson ST, Watt M. Use of autologous blood in total hip replacement. *J Bone Joint Surg [Am]* 1991;73-A:76-80.

75. Stehling LC, Zauder HL, Rogers W. Intraoperative autotransfusion. *Anesthesiology* 1975;43:337-45.

76. Williamson KR, Taswell HF. Intraoperative blood salvage: a review. *Transfusion* 1991;31:662-75.

77. Baussand V, Mentec H, Fourcade C. Hemolysis after autologous transfusion. *Ann Intern Med* 1996;124:931-2.

78. Cregan P, Donegan E, Gotelli G. Hemolytic transfusion reaction following transfusion of frozen and washed autologous red cells. *Transfusion* 1991;31:172-5.

79. Domen RE. Adverse reactions associated with autologous blood transfusion: evaluation and incidence at a large academic hospital. *Transfusion* 1998;38:821-2.

80. Carson JL, Chen AY. In search of the transfusion trigger. *Clin Orthop* 1977;339:132-9.

81. Hansen E, Knuechel R, Altmeppen J, Taeger K. Blood irradiation for intraoperative autotransfusion in cancer surgery: demonstration of efficient elimination of contaminating tumor cells. *Transfusion* 1999;39:608-15.

PREVENTION OF INFECTION IN ORTHOPAEDIC SURGERY

GEERT H. I. M. WALENKAMP

From the Academic Hospital, Maastricht, The Netherlands

PATHOPHYSIOLOGY OF ORTHOPAEDIC WOUND INFECTIONS

Infection of a wound will occur when the bacterial contamination exceeds the minimum infective dose. In experimental studies in healthy volunteers this appeared to be 2 to 8 million organisms of *Staphylococcus aureus* when injected intradermally. When a foreign body (e.g., a stitch) was introduced, however, the minimum infective dose was reduced by 10 000 times.[1]

The extensive use of biomaterials in orthopaedics requires a better understanding of the pathophysiology of musculoskeletal sepsis, especially the molecular mechanisms. Microbial adhesion to inert substrates causes colonisation of biomaterials and damaged tissues. This adhesion is due to the chemical bonding of bacterial extracapsular structures to the surface of the implant or bone.[2] Bacteria and substrates are anionic and repel each other. The dipoles of the surface molecules, however, create electromagnetic 'Van der Waals' forces, and bacterial cells and biomaterials will bond. A strong connection is then created by fimbriae and exopolysaccharides.

A biofilm consists of exopolysaccharide polymers, produced by the bacteria, and it varies with local conditions and bacterial species.[3] It protects bacteria against several mechanisms of host defence and antibiotics, and serves as an adhesive device for the bacteria on a passive substrate, with the help of proteins such as fibronectin, osteonectin, fibrogen, collagen and others. Devitalised bone can act as the passive substrate, as can all biomaterials such as heart valves, endotracheal tubes, Hickman catheters and joint prostheses. It appears that in the case of biomaterials containing polymers, the principal isolate is *Staphylococcus epidermidis,* whereas *Staph. aureus* is found mainly in conjunction with metals, compromised tissues, surgical wounds and bone infections.

At the time of implantation a biomaterial will attract cells to its surface because of sites of free energy. These will be bound within a few hours either by the patient's own host-tissue cells or by bacteria: the 'race for the surface' (Fig. 1).[4] Once the biofilm with bacteria is formed, it creates a microenvironment of its own as regards pH, ions and nutrients; the bacteria multiply and the infection is established. In conjunction with the adverse effects of the relative hypoxia of the tissues in chronic osteomyelitis, this mechanism of adhesion and biofilm protection provides an explanation for the ability of bone infections to remain dormant for very long periods, the ineffectiveness of antibiotic treatment in the presence of dead bone and biomaterials, and the pathogenicity of organisms of low virulence such as *Staph. epidermidis* and some anaerobes.[5]

Another mechanism which could explain why orthopaedic infections can be difficult to treat and may relapse after a number of years is that *Staph. aureus* can form small-colony variants (SCV), especially when subinhibitory concentrations of antibiotics are present. These SCVs can persist in endothelial cells and cause persistent and antibiotic-resistant infections in man.[6,7]

Bone resorption in infection is induced by cytokine-stimulating osteoclasts and by the direct resorptive effects of inflammatory cells such as macrophages and granulocytes. In osteomyelitic bone the prostaglandin activity appears to be 5 to 30 times higher than in normal bone. In septic arthritis the destruction of cartilage seems to be caused mainly by the release of destructive enzymes by the synovium, and also by focal adherence and invasion of bacteria into the cartilage resulting in destruction of its integrity with loss of collagen and proteoglycan.[5]

PREVALENCE AND INCIDENCE OF ORTHOPAEDIC WOUND INFECTIONS

Hospital or nosocomial infections are mainly caused by bacteria and involve not only wound infections from surgery, but all types of infection acquired during a hospital stay. In 'prevalence' studies of nosocomial infections, new as well as previous infections are included. The numbers of infections in prevalence studies are determined in a hospital during a short period of time, and therefore may vary widely. In hospital inpatients in 14 European countries, the prevalence of nosocomial infections ranged from 3% to 21%, with a mean of 8.4%. The 'incidence' of all hospital infections is about 5%. Of these patients, 45% have a urinary infection, 29% a wound infection, 19% pneumonia,

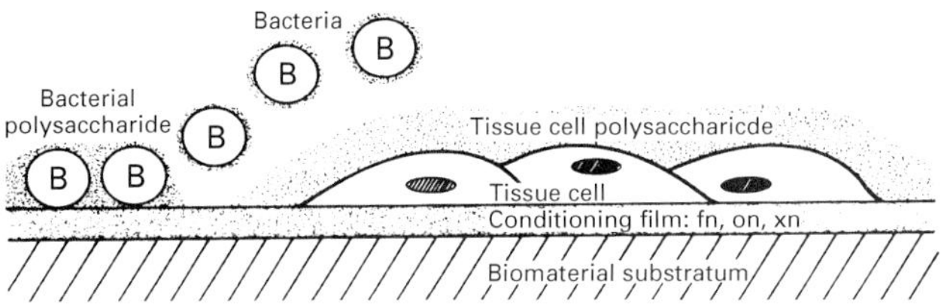

Fig. 1

Diagram of the concept of Gristina et al[4] of bacteria binding to a biomaterial. Reprinted with permission from Gristina AG, Barth E, Webb LX. Microbial adhesion and the pathogenesis of biomaterial centered infections. In: Gustilo RB, ed. *Orthopaedic infections: diagnosis and treatment.* Philadelphia: WB Saunders, 1989:325.

2% sepsis (with positive blood cultures) and 6% another type of infection. About 10% of the patients with a hospital infection die during the period of the infection, and 1% directly because of it.[8,9]

Data from the USA are available from the National Nosocomial Infections Surveillance (NNIS) system of the Center for Disease Control and Prevention (CDC). Wound infections from surgery accounted for 38% of the nosocomial infections in the surgical patients. Between 1986 and 1996 in the USA, 15 523 wound infections were reported from 593 344 operations,[10] an overall surgical site infection (SSI) rate of 2.6%.

The incidence of wound infections depends largely on the classification of the surgical wound which expresses the degree of contamination of the wound during surgery. This widely accepted CDC classification divides wounds into clean, clean/contaminated, contaminated or dirty, and can be used as an index of risk. In clean wounds the post-operative rate of wound infection in large series is about 2%; after dirty operations, when, for example, the operation takes place in an infected area, the rate of infection may rise to about 40%.[11] Results of infection surveys in orthopaedics confirm that the classification of surgical wounds is a valuable index for the SSI risk.[12-14]

The NNIS system has refined the classification by adding the duration of the operation and the ASA classification: the NNIS risk index (Table I). In surveillance reports, other risk factors associated with SSI can be classified as definite, likely and possible, and they are host- or procedure-related (Table II).[10]

DEFINITION OF WOUND INFECTION

The use of generally accepted definitions is crucial to compare reports of wound surveillance and to decide if preventive measures are effective. The definition of surgical wound infection (SWI) most widely used is that of the NNIS system of the CDC.[15] Since 1992 this definition has been changed: SWI is now named surgical site infection (SSI), and is subdivided into incisional (further divided into superficial and deep) and organ/space SSI (Fig. 2). The superficial layers are the skin and subcutaneous tissue, and the deep soft tissues are, for example, fascia and muscles.

Table I. NNIS risk index[10]: one point is given for each criterion

1) Class of wound is contaminated or dirty
2) Length of operation is ≥75 percentile of the duration of that procedure
3) ASA score > 3

Table II. Risk factors associated with SSI[10]

Host-related risk factors	Procedure-related risk factors
Definite	Definite
Age	Preoperative hair removal
Obesity	Type of procedure
Disease severity	Antibiotic prophylaxis
ASA score	Duration of surgery
Likely	Likely
Malnutrition and low serum albumin	Multiple procedures
Diabetes mellitus	Tissue trauma
Possible	Possible
Malignancy	Preoperative showers
Immunosuppressive therapy	Emergency surgery
Breast size in women	Drains

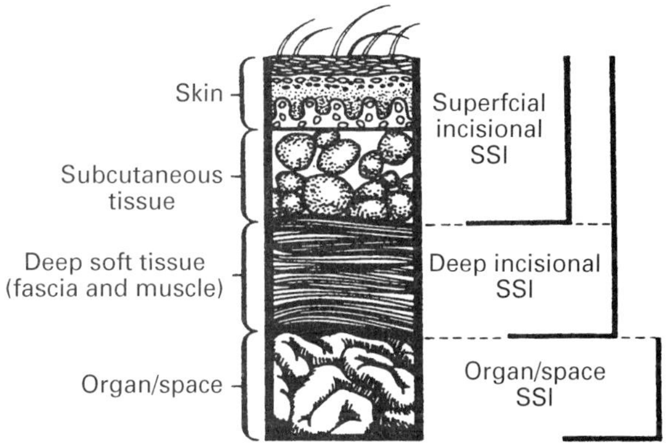

Fig. 2

Diagram of a cross-section of the abdominal wall depicting the CDC classification of surgical site infection.[15]

Organ/space SSI involves any part deeper than the incised layers of the body wall, including cavities, and is especially defined for use in, for example, thoracic and abdominal surgery, in which deep infections can occur without infection of the site of the incision in the thoracic or abdominal wall. An SSI is present when diagnosed within 30 days of the operation or within one year of when an implant is used. Stitch abscesses are not regarded as SSI, nor are infected burn wounds. A deep SSI is diagnosed when one of the following symptoms is present: pus within the deep soft-tissue layers; spontaneous or surgical dehiscence of the deep layers with a positive culture and fever (>38°C) or local pain; an abscess or other infection in deep tissues seen by direct observation at reoperation, radiology or histology; or when diagnosed by a surgeon or physician.

The diagnoses for superficial and organ/space SSI are comparable to those for deep SSI. In both cases the doctor may decide that a wound infection is present, without other objective signs. According to the CDC guidelines, the following deep postoperative orthopaedic infections could be classified as organ/space SSI: spondylodiscitis, arthritis, bursitis and osteomyelitis. Infection of a prosthesis may be regarded as arthritis or osteomyelitis. In surveillance reports in orthopaedic surgery the concept of organ/space SSI is hardly used, and most infections are classified as deep SSI.

SOME PREVENTIVE MEASURES FOR SSI

Risk factors associated with SSI in all types of surgery can be divided into host-related and procedure-related. These can then be classified as definite, likely or possible (Table II).[10] Some patient characteristics which may increase the risk of postoperative infections in clean operations are, for example, advanced age, a high ASA classification, diabetes (up to 10.7%), obesity (13.5%) and malnutrition (16.6%).[10,11,15] Rheumatoid arthritis was not found to be related to higher rates of infection in total hip replacement.[16]

The recommendations for prevention are related to known risk factors and should be based on scientific data, on theoretical rationale and the applicability of the preventive measures. Several such recommendations are described in the most recent guidelines for prevention of SSI.[15] Other reviews have been published from the Cochrane Collaboration, describing the evidence base of some preventive measures.[17] Important conclusions can also be drawn from some publications derived from arthroplasty registers, since they are based on a huge number of patients who have been followed up prospectively.[18-20]

Malnutrition. A reduced serum albumin and loss of body-weight are related to a higher rate of infection. In elective surgery, patients with malnutrition are much more likely to have postoperative complications including death. These patients could be identified by determining those who had a 10% loss of body-weight during the six months before operation. They can be supported in cases of elective surgery with extra nutritional treatment during the ten days before operation.[21] In orthopaedic surgery these patients are not frequently seen. Malnourished patients are mostly those who sustain a fracture of the proximal femur or hip and they can be given supplementary nutrition after operation. The catabolic stress response of the operation and the temporary decrease in the immune response postoperatively make supplementation with specific nutritional components attractive; a beneficial effect is suggested in animal experiments. Prospective studies, however, are needed, especially in orthopaedics.

Immune capacity. In orthopaedic patients with infections the immune response may be inadequate, for unknown reasons. Studies in patients with osteomyelitis indicate that in these patients immunoglobulins do not increase despite infection.[22] The phagocytic activity is also diminished and the amount of T-cells and helper T-cells decreased.[23]

Improving the immune response by preoperative vaccination for the prevention of SSI has been tried for many years,[24] but without much success. Experimental studies are published on prophylactic vaccines against infections in animal experiments with, for example, *Pseudomonas* and *Staph. aureus.* A very recent experimental study has been the local application of, for example, human IgG, in the prevention of biomaterial-related bacterial infection, by reduction of adherence of bacteria.[25,26] Surgical irrigation with pooled human IgG reduced postoperative spinal infection in rabbits.

Clinical studies are now in progress. Vaccines are being used as supplements to other surgical therapeutic measures for infections.[27]

Preoperative hospital stay. A long preoperative hospital stay is often suggested to be a risk factor for SSI in that patients are increasingly colonised with *Staph. aureus* and other hospital bacteria and are at risk because of this. The length of the preoperative hospital stay, however, is related to the severity of the illness of the patient and comorbidity, requiring evaluation or therapy before operation.[15]

Nasal carriage of *Staph. aureus.* In the general population the mean nasal carriage of *Staph. aureus* is about 37%.[28] Nasal carriers have an increased risk of developing SSI, and these are caused in 50% to 61% by the same bacteria as found in their noses. In some studies nasal carriers have wound infections 2 to 17 times more frequently than non-carriers.[29] Preoperative carriage of *Staph. aureus* in cardiothoracic operations was a powerful independent risk factor for SSI. Preoperative application of mupirocine nasal ointment was recommended for these patients,[30,31] but in this study the control was a historical patient group. In orthopaedic surgery there is an indication that nasal carriage may play a comparative role: the risk ratio for SSI was 8.9% (confidence interval (CI) 1.7 to 45.5).[28] The prophylactic use of mupirocine nasal ointment in orthopaedic patients was evaluated in two Dutch studies. A reduction of the incidence of wound infection was suggested,[31] but the effectiveness of the prophylaxis could not be proven in a randomised controlled trial.[32] In our own hospital and department, the incidence of nasal carriers in patients is considerably lower than in the literature, making a randomised controlled trial impossible and prophylaxis probably not cost-effective.

Preoperative skin preparation. The goal of preoperative preparation of the skin by washing, shaving and disinfection is to reduce the cutaneous bacterial load. Washing the skin with disinfecting soap may only be necessary in patients who are hospitalised preoperatively for more than two to three days. Special soap containing 4% chlorhexidine has to be used repeatedly. There is evidence that this reduces the degree of colonisation of the skin. Removal of hairs from the bodily region to be operated on is mainly necessary for practical reasons to avoid them coming in contact with the wound. There is no evidence that removal is necessary for the prevention of infection and bacteria are more prolific in the follicles of the hair than on the hairs themselves. Shaving has a negative effect on the prevention of wound infection in that, when a knife is used, small skin lesions are produced, facilitating bacterial growth. The longer these lesions exist, the heavier is the skin colonisation and the more the risk increases for infection. Therefore, if shaving is done, it should be carried out as close to the time of the operation as possible. Better methods are the use of hair-clippers or depilatory creams because they leave the skin intact. Disinfection of the skin is performed immediately before operation in the operating theatre. The skin must first be freed from gross contamination. The most effective disinfectants are 1% iodine in 70% alcohol or 0.5% chlorhexidine in 70% alcohol (ethanol or isopropanolol).[15] The advantage of chlorhexidine is that it sticks to the skin, making it effective for six hours. The effectiveness is decreased by soap, but not by blood. Iodine has the advantage that it also kills bacterial spores. Some clinics therefore apply towels with iodine to the operative area some hours before operation. Povidone-iodine is iodine in water: solutions of 0.1 to 10% are used as disinfectant, especially in wounds or mucous membranes, but blood and proteins may inactivate iodophors. Operative adhesive drapes impregnated with iodine may be used.

SYSTEMIC ANTIBIOTIC PROPHYLAXIS

Antibiotic prophylaxis has proved to be very effective in reducing deep as well as superficial postoperative infections. In total hip surgery the reduction is about 75%; in surgery for closed fractures a reduction of the rate of infection of 5% to less than 1% is claimed,[17] and the mean risk reduction for deep infection in closed fractures is 2.8% (95% CI 1.3 to 4.3).

In recent years the duration of prophylaxis has gradually decreased to one day. A large study investigated the possibility of using only one dose in total hip replacements.[16] No significant difference was found between one dose of cefuroxime and use for one day. This particular study, however, did not prove that there was no difference; the trend was that prophylaxis of only one dose was two times less effective than that of use for one day. Other studies indicate that a one-dose regime can be worse because an antibiotic may not have the appropriate pharmacokinetics. The minimal inhibitory concentrations for the causative bacteria must be exceeded throughout the period that the wound is open, and the antibiotic should therefore have a half-life which is long enough. It therefore appears, at the present time, that it is safer to use a schedule of prophylaxis for 24 hours in orthopaedic surgery.

The choice of antibiotic to be used for prophylaxis should be based on the expected causative bacteria. If biomaterials are implanted, the antibiotic must have a bactericidal effect against *Staph. aureus* and *Staph. epidermidis.* Many authors therefore advise a first-generation cephalosporin or a penicillin active against β-lactamase-producing bacteria, such as flucloxacillin. In arthroplasty anaerobic bacteria may play an important role in low-grade infections, and therefore they should also be covered: metronidazole should be added or amoxicillin-clavulanic acid. If antibiotics are given to prevent a relapse of infection after an operation, then they must also cover the causative organism of the former infection.

Prophylaxis must start not later than half an hour before the operation, and is given intravenously. In the case of a bloodless field with an Esmarch bandage, the antibiotic must be given at least ten minutes before the bandage is applied. If bacteriological samples must be taken, as in prosthesis revisions, the antibiotic must not be given before material from the deep tissues has been taken for evaluation.

Systemic antibiotic prophylaxis is indicated in orthopaedics when the risk of infection is relatively high, or when an infection is likely to result in serious consequences, e.g., with implantation of joint replacement prostheses, osteotomies and arthrodeses of large bones or joints, hip operations, spondylodeses, operations lasting longer than two hours, and operations on patients with decreased immunity.

ANTIBIOTIC-LOADED BONE CEMENT

In vitro pharmacokinetics. Although many types of antibiotic have been admixed to various bone cements, sufficient release from the cement is not always achieved. A combination should only be used if adequate test results are available which show that the release is sufficient. It is a diffusion process in which antibiotics are exchanged against water. The centre of a bone-cement block loaded with antibiotic may still have the same concentration of antibiotic after several years since release is mostly from a few millimetres of the superficial layer of the cement. Several prerequisites are important in choosing the antibiotic. It must be water-soluble to diffuse into a haematoma. Because of the elevation of temperature during the polymerisation of cement, it must also be heat-stable. The bacteriological spectrum of the antibiotic should be wide and bactericidal. Tetracycline, chloramphenicol and polymyxin are not released from bone cement; cephalosporins are poorly released. If gentamicin is chosen Palacos has had the best release.[33] The new antibiotic in which gentamicin is combined with clindamycin (Copal) gives a greater release of the gentamicin. It is suggested that bone cements should release >0.2 mg of gentamicin per gram of bone cement in seven days in a standardised test in vitro.[34] Other new antibiotic-cement combinations with tobramycin, clindamycin and vancomycin are commercially available.

The release of the antibiotic results in a relatively high concentration in the tissues immediately around the cement, but the diffusion into the rest of the body is low, resulting in concentrations in the serum which are too low to be measured, and with no toxic side-effects.[35] The concentration of antibiotic in the exudate present in the joint space around a prosthesis has had wide variation in published reports. This can be explained by variation in the surface of the bone cement which comes into contact with the haematoma, and therefore the variation of the diffusion.

Prophylactic effectiveness in animal experiments. In animal experiments the evidence for prophylactic effectiveness of antibiotic-loaded bone cement is well documented. It protects against early peroperative contamination and postoperative haematogenous infection. Gentamicin was found effectively to prevent haematogenous infection of a cement plug in rat tibiae with *Staph. aureus, Pseudomonas, Proteus* and group-G streptococcus when bacteria were injected intravenously half an hour after operation, but not when the injection was given six weeks after surgery.[36] In a knee arthroplasty model in the rat,[37] a protective effect was also shown, but it lasted for only six weeks. However, this may be as important as the peroperative and immediate postoperative period. In the early postoperative weeks patients often have urinary infections, pneumonia and decubitus ulcers, and require continuous prophylaxis.

Prophylactic use in patients. The clinical use of antibiotic-loaded bone cement started in 1969 when Buchholz used it as a prophylactic measure in primary total hip arthroplasty. After penicillin and erythromycin, he used gentamicin with more success from about 1972. The reduction of the rate of infection in primary hip replacement in his clinic was confirmed by others: in non-randomised cohort studies the reduction of deep infections was from 3% to 6% to about 1% (Fig. 3). In a large randomised, prospective study of 1688 total hip arthroplasties, Josefsson and Kolmert[38] found a significant reduction of deep infections using gentamicin-containing cement. The reduction was still significant at follow-up at two and five years, but not at ten years.

This prophylactic effect was later confirmed in the large Swedish Hip Register cohort study of about 150 000 total hip arthroplasties.[18] Gentamicin-containing Palacos had the most pronounced association with prevention of infection, with a risk ratio of 0.61 (CI 0.50 to 0.74). A very interesting finding in this register was that antibiotic-loaded bone cement was also associated with a reduced rate of aseptic loosening. It is probable that this is related to unrecognised low-grade infections owing to false-negative peroperative cultures, or to absence of cultures. In the Norwegian Arthroplasty Register, it was shown that the lowest probability of revision for infection of a total hip arthroplasty was found in patients who received systemic antibiotics in combination with antibiotic-loaded cement. This benefit was highest in the first and second postoperative years. If only systemic antibiotics were used without antibiotic cement, the risk was 4.3 times higher.[19] Also, in the Swedish Hip Register, the cost-benefit analysis of prophylaxis showed that the best and most cost-effective combination was antibiotic-loaded bone cement in combination with systemic antibiotics.[20]

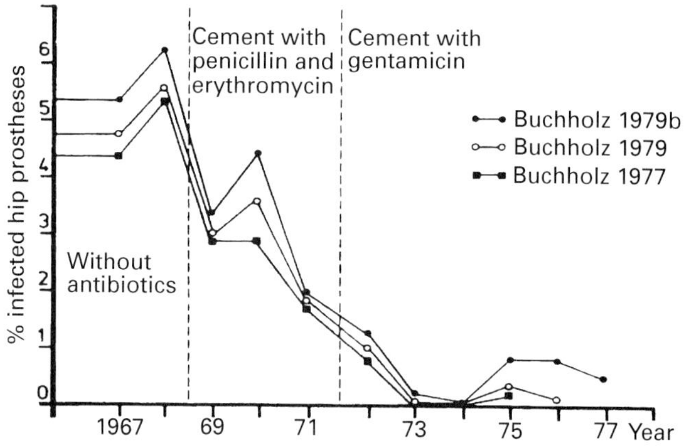

Fig. 3

Graph showing the beneficial effect of mixing antibiotics with bone cement, as reflected by the decrease of the percentage of infections of primary THRs. The graph also shows the increase of these percentages of infections when the length of the follow-up increased, as published in three consecutive publications.[45] Reproduced by permission from Walenkamp GH. Prevention and treatment of infection in orthopaedic surgery and traumatology. Editions Scientifiques et Médicales Elsevier SAS (Paris). All rights reserved. *Surgical Techniques in Orthopaedics and Traumatology.* 55-010-C-10, 2000, 11p.

In conclusion, antibiotic-loaded bone cement was found to be effective in studies in vitro, in animal experiments and in clinical prospective, randomised and cohort studies. There is no evidence that using gentamicin-loaded bone cement is related to an increased incidence of resistant *Staph. epidermidis*. It would seem wise, however, not to use vancomycin-admixed bone cement routinely, not even in clinics where gentamicin resistance is common. Vancomycin is now a last-resort drug, and should not be used in routine prophylaxis.

THE OPERATING THEATRE: REDUCED AIR CONTAMINATION

In the continuous prophylactic battle against bacteria, the use of antibiotics may lead to the development of more resistant organisms. Antibiotics may have toxic side-effects and may sometimes not be effective. It is more logical to prevent bacteria entering the wound after operation.

Of the bacteria entering the wound peroperatively, 98% come from the air in the operating theatre (OP) and 2% from the patient. Bacteria in the OP do not float free in the air, but are carried by particles of varying size, mainly skin cells of the individuals present. An individual sheds about 10^9 skin cells per day with a mean size of 20 μm; about 7% are less than 7 μm,[39] and one in every 100 to 5000 cells carries a bacterium.

The size of the bacteria-carrying particles is over 3 μm, with a mean of 12 to 14 μm. The larger particles with bacteria which enter the wound fall directly downwards from the heads of the surgical team. The smaller ones follow the airstream and thus contaminate the wound or instruments and the hands of the surgical team. Bacteria found in the wound have entered via the air of the OP in 30% of cases, and via hands and instruments in 70%. The latter have also been contaminated by the OP. There are two important conclusions from this. First, the air in the OP has a decisive role in the contamination of the wound and in the prophylaxis of wound infection. Secondly, the main source of contamination is the bacteria on the skin cells of workers in the OP. This is confirmed by the relationship found, in several studies, between the concentration of bacteria in the air and the number of persons present in the OP, the activity of these individuals (highest at the start and the end of the operation), the use of occlusive operating gowns, the use of helmets ('aspiration suits') and the 'ultra-clean-air' installations.

Infection and increased wound contamination are related to the duration of exposure to air contamination in the OP, especially when longer than two hours.

More bacteria in the air result in greater bacterial contamination of the wound[40] which gives more wound infection.[1] The direct relationship, however, between air contamination and the rate of postoperative wound infection could only be proven in a large multicentre study.[41] General measures to reduce the bacterial load of the OP air are effective and include reduction in the number of people in the OP, the wearing of proper head cover and masks, reduction in movement, i.e., walking slowly and not too close to the tables, speaking only if necessary, the wearing of clothes which reduce the shedding of their skin scales, the barring of persons with skin diseases from work if they have increased shedding or have *Staph. aureus* skin infections, and exposure of instruments to the air only when air contamination is reduced after preparing the patient.

An important factor is the reduction of shedding. Good clothing systems can reduce the airborne bacterial counts by 5 to 10 times. Clothes with an open structure do not prevent bacterial dispersion; ordinary cotton is woven with a pore size of >80 μm and therefore bacteria on skin scales can pass through easily. A reduction of the pore size is possible when fabric is woven very tightly, or when the clothes are made of semi- or impermeable material. When these materials are used as a gown over cotton clothing they give no reduction in shedding. Since the material is impermeable to air, skin debris is pumped out from the neck opening. These materials should be used as a suit with effective seals at the neck, trousers and waist, and are then 1000 times more effective than open cotton clothing.[39] Unfortunately, such a design is uncomfortably warm. When air-exhaust systems are used under impermeable gowns the heat may be reduced, as well as the dispersion of skin scales carrying bacteria.

AIR-HANDLING SYSTEMS IN THE OPERATING THEATRE: REMOVAL OF BACTERIA

The role of the air-handling system is to supply the OP with sterile, fresh air, and to remove the polluted air, e.g., narcotic gases and particles with bacteria. Not all air-handling systems can do these tasks well. Broadly, there are two systems: mixing and non-mixing.

In the older mixing systems, fresh, clean air is introduced into the OP with the objective of reducing the contamination of the air by dilution (Fig. 4). It appears that it has no additional effect when more than 20 times the content of an OP is refreshed. In a regular OP of 100 m^3 this results in an air supply of 2000 m^3/hour which applies to most of the OPs built in The Netherlands in former years. Instructions for architects and the budgets were based on this calculation. This type of mixing system, however, provides no special direction of the air towards the OP table, and is not designed to move germs away from the OP field; the airflow is turbulent.

In non-mixing systems, the insufflated air itself is used to drive away the polluted air (Fig. 5). These systems deliver sterile laminar flow, directed to the wound and must be capable of taking away contaminated particles via the outlet openings. It has been proved that downflow laminar systems are more effective than horizontal flow systems, which are often used in rebuilding situations. The OP lamp forms the greatest obstruction to an effective downflow, and the heat produced also causes an upward convection force

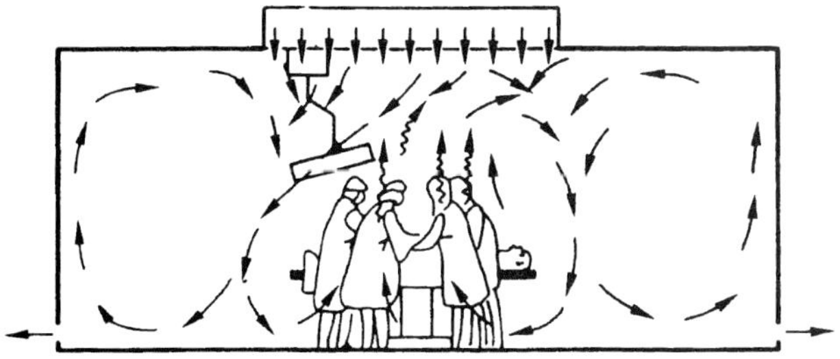

Fig. 4

Diagram showing the mixing type of an OP air-handling system: the system is not capable of directing the airstream from clean to contaminated zones.[46] Reproduced by permission from Walenkamp GH. Prevention and treatment of infection in orthopaedic surgery and traumatology. Editions Scientifiques et Médicales Elsevier SAS (Paris). All rights reserved. *Surgical Techniques in Orthopaedics and Traumatology.* 55-010-C-10, 2000, 11p.

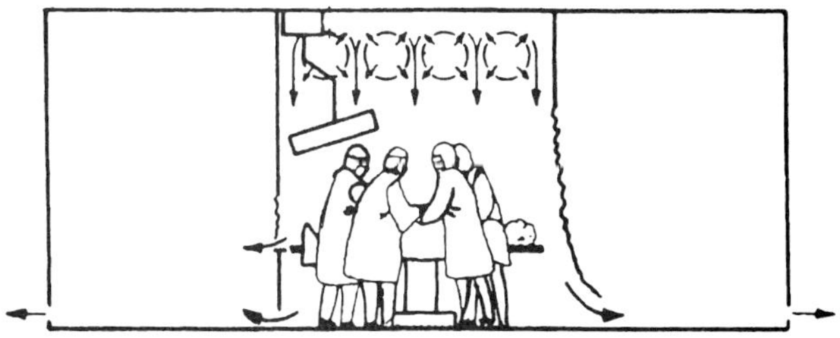

Fig. 5

Diagram showing the non-mixing type of an OP air-handling system: clean air does not mix with contaminated air, but is able to push it away, in this case with the help of curtains and laminar flow.[46] Reproduced by permission from Walenkamp GH. Prevention and treatment of infection in orthopaedic surgery and traumatology. Editions Scientifiques et Médicales Elsevier SAS (Paris). All rights reserved. *Surgical Techniques in Orthopaedics and Traumatology.* 55-010-C-10, 2000, 11p.

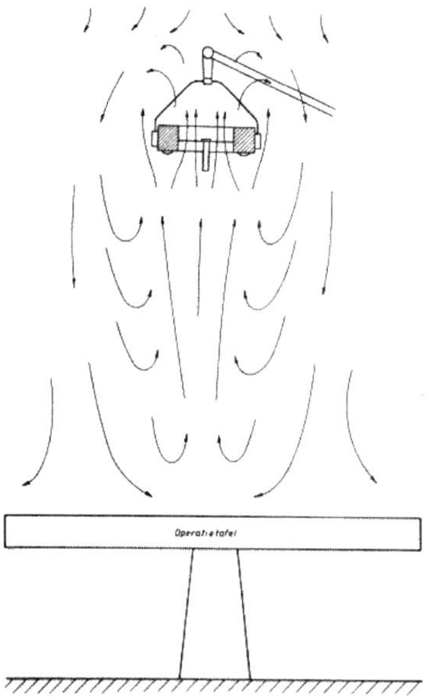

Fig. 6

Diagram showing how OP lamps must be designed to minimise the obstruction of the downward air flow, and to produce minimal convection so that the downflow is not hindered.[46] Reproduced by permission from Walenkamp GH. Prevention and treatment of infection in orthopaedic surgery and traumatology. Editions Scientifiques et Médicales Elsevier SAS (Paris). All rights reserved. *Surgical Techniques in Orthopaedics and Traumatology.* 55-010-C-10, 2000, 11p.

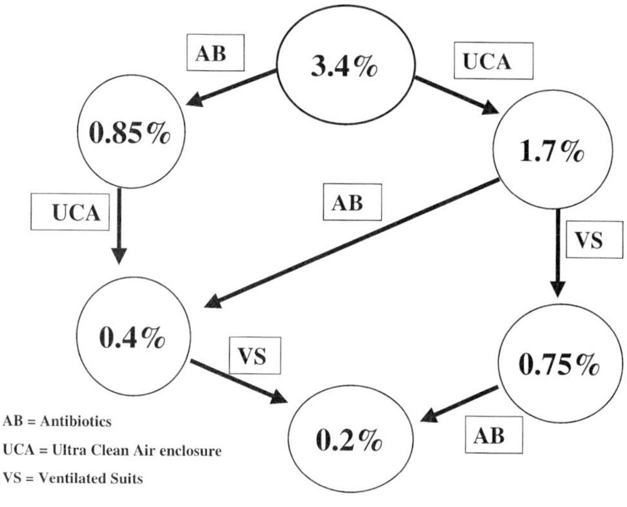

Fig. 7

Diagram showing reduction of postoperative deep infections in 8052 joint replacements by several prophylactic measures.[42] The effect of antibiotic-loaded cement could not be evaluated in this study. Reproduced by permission from Walenkamp GH. Prevention and treatment of infection in orthopaedic surgery and traumatology. Editions Scientifiques et Médicales Elsevier SAS (Paris). All rights reserved. *Surgical Techniques in Orthopaedics and Traumatology.* 55-010-C-10, 2000, 11p.

(Fig. 6). In practice, the speed of downflow of the air must be about 45 cm/second at the plenum, and the best inlet temperature is 19°C; in general it should be at least 2°C lower than the air outlet temperature (ΔT) to be able to create a downflow.

To maintain the downflow for as long as possible, side walls can be used hanging from the ceiling around the plenum. For practical reasons these walls should end 2 metres above the floor in order to allow individuals and image intensifiers to pass through. In the well-known 'greenhouse', as designed by Charnley-Howorth or Weber-Meierhans, these walls come down to 10 cm above the floor. In such ultraclean air installations large volumes of air are used, up to 12 000 m^3/hour, with up to 600 exchanges per hour. In the best situation these air systems are combined with 'body-exhaust suits' which are impermeable gowns and helmets, suctioning the air away. In such an operating environment the infective bacterial dose of the wound via hands, instruments and air is reduced to the absolute minimum. The influence of the operating time, the number of persons in the OP and other factors is largely reduced. Reduction of the rate of deep postoperative infection in primary total hip replacement (THR) is 50% with an ultraclean air installation, and also 50% with a body-exhaust suit. Because these reductions act independently of each other, their combination gives a reduction of 75%. In combination with the 75% reduction of infection provided by systemic antibiotics, the rate of infection can be reduced from 3.4% to 0.2% (Fig. 7). In the study of Lidwell et al[42] the influence of antibiotic-loaded bone cement could not be demonstrated; the number of more than 8000 prostheses assessed did not reach significance. The same calculation, however, was undertaken by Persson et al,[20] based on data from almost 150 000 total hip prostheses, registered with the Swedish National Register (Fig. 8). They were also able to evaluate the influence of antibiotic-loaded cement, and calculate the costs of the various prophylactic measures. When the costs of hip revision were taken into account, the most cost-effective strategy of prophylactic measures could be calculated. The best combination appeared to be gentamicin-loaded bone cement in combination with systemic antibiotics, as in the study of Josefsson and Kolmert[38], which resulted in a reduction of the postoperative percentage of infection from 3.4% to 0.24%. The use of ultraclean air in combination with antibiotic-loaded bone cement and systemic antibiotics further reduced the risk in this register to 0.19%.[20] This percentage is fully comparable with that in the study of Lidwell et al[42] if ultraclean air and ventilated suits are used (compare Figs 7 and 8). In the calculations of Persson et al,[20] the extra costs of such a sterile enclosure depend on the number of total hips implanted a year; from 157 US dollars for 100 THRs/year to 66 US dollars for 250 THRs/year. There is no good explanation as to why in this study ventilated exhaust suits

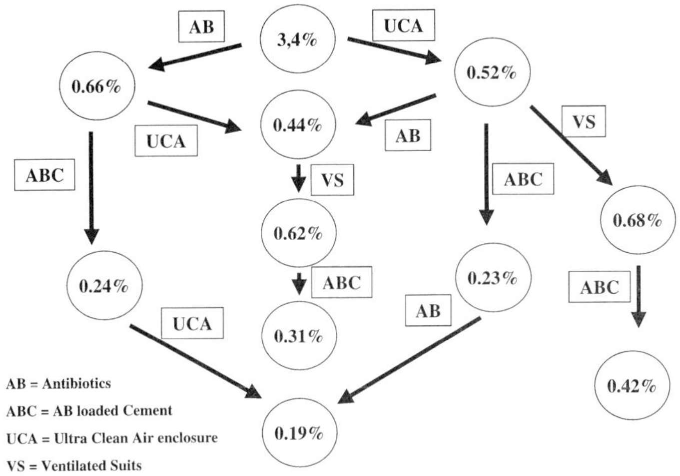

Fig. 8

Diagram showing the reduction of deep infections by several prophylactic measures in 148 359 THRs,[20] including the kind of bone cement. Reproduced by permission from Walenkamp GH. Prevention and treatment of infection in orthopaedic surgery and traumatology. Editions Scientifiques et Médicales Elsevier SAS (Paris). *Surgical Techniques in Orthopaedics and Traumatology*. 55-010-C-10, 2000, 11p

always had a negative effect when combined with any other prophylactic measure.

In these calculations only the direct medical cost of an uncomplicated revision of the infected prosthesis was used; which in 1996 was 17 600 US dollars for a two-stage revision.[20] No indirect costs were taken into account such as social insurance payments for disability and costs to be paid by patients for various kinds of help. These calculations may be comparable for all other types of prosthesis, especially when the benefit of ultraclean air installations is studied. In terms of cost-effectiveness, all prostheses may be counted together.

In OPs where operations which are more prone to infection such as implantation of prostheses and repair of hip fractures are performed, the suggested standard for the bacteriological quality of the air should be <10 colony-forming units/m^3. Other types of operation, as well as day-care treatment, can be performed in OPs with a maximum air contamination of 100 to 200 colony-forming units/m^3, if cost-effectiveness is a matter of concern.

WHICH PROPHYLACTIC MEASURES ARE JUSTIFIED?

All prophylactic measures reduce the rate of infection independently, and their individual rates can be combined. The combination to be chosen is up to the surgeons, their administrators and health-care providers, depending on budgets and local and national consensus documents. It is the responsibility of orthopaedic surgeons to be involved in the formulation of national consensus texts, because these have an impact on local decisions and budgets. In the choice of prophylactic measures, the orthopaedic surgeon has to weigh up the maximal effects and cost for an individual patient against a cost-effective choice for the population of patients. Arguments should be based on scientific evidence in the international literature, national and local SSI surveillance data, and calculations of costs including indirect costs of infections and the resulting disability.

Based on the above, the logical choice in the implantation of prostheses indicates that we should:

1) always use systemic antibiotics;

2) optimise the OP air-handling system (downflow, laminar, clean) and clothing; and

3) use antibiotic-loaded bone cement if most of the bacteria in the hospital are susceptible to gentamicin.

If an ultraclean air system is available, plain bone cement can be considered without antibiotic admixture. The saving of not using the antibiotic-loaded bone cement may be used for the payment of the ultraclean air installation and its maintenance. Other arguments, however, in favour of the use of antibiotic-loaded cement must also be taken into account. The installation of an ultraclean air enclosure is more cost-effective when more prostheses are implanted, and should be considered when >200 prostheses are introduced per year and also when there is a higher risk of contamination than normal, such as in university hospitals with more crowded operating theatres.

SURVEILLANCE OF SSI

A major aim of postoperative surveillance programmes is to be informed about SSI results, which give the surgeon feedback, and can be related to the results of other departments in the same hospital, nationwide and worldwide. The primary aim of surveillance is to reduce the rate of SSI, and in this way the morbidity and mortality for the patient and, secondarily, to save costs for the hospital and reduce the national health-care budget. A surveillance programme could reduce the overall rates of all nosocomial infections by up to 32%. Feedback to the surgeons is an indispensable component of this. A good surveillance programme, however, requires the involvement of all staff and is only reliable with considerable effort. Several methods have been described to collect the data but these will

Table III. Dutch reference data on the incidence of surgical site infections[44]

Procedure	Number	All SSI (%) (95% CI)	Deep SSI (%) (95% CI)	Median duration of surgery (min)	Number of hospitals
Total hip prosthesis	12588	*3.4* (*3.0* to *3.7*)	*0.8* (*0.6* to *1.0*)	85	52
Revision of total hip replacement	878	*8.1* (*6.4* to *10.1*)	*1.8* (*1.1* to *3.0*)	130	41
Hemiprosthesis	1845	*6.2* (*5.2* to *7.5*)	*2.0* (*1.4* to *2.7*)	65	45
Osteosynthesis of femoral neck fracture	1376	*3.9* (*2.9* to *5.0*)	*1.2* (*0.7* to *1.9*)	60	35
Osteosynthesis diaph. + distal femoral fracture	377	*5.8* (*3.8* to *8.8*)	*1.1* (*0.3* to *2.9*)	90	29
Osteosynthesis pertroch. Femoral neck fracture	730	*2.7* (*1.7* to *4.3*)	*0.7* (*0.3* to *1.7*)	70	30
Total knee prosthesis	4502	*2.2* (*1.8* to *2.7*)	*0.8* (*0.6* to *1.1*)	95	45

be influenced by personnel, financial resources and the limitations of information technology. Surveillance can be performed by direct observation of the surgical site by a doctor or nurse, or indirectly by reviewing records and reports.[10]

The percentage of infections is constructed by producing a nominator and a denominator. The nominator is the number of infected wounds (SSI). The best method of collecting these data is by direct observation of surgical sites by the doctors themselves. Wounds are observed over 30 days, but when a prosthesis is implanted, they must be followed up for one year postoperatively. It is estimated that currently 75% of the operations performed in the USA are in outpatient settings, and day surgery or shorter hospital stays are encouraged. This is the reason why an increasing number of SSIs are detected after discharge from hospital (now 12% to 84%), and postdischarge surveillance is increasingly important. The facilities for this depend on the organisation of the health-care in the country, and may present difficulties.

To achieve a complete and reliable registration, all wounds must be judged, and therefore the registration of undisturbed wound healing is as important as that of the infected wounds themselves. The total number of undisturbed wounds plus the number of SSIs is the number of registered wounds. Ideally, this should be the same number as the denominator (the total number of operations): it reflects the response rate of the surveillance system. The data on the total number of operations and the patients may be downloaded, if possible, from the hospital information system.

In our department surveillance is performed by the surgeons themselves by completion of a registration form with a minimum of data. They record the type of operation, classification of the wound on the day of operation, and the judgement of wound healing postoperatively. A system of distributing and collecting such registration forms must be tailored to every department. One of the members of staff must be involved to oversee the process of completion of the forms, to correct errors and to motivate colleagues. The bottleneck of data entry in wound surveillance may be solved by automatic scanning. Regular feedback to the surgeons is important to keep the motivation at the level required.

A choice has to be made as to whether the surveillance is performed for all operations or only for a selection, e.g., total hip and knee replacements. The advantage of registering total hip and knee prostheses is the relative uniformity of the procedure all over the world, making it useful for comparison. The disadvantage is the relatively low SSI rate. Higher rates of infection are recorded in, for example, femoral neck fractures and foot surgery.

In The Netherlands over five years (1995 to 1999) in a national registration project, data on 72 720 operations in 70 of the 114 Dutch hospitals were collected, after which 2493 SSIs were reported.[43] Altogether 35 520 (53%) of the operations were orthopaedic, which illustrates the relatively high interest of orthopaedic surgeons in surveillance in The Netherlands. Some of the results are given in Table III.

CONCLUSION

A surveillance programme may be helpful in reducing the rate of infection and is an important tool in evaluating the effectiveness of preventive measures.

REFERENCES

1. **Elek SD, Conen PE.** The virulence of *Staphylococcus Pyogenes* for man: a study of the problems of wound infection. *Br J Exp Pathol* 1957;38:573-86.
2. **Gristina AG, Naylor PT, Myrvik QN, Esterhai JL, GAPR eds.** *Musculoskeletal infection.* Park Ridge: American Academy of Orthopaedic Surgeons, 1992:13-28.
3. **Schurman DJ, Smith RL, Esterhai JL, GAPR eds.** *Musculoskeletal infection.* Park Ridge: American Academy of Orthopaedic Surgeons, 1992:133-47.
4. **Gristina AG, Barth E, Webb LX, Gustilo RB, GRTD eds.** *Orthopaedic infections: diagnosis and treatment.* Philadelphia: Saunders, 1989:3-25.
5. **Norden C, Gillespie WJ, Nade S.** *Infections in bones and joints.* Oxford: Blackwell, 1994.
6. **Proctor RA, Balwit JM, Vesga O.** Variant subpopulations of Staphylococcus aureus as cause of persistent and recurrent infections. *Infect Agents Dis* 1994;3:302-12.
7. **Von Eiff C, Bettin D, Proctor RA, et al.** Recovery of small colony variants of Staphylococcus aureus following gentamicin bead placement for osteomyelitis. *Clin Infect Dis* 1997;25:1250-1.
8. **Haley RW.** Surveillance by objective: a new priority-directed approach to the control of nosocomial infections. *Am J Infect Control* 1985;13:78-89.

9. **Haley RW, Culver DH, White JW, et al.** The efficacy of infection surveillance and control programs in preventing nosocomial infections in US hospitals. *Am J Epidemiol* 1985;121:182-205.

10. **Smyth ETM, Emmerson AM.** Surgical site infection surveillance: review. *J Hosp Infect* 2000;45:173-84.

11. **Cruse PJE, Foord R.** A five-year prospective study of 23 649 surgical wounds. *Arch Surg* 1973;107:206-10.

12. **Vasey H, GEEIOA eds.** *L'infection en chirurgie orthopédique.* Paris: Expansion Scientifique Francaise, 1974:127-46.

13. **Lidgren L, Lindberg L.** Postoperative wound infections in clean orthopaedic surgery: review of a 5-year material. *Acta Orthop Scand* 1974;45:161-9.

14. **Gastrin B, Lovestad A.** Postoperative wound infection: relation to different types of operation and wound contamination categories in orthopaedic surgery. *J Hosp Infect* 1989;13:387-93.

15. **Mangram AJ, Horan TC, Pearson ML, Silver LC, Jarvis WR.** Guidelines for prevention of surgical-site infection, 1999: The Hospital Infection Control Practices Advisory Committee. *Infect Control Hosp Epidemiol* 1999;20:247-78.

16. **Wymenga AB.** *Joint sepsis after prophylaxis with one or three doses of cefuroxime in hip and knee replacement surgery.* Thesis, Katholieke Universiteit, Nijmegen, 1991.

17. **Gillespie WJ, Walenkamp G.** *Antibiotic prophylaxis in patients undergoing surgery for proximal femoral and other closed long bone fractures.* Cochrane Library. Issue 2. Oxford: Update Software, 1998.

18. **Malchau H, Herberts P.** *Prognosis of total hip replacement: revision and rerevision rate in THR: a revision risk study of 148 359 primary operations. In: JRUDoOUoGS, ed.* The National Hip Arthroplasty Registry of Sweden, 1998.

19. **Espehaug B, Engesaeter LB, Vollset SE, Havelin LI, Langeland N.** Antibiotic prophylaxis in total hip arthroplasty: review of 10,905 primary cemented total hip replacements reported to the Norwegian arthroplasty register, 1987 to 1995. *J Bone Joint Surg [Br]* 1997; 79-B:590-5.

20. **Persson U, Persson M, Malchau H.** The economics of preventing revisions in total hip replacement. *Acta Orthop Scand* 1999; 70:163-9.

21. **Von Meyenfeldt MF, Meijerink WJH, Rouflart MMJ, Buil-Maassen MTHJ, Soeters PD.** Perioperative nutritional support: a randomised clinical trial. *Clin Nutr* 1992;11:180-6.

22. **Bansal VP, Mittal PK, Ashokraj G.** Humoral immune responses in osteomyelitis. *Int Orthop* 1992;16:297-301.

23. **Peters KM, Koberg K, Zwadio-Klarwasser G, Zilkens KW.** Immune reactions in chronic post-traumatic osteomyelitis: current status determination. *Z Orthop Ihre Grenzgeb* 1991;129:313-8.

24. **Weber BG, Chapchal G.** *Arthroplasty of the hip: 5th International Symposium in 1972 in Nijmegen, Netherlands.* Stuttgart: Thieme, 1973:206-9.

25. **Poelstra KA.** *Local application of human IgG to prevent biomaterial-centered bacterial infection.* Thesis, Rijksuniversiteit Groningen, 2000.

26. **Poelstra KA, Barekzi NA, Slunt JB, Schuler TC, Grainger DW.** Surgical irrigation with pooled human immunoglobulin G to reduce postoperative spinal implant infection. *Tissue Eng* 2000;6:401-11.

27. **Morandi M, Zembo MM, d'Ambrosia R.** *Orthopaedic infections.* New Jersey: Slack, 1989;9:163-90.

28. **Kalmeijer MD, van Nieuwland-Bollen E, Bogaers-Hofman D, de Baere GAJ.** Nasal carriage of Staphylococcus aureus is a major risk for surgical-site infections in orthopaedic surgery. *Infect Control Hosp Epidemiol* 2000;21:319-23.

29. **Casewell MW.** The nose: an underestimated source of Staphylococcus aureus causing wound infection. *J Hosp Infect* 1998;40:3-11.

30. **Kluytmans JAJW.** *Nasal carriage of Staphylococcus aureus: the key to preventing staphylococcal disease.* Erasmus Universiteit Rotterdam, Thesis, 1996.

31. **Gernaat-van der Sluis AJ, Hoogenboom-Verdegaal AMM, Edixhoven PJ, Spies-van Rooijen NH.** Prophylactic mupirocin could reduce orthopedic wound infections: 1044 patients treated with mupirocin compared with 1260 historical controls. *Acta Orthop Scand* 1998;69:412-4.

32. **Kalmeijer MD, Coertjens H, van Nieuwland-Bollen E, et al.** Surgical site infections in orthopaedic surgery: the effect of a double-blind, randomised, placebo-controlled study with mupirocin nasal ointment. 2000;in press.

33. **Wahlig H, Willert HG, Buchhorn G.** *Knochenzement.* Stuttgart; Hubert, 1987:221-5.

34. **Kuhn K-D.** *Bone cements: up-to-date comparison of physical and chemical properties of commercial materials.* Berlin, Springer, 2000.

35. **Walenkamp GHIM, Vree TB, van Resn TJG.** Gentamicin-PMMA beads: pharmacokinetic and nephrotoxicological study. *Clin Orthop* 1986;205:171-83.

36. **Elson RA, Jephcott AE, McGechie DB, Verettas D.** Bacterial infection and acrylic cement in the rat. *J Bone Joint Surg [Br]* 1977; 59-B:452-7.

37. **Blomgren G.** Hematogenous infection of total joint replacement: an experimental study in the rabbit. *Acta Orthop Scand Suppl* 1981; 52:1-64.

38. **Josefsson G, Kolmert L.** Prophylaxis with systemic antibiotics versus gentamicin bone cement in total hip arthroplasty: a ten year survey of 1688 hips. *Clin Orthop* 1993;292:210-4.

39. **Whyte W.** The role of clothing and drapes in the operating room. *J Hosp Infect* 1988;11:2-17.

40. **Whyte W, Hodgson R, Tinkler J.** The importance of airborne bacterial contamination of wounds. *J Hosp Infection* 1982;3:123-35.

41. **Lidwell OM, Lowbury EJ, Whyte W, et al.** Effect of ultraclean air in operating rooms on deep sepsis in the joint after total hip or knee replacement: a randomised study. *Br Med J* 1982;285(6334):10-4.

42. **Lidwell OM, Elson RA, Lowbury EJ, et al.** Ultraclean air and antibiotics for prevention of postoperative infection: a multicenter study of 8052 joint replacement operations. *Acta Orthop Scand* 1987;58:4-13.

43. **Geubbels ELP, Mintjes-de Groot AJ, Wille J, et al.** *PREZIES; Preventie van Ziekenhuisinfecties door surveillance: component post-operatieve wondinfecties III, 1997-1999.* Bilthoven: RIVM, 2000:RIVM 210601001.

44. **Guebbels ELP, Mintjes-de Groot AJ, Wille J, et al.** *Dutch reference data on the incidence of surgical site infection after orthopaedic surgery.* 2000;in press.

45. **Walenkamp GHIM.** *Gentamicin PMMA beads: a clinical, pharmacokinetic and toxicological study.* Thesis Katholieke Universiteit Nijmegen, 1983.

46. **Walenkamp GHIM, GEEIOA.** L'infection en chirurgie orthopédique. Paris: Expansion Scientifique Francaise, 1990:14-21.

GENE THERAPY IN CARTILAGE REPAIR

ANDREAS B. IMHOFF AND VLADIMIR MARTINEK

From the Technical University, Munich, Germany

Lesions of the articular cartilage in the knee are common sports-related injuries.[1] In a review of more than 30 000 knee arthroscopies, lesions of the hyaline cartilage occurred in about 63% and most were located on the medial femoral condyle.[2] Such injuries are frequently associated with rupture of the anterior cruciate ligament (ACL). MRI has demonstrated bone bruises in 68% of patients with acute tears of the ACL.[1] While no relationship can be shown directly between bone bruises and osteochondral lesions, a significantly higher prevalence of articular chondromalacia was seen in patients with untreated injuries of the ACL.[1]

Articular cartilage has only a limited capability to regenerate. In most cases premature osteoarthritis will develop in the knee after trauma to the articular cartilage.[3] Although current concepts of treatment for injuries of the articular cartilage are promising, none can yet give complete restoration of the hyaline cartilage and the subchondral bone to a normal status.[4,5]

The advent of gene therapy has promoted new strategies for the treatment of osteochondral injuries. Significant contributions have been made in the last two decades in the understanding of the biology of articular cartilage and towards new approaches to treatment. The delivery of growth factors, cells, scaffolds, and therapeutic genes to lesions of the articular cartilage promises to change a field which historically has been limited to frustrating outcomes. Despite significant progress in the treatment of osteochondral lesions, however, many questions remain. This review focuses on the principles underlying gene therapy and describes the current state of gene transfer for disorders of the articular cartilage.

HEALING OF CARTILAGE

In adults articular cartilage lacks a blood supply, lymphatic drainage, or neural elements. The chondrocytes are protected from the nutritional synovial fluid and reparative recognition by their extracellular matrix. Only in situations of minor mechanical damage and limited loss of the matrix components are chondrocytes able to synthesise new proteoglycans and restore cartilage.[6] After considerable mechanical destruction of the cells and collagen scaffold, regeneration of articular cartilage is very limited.[7]

A particular requirement for the healing of defects of cartilage is the involvement of the underlying vascularised subchondral area. When the articular lesion reaches the subchondral marrow, a process of repair can be initiated by resident progenitor and blood cells which occupy the chondral defect. This new reparative tissue, however, which often contains fibrous elements, undergoes relatively fast degeneration and fails to function as hyaline cartilage.[7]

CONCEPTS OF TREATMENT

Based on knowledge of the pathophysiology of articular cartilage, many clinicians have attempted to improve healing by drilling, abrasion or microfracture of the subchondral bone.[8-10] The goal of these techniques was to recruit bone-marrow stem cells to stimulate the formation of fibrocartilaginous repair tissue. Although decreased pain is reported in patients treated by these techniques, the clinical value is uncertain.[6]

The transplantation of articular cartilage by autologous and allogenic osteochondral grafts has shown promising results in the treatment of circumscribed cartilage lesions.[5,11,12] Compared with the outcome of penetration of subchondral bone, osteochondral grafts provide repair with a fully-formed matrix of articular cartilage and viable chondrocytes potentially capable of maintaining the matrix.[6,8-10] Reports of recent clinical studies indicate that these techniques can restore the articular surface of the joint. The potential morbidity of the donor sites, however, is a major limitation of this approach.

Periosteal or perichondral soft-tissue grafts can also be used to deliver osteochondral progenitor cells to the sites of the cartilage defect.[13] These mesenchymal cells are capable of a broad range of chondrogenic expression and of producing new cartilage. Studies reporting small groups of patients with osteochondral lesions treated by periosteal and perichondral grafts suggest that improvement in symptoms can be achieved for a short time. The long-term durability of these graft materials, however, remains uncertain because of poor integration, and degeneration over time.[13]

Table I. Growth factors which have an effect on the metabolism of chondrocytes

Growth factor	Proliferation	Differentiation	Migration	Matrix synthesis
IGF-1	+			+
bFGF	+		+	+
EGF	+			+
TGF-β		+		+
BMP2		+		+
CDMP (1 to 3)		+		

A newly-introduced approach for the treatment of osteochondral lesions is implantation of autologous chondrocytes.[14] This technique of treatment uses standard cell-culture techniques for autologous chondrocytes, which are injected underneath a periosteal flap sutured over the articular defect. The clinical results of this treatment are good or excellent in 85% of patients after three years, but the correlation with the histological findings of a 'hyaline-like cartilage' is lacking.

GROWTH FACTORS

Growth factors are cytokines with key functions for the healing of tissues of the musculoskeletal system. They are small peptides synthesised both by the resident cells at the site of injury, such as mesenchymal stem cells or chondrocytes, and by the infiltrating inflammatory cells which stimulate proliferation, migration, synthesis of matrix, and differentiation of the cells.[6,15] Many of these growth factors, including insulin-like growth factor (IGF-1), transforming growth factor-β (TGF-β), basic fibroblast growth factor (bFGF), bone morphogenetic proteins (BMPs), epidermal growth factor (EGF), platelet-derived growth factor (PDGF), and cartilage-derived morphogenetic proteins (CDMPs) can affect the metabolism of chondrocytes (Table I).[15]

Several growth factors have been shown to improve the healing of cartilage in vivo.[16,17] Hunziker and Rosenberg[16] investigated the repair of partial-thickness defects of the articular cartilage using several growth factors, fibrin clots and digestive enzymes. Although the findings did not result in a normal articular cartilage, the study showed a positive effect of TGF-β and of enzymic digestion of the articular surface on the healing of cartilage. BMP-2 appears to be involved in the growth and differentiation of mesenchymal cells to chondroblasts and osteoblasts. Sellers et al[17] used recombinant human BMP-2 for the treatment of full-thickness defects of articular cartilage in rabbits and found an accelerated formation of new subchondral bone and an improved histological appearance of the overlying articular surface. Neidel[18] found no effect on the healing of articular cartilage after intra-articular injections of FGF, IGF-1 or EGF in adult rabbits.

Although the direct application of specific growth factor proteins has some beneficial effect on the healing process of cartilage in vivo, it is uncertain if single applications of growth factors can obtain the optimal effect of repair of the complex cartilage tissue.[16-18] Because of the relatively short biological half-life, high dosages and repeated injections of growth factors will probably be required to reach the optimum in the treatment of osteochondral defects.[19] Various strategies, including carrier matrices, pumps and heparin, have been investigated to achieve constant levels of growth factors at injured sites. Despite the fact that these approaches have been capable of improving the local persistence of the growth factor proteins, the results of these delivery techniques remain limited and often clinically irrelevant. Of the different methods developed for the local administration of growth factors, gene-transfer techniques have proved to be the most promising.[20]

GENE THERAPY

Gene therapy is a technique which relies on the alteration of cellular genetic information, and is applicable to the treatment of lesions of cartilage by transferring genes, encoded for specific growth factors, into chondrocytes or progenitor cells. For gene expression, the transferred DNA material must enter the nucleus where it can be transcripted. After this, the generated mRNA is transported outside the nucleus, serving as a matrix for the production of proteins, such as growth factors, in the ribosomes (Fig. 1).

Viral and non-viral vectors can be used for the delivery of genetic material into cells. The non-viral gene-transfer systems including liposomes, naked DNA, and DNA ligands, are usually easier to produce and have lower toxicity and immunogenicity, but the efficiency of their gene delivery is hindered by a low rate of infection unless the transduced cells are selected.

Currently, viral gene vectors, such as retrovirus, adenovirus, adeno-associated virus, and herpes virus, present a more efficient method for gene transfer.[19] Gene delivery into the cartilage and the subchondral bone is potentially possible by an ex-vivo or in-vivo approach. Either the vectors can be directly injected into the host tissue (in vivo) or the cells from the injured tissue are removed, genetically altered in vitro, and reinjected in the injury site (ex vivo). While the direct method is less technically demanding, indirect gene delivery is safer, because the genetic engin-

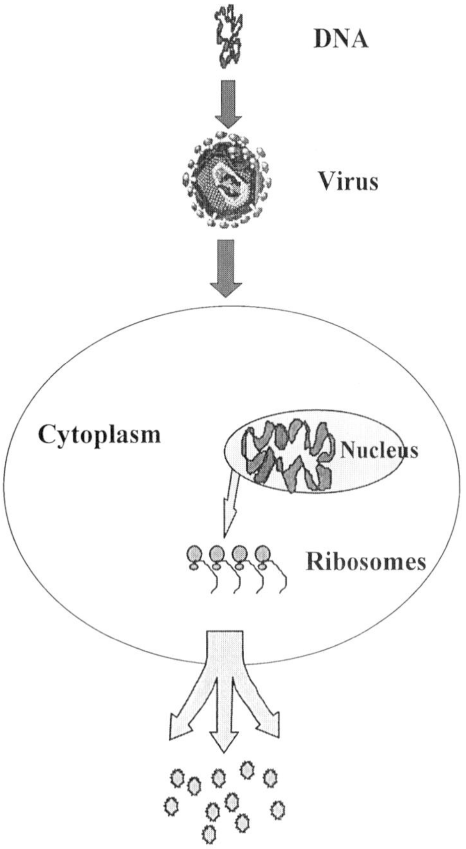

Fig. 1

Principles of gene transfer with viral vectors.

eering takes place under controlled conditions outside the organism. With the ex-vivo approach, growth factors can be delivered with endogenous cells capable of responding to the stimuli and participating in the healing process in the injured tissue.

For the treatment of defects of cartilage, the major concern in the use of gene therapy is safety. While gene therapy may represent a 'last chance' treatment option for severe disorders such as malignancies or Duchenne's muscular dystrophy, the risks of side-effects and potential consequences may be unacceptable in elective orthopaedic surgery. Viral vectors integrating into the genome of the cells bear the risk of insertional mutagenesis.[21] Possible abnormal regulation of cell growth, toxicity due to chronic overexpression of the growth factor protein, and the development of a malignancy are theoretically conceivable, although cases have not been reported.

Gene-transfer techniques for clinically applicable treatment of osteochondral lesions are still not available. Feasibility studies, however, have demonstrated the capability of chondrocytes to be transduced with marker genes in vitro and in vivo.[22-24] Doherty et al[23] showed that chondrocytes transduced with the β-galactosidase gene are able to bind to cartilage explants in vitro and to express the transgene up to seven weeks. These findings raise the possibility of rebuilding cartilage by resurfacing with genetically-modified chondrocytes. The first successful delivery of potentially therapeutic genes was demonstrated by Ikeda et al.[24] They administered TGF-β gene into the joints of Hartley guinea-pigs using an adenoviral vector, but the effect on the turnover of cartilage was not reported in this study.

Although progress is evident with gene therapy, it still cannot be considered as an established technique. Many laboratories focus their effort on the development of viral and non-viral vectors to deliver therapeutic genes and, consequently, major advances in vector development can be expected in the near future.[25]

TISSUE ENGINEERING

Tissue engineering is a technique based on the development of biological substitutes for the repair, reconstruction, regeneration, or replacement of biological tissues.[26] The

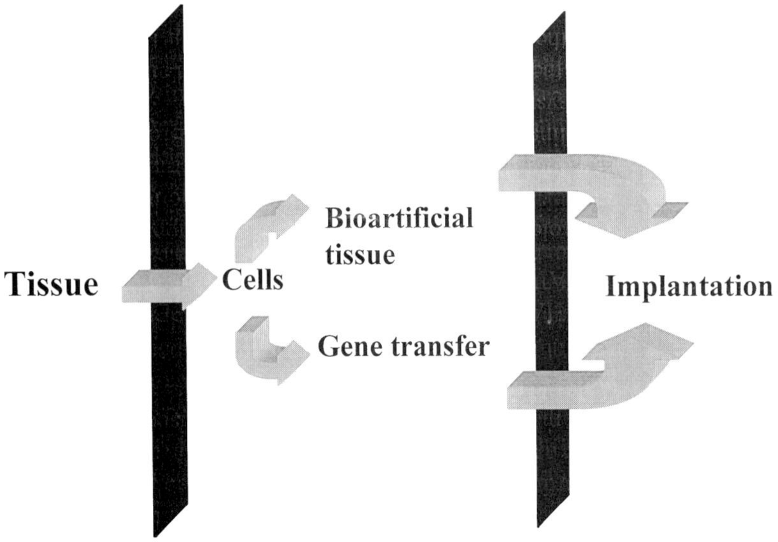

Fig. 2

Principle of tissue engineering.

Table II. Experimental treatment of chondral and osteochondral lesions

Matrix/scaffold*	Cells/growths factors*	Species	Follow-up	Healing
Cartilage allograft	Chondrocytes/GP	Rabbit	1 yr	29% to 80%
Collagen gel	Chondrocytes/ALLO	Rabbit	24 wks	80%
Fibrin	Chondrocytes/ART	Horse	35 wks	Improved
Collagen gel	Chondrocytes/ALLO	Rat	52 wks	94%
PGA matrix	Chondrocytes/ART	Rabbit	7 wks	Improved
Collagen scaffold	Chondrocytes/ART	Horse	35 wks	Improved
PDLA matrix	Perichondrocytes	Rabbit	6 wks	96%
Carbon-fibre pads	Chondrocytes/ART	Rabbit	52 wks	Improved
Fibrin clot	bFGF, TGF-β, IGF-1	Rabbit	48 wks	Improved
PLG polymers	TGF-β	Goat	16 wks	Improved
2-layer collagen	Chondrocytes/ART	Rabbit	24 wks	Improved
Collagen sponge	BMP-2	Rabbit	24 wks	Improved
PLA matrix	Perichondrocytes/ALLO	Rabbit	52 wks	85%
Hydroxyapatite	Chondrocytes/ART	Goat	52 wks	Poor
Collagen matrix	Chondrocytes/ART	Dog	15 wks	Improved
Collagen gel	Mesenchymal cells	Rabbit	24 wks	Improved
Agarose gel	Chondrocytes/ALLO	Rabbit	1.5 yrs	47%
Fibrin	IGF-1	Horses	24 wks	Improved

* ART, articular; GP, growth plate; ALLO, allografts; PDLA, D,D-L,L-polylactic acid; PGA, polyglycolic acid; PLG, polylactide/-glycolide

goal is to construct biomaterials which are biocompatible, biodegradable, and capable of integrating molecules, such as growth factors, or cells. Generally, the tissue of interest can be used to obtain cells for the construction of bio-artificial tissue or for genetic engineering (Fig. 2). Meanwhile, various ceramics, polymers of lactic and glycolic acid, collagen gels, and other polymers have been tested in vitro and applied in vivo in experimental situations (Table II).

The application of tissue engineering to defects of the articular cartilage necessitates the transplantation of viable cells in an appropriate supportive vehicle. In general, two different principles are used in the choice of cells for the repair of articular defects. Either fully-differentiated chondrocytes are used or less differentiated pluripotential cell lines, so called mesenchymal stem cells, are chosen for cartilage engineering in the restoration of articular defects.[27-32] Differentiated articular chondrocytes are able to produce cartilage under appropriate conditions. They are probably optimal if the lesion of the joint surface is limited to the articular cartilage, but they are not capable of restoring the subchondral bone. Many defects, however, involve the subchondral bone, and in these cases pluripotential stem cells capable of forming bone are a better choice for the repair of osteochondral lesions.

Today, the most popular method of articular cartilage engineering is the transplantation of autologous chondrocytes which was developed for clinical use by Brittberg et al.[4] Chondrocytes are isolated from biopsy specimens and grown in a monolayer culture to increase the cell population. The cultured cells are resuspended in a liquid medium and placed underneath a periosteal flap sewn over the cartilage lesion. This method of treatment has received much attention and has been applied in small groups of patients worldwide, but there is some controversy regarding the disparity between the subjective and objective results, and the long-term effects. The role of the periosteum, containing pluripotential stem cells with chondrogenic potency, is also not clear.

Scaffolds and matrices are the supportive components in cartilage engineering. Their role is not confined to retaining chondrocytes or other chondrogenic cells in the articular defect. There is evidence that at least some types of bio-matrix can contribute to the repair of articular cartilage.[6] Fibrin has been used as an implant which allows the timed release of growth factors.[16,33] Among the numerous biological and synthetic materials, biodegradable matrices are thought to possess the most promising potential for the repair of osteochondral defects. The ideal scaffold for cartilage engineering has not yet been identified, however, and new biomatrices are being developed.

In recent studies, the scaffolds were seeded with growth factors to stimulate locally the repair of articular cartilage and to attract the chondroprogenitor cells from the bone marrow or from the articular synovium.[16,17,34] Athanasiou et al[34] have demonstrated in goats that polylactic acid-polyglycolic acid implants can be used to deliver TGF-β to large osteochondral defects. Although the regenerated new cartilage did not fill the defects completely, the implants with TGF-β resulted in better structural integrity. Hunziker and Rosenberg[16] have treated partial-thickness defects in articular cartilage in rabbits with fibrin clots and mitogenic

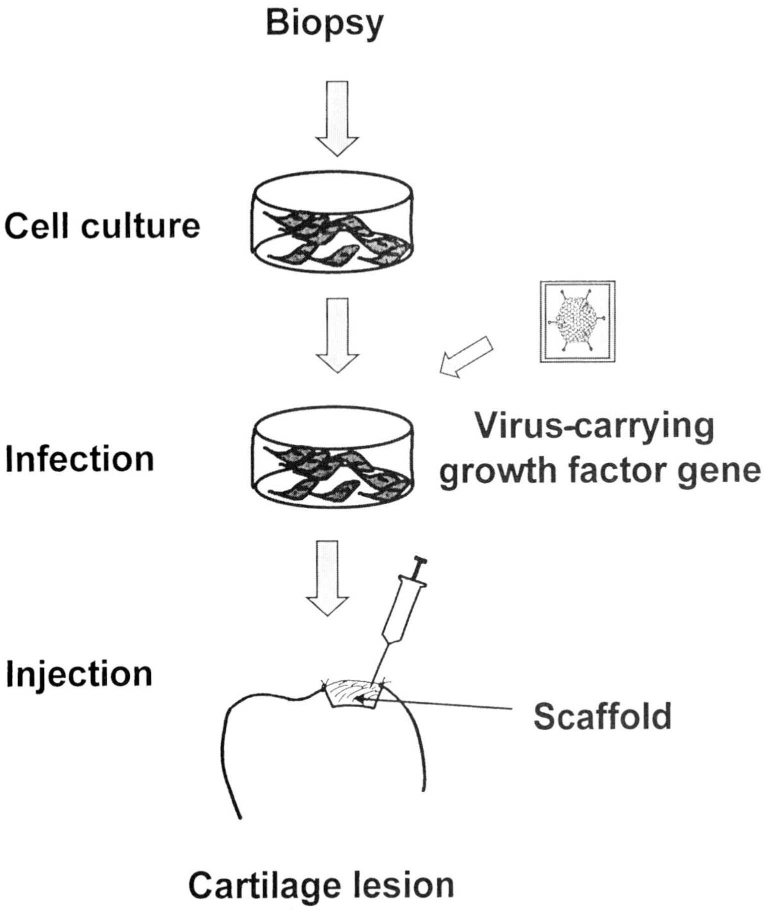

Fig. 3

Diagram of cell-based gene therapy and tissue engineering in the treatment of osteochondral lesions.

growth factors after digesting the surface of the defect with chondroitinase ABC or trypsin. They were able to show that under these conditions the mesenchymal cells originating from the synovium participated in the repair of the articular defect. Sellers et al[17] reported the improved repair of osteochondral defects treated with a collagen sponge impregnated with BMP-2. They observed not only an accelerated formation of the subchondral bone, but also an improved histological appearance of the overlying articular cartilage.

FUTURE PERSPECTIVES

Future research will investigate the optimal combination of scaffolds, matrices, cells, adhesives and growth factors to repair defects of the articular cartilage. The combination of gene-transfer techniques and tissue engineering is one of the promising new strategies for the treatment of osteochondral injuries. The potential advantage of gene transfer into the chondrogenic cells relies on sustained levels of growth factors, which can be reached through transgene expression in situ.

Recently, studies have been performed to demonstrate the feasibility of viral transduction of chondroprogenitor cells in vivo.[35] Using rabbit mesenchymal stem cells embedded in polymer scaffold grafts and transduced with a retroviral vector encoded for the marker gene lacZ, β-galactosidase-positive cells have been detected up to eight weeks after implantation into osteochondral defects in rabbit femora.[35] In an experiment ex vivo, Grande et al[36] used autologous periosteal cells retrovirally transduced with BMP-7 to repair osteochondral defects in rabbits. Rapid reconstitution of the subchondral bone and predominantly hyaline-like tissue were found in the samples implanted with transduced periosteal cells. Generally, cells from different tissues, including mesenchymal stem cells, muscle-derived cells and dermal fibroblasts, can be used to deliver genes into cartilage (Fig. 3).

REFERENCES

1. **Dimond PM, Fadale PD, Hulstyn MJ, et al.** A comparison of MRI findings in patients with acute and chronic ACL tears. *Am J Knee Surg* 1998;11:153-9.
2. **Curl WW, Krome J, Gordon ES, et al.** Cartilage injuries: a review of 31 516 knee arthroscopies. *Arthroscopy* 1997;13:456-60.
3. **Mankin HJ.** The response of articular cartilage to mechanical injury. *J Bone Joint Surg [Am]* 1982;64-A:460-6.
4. **Brittberg M, Lindahl A, Nilsson A, et al.** Treatment of deep cartilage defects in the knee with autologous chondrocyte transplantation. *N Engl J Med* 1994;331:889-95.
5. **Hangody L, Kish G, Karpati Z, et al.** Arthroscopic autogenous osteochondral mosaicplasty for the treatment of femoral condylar articular defects: a preliminary report. *Knee Surg Sports Traumatol Arthrosc* 1997;5:262-7.
6. **Buckwalter JA, Mankin HJ.** Articular cartilage: degeneration and osteoarthritis, repair, regeneration, and transplantation. *Instr Course Lect* 1998;47:487-504.

7. **Shapiro F, Koide S, Glimcher MJ.** Cell origin and differentiation in the repair of full-thickness defects of articular cartilage. *J Bone Joint Surg [Am]* 1993;75-A:532-53.

8. **Dzioba RB.** The classification and treatment of acute articular cartilage lesions. *Arthroscopy* 1988;4(2):72-80.

9. **Friedman MJ, Berasi CC, Fox JM, et al.** Preliminary results with abrasion arthroplasty in the osteoarthritic knee. *Clin Orthop* 1984;182:200-5.

10. **Steadman JR, Rodkey WG, Briggs KK, Rodrigo JJ.** The microfracture technique in the management of complete cartilage defects in the knee joint. *Orthopade* 1999;28:26-32.

11. **Meyers MH, Akeson W, Convery FR.** Resurfacing of the knee with fresh osteochondral allograft. *J Bone Joint Surg [Am]* 1989;71:704-13.

12. **Outerbridge HK, Outerbridge AR, Outerbridge RE.** The use of a lateral patellar autologous graft for the repair of a large osteochondral defect in the knee. *J Bone Joint Surg [Am]* 1995;77:65-72.

13. **Chang PC, Pradhan RM, Mitra AK, Sim CS, Tay BK.** The results of autogenous tibial periosteal transplants for full thickness cartilage defects in the knee joints of pigs. *Ann Acad Med Singapore* 1999;28:8-14.

14. **Brittberg M, Nilsson A, Lindahl A, Ohlsson C, Peterson L.** Rabbit articular cartilage defects treated with autologus cultured chondrocytes. *Clin Orthop* 1996;326:270-83.

15. **Trippel SB.** Growth factors as therapeutic agents. *Instr Course Lec* 1997;46:473-6.

16. **Hunziker EB, Rosenberg LC.** Repair of partial-thickness defects in articular cartilage: cell recruitment from the synovium. *J Bone Joint Surg [Am]* 1996;78-A:721-33.

17. **Sellers RS, Peluso D, Morris EA.** The effect of recombinant human bone morphogenetic protein-2 (rhBMP-2) on the healing of full-thickness defects of articular cartilage. *J Bone Joint Surg [Am]* 1997;79-A:1452-63.

18. **Neidel JJ.** No improvement of joint cartilage healing after trauma by the administration of insulin-like growth factor I, epidermal growth factor and fibroblast growth factor in rabbits. *Z Orthop Ihre Grenzgeb* 1992;130:73-8.

19. **Evans CH, Robbins PD.** Possible orthopaedic applications of gene therapy. *J Bone Joint Surg [Am]* 1995;77-A:1103-14.

20. **Mulligan RC.** The basic science of gene therapy. *Science* 1993;260:926-32.

21. **Crystal RG.** Transfer of genes to humans: early lessons and obstacles to success. *Science* 1995;270:404-10.

22. **Arai Y, Kubo T, Kobayashi K, et al.** Adenovirus vector-mediated gene transduction to chondrocytes: in vitro evaluation of therapeutic efficacy of transforming growth factor-beta 1 and heat shock protein 70 gene transduction. *J Rheumatol* 1997;24:1787-95.

23. **Doherty PJ, Zhang H, Tremblay L, Manolopoulos V, Marshall KW.** Resurfacing of articular cartilage explants with genetically-modified human chondrocytes in vitro. *Osteoarthritis Cartilage* 1998;6:153-9.

24. **Ikeda T, Kubo T, Arai Y, et al.** Adenovirus mediated gene delivery to the joints of guinea pigs. *J Rheumatol* 1998;25:1666-73.

25. **Robbins PD, Ghivizzani SC.** Viral vectors for gene therapy. *Pharmacol Ther* 1998;80:35-47.

26. **Freed LE, Vunjak-Novakovic G, Biron RJ, et al.** Biodegradable polymer scaffolds for tissue engineering. *Biotechnology (NY)* 1994;12:689-93.

27. **Aston JE, Bentley G.** Repair of articular surfaces by allografts of articular and growth-plate cartilage. *J Bone Joint Surg [Br]* 1986;68-B:29-35.

28. **Frenkel SR, Toolan B, Menche D, Pitman MI, Pachence JM.** Chondrocyte transplantation using a collagen bilayer matrix for cartilage repair. *J Bone Joint Surg [Br]* 1997;79-B:831-6.

29. **Nehrer S, Breinan HA, Ramappa A, et al.** Chondrocyte-seeded collagen matrices implanted in a chondral defect in a canine model. *Biomaterials* 1998;19:2313-28.

30. **Sams AE, Nixon AJ.** Chondrocyte-laden collagen scaffolds for resurfacing extensive articular cartilage defects. *Osteoarthritis Cartilage* 1995;3:47-59.

31. **Wakitani S, Kimura T, Hirooka A, et al.** Repair of rabbit articular surfaces with allograft chondrocytes embedded in collagen gel. *J Bone Joint Surg [Br]* 1989;71-B:74-80.

32. **Robinson D, Efrat M, Mendes DG, Halperin N, Nero Z.** Implants composed of carbon fibre mesh and bone-marrow-derived, chondrocyte-enriched cultures for joint surface reconstruction. *Bull Hosp Jt Dis* 1993;53:75-82.

33. **Kawabe N, Yoshinao M.** The repair of full-thickness articular cartilage defects: immune responses to reparative tissue formed by allogeneic growth plate chondrocyte implants. *Clin Orthop* 1991;268:279-93.

34. **Athanasiou KA, Korvick D, Schenck R.** Biodegradable implants for the treatment of osteochondral defects in a goat model. *Tissue Eng* 1997;3:363.

35. **Mason JM, Grande DA, Barcia M, et al.** Expression of human bone morphogenic protein 7 in primary rabbit periosteal cells: potential utility in gene therapy for osteochondral repair. *Gene Ther* 1998;5:1098-104.

36. **Grande DA, Mason J, Paulino C, et al.** Gene enhanced tissue engineering for repair of osteochondral defects. Procs 45th Annual meeting of the Orthopaedic Research Society, 1999.

ENHANCEMENT OF THE HEALING OF FRACTURES

DAVID I. ROWLEY

From the University of Dundee, Scotland

The healing of fractures is a unique phenomenon, which so far has defied a full and logical explanation, based upon biological and mechanical factors that can be linked together in a coherent fashion. Further understanding of this is of importance because it may help us to optimise healing and provide information on which to base judgements when assessing different regimes of the management of fractures.

The fact that bones do heal is in itself remarkable; as Marsh and Li[1] have pointed out, they do not so much heal as regenerate. In most cases after a fracture has undergone the repair, within a few years, there are no obvious physical or functional signs that the bone was broken. This makes bone a very special type of connective tissue. The terminology which we use for the process of bone healing, may be summarised as a 'regenerative repair process'. Even more remarkably, this facility of bone is not dependent upon the tissue itself, but also on the surrounding soft tissues, especially the capillaries and the totipotential cells, which they import to the site of the fracture. The role of cells and bony and other tissues will be explored later.

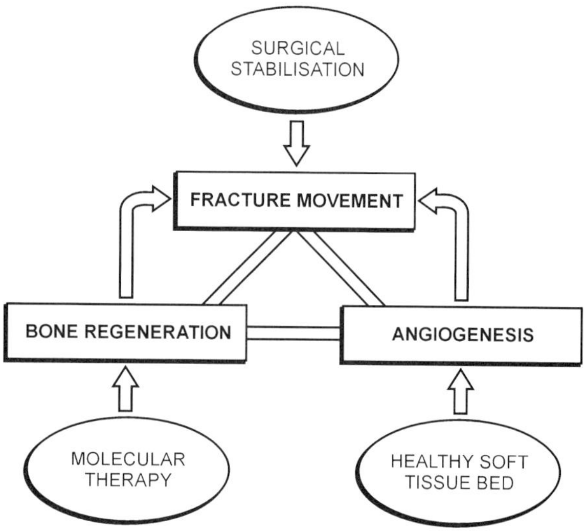

Fig. 1

Diagram of Marsh and Li's[1] triad of inter-relationships in the regenerative repair of fractures.

THE 'HOWS' AND 'WHYS' OF THE HEALING OF FRACTURES

Apley used to give a celebrated lecture called 'Choices'. In this talk he explored why groups of surgeons decide to choose to manage fractures in different ways, usually with similar results. If he was being unkind, he would point out that "fixation is fun" and would describe how when given a drill, a gleam would come into the surgeon's eye.

More significantly he asked "Why do fractures heal?". Some interesting facts flow from this apparently naïve question. For instance, we observe that in an amputated limb the divided bone end makes no attempt to repair. In other words the bone 'knows' that the other end is no longer there; how does it 'know'? The implication is that there are signals of some kind, and we are beginning to appreciate that these are cellularly mediated, initially in association with the body's response to injury, and subsequently in ways which are dependent on the changes in the mechanical and biological environment of the site of the fracture.

The exploration of responses at the cellular level offers us insights into the physiological processes and how we may manipulate them.

Apley made another key observation in that "fracture healing is like making love . . it brings two things together and a little bit of movement helps". Broken bones heal because they are no longer stiff, and as they stiffen up the healing process changes. The rate at which stiffness occurs affects the process and *vice versa*. A major breakthrough in understanding healing is to appreciate the relationship between stiffness and function rather than between strength and function. Bones are naturally much stronger than they need to be for ordinary function and they are in a sense, 'overly engineered'. It is clearly an evolutionary advantage to be able to overcome the natural violence that occurs from falls. Marsh and Li[1] have summarised this eloquently in a relationship between movement, soft-tissue response and bone regeneration (Fig. 1). We can summarise here as only Apley could: "Bones heal because they are broken".

THE 'HOW'S' AND MODERN UNDERSTANDING OF HEALING

In general, we will concentrate on the healing of long bones because the biology and mechanics are more comprehensible. We need to assume that natural healing relies on an adequate blood supply and so 'damage', in this discussion, must be assumed to be of the low-energy type.

The formation of a haematoma and local bone death at the site of a fracture occur immediately after injury. The haematoma is believed to be more than a passive stage and is the first opportunity for repair to begin. Platelets, in particular, release a variety of products. Growth factors, especially platelet-derived growth factor and transforming growth factor beta (TGF-β), trigger a sustained inflammatory response which results in a cytokine cascade and attracts relevant repair cells to the site of the fracture.

It seems pertinent to ask what are the consequences of interfering with the haematoma or what are the surgical consequences of avoiding such a natural event?

The next crucial step is the re-establishment of a fresh blood supply to the necrotic area and the formation of cartilage, fibrous tissue and bone (provisional or the formation of soft callus). This seems to require the "little bit of movement" mentioned by Apley and if movement is excluded this type of healing will not occur. This has profound consequences for stable fixation and leads to a form of direct cortical union, more akin to remodelling, which is the slower last phase of the natural healing of fractures.

With fixation we also artificially restore stiffness at the site of the fracture as a consequence of restoring continuity; in doing so, however, we do not make the bone strong enough to stand up to all activities and it takes time for the load share between bone and implant to become predominantly that of the bone. What we have done is to 'short-circuit' the natural progression to stiffness which occurs through the formation of callus and we must realise that we do so at our peril, given the current state of knowledge.

Callus may also form on the inside surface of bones, so-called endosteal callus. This is seen by some as a late[2] and by some as an early[3] event. Marsh and Li[1] point out that as healing is a function of increasing stiffness associated with the restoration of blood supply, in relatively stable, but not rigid, situations, endosteal callus, facilitated via a largely intact intramedullary blood supply, is a significant contributor to early bone healing. This, they claim, may be the reason why fine-wire external fixators facilitate rapid healing in low-velocity injuries and allow prompt healing in high-velocity states because they restore sufficient stability to allow formation of endosteal as well as soft callus and prejudice the blood supply minimally beyond the initial damage from the injury.

The conversion of soft to hard callus is a continual process whereby bone is either formed directly from mesenchymal tissue or via cartilage. It is this progression to bone which provides the stiffness that allows function. The resulting stage is of a stiff construct, but with woven bone of random orientation.

It is now possible for remodelling to take place to restore the old structure. This is normally a process of laying down a new extracellular matrix built on a collagen framework which changes with time and is significantly influenced by the presence of osteonectin.

HEALING IN SUMMARY

Referring back to Figure 1 we can sum up some aspects of natural healing and begin to understand some of the underlying processes and how we may influence them. Bones respond to fracture through a process associated with detecting changes in stiffness. The initial healing of the fracture requires an early restoration of stiffness, and it is equally important as the restoration of the blood supply. The initial haematoma[4] and inflammatory response start the process, and only with increasing stiffness will an optimal blood supply be restored. There is therefore a fine balance between stiffness, blood supply and progressive healing. Both mechanical and cellular responses contribute to this complex process.

MECHANICAL MODIFICATIONS TO FRACTURE HEALING

The reasons for fixing fractures are many. In multiple injuries we do so to minimise a life-threatening pathophysiological response to injury. This has been a major factor in reducing mortality and morbidity. However, it is one thing to say that it works in multiple injury and another that it should work even better in injury to single bones.

In the latter we are able to establish that the degree of energy transfer and the damage to the soft tissues are major factors in determining outcome. From the description above it should be clear that there is a critical time for achieving adequate stiffness before angiogenesis is able adequately to sustain healing. If stiffness is delayed, the degree of development of new blood vessels may also be retarded and the cascade of healing interrupted.[5] Marsh[6] indicates that without the cells associated with the importation of new capillaries, the callus would not progress.

Let us look in particular at the function of the soft-tissue element of an injury. I was involved in a series of studies in association with the International Committee of the Red Cross in Afghanistan and Sudan. My remit was to investigate the treatment of bone wounds caused by high-velocity missiles, predominantly bullets from assault rifles.[7,8] Observations on successfully treated bullet wounds of the femur were remarkable. Provided that the wound track was appropriately excised and allowed to heal by skin grafting or delayed primary closure, the underlying rate of bone healing was much shorter than would be expected from a similar bone injury experienced in civilian blunt trauma. Figure 2 illustrates a bone wound from a high-velocity

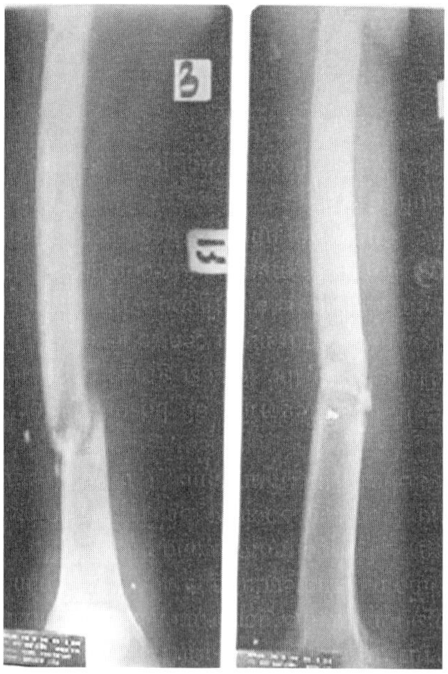

Fig. 2

Radiographs showing a femoral fracture caused in warfare by a high-velocity stable bullet. This fracture went on to heal in four weeks.

injury which if experienced in civilian life would have been a major challenge to a trauma surgeon. In an Afghan study[7] the mean time on traction was only four weeks, followed by early mobilisation either in a simple thin cast gaiter or merely with crutches. Clinically, the fractures were stiff and many of the patients went back to their homes within a few days of mobilising, because of the exigencies of war and scarce resources.

In order to explain this phenomenon we examined the circumstances and in particular the wound ballistics more carefully. We were able to demonstrate that high-velocity bullets would produce intense areas of local damage to the soft tissues with very little energy transfer to the broader soft-tissue envelope. It is common experience that in blunt trauma the degree of soft-tissue damage is likely to be more diffuse. Perversely, these war wounds gave a type of controlled understanding of energy-transfer mechanisms. Figures 3 and 4 show a laboratory simulation of the situation shown in Figure 2. It is clear that local disruption is limited to the bone and the immediately adjacent soft tissues.

Although circumstantial, this evidence supports the connection between the degree of damage to the local blood supply and its effect on fracture healing. Put simply, the less the local tissue damage is, the more rapid the healing. It also supports the earlier observation that less extensive damage to the soft-tissue envelope will render the fracture stiffer than if these tissues are extensively stripped. This in turn supports the benefits of early stability being important in allowing the rapid contribution of endosteal callus to the healing process.

Kenwright et al[9] demonstrated a clear association between movement at the site of the fracture (properly expressed as strain) and healing. Early on[9] it was shown that strain applied for even short periods of time was adequate to induce healing when compared with no perceived movement. More recently, Goodship, Cunningham and Kenwright[10] have refined this to illustrate that the rate of strain affects healing by the formation of callus directly. High rates of strain were more effective in producing callus than were low rates. Furthermore, the quality of callus as measured by densitometry was improved if the strains were applied shortly after fracture as opposed to after a period of rest. We already know from earlier work by Sarmiento et al[11] that early bracing is associated with good rates of healing. All this, as yet circumstantially, supports the notion that changing the strain at the site of fractures is intimately associated with changes in healing. The mediating factors are likely to be cellular as will be discussed below. As yet the link between these observations and the cellular activity

Fig. 3a

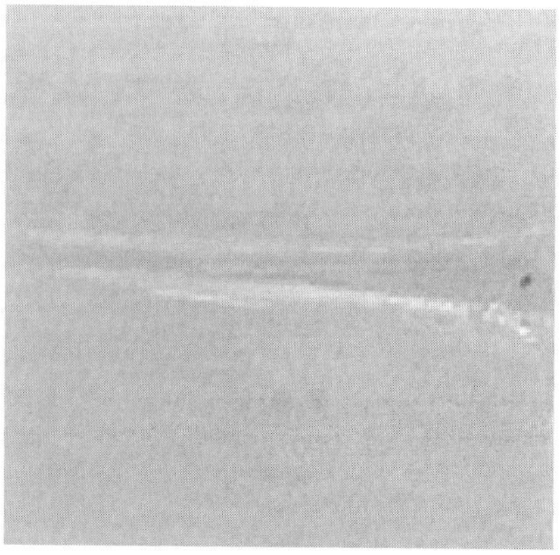

Fig. 3b

Photograph showing an identical simulated fracture to that in Figure 2, created in plastic bone by firing a high-velocity bullet such that it entered the gelatine block (a) in stable flight. When a bullet is fired in identical circumstances through a paraffin block (b), the degree of energy transfer is small, as illustrated by the minimal displacement of the paraffin.

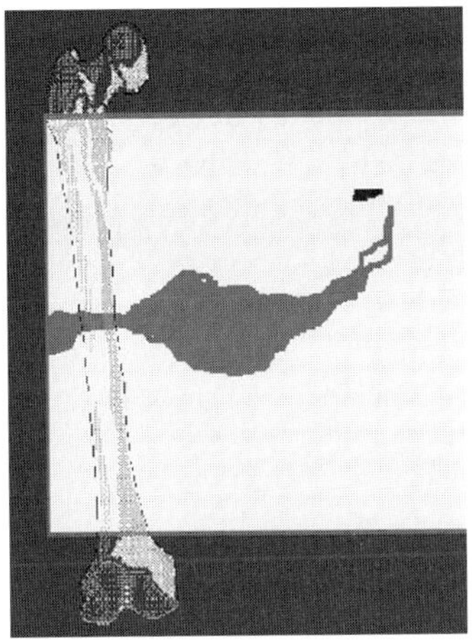

Fig. 4

A diagram showing the bullet track and its energy transfer to the soft-tissue envelope. The superimposed femur illustrates how a simple transverse fracture like that in the radiograph could be produced with surprisingly little damage to the blood supply.

and mediators still has to be elucidated in any depth. The implication that strain applied early is more favourable than the same forces applied later accords with clinical experience, although we can only speculate as to why the healing process is so dependent on time.

Using this information we can now begin, if not to enhance natural healing, at least to avoid inhibiting it. Early movement at strain rates of a higher frequency can be induced as an adjunct to stiff systems, such as with biaxial beam external fixators or with more strain-permissive systems such as the Ilizarov fixator. In the latter we now have strong supportive evidence as to why, if not how, such systems are so effective in allowing natural healing. Goodship et al[10] also provide support for earlier observations that stable fixation delays union by restoring continuity without a transitional phase of relative lack of stiffness.

How does that help us look at ways of modifying, by optimising, rather than enhancing the healing of fractures? We have observed the remarkable work of Ilizarov, whereby the healing of fractures in the most adverse circumstances appears to be more effective when fine-wire fixators are used. This principle has been extended in more routine fracture management (Atkins, personal communication) whereby a degree of stability is restored which seems to create the right blend of 'a little bit of movement' and sufficient stiffness[12] to optimise healing, particularly because the fine wires have been inserted without effect on the local blood supply and perhaps also because the fracture haematoma was not interfered with. It may well be that this situation of treating closed, lower-velocity injuries by the Ilizarov method will open up significant possibilities for studying cell-mediated responses to the normal healing of fractures. It seems a pity to miss this opportunity to extend our knowledge, but as yet it would appear that there is no economic justification for changing to such radical interventions for the treatment of routine fractures. We must continue to use cost-effective casting and bracing technology which has been shown to be so effective in low-velocity trauma.[11]

UNDERSTANDING THE CELLULAR RESPONSE

Following on from the preliminary observations above, we can fit together the roles of some well-known intercell messengers in terms of growth factors and cytokines. These may be summarised in a list which matches our empirical knowledge, but the following may not necessarily be the true sequence and pattern of events.

TGF-β is released by platelets as part of the initial inflammatory response which suggests that it may be the principal regulator of healing.[13]

In animal models we know that bone morphogenetic proteins (BMP), especially BMP-2 and BMP-4, are present early in the healing process and that they are associated with the rapid proliferation of mesenchymal cells. We also know that as these cells move from proliferation to hypertrophy and differentiation, the concentration of BMPs declines. We may conclude that these osteoconductive substances induce the formation of callus. Jin and Yang[14] feel that some bone cells produce BMPs, which in turn make other cells lay down callus. This pattern is clearer in intramembranous ossification than in enchondral ossification.

The role of BMPs in enchondral ossification thus remains unclear. BMP-7 is also present during healing but occurs later in the process, and is seen in chondroprogenitor cells and chondrocytes. Its role seems to be synergistic and complementary to the other BMPs but in ways not yet understood.

There are now about a dozen BMPs described in various animal models of fracture healing. It is perplexing to contemplate what this means for the practising orthopaedic surgeon. We need to be cautious before taking the therapeutic implications of these substances into common practice without properly conducted, statistically powerful, randomised controlled trials.

A simplistic summary may be that TGF-β stimulates cells to make and react to BMPs and other factors in a synergistic cascade which, given the right mechanical conditions, in the presence of a new blood supply, leads to regenerative bone repair. As pointed out by Bostrom and Asnis,[13] it is tempting to contemplate therapeutic effects especially from TGF-β, as observations clearly demonstrate that, in its presence, the formation of bone in animal models is augmented.[15]

ENHANCING AND SUPPLEMENTING HEALING

Many authors have discussed the ethics and cost-benefits of interventions in the process of fracture healing. We would all accept that some fractures do not heal and others take longer to heal than the statistical norm. Einhorn and Lane[16] imply that between 5% and 10% of fractures have some difficulty in healing. This figure seems somewhat high, but even taking an overall rate of nonunion of 2%, when considering the over 6 million fractures per annum in the USA this represents a high level of morbidity.

It seems unreasonable to suggest in these times of scarce resources, and against this evidence, that we should seek to accelerate or even anticipate in a blanket fashion, problems with healing by trying to enhance or supplement all healing. However, given useful and practical guidelines, it is reasonable to attempt to find ways to anticipate difficult problems of union and to seek appropriate treatment. These techniques, however, must be subjected to appropriate double-blind trials.

THE METHOD OF CHOICE

Given that most fractures unite eventually, judgement of a successful intervention is difficult. It requires the utmost scientific rigour to be certain that progress to union has been influenced by a method of treatment. Our task is further made difficult because an all-embracing definition of union eludes us. On the whole, we now acknowledge that reaching a level of stiffness indicates union, but, until cortical architecture is restored, we are never really confident of definitive repair. We must, therefore, accept that we have to take some claims with healthy scepticism, while retaining a degree of pragmatism.

What is the method of choice? Cancellous autograft supplied in large amounts to a well vascularised bed is known to be osteogenic.[17] The advantages of immunocompatibility of autograft are obvious. Some cells survive, especially surface-based osteoblasts. The bodily reaction to autograft is similar to the physiological process of repair. As with normal healing, the incoming new blood vessels are important and so a well-vascularised bed for the graft is vital, to such a degree that in poorly vascularised areas the importation of new blood supply via free flaps should be considered an integral part of management. Cancellous graft, however, has no intrinsic strength for many months and so supplementary support is required, bringing in confounding factors to the degree of overall stiffness of the nonunion-graft-fixation construct. Even allowing for this, it is reasonable to judge new modes of treatment against this standard of autografting of internally fixed delayed union or nonunion.

ELECTROMAGNETIC INTERVENTIONS

Since the original observations of Fukada and Yasuda,[18] Bassett, Pawluk and Pilla[19] have championed the use of electromagnetic fields in the management of nonunion and delayed union. Strain is thought to be a stimulus to the generation of electromagnetic fields although how this is effectively mediated is not known. It is particularly difficult to separate this electromagnetic effect from a cell-mediated chemical response, which is better understood and seems to be the mechanism which is most likely to regulate normal healing of fractures.

Despite this, Ryaby[20] has completed a useful review of the evidence which he concludes supports, in general, the view that electromagnetic effects can enhance healing in nonunion. He does point out that this area of science is plagued by the problems of applying true scientific rigour to the process, and suggests that a set of criteria must be applied to all trials looking at intervention as follows: 1) the nonunion should have been monitored for three months before the intervention to ensure no background of low-rate progression of healing; 2) there should have been no surgical interventions in that three-month period; and 3) radiological assessment must be blinded.

In terms of the intervention, ideally trials should be double-blinded, randomised against a placebo, with an analysis of intent to treat.

The only trial in the literature meeting these criteria for electromagnetic intervention is by Scott and King[21] who examined 21 of 23 cases of nonunion of long bones in patients who had completed treatment. In addition, many of the patients in the placebo group chose to continue with the same regime with active devices. A total of 60% of the original active group healed in 21 weeks and none of the inactive group healed in the same period. In the second group, four of the six who elected to continue the active regime went on to show signs of healing. Analysis of intention to treat confirmed that the technique of using capacitatively coupled electric fields, applied for 24 hours a day, showed a positive effect.

The other trials reported by Ryaby, which did not meet all the criteria, tended at least circumstantially to support electrical stimulation. He indicated, however, that the work done so far, despite 40 years of effort, provides more questions than answers and we are still not certain precisely which technique to use, in terms of voltage and current pattern, and to which fractures we may apply it.

Comparisons with bone grafting became impossibly difficult as the criteria defined above can clearly not be applied simply to surgical interventions.

ULTRASOUND

Sound is another modality whereby energy can be transferred. Pulsed low-intensity ultrasound appears to enhance the healing of fractures.[22] The mechanism is entirely unknown, although indirect evidence seems to support a cell-mediated mechanism and many of these processes are temperature-sensitive. It may well be that ultrasound is converted to heat, resulting in local changes in temperatures which in turn stimulate genetic expression of cell mediators such as TGF-β.

Most of the clinical trials reported are of accelerated healing in normal fractures or considering healing rates in groups known to be at risk, such as smokers or diabetics.[23] Although double-blind, many of these studies do not met our earlier criteria strictly and so the evidence is circumstantial. There is a large registry of fractures treated by ultrasound, showing 91% healing in 1700 cases of delayed union and 85% union in established nonunion,[22] but these are open non-consecutive studies on a variety of patients. These data are impossible to interpret with confidence. A proper double-blind trial would be relatively easy to devise. The cost-effectiveness of this type of intervention is attractive.

CELLS AND GENETICS

From our earlier descriptions it must be concluded that we only have an outline understanding of the cascading factors which influence regenerative repair of fractures at the cellular level. There is strong evidence to suggest that we can import or generate growth factors. In particular BMP-2 and BMP-7 and TGF-β seem to work in animal models. Cells, in particular osteoprogenitor stem cells from bone marrow, can also enhance healing and we therefore have the prospect of extracting cells, reproducing them in culture and reimplanting them later. Both these techniques are likely to remain very expensive. Recombinant techniques will provide growth factors, which are required in large amounts at the site of the fracture, but there are practical difficulties in delivering and maintaining them in the locality of the fracture for a sufficient period of time to have an effect.

An alternative approach is to induce cells already present to produce proteins which enhance the healing process. Gene therapy implies the manipulation of the cell's own genetic environment. Essentially, this involves infecting cells with viral vectors or plasmids[24] which contain genetic information and which induce cells to produce growth factors at an appropriate time during healing. The viral factors can be injected in vivo, or into cells that are removed, infected and then returned. The latter appears to offer more promise in terms of the control of the process. There are other techniques of the direct injection of DNA at sites of fracture attached to a collagen matrix, but as yet these are experimental.

Cellular transfer has been tested in animal models but there are no reports of human clinical trials. Niyibizi et al[25] have described preliminary animal experiments on gene transfer but, clearly, this theoretically attractive concept is at its very early stages. Similarly, TGF-β has undergone some animal experimentation and shows great promise both in terms of enhanced enchondral ossification and in promoting the filling of larger cortical defects. This compound is also thought to be potentially beneficial in encouraging osseo-integration on the surface of implants.[26]

Perhaps the most advanced clinical trials are in the use of BMPs, particularly BMP-2 and BMP-7. Open trials have shown that they are safe in human usage. The protein is adsorbed onto a collagen matrix and placed at the site of the fracture. Unfortunately, this was carried out on a mixed group of patients in which some had intramedullary nailing and some external fixation. Three of the 12 cases required further intervention and the results are thus only preliminary.

Early results of a multicentre trial of BMP-7 are available[27] which compare nonunion treated by surgery plus graft or plus BMP-7. The results were similar in both treatment groups but in neither was 100% union assured. Another human trial by Geesink, Bulstra and Hofnagels[28] has used a fibular osteotomy model, whereby fibular defects created at the time of high tibial osteotomy were used. In this interesting study, the bone gap received either no treatment, collagen carrier alone, decorticated bone or BMP-collagen matrix. In the group receiving a bone graft and the group treated with BMP, five of six healed; in the other two control groups, none healed.

All these studies justify continued randomised blind trials using our well defined criteria.

CONCLUSIONS

Surgeons need to study the literature carefully. We continue to understand how we must manage the physical environment around fractures and to carry out research which seeks to clarify the complexities of the regenerative process of repair of fractures. Only by understanding the timing and the critical relationship between the cellular response, stiffness and strain, and blood supply can we begin to manipulate the environment of the fracture appropriately.

The definitive tests must be randomised, controlled and, where possible, blinded trials which must include analysis of intention to treat. Surgeons must be able to express certainties in their management so that they can comfortably explore uncertainties. Trials which dabble are unhelpful, as shown by the confusion which has dogged research in electromagnetic fields. We must avoid such equivocation as we explore the ways in which we can, as yet uncertainly, manipulate the cell biology of the repair of fractures. Although we welcome the emerging safe and ethical human trials, especially those concerned with BMPs, most of us must be patient. This is not an area for registries of activity, but solely for randomised, controlled trials. When small groups of experts report on work of true rigour, then wider, clinical user trials may commence.

Alan Apley began to ask real and searching questions in the second half of the 20th century. In the 21st century it is almost certain that we will understand fracture repair sufficiently to manipulate it and so be able to some day to answer his questions with more concrete information than "because the bone is broken". In the meantime surgeons and industry will continue to observe that "fixation is fun," if expensive.

REFERENCES

1. **Marsh DR, Li G.** The biology of fracture healing: optimising outcome. *Br Med Bull* 1999;55:856-69.

2. **McKibbin B.** The biology of fracture healing in long bones. *J Bone Joint Surg [Br]* 1978;60:150-61.

3. **Rhinelander FW.** Tibial blood supply in relation to fracture healing. *Clin Orthop* 1974;105:34-81.

4. **Grudnes O, Rickeras O.** The importance of haematoma for fracture healing in rats. *Acta Orthop Scand* 1993;64:340-2.

5. **Clemens TL.** Vasoactive agents and bone metabolism. In: Bilezikian JP, Raisz LG, Rodan GA, eds. *Principles of bone biology.* San Diego, CA: Academic Press, 1996:597-601.

6. **Marsh DR.** Concepts of fracture union, delayed union and nonunion. *Clin Orthop* 1998; Supp355:22-30.

7. **Rowley DI.** The management of war wounds involving bone. *J Bone Joint Surg [Br]* 1996;78-B:706-9.

8. **Coupland RM, Kneubuehl BP, Rowley DI, Bowyer GW.** Wound ballistics, surgery and the law of war. *J Trauma* 2000;2:1-10.

9. **Kenwright J, Richardson JB, Goodship AE, et al.** Effect of controlled axial micromovement on healing of tibial fractures. *Lancet* 1986;ii:1185-7.

10. **Goodship AE, Cunningham JL, Kenwright J.** Strain rate and timing of stimulation in mechanical modulation of fracture healing. *Clin Orthop* 1998;Supp355:105-15.

11. **Sarmiento A, Mullis DL, Latta LI, Tarr RR, Alvarez R.** A quantitative comparative analysis of fracture healing under the influence of compression plating vs closed weight-bearing treatment. *Clin Orthop* 1980;149:232-9.

12. **Kay P, Edwards J, Taktat A, Laycock D.** Measurement of fracture healing by simple bending and vibration. *J Bone Joint Surg [Br]* 1992;74-B:Suppl II:230.

13. **Bostrom MPG, Asnis P.** Transforming growth factor beta in fracture repair. *Clin Orthop* 1998;Suppl355:124-31.

14. **Jin Y, Yang LJ.** The relationship between bone morphogenic protein and neoplastic bone diseases. *Clin Orthop* 1990;259:233-8.

15. **Neilsen HM, Andreassen TT, Ledet T, Oxlund H.** Local injection of TGF-beta increases the strength of tibial fractures in the rat. *Acta Orthop Scand* 1994;65:37-41.

16. **Einhorn TA, Lane JM.** Significant advances have been made in the way surgeons treat fractures. *Clin Orthop* 1998:Suppl355:2-3.

17. **Stevenson S.** Enhancement of fracture healing with autogenous and allogenic bone grafts. *Clin Orthop* 1998;Suppl355:239-46.

18. **Fukada E, Yasuda I.** On the peizoelectric effect of bone. *J Physiol Soc Japan* 1957;12:121-8.

19. **Bassett CAL, Pawluk RJ, Pilla AA.** Augmentation of bone repair by inductively coupled electromagnetic fields. *Science* 1974;184:575-7.

20. **Ryaby JT.** Clinical effects of electromagnetic and electric fields on fracture healing. *Clin Orthop* 1998;Suppl355:205-15.

21. **Scott G, King JB.** A progressive double-blind trial of electrical capacitative coupling in the treatment of nonunion of long bones. *J Bone Joint Surg [Am]* 1994;76-A:820-6.

22. **Hadjiargyrou M, McLeod K, Ryaby JP, Rubin C.** Enhancement of fracture healing by low intensity ultrasound. *Clin Orthop* 1998;Suppl355:216-29.

23. **Cook SD, Ryaby JP, McCabe J, et al.** Acceleration of tibia and distal radius fracture healing in patients who smoke. *Clin Orthop* 1997;337:198-207.

24. **Rosier RN, O'Keefe RJ, Hicks DG.** The potential role of transforming growth factor beta in fracture healing. *Clin Orthop* 1998;Suppl355:294-300.

25. **Niyibizi C, Baltzer A, Lattermann C, et al.** Potential role for gene therapy in the enhancement of fracture healing. *Clin Orthop* 1998;Suppl355:148-53.

26. **Lind M, Overgaard S, Nguyen T, et al.** Transforming growth factor-beta stimulates bone ongrowth: hydroxyapatite-coated implants studied in dogs. *Acta Orthop Scand* 1996;67:611-6.

27. **Friedlander G.** Treatment of established tibial nonunions using recombinant human mophogenic protein. Second International OP - 1 Conference. Boston, MA: Abstract, 1977.

28. **Geesink RGT, Bulstra SK, Hofnagels NHM.** Fibula defect repair using OP - 1 device versus sham treatment carrier on demineralised bone in patients undergoing tibial osteotomy. Second International Conference of BMPS, Sacramento, CA 2: abstract 137, 1997.

THE TRAUMA CENTRE IN 2000

N. P. HAAS

From Humboldt University, Berlin, Germany

The 20th century has been remarkable for its revolutionary innovation. At the beginning of the last century messages were carried on horseback, but now we are able to transmit gigabytes of information in only a few seconds. We communicate in real time via the Internet. We have entered into a new world of a digital network, even although we cannot calculate mechanical clockwork invented in the 17th century.[1] If we replace the linear movement of a simple pendulum with the complex movements of a three-part pendulum, the most powerful computers are not able to calculate the complex movements for more than 20 seconds. Because we cannot perform the calculations for complex non-linear systems we are still unable to predict the future.

In 1904 Mercedes-Benz ordered a study to investigate the future of the automobile market. The prediction was that no more than 70 000 new cars would be needed each year. It was thought that a technician would be required for every car to facilitate its use, and there were then only 70 000 technicians in the world.[1]

In 1980 the IBM board discussed whether the personal computer (PC) or the megacomputer would be the future requirement. They agreed that ordinary people would not be able to use such a sophisticated machine as a PC.[1]

These examples show the difficulty in making predictions. Nevertheless, we have to think about the future since we live in a world of such rapid change. With this in mind we have to examine the demands on and need for trauma centres in Europe. We need to ensure that they bring high-quality care in an economical way.

In spite of the economic pressures and rising costs European citizens expect a high level of efficiency in modern medicine. Trauma centres will be judged by their ability to manage polytrauma. This is of a particularly high standard in Germany and is based on an outstanding system for the transport of the injured.[2,3]

THE FREQUENCY OF POLYTRAUMA IN GERMANY

Between seven and eight million accidents occur in Germany each year; 60.5% are in the home or at sport, 27% at work, 8.5% in road-traffic accidents and 4% are due to direct violence or suicide.

Traffic accidents cause the most severe injuries. A person is injured in a traffic accident every 15 seconds. More than 395 000 accidents resulting in injury to persons occurred in 1999, 7749 people died (0.6% less than 1998) and 521 000 were injured.

More than 70% of polytrauma was caused by traffic accidents followed by those at home (20%) and at work (10%).[4] The number of polytrauma patients can only be estimated because there is not a complete register. Registration depends on the severity of injury and the scoring system used to describe it. The 'Polytrauma Schlüssel' (PTS)[5] is established in German-speaking countries, whereas the 'Injury Severity Score' (ISS)[6] is predominantly used in the English-speaking world.

The number of polytrauma patients with a PTS score of III or IV in Germany is estimated at 20 000 per year.[7] This rises to 100 000 if the PTS score II is included.[8] These figures correlate with police statistics concerning persons injured in traffic accidents and treated in hospitals.

The combination of home and work accidents and the increasing number of acts of violence and suicide attempts produce about 32 500 polytrauma patients with a PTS score of III or IV in Germany each year.

TRAUMA CENTRES IN GERMANY

The treatment of polytrauma patients is carried out in hospitals with different levels of facility. A profile of the requirements for trauma departments in German hospitals is found in the recommendations of the German Society of Traumatology.[9] The definitions and needs follow the guidelines of the German Society of Traumatology and the American College of Surgeons (ACS) Committee on Trauma.[10]

We have three categories of hospitals for trauma in Germany. Those with the lowest grade of facilities correspond to the American trauma centre level IV. The head of the department should be a surgeon with a specialisation in traumatology and there must be a recognised department of surgery. The ability to undertake surgery throughout 24 hours is required.[9]

The hospital on the next higher level, similar to the ACS

trauma level III, needs an independent department for traumatology with its own budget and an autonomous service plan. It must have the capacity for 24-hour trauma surgery, its own emergency room, separate beds in an intensive-care unit and the full access to the system for the primary evacuation of injuries.

Hospitals at the highest level, similar to ACS level II or I, provide a 24-hour service with full specialist cover for the treatment of polytrauma patients. All departments and subspecialities are available.

An overview of the different categories is shown in Table I. It describes the different roles played by the varying types of hospital in the treatment of polytrauma. It shows that hospitals at level III or IV should only stabilise the vital parameters of the patient who should then be transferred to the next most suitable hospital. Level-II hospitals should only undertake measures which are within their ability. The level-I trauma centre must guarantee the availability of all personal and the structural requirements for the full treatment of polytrauma.

ECONOMIC ASPECTS OF TRAUMA

The costs of the treatment and rehabilitation of patients after injury are high and must be appreciated when considering the economics of a trauma centre. The national accident insurance companies insure 29.7 million people. The total expenses including follow-up treatment pensions and indemnity are 17.6 billion DM for victims of accidents.[11] Although under 11% of the patients have multiple injuries they are responsible for 25% of the total expenditure,[12] approximately 4.4 billion DM.

For the German economy the consequences of accidents produce a yearly loss of 620 000 living years and 520 000 working years.[13]

The victim of an accident costs an average of 98 000 DM, which increases to up to 500 000 DM with lifelong disablement.[14] If we consider the 32 500 multiply injured patients and calculate that 15 000 have consequent problems and 17 500 do not, the cost to the public economy is nearly 10 billion DM per year.

In an individual case of a multiply injured person there are three current estimates in Germany, which calculate the primary costs of managing a polytrauma patient. Ruchholtz et al[15] state that the average cost is 64 000 DM whereas Kinzl[16] quote a figure of 62 000 DM and Obertacke et al[17] 104 000 DM. When the marginal costs are included the figure rises to between 100 000 and 150 000 DM per person. The studies from Munich[15] and Ulm[16] divide the costs into the emergency room (5%), the operating room (20%), intensive care (65%) and the ward (10%).

ECONOMIC ASPECTS OF A TRAUMA CENTRE

The costs of a single trauma centre can be illustrated by those for the trauma centre Charité Campus Virchow at the Humboldt University, Berlin.

Between May 14, 1995 and May 14, 1996, 17 211 victims of an accident received clinical treatment; 2077 had been brought in by ambulance and 1186 (53.7%) as an emergency. Of those admitted as emergencies, 154 (13%) had an ISS score >16. There were 104 patients (8.8%) with a PTS score of III or IV. Basing the calculation of primary costs for multiply injured persons on the number of severely traumatised patients and the primary costs as stated by Ruchholtz et al[15] at 64 000 DM, the primary treatment costs for the multiply injured patients were 104 × 64 000 = 6 656 000 DM.

It is important to look at this figure in relation to the primary costs of clinical treatment for all emergency patients which is based on the primary total costs of the emergency room, operating unit, intensive-care unit and the normal ward as shown in Table II.

These figures include the primary costs of treatment of all traumatological patients, the primary costs of medical equipment and those for other departments. The amounts for the buildings, their maintenance, cleaning, catering and management are not included.

The primary costs for all forms of clinical treatment for both elective and emergency patients are assessed by a factor for their distribution. The primary costs of the trauma centre were weighted as follows. For the emergency room (ER), with 17 000 patients per year for ambulant treatment, we define 0.7 as the factor, because the costs for patients who were admitted, especially those with multiple injuries, take the major part. For the operating theatre we have chosen a factor of 0.6 since emergency operations are more expensive than elective procedures. The intensive-care unit does not deal with the immediate postoperative patient, and hence the

Table I. Requirements for hospitals treating severely injured persons: +, necessary; (+), desirable; and -, not necessary

Criteria for the departments	Level I or Level II	Level III	Level IV
Independent	+	+	-
Trauma surgery/surgery	+	+	+
Neurosurgery, etc.	+	(+)	-
Heart surgery	+	-	-
Anaesthesia	+	+	+
Radiology	+	+	(+)
Urology	+	(+)	-
Replantation medicine	+	-	-
Complete infrastructure	+	(+)	-

Table II. Costs of treatment (DM) of all emergency patients (marginal costs in parentheses)

Emergency room	2 104 000 (600 000)
Operation unit	5 000 000 (3 044 000)
Intensive-care unit	4 560 000 (2 400 000)
Normal ward	4 824 000 (1 132 000)

Table III. Primary costs (DM) of treatment for emergency patients at the trauma centre of Charité Campus Virchow

Emergency room	2 104 000 × 0.7	= 1 472 800
Operation unit	5 000 000 × 0.6	= 3 000 000
Intensive-care unit	4 560 000 × 0.9	= 4 104 000
Normal ward	4 824 000 × 0.65	= 3 135 600
Total		11 712 400

Table IV. The infrastructure for the treatment of polytraumatised patients in Europe

Country	Inhabitants (million)	Area (km^2)	Trauma centres	Polytrauma patients treated per year
Germany	81.0	356 970	90	100 to 200
Austria	8.0	83 850	12	100 to 200
Switzerland	7.1	41 290	7	6<100, 1>200
France (Paris)	14.0	10 000	15	100 to 200
Finland	5.1	305 470	5	100 to 200
Sweden	8.8	410 928	7	100 to 200
The Netherlands	15.4	33 920	12	4<100, 8>100
Portugal	10.5	91 649	4	>1000 (Lisboa)
Croatia	4.7	56 410	4	>200

costs are mostly for emergency patients, particularly those with multiple injuries. We therefore allocated a factor of 0.9. Because of the increased time spent by emergency patients in hospital we calculated the cost factor for the normal ward as 0.65, slightly higher than the average of 53.7%.

Taking these factors into account the primary costs of the clinical treatment of emergency patients at the trauma centre Charité Campus Virchow are shown in Table III. These amount to nearly 12 million DM. The primary treatment costs for polytrauma patients were calculated as 6.6 million DM, 56.8% of the overall sum. To calculate the total costs of a trauma centre, allowance must be made for depreciation of medical equipment and buildings, maintenance and cleaning, catering and laundry. The department of finance has the job of identifying these additional figures but they are probably equal to the primary costs, giving an overall figure of 24 million DM. From these statistics we can calculate the running costs for the polytrauma treatment. The following formula was developed:

$$\text{whole primary treatment costs} \times 0.7 - \text{costs for objects} \times 0.9$$

A major part of the costs is for staff. Every part of their working time can be used for the treatment of outpatients; their presence at the hospital is always necessary in order to treat polytrauma patients as required.

ANALYSIS OF GERMAN AND EUROPEAN TRAUMA CENTRES (TABLE IV)

When planning centres for the treatment of polytrauma patients, the overall population must be considered together with its density and geographical spread.

There are about 90 level-I trauma centres in Germany corresponding to American level-I or level-II centres. Germany has a population of 81 million occupying an area of 356 000 km^2.[18] The average centre receives between one and two hundred polytrauma patients per year. Theoretically, each of the 90 trauma level-I centres should treat 361 such patients per year, but only about half of all polytrauma patients are treated in a centre of the highest level. This trend can be seen elsewhere in Europe. For instance, in Austria between 100 and 200 patients are seen in each level-I centre per year. There are 12 centres and 8 million inhabitants. In Switzerland which has 7.1 million inhabitants, there are seven trauma centres, but six treated less than 100 patients per year and only one more than 200. In the Paris area of France there are 15 trauma centres, four of level-I and 11 of level-II for 14 million inhabitants. There is a similar relation of population and trauma centres in the sparsely populated Scandinavian countries: five centres for 5.1 million people on 305 470 km^2 in Finland and seven for the 8.8 million inhabitants of Sweden.

In Portugal, with a population of 10.5 million, there are only four trauma centres but that in Lisbon treats 1300 patients per year.

In The Netherlands the figures correspond to the European average, while in Croatia there are four centres for 4.67 million people.

Collection of these data has demonstrated the lack of centres undertaking documentation of trauma care in Europe. Such organisations are necessary in order to plan the proper development of the appropriate management of trauma. On the basis of our data we found a requirement for one level-I centre per one million population.

THE AIR-RESCUE SYSTEM

The facilities for the transport of the injured to a trauma centre require proper consideration. In Germany in 1994 there were 854 locations for emergency physicians and 51 bases for air rescue. These were co-ordinated by 442 central rescue offices involving both private and public organisations. A rescue helicopter with an average flight radius of 50 km can service an area of 7850 km^2. The 51 rescue helicopter centres cover nearly the whole area of Germany. In Switzerland, because of the high mountains, there are 15 helicopters in operation although, theoretically, only six would be needed to cover the area.

The need for the availability of a secondary system of helicopters for the transfer of severely injured patients from small hospitals to level-trauma centres is increasing.

EUROPEAN TRAUMA CENTRES IN THE NEXT CENTURY

In order to describe the future of trauma centres in Europe it is helpful to include the American experiences and figures. The Committee on Trauma of the ACS has defined the categories of I to IV of trauma centres and the number of patients which they should treat. They considered that on the basis of one level-I centre per million inhabitants, each would treat between 800 and 1000 severely injured patients per year. Each trauma surgeon would deal with about 50 patients per year, a minimum of one per week. This number of cases is necessary to maintain proper skills.

An overall balance of quality of cases related to costs suggests that an average of 300 to 400 patients per centre per year would be ideal. This would give one multiply injured patient per day at each centre. However, the reality is far from this ideal situation. In Europe more than half of all polytrauma patients were treated in level-III or level-IV centres. The first phase of treatment in the emergency room costs only about 5% of the whole costs. The major part of the costs is the intensive-care unit and the many operative procedures. Costs increase with permanent improvement in the quality of patient care. The overall costs of treatment can be made less by avoiding the entire management of polytrauma at level-III or level-IV centres. In order to guarantee the treatment of severely injured persons at a high-quality level in an economical way it is necessary that a hospital of a lower level does the primary treatment, stabilises the vital parameters and then transfers the patient to the next level trauma centre.

OUTLOOK

Accepting the need for one level-I trauma centre per one million people, there are already enough centres for the population across Europe. However, too many patients are treated in hospitals which are inappropriate. We need a further shift in favour of level-I trauma centres, with one per one million inhabitants treating 300 to 400 patients per year. The ACS guidelines demand that a trauma surgeon treats 50 polytrauma patients per year. Hospitals at trauma level-III or level-IV should treat the severely injured patients primarily and stabilise the vital functions and then transfer the patient to a level-I or level-II centre. The infrastructure for the treatment of polytrauma is available in Europe. We should concentrate on the better use of the given resources and the permanent development of a system for the treatment of these patients.

REFERENCES

1. **Kroy W.** The business of the future, 1995.
2. **Trunkey DD.** Trauma. Accident and intentional injuries account for more years of life lost in the US than cancer and heart disease: among the prescribed remedies are improved preventive efforts, speedier surgery and further research. *Sci Am* 1983;249:28-35.
3. **Tscherne H, Regel G, Sturm JA, Friedl HP.** Schweregrad und Prioritäten bei Mehrfachverletzungen. *Chirurg* 1987;58:631-40.
4. **Heiss MM, Jauch K-W, Madler C.** Polytrauma. In: Madler C, Jauch K-W, Werdan K, eds. *Das NAW Buch.* München: Urban & Schwarzenberg, 1994:570-86.
5. **Oestern HJ, Tscherne H, Sturm J, Nerlich M.** Klassifizierung der Verletzungsschwere. *Unfallchirurg* 1985;88:465-72.
6. **Baker SP, O'Neill B, Haddon W, Long WB.** The injury severity score: a method for describing patients with multiple injuries and evaluating emergency care. *J Trauma* 1974;14:187-96.
7. **Ott R, Holzer U, Spitzenpfeil E, et al.** Quality of life after survival of severe trauma. *Unfallchirurg* 1996;999:267-74.
8. **Haas NP, Hoffmann RF, Mauch C, von Fournier C, Südkamp NP.** The management of polytraumatized patients in Germany. *Clin Orthop* 1995;318:25-35.
9. **Haas NP.** Recommendations for structures, organization and outfitting preclinical and clinical patient care in trauma surgery departments of German hospitals. *Unfallchirurg* 1997;100:2-7.
10. **ACS.** *Resources for optimal care of the injured patients.* American College of Surgeons, Chicago, 1995.
11. **BG.** BG-Statistiken für di Praxis, 1993.
12. **MacKenzie EJ, Morris JA Jr, Smith GS, Fahey M.** Acute hospital costs of trauma in the United States: implications for regionalized systems of care. *J Trauma* 1990;30:1096-101.
13. Statistisches Jahrbuch für die Bundesrepublik Deutschland, 1991.
14. **Schaefer A, Neugebauer E, Bouillon B, Tiling T, Troidl H.** Instruments for measuring the quality of life of severely injured patients. *Unfallchirurg* 1994;97:223-9.
15. **Ruchholtz S, Nast-Kolb D, Waydhas C, et al.** Cost analysis of clinical treatment of polytrauma patients. *Chirurg* 1995;66:684-92.
16. **Kinzl L.** Polytraumakosten, 1996.
17. **Obertacke U, Neudeck F, Wihs HL, Schmit-Neuerberg KP.** Cost analysis of primary care and intensive care treatment of multiple trauma patients. *Unfallchirurg* 1997;100:44-9.
18. **Strassenverkehrsunfallbilanz 1999 (2000).** Internet: http://www.statistik-bund.de (accessed 20th December 2000).

EXTERNAL FIXATION IN TRAUMATOLOGY

MANVILIUS KOCIUS

From the University of Vilnius, Lithuania

The last 20 years have opened a new era of trauma care. Rapid advances have been made in the development of systems for internal and external fixation of fractures. Improvements in technology and surgical technique have allowed reduction and fixation of fractures to be achieved with less invasive surgical approaches and by external fixation.

This article represents an attempt to define the current status and application of external fixation in the treatment of fractures, but omits the treatment of late sequelae such as nonunion and delayed union, bone defects and osteomyelitis. New designs and configurations of frames have given us the opportunity to re-examine external fixation in the light of current needs. Knowledge of existing systems, understanding of the fundamental principles of external fixation and the establishment of indications for the method are essential for obtaining better results in the treatment of severely injured patients.

This article describes the author's 20 years of clinical experience in external fixation of fractures based mainly on the use of the circular Ilizarov and Kalnbers devices. In the last ten years mono or bilateral frames (AO/ASIF and Wagner) and hybrid fixators have also been used. The author has operated on more than 500 fractures of the tibia, about 250 of the femur, 50 of the forearm, 35 of the humerus and 32 of the pelvis using different external fixation devices in the Latvian Institute for Traumatology and Orthopaedics (1979-1986) and the Vilnius University Clinic of Traumatology and Orthopaedics (1987-2000).

HISTORICAL REVIEW

The concept of external fixation appears in the works of Malgaigne in the mid-19th century. The practical realisation of external fixation is ascribed to an American surgeon Clayton Parkhill and Albin Lambotte from Belgium. Both incorporated the introduction of pins or screws into fracture fragments with an external linkage assembly. With ideas borrowed from Malgaigne, Parkhill and Lambotte, many other external fixation systems have been introduced. A number of these devices have been used only rarely, and some of them have required additional fixation by a plaster cast. Numerous problems were encountered with pin-track infection, inadequate stability and difficulties in realignment of the fragments. Because of the high incidence of significant complications associated with external fixation, the method fell into disrepute. Later improvements realised by Roger Anderson, Raoul Hoffmann, Robert and Jean Judet, Jacques Vidal, and many others renewed interest in the technique.

After World War II, Ilizarov developed the original circular fixation system based on rings and tensioned wires. These devices generally use four pairs of crossed Kirschner (K-) wires (diameter 2 mm or less) which are held under high tension by screws on circular frames. The standard circular frame provides good stability and allows compression, distraction or neutralisation of bone fragments. The original circular frame described by Ilizarov has undergone several modifications over the last few years, with the introduction of carbon fibre rings and hybrid frames, making the system more versatile. Distraction osteogenesis according to the principles of Ilizarov has become extremely popular in recent years and is considered by many to be the current standard treatment for bone defects, limb shortening and other difficult orthopaedic cases.[1-4] But what is the place of external fixation in fracture management?

The Ilizarov method for external fixation of fractures has been widely used in the former Soviet Union for 40 years and is rapidly gaining acceptance in other countries. In western Europe external fixators have been used mainly to allow soft-tissue healing in severe open fractures, but in countries of the former Soviet Union the indications for their use have been expanded considerably. The Ilizarov, Kalnberz, Volkov-Oganesian and other circular devices have been used extensively in the treatment of a wide variety of fractures mainly because of the efficacy of the method and the limited opportunities for using appropriate implants for internal fixation. In Lithuania ten years ago external fixators were used even for treating simple closed fractures. The indications for external fixation became more realistic only after the restoration of independence, when implants for fracture fixation became generally available. The distribution of the different methods of fixation of fractures of the long bones in Lithuania is shown in Figure 1.[5]

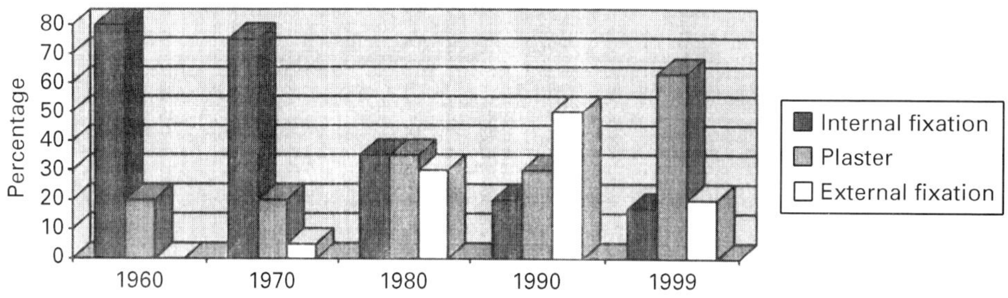

Fig. 1

The management of fractures of the long bones in Lithuania from 1960 to 1999.

CLASSIFICATION

Numerous varieties of external fixator are in use. There is a need for a single classification system which can adequately describe all types. Although no one classification system is ideal, that proposed by Vidal[6] is in our opinion, the most comprehensive. According to the geometrical configuration of the frame, he describes six different models: unilateral, bilateral, quadrilateral, half-circular, circular and triangular. A very simple classification system based on the appearance of the external configuration was proposed by Chao, Kasman and An.[7] They describe two main groups of external fixator, linear and circular, with the difference being related to the external appearance and the placement of the fixation elements in two (linear) or more than two (circular) planes. In our opinion, however, this classification cannot clearly describe all existing devices. New external fixators have been introduced with mechanical principles not considered above. Some circular fixators use combinations of pins and wires for bone fixation, which means that they cannot readily be described as circular fixators making the term confusing.[8] We have simplified Vidal's system to four basic configurations: monolateral, bilateral, semicircular and circular (Fig. 2).

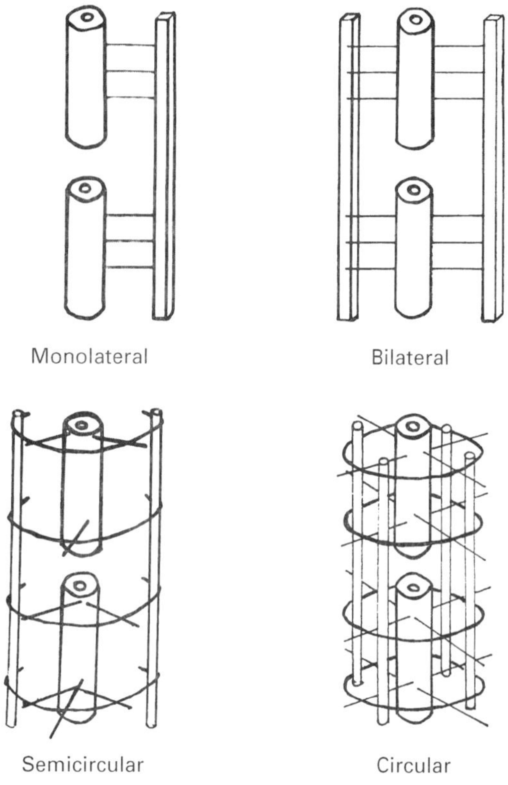

Fig. 2

Diagram showing configurations of external fixators.

1) The monolateral frame is the simplest configuration. Such fixators place pins in one plane and connect them to a rigid bar (Lambotte, Hoffmann, AO/ASIF, Wagner devices).

2) The bilateral frame employs simple or double rigid bars on both sides of the limb connected to full pins which transfix the bone (Charnley, Vidal-Adrey, Roger-Anderson).

3) The semicircular fixator places pins and wires in two or more planes and connects it to half-rings or a triangular frame (Fischer, Hoffmann-Vidal, Guduschauri).

4) The circular fixator uses rings which completely encircle the limb. Thin tensioned wires or full transfixing pins are used. Compression or distraction is achieved by turning the nuts of the rods connecting the rings (Ilizarov, Kalnberz, Volkov-Oganesian, Kronner, Monticelli-Spinelli).

According to the classification of Chao et al,[7] unilateral and bilateral frames are termed linear, but both circular and half-circular ones are termed circular.

Hybrid frames have now become popular. They cannot be assigned to any configuration mentioned above, because they usually have elements of circular, semicircular and monolateral frames. Linear, circular and hybrid fixators have a different qualitative mechanical performance.[8]

THE BIOMECHANICS OF EXTERNAL FIXATION

Many factors influence the application of an external fixator once this has been selected as the mode of treatment. The optimum application of the device requires an understanding of the influence of various configurational parameters on the fracture stabilisation characteristics of an external fixator.

The rigidity which is achieved by linear external fixation depends on several factors, including: a) the number and size of the pins; b) the proximity of the fixator to the bone; c) the stiffness of the frame; and d) the position of the pins between and within the components of the fracture.[7-10]

Because the pins are more flexible than the sidebar, they govern the rigidity of fixation. The stiffness of the pin is proportional to the cube of its length.[7] When the sidebar/bone distance increases, the length of the pins is increased, and the axial stiffness of a single-sided frame decreases. For a similar reason, the anteroposterior bending stiffness decreases with a larger sidebar/bone distance. Increasing the pin separation across the fracture gap also affects stiffness, decreasing bending rigidity as the distance increases. Separation of the pins close to the site of the fracture creates a larger span of the sidebar, and the stiffness of the sidebar is proportional to the cube of its unsupported length. A triangulated fixator using two half-pin frames was found to be 66% as stiff as the intact tibia in anteroposterior bending, 95% in mediolateral bending, 65% in axial compression, and 51% in torsional loading. A single half-pin frame, by comparison, has relative stiffness of about 18%, 12%, 12% and 20%, respectively.[10] In general, bilateral configurations using full pins have 50% higher overall rigidity than unilateral configurations. Unilateral external fixators with increased pin diameter or with two plane geometries, however, can provide stiffness characteristics comparable with bilateral configurations.[7]

The mechanical behaviour of the circular external fixation device using thin, pretensioned wires is difficult to predict, because the individual elements, such as rings, rods and wires, can be assembled in a large variety of configurations. Biomechanical experience has indicated that the rigidity of the circular frame device with K-wires is dependent on: a) wire tension; b) the wire crossing angle; c) the wire group separation on either side of the fracture; and d) ring diameter.[1,11-16]

These variables have different effects on the axial, bending and torsional stiffness, and by varying these key parameters it is possible to achieve the desired stability of the fracture. The standard Ilizarov circular configuration is four rings, two for each bone fragment, connected by four threaded rods. To provide the best stability, the ring diameter should be as small as possible. The distance between two rings of each fragment should be as great as possible. Each ring is fixed to the bone by two crossed K-wires, tensioned to between 1000 and 1200N. The K-wires should be placed perpendicular to the long axis of the bone and the angle between them should be as great as possible; the optimal angle is 90°.

There is increasing information available, concerning the stability of circular external fixation.[8,15,16] Pugh et al[15] in a comparative biomechanical study, tested nine different external fixation constructs and found that a four-ring Ilizarov frame was the stiffest configuration in all modes of testing.

Optimisation of stability of the fracture site is surgically possible by pin placement and frame orientation. These are under the control of the surgeon, within limits imposed by the injury and the design of the fixator. The findings of experimental studies emphasise that the axial rigidity of the bone-fixator system is dependent not only on the stiffness of the frame, but on the fracture pattern and the quality of reduction.[16]

The type of fixator and the mechanical performance may influence the complications seen during treatment. For instance, for linear fixators the pin-bone interface is critical for the mechanical performance, while for circular fixators the mechanical characteristics are more dependent on accurate wire tension than on the wire-bone interface.[8]

Dynamisation. External fixators have been considered to be too stiff in axial compression and thus cause stress shielding.[7,11] Dynamisation has therefore been proposed for reduction of the axial stiffness. The influence of dynamisation on bone healing has been shown in the excellent biomechanical study of Claes et al.[11] They evaluated metatarsal osteotomies in 12 sheep. The osteotomy with a 0.6 mm gap was stabilised by a specially designed high bending and torsionally stiff external ring fixator. Osteotomies in six sheep were stabilised rigidly and in six sheep dynamically. After nine weeks the sheep were killed and the healed bones were investigated biomechanically and histomorphologically. Compared with the rigidly fixed osteotomies, the dynamised osteotomies showed 41% greater ($p < 0.05$) formation of callus and 45% greater tensile strength of the newly formed bone in the cortical osteotomy gap.

External fixation has the unique feature of allowing a controlled adjustment of the rigidity of fixation during the progress of fracture healing. Dynamisation of external fixation is currently achieved by rigid fixation at the beginning and flexible fixation at the end of treatment. The rigidity of external fixation can be gradually decreased by removing pins, wires, side bars or even separate rings as the healing progresses.

ADVANTAGES AND DISADVANTAGES OF EXTERNAL FIXATION

Each method of fixation of fractures, either internal or external, has its specific advantages and disadvantages according to its original developmental concept and specific indications.

The main *advantages* of external fixation are as follows.

1) Unlike internal fixation, mechanical control and stabilisation of the bony elements at the site of injury are achieved without additional damage to the vital soft-tissue envelope.

2) External fixation is minimally invasive and does not cause additional blood loss.

3) The method provides rigid fixation of the bones in cases

in which other forms of stabilisation are inappropriate. This is most useful in severe open type-II and type-III fractures in which internal fixation would additionally devitalise soft tissues and bone, and might significantly increase the risk of infection.
4) Closed reduction is possible. In many cases a near anatomical reduction can be achieved by simple distraction alone. If fragments are not well aligned during surgery most external frames allow for progressive reduction without the need for further intervention. Different methods of reduction of bone fragments by circular devices are shown in Figure 3.
5) After differing initial periods of fixation, adjustment of the rigidity of axial fixation is possible at any time during the course of healing of the fracture.
6) The external frame allows direct surveillance of the limb and wound. Associated treatment such as dressing changes, skin and bone grafting, and irrigation is possible without disturbing the fixation. External fixation allows aggressive and simultaneous treatment of bones and soft tissues.
7) External fixation, especially with circular devices, allows elevation of the limb without pressure on the posterior soft tissues.
8) Immediate movement of the proximal and distal joints is allowed. This facilitates reduction of oedema and nutrition of articular surfaces and retards capsular fibrosis, joint stiffening, muscle atrophy and osteoporosis.
9) Patients are mobilised early by external fixation. In stable, uncomminuted fractures, early walking with partial or even full weight-bearing is usually possible.
10) Rigid external fixation can be used in infected fractures or pseudarthroses. Ilizarov taught that "infection burns in the fire of the regenerate".[17]

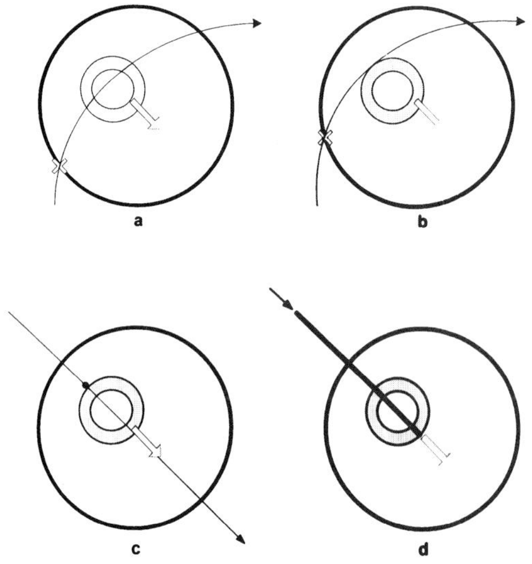

Fig. 3

Diagram showing reduction of bone fragments with: a) a convex transosseous wire with one end fixed to the ring, the other tensioned; b) a convex paraosseous wire; c) an olive wire; and d) a half-pin.

11) The method is relatively inexpensive because the components of the external frame (rings, rods) may be re-used many times.
12) External fixation of fractures is associated with a reduced length of hospitalisation and of hospital costs.[18]

The main *disadvantages* of external fixation are as follows:
1) A meticulous technique of pin insertion and daily care of the skin and pin sites are required to prevent pin-track infection.
2) Considerable surgical and engineering skill and experience are required. The pin and fixator frame may be mechanically difficult to assemble by the uninitiated surgeon.
3) The postoperative care is time-consuming.
4) The frame may be cumbersome, and the patient may reject it for aesthetic reasons.[19]
5) The non-compliant patient may disturb the adjustments of the appliance.
6) Joint stiffness may occur if the fracture requires that the fixator immobilise the adjacent joint. This is most common with fractures involving the proximal or distal aspects of the bone, with the major fragment affording insufficient pin purchase and requiring a set of pins and a frame above the joint.
7) Refracture may occur after removal of the frame unless the limb is adequately protected until the underlying bone can again become accustomed to stress.[19]

Linear fixators offer some advantages when compared with circular fixators. In the postoperative period they allow a wider range of movement because less muscles are transferred.

The hybrid constructions are less bulky, lighter and with less transfixation elements but still provide similar stiffness to the standard circular configurations.[14]

COMPLICATIONS

Pin-track infection. Problems with the pin track remain one of the potential drawbacks in modern techniques of external fixation. The pathophysiology of pin loosening, often complicated by pin-track infection, is still controversial. One of the basic questions concerns the time sequence of events in pin-track sepsis. Undoubtedly, mechanical loosening of a pin as a result of thermal bone necrosis or mechanical cortical bone failure carries a risk of subsequent pin-track infection. However, bacterial colonisation from the pin-skin interface to the pin-bone interface may lead to resorption of bone and subsequent pin loosening.[12]

The reported rate of pin-track infection varies from 0% to 100%.[17,20-26] The data differ because each author, with individual ideas about pin sepsis, views the problem differently. Some calculated the number of pins infected per total number of pins used rather than by patient occurrence. For this reason, Green[21] introduced the concept of major and minor pin-track sepsis in which a major infection produces

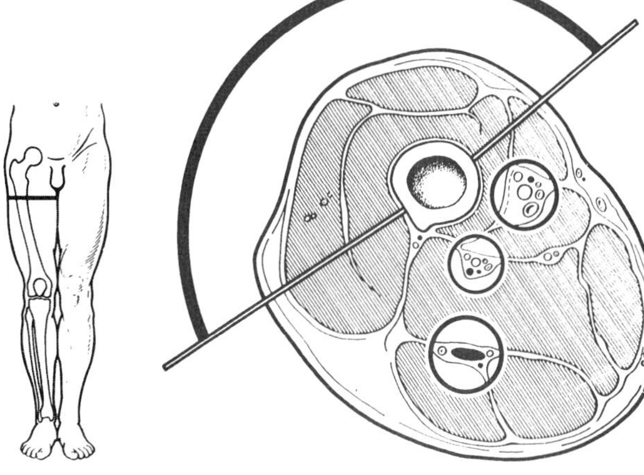

Fig. 4a

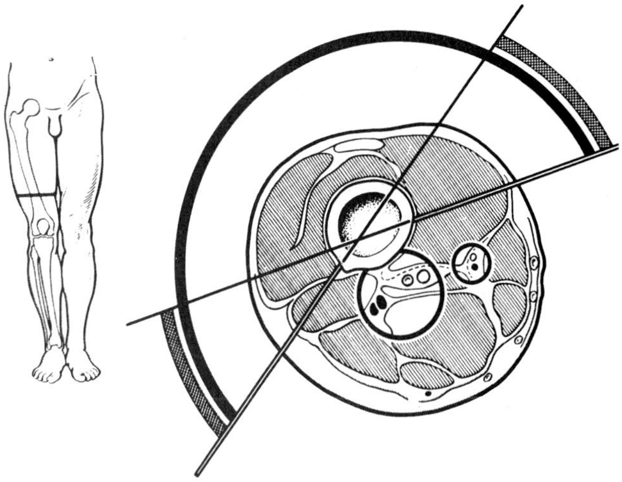

Fig. 4b

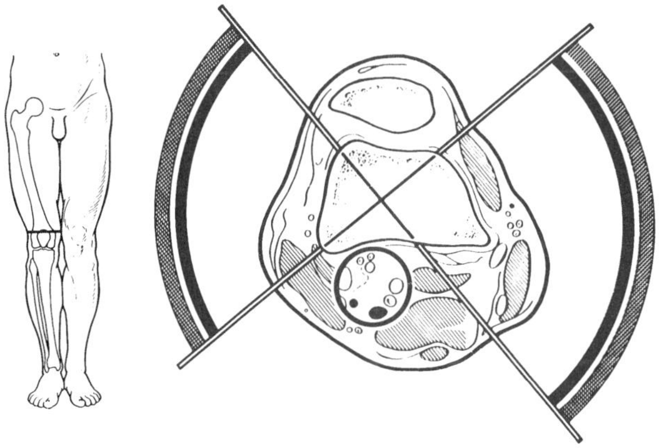

Fig. 4c

Diagram showing safe and danger zones for pin and wire insertion in the right thigh. Cross-sectional anatomy of the right thigh in proximal (a), middle (b) and distal (c) areas as viewed from a distal perspective.

sufficient redness, pain, or drainage to require hospital admission for either parenteral antibiotic therapy, pin removal, or removal of the entire fixator. Any other reaction is defined as minor, even that with a purulent discharge.

We believe that pin-track infection occurs in all cases (100%) of external fixation unless this is used on a temporary basis only. During the period of fixation at least one wire or pin will have adjacent redness, swelling or even drainage. In our experience the rate of major pin-track sepsis was 7.3% (16/217 patients) for the tibia and 11.0% (12/109 patients) for the femur.

Key elements in the prevention of pin-track complications are: a) reduction of the fracture before insertion of the pins; b) avoidance of skin, muscle and bone necrosis; c) insertion of the pin through the maximum diameter of the bone after low-speed predrilling through the drill guide; d) sufficient soft-tissue release around the pins; e) proper care of the limb after application of the frame to decrease oedema; f) regular cleaning of the pin exits; and g) reduction of soft-tissue movement, particularly in the thigh.

Pin reactions should be treated aggressively. Treatment should begin at the earliest sign of pain, erythema, or drainage. With minor erythema around the pins patients are advised to wash around the pin holes twice daily with antiseptic solutions. Minor drainage usually responds to a few days of rest, elevation, and oral antibiotic therapy. Significant redness, associated with pain or swelling around the pins, frequently requires hospital admission, enforced bed rest and parenteral antimicrobial agents. Continuous purulent drainage around a pin usually requires incision of the surrounding skin or removal of the pin.

Neurovascular injury. Reports of fixator-related injuries to nerves or vessels are rare.[21,27] The radial nerve in the distal part of the upper arm and proximal part of the forearm, the dorsal sensory radial nerve just above the wrist, the anterior tibial artery and the deep peroneal nerve in the leg are the structures most often involved. Vessel penetration, thrombosis, late erosion and the formation of aneurysms have also been observed.[21,25] Iatrogenic injuries of main arteries or nerves have not been seen in our experience, but we have noted late erosions and transitory nerve palsy, especially in cases of inadequate distraction and progressive reduction.

The surgeon must be familiar with the cross-sectional anatomy of the limb, the relatively safe zones and the danger zones for pin insertion. Transfixing wires are more dangerous than half pins, because they have two entries. Therefore K-wires and full pins should be inserted from the at-risk side of the limb (Fig. 4).

The safest localisation for external fixation is the tibia. The narrowness of the safe corridor in most other parts of the body limits the choice of safe frames to one-plane unilateral or hybrid configurations.[21]

Muscle tethering by pins and joint stiffness. Tightness of the soft tissues, joint stiffness and loss of range of movement at the distal joints are common problems in patients treated by an external fixator. Imbalances between the forces in the anterior and posterior muscle groups causes contractures, particularly in muscles which cross two joints. Transfixation of the musculature causes local pain, drainage and cellulitis. Tethering of the muscles results in stiffness of the distal joints and persistent discomfort when attempting to mobilise distal joints. To minimise this adverse effect of muscle tethering, during the operation we push the wire through the posterior muscle group with the leg straight and through the anterior muscle group with the leg flexed (Fig. 5).

Pressure necrosis from the fixator. This complication can occur when the components of the frame are too close to the skin, allowing insufficient space for swelling of the limb. It is most likely to occur in the posterolateral calf and upper lateral thigh. Clearance of 2 to 3 cm should be allowed between the skin and fixator in these regions.

Septic arthritis. Following application of external fixation by a circular ring septic arthritis has been reported.[20,22] The knee is especially prone to this complication. To achieve two planes of fixation in the proximal tibia, many surgeons tend to place the crossing wires close to the joint. It has been stated that pins placed through the lateral aspect of the proximal tibia are at greater risk of intra-articular placement because of the more distal reflection of the knee capsule and possible synovial communication.[22]

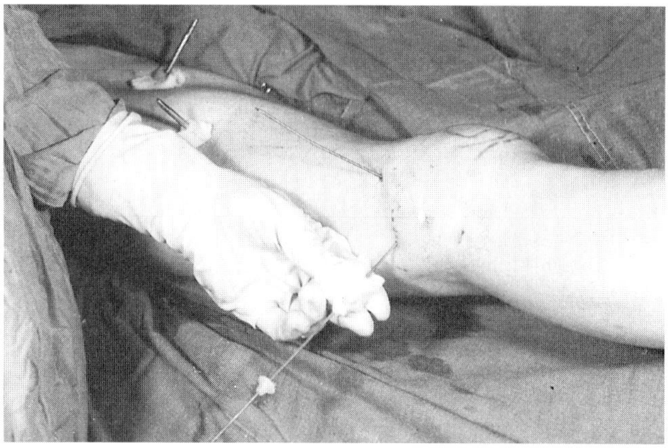

Fig. 5a

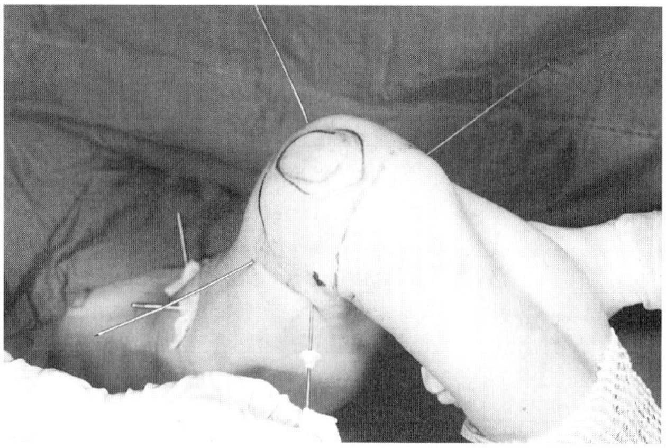

Fig. 5b

To prevent contracture of the knee, when pushing the wire through the posterior muscle group the leg is straightened (a) and when through the anterior group the leg is bent (b).

INDICATIONS

No single method or device can be so universal as to be applicable to every type and location of fracture. It is therefore logical to select the best treatment and fixation device according to the lesion and the clinical condition of the patient.

The indications for external fixation are relatively specific and infrequent, but there are no absolute indications. Each fracture must be individualised. Routine use of external fixation in patients in whom other conventional methods are better applicable is not justified.

The main indications for external fixation are described as follows.

Open fractures. The treatment of open fractures often has associated difficulties. The fractures tend to be more comminuted and accompanied by cortical bone defects.

The optimum treatment involves appropriate initial evaluation with the administration of antibiotics, urgent operative debridement and skeletal stabilisation. External fixation offers several advantages in treatment. It decreases the risk of infection because of the minimally invasive approach. Most modern external fixation frames provide acceptable stability for such fractures, even in cases of bone loss. There is good access to the soft tissues and most forms of external fixation do not substantially impair the range of movement of surrounding joints. In some cases external fixation may offer the best chance of avoiding amputation.

Early bone grafting is recommended for fractures with a loss of more than 50% of the circumference of the bone or areas of segmental loss.[28] The introduction of distraction osteogenesis, as recommended by Ilizarov, has led to the development of an ingenious protocol to deal with both the soft-tissue and bone defects. Primary shortening of the limb is carried out at the time of the initial debridement and external fixation. This facilitates closure of the soft-tissue defect without the need for local rotational or distant free flaps. Once a stable soft-tissue envelope has been achieved a corticotomy is performed and the limb is then gradually returned to its original length. This may have to be combined with linking the intervening segment with the distal main fragment if contact has not been achieved at the time of the initial shortening. There are many reports of this technique in the literature.[1,3,17,29]

Polytrauma. Studies of polytrauma patients with fractures of long bones have demonstrated that immediate stabilisation of the long bones may be a life-saving measure. Although the method of fracture stabilisation in multiply-injured patients is still controversial, most clinicians agree that early fixation offers many benefits, including early mobilisation, improved pulmonary toilet, decreased cardiovascular risk and improved psychological well-being.[9,30,31]

External skeletal fixation is theoretically the ideal choice; it is the least invasive and the least traumatising because fixation of the bone is secured at a distance from the zone of injury and there is no additional blood loss. Depending on the general state of the patient, application of the external fixator can be divided into two steps: primary temporary immobilisation and later definitive fixation. External fixation may be an alternative in polytrauma patients with fractures which could be managed singly by traction, casting or open reduction and internal fixation but which may be difficult to treat in combination. In multiply-injured patients external fixators can be applied in different places at the same time by separate teams of surgeons. This reduces the time of operation and anaesthesia, as well as surgical risk (Fig. 6).

Articular fractures. Fractures around the joints, particularly the knee and ankle, are frequently associated with soft-tissue trauma, which necessitates a delay in internal fixation to prevent wound complications or may make internal fixation impossible. During this time, temporary or definitive stabilisation is required. External fixation offers the advantage of stability, control of length and alignment, access to the soft tissues and patient mobility.

If the joint segment is too small to allow adequate purchase for the fixator, the joint is bridged and distraction applied.[32] It permits the reduction and fixation of comminuted epiphyseal fractures by creating a strong distraction on both sides of the joint, placing tension on capsuloligamentous structures and aligning the fracture fragments. Vidal[6] has called this "ligamentotaxis".

Comminuted fractures. The operative treatment of comminuted fractures with the associated severely compromised soft tissues should avoid additional intraoperative trauma. It is thought that for comminuted fractures early revascularisation is more important than stable fixation.[30,33] The less invasive external fixation of these fractures has become increasingly popular. In a comminuted fracture model in sheep, Claes et al[33] showed that less invasive bridging techniques, with an external fixator or a *fixateur externe* bridging plate give earlier and better osteogenesis of the bone than compression plate fixation.

The decision to use external fixation must be based on the severity of the soft-tissue injury and the localisation and pattern of the fracture.

The tibia. Diaphyseal fractures of the tibia are widely acknowledged to be the commonest shaft fracture. The management remains controversial despite advances in both non-operative and operative care.[5,9,28,34] There is no perfect method for treating all tibial fractures. Different circumstances demand differing approaches to the same problem.

The tibia is the prime area of application of external fixation. Tibial external fixation offers all the advantages of this method with minimal drawbacks. The tibial external fixator is relatively easy to apply, allows for optimal soft-tissue treatment, and promotes rapid mobilisation of the limb and the patient.

The safe soft-tissue corridor in the lower leg through which pins and wires can be inserted without injuring the main vessels, nerves and musculotendinous units, lies anteromedially and varies in size from an arc of 220° close to the tibial plateau to one of 120° just above the ankle.

External fixation has been the method of choice to stabilise fractures of the tibial shaft with associated soft-tissue injury. Healing rates in the fixator group of up to 88% have been reported.[29] The external fixator has the advantage of definitive and immediate stabilisation of the fracture with easy repeated access for surgery to the soft-tissue envelope.

External fixation in fractures of the tibial shaft can be used as a modern, minimally invasive alternative to internal fixation not only in severe open fractures, but also in more simple cases.

A half-pin frame placed anteriorly is the simplest form of tibial external fixation. The pins traverse the safe anteromedial corridor and so avoid transfixation of musculotendinous and neurovascular structures. Unfortunately, this form of configuration does not stabilise comminuted fractures and fractures with bone loss. Thus, unilateral configuration is indicated for simple open and closed diaphyseal fractures as a temporary or a definitive type of fixation, and for fractures with skin loss if skin cover is needed.

Circular four-ring configuration is indicated for open comminuted fractures and fractures with bone loss as a definitive type of fixation, and for comminuted fractures of the tibial plateau (minimal internal fixation and/or femoral frame extension), as temporary fixation.

Most external fixators for fractures of the tibial shaft can be applied without crossing a joint. This allows physiotherapy for active and active-assisted range of movement exercises to the knee and ankle. In order to prevent a plantar flexion contracture of the foot, a special slipper, fixed to the external device by rubber bands, is used for the first two months after surgery.

Periarticular tibial fractures around the knee and ankle are frequently associated with soft-tissue trauma. Monolateral fixators as well as circular or hybrid devices have been shown to be effective.[24,26,32,34] Monolateral fixators, used as a temporary form of stabilisation, usually require

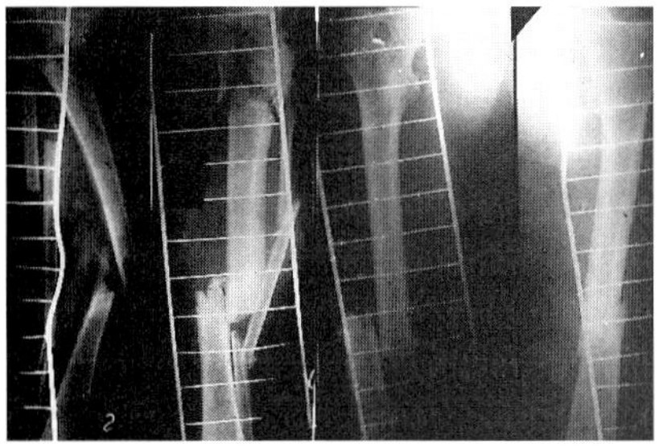
Fig. 6a

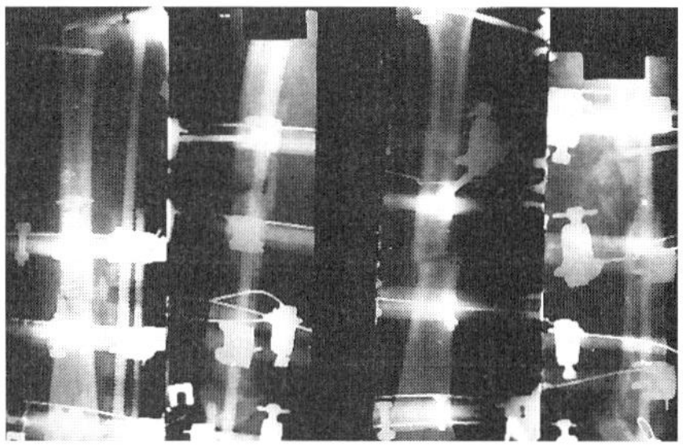
Fig. 6b

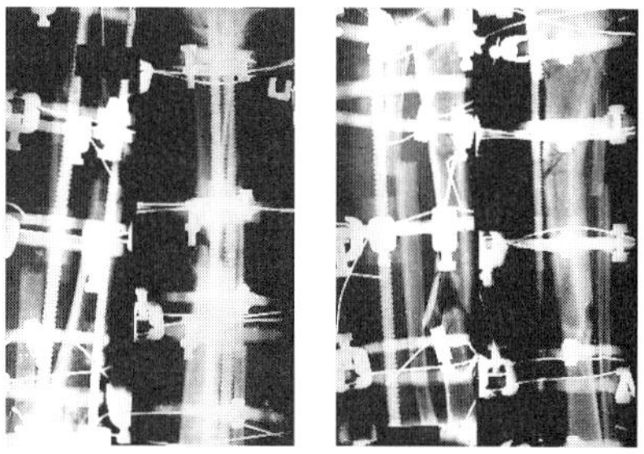
Fig. 6c

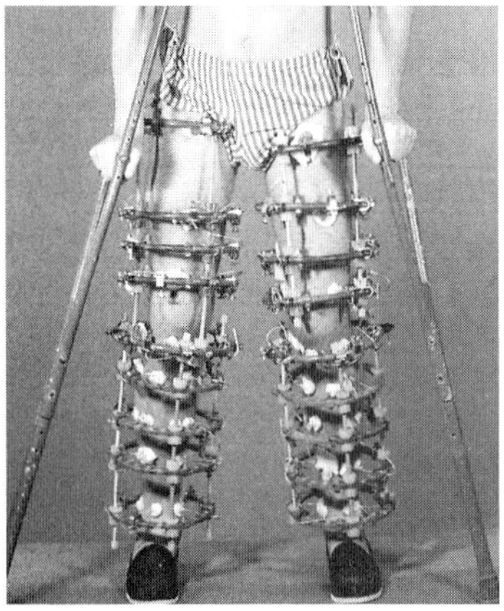
Fig. 6d

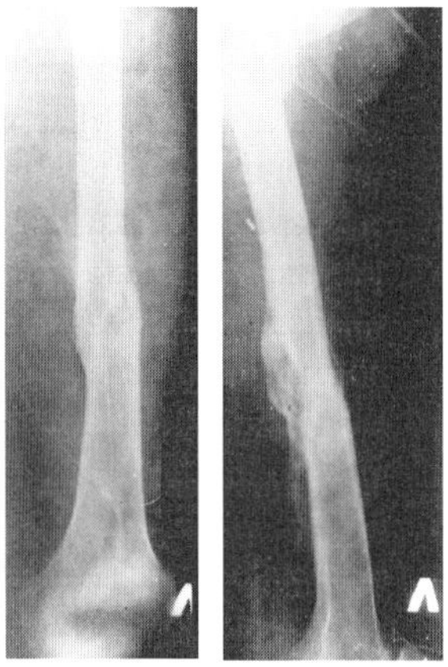
Fig. 6e

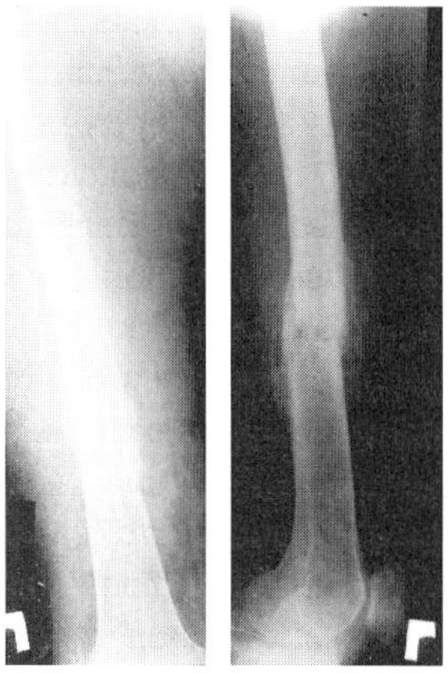
Fig. 6f

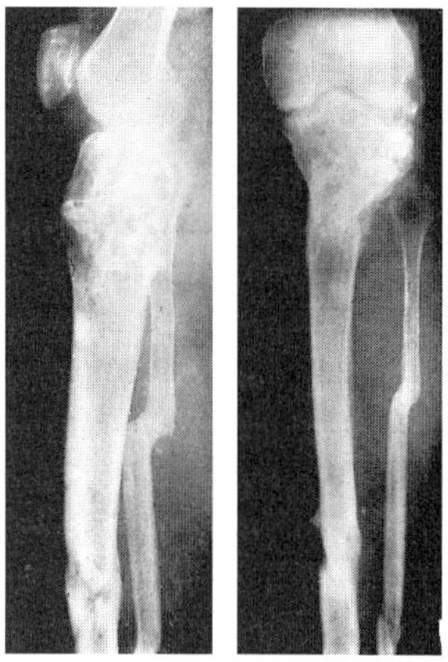
Fig. 6g

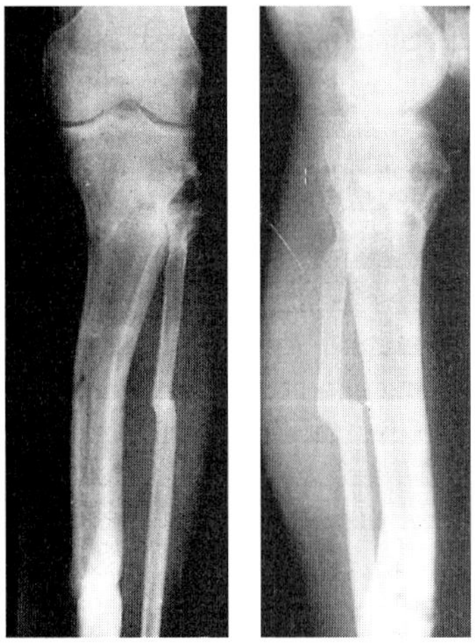
Fig. 6h

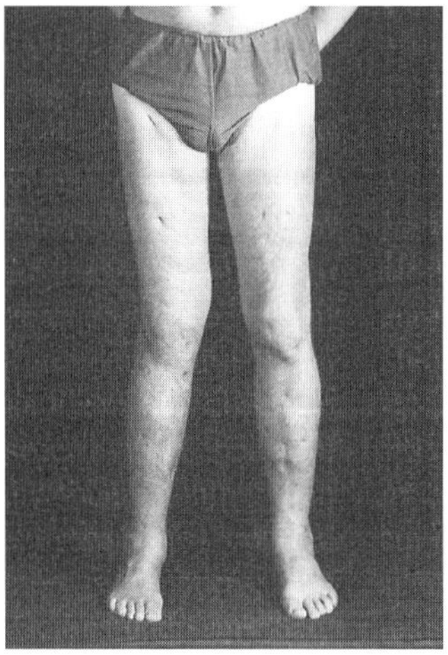
Fig. 6i

A patient with four-segment Kalnberz external fixation. Figure 6a – AP radiographs showing a comminuted extra-articular fracture of the left tibia, and a comminuted intra-articular fracture of the right tibia (both open), and fractures of the shafts of the left and right femur. Figures 6b and 6c – Radiographs of the left and right femur and the left and right tibia during fixation. Figure 6d – Photograph of the patient eight weeks after injury with four externally fixed segments. Figures 6e to 6h – Radiographs showing consolidation of all fractures. Figure 6i – Photograph of the patient 16 months after injury.

temporary transfixation of the joint. Surgeons, using this kind of fixation, believe that temporary transarticular fixation of the knee or ankle has little morbidity and can safely be used to decrease the incidence of wound complications associated with early internal fixation through damaged soft tissues.[32] Combinations of external fixation with limited internal fixation have been used effectively in the treatment of intra-articular fractures of the tibial plateau and plafon fractures.[9]

For condylar fractures we use the traditional four-ring (sometimes three-ring) circular fixator and, if needed, olive wires to lag the condyles together. Proximal transfixation wires are generally placed through the tibial metaphysis as close to the subchondral bone as possible without violating the articular surface and joint capsule. Because of the short proximal fragment, three transmetaphyseal wires are placed proximally, one of them through the fibular head. Solid fixation of tensioned fine wires in the fragments of the metaphyseal fracture allows early movement which prevents joint stiffness and improves fracture healing.

In the recent literature several types of hybrid external fixators have been described.[14,15,24] These stabilise the tibial plateau with two or three tensioned wires, which penetrate the subchondral bone just distal to the articular surface. The wires are connected to a ring construct which is in turn fixed to the distal tibial fragment by half-pins.

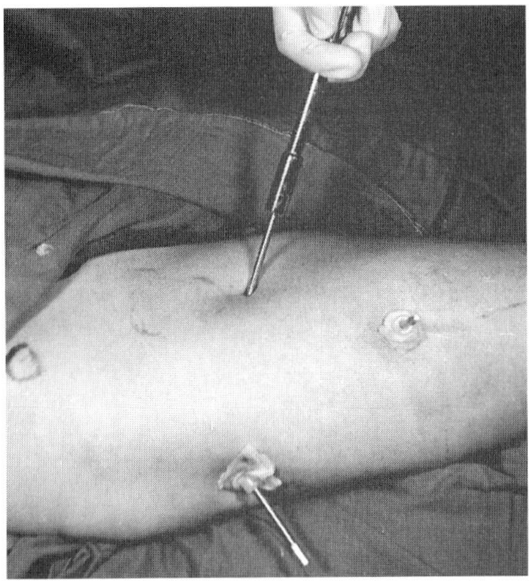

Fig. 7a

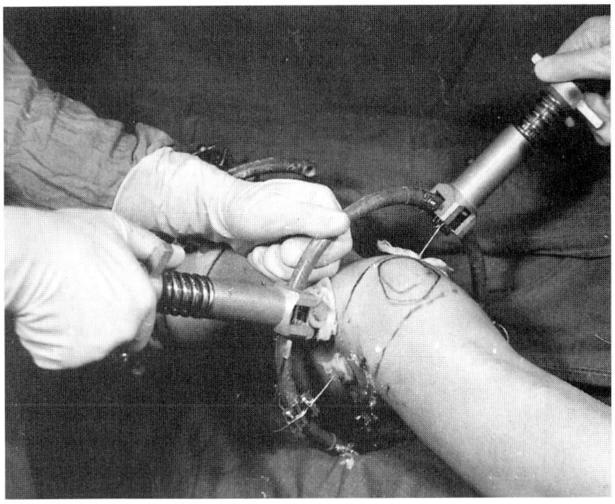

Fig. 7b

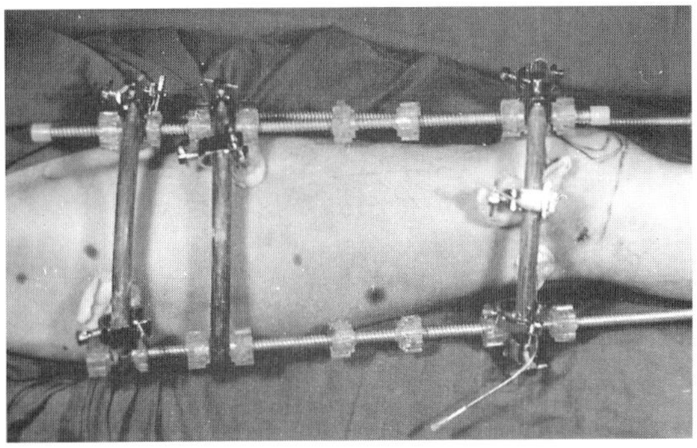

Fig. 7c

The configuration for femoral external fixation with the Kalnberz device. Figure 7a – Placement of the proximal half-pins. Figure 7b – The distal fragment is fixed by two tensioned 2 mm wires. Figure 7c – Two half-rings are assembled proximally and one full ring distally; after fluoroscopy two K-wires and one full ring will be added.

Some authors suggest using olive wires even for fractures of the shaft.[16,28] In our experience we have observed that these sometimes lead to osteolysis and the formation of ring sequestra. Catagni[17] reports the same complications. DiCicco, Ostrum and Martin[35] have noted that fixators with olive wires should be removed in the operating room. We therefore prefer to use the olive wires as reduction devices only. When the reduction has been obtained, we place a standard wire or pin and then remove the olive.

The femur. Fractures of the femoral shaft are the result of high-energy trauma. Open injuries are comparatively common. Intramedullary nailing has become a superior technique for treating closed fractures of the femoral shaft. Comminution and the extent of disruption of the diaphysis determine the choice of locking and non-locking types of nail.[9] Unlike the lower leg, the femur is covered circumferentially with a thick soft-tissue sleeve and therefore does not provide ideal corridors for pins and particularly for transfixing K-wires (Fig. 4).

Several authors have clinically evaluated external fixation for femoral fractures[23,25] and some have compared external fixation with other techniques. Nork and Hoffinger[18] found that external fixation of fractures of the femoral shaft in children resulted in decreased hospital costs and length of hospitalisation. Although a few authors have reported good results from the treatment of femoral fractures with external fixation, the method is mainly used in severe fractures with extensive soft-tissue injury, infected pseudarthroses previously treated by internal fixation, or in patients with severe polytrauma. Use is restricted because external fixation of the femoral fractures is more difficult and carries potentially serious complications such as deep pin-track infection, stiffness of the knee and the risk of nonunion.

In accordance with Rööser et al,[25] we believe that external fixation can be used in grade-III open fractures, with bone loss and in closed fractures when a multiply-injured patient is critically ill. A fast and atraumatic fixation of the fracture is mandatory. We do not agree, however, with this and many other reports[9,18] which suggest that the best configuration for femoral fixation is a monolateral frame. In our opinion, the stiffness of a linear frame is not sufficient for neutralisation of these fractures. For stabilisation of fractures in the proximal and middle femoral shaft circular or hybrid configurations should be used. Since 1980 we have preferred to use the Kalnberz circular device with one half-ring in the proximal part with two threaded pins at 90° to each other, one full or half-ring with one or two pins in the distal part of the proximal fragment and two full-rings with two tensioned 2 mm transfixation wires each in the distal fragment (Fig. 7). Distal femoral fractures can be stabilised by a standard circular four-ring device. For temporary stabilisation in a patient in a critical condition, the use of a temporary external fixator consisting of a monolateral frame should be considered.

The humerus. External fixators, both monolateral and circular, have been used in the treatment of fractures of the humerus.[1,2,9,36] The monolateral fixator is preferred for the treatment of complex humeral fractures since it gives sufficient stability and is well tolerated by the patient. The only indication for the application of the circular fixator in a humeral fracture is a fracture with bone loss, or in some special cases in which pin fixation is impossible due to the small fragments. In such cases we prefer a hybrid frame using K-wires and circular rings in the distal part and self-tapping pins and half-rings in the proximal portion leaving the axilla free and allowing the patient movement of the shoulder and elbow. We believe that the hybrid frame offers the advantages of both configurations: the use of a circular frame with thin wires in the distal fragment of the fracture where half-pins may be too large, and the less bulky monolateral fixator at the upper arm.

The anatomy of the arm is not very suitable for external fixation. Careful consideration must be given to neurovascular anatomy during application of the fixator, especially with respect to the ulnar and radial nerves. Distal transfixing wires are the most dangerous. These should both engage the medial epicondyle, be anterior to the ulnar nerve, orientated near the coronal plane, and separated by approximately 30°.

The forearm. In the forearm shaft, external fixators are generally used for open fractures as temporary devices until an open or infected lesion is covered by healthy soft tissue. The frames are then replaced by internal fixation.[9] Isolated fractures of the ulna can be managed by a monolateral fixator with the pins placed through the dorsal subcutaneous border. In some complex forearm injuries, separate monolateral fixators for the ulna and radius can be used, thus creating bilateral fixation of the forearm. External fixation of isolated fractures of the shaft of the radius should be avoided because of the danger of injury to the radial nerve. The use of a circular fixator is limited to open and severely comminuted fractures that cannot be reduced or sufficiently stabilised by a monolateral fixator. At least one wire should be placed through both bones.

Treatment of fractures of the distal radius using external fixation has been reported by several authors.[9,27,37] Huch et al[27] in a series of 40 patients with an average age of 58 years, reported good or excellent results in 82.5% for the treatment of comminuted intra-articular fractures of the distal aspect of the radius (AO type C2 or C3). They concluded that external fixation of these fractures results in good recovery for young patients, and elderly patients with osteoporosis. The procedure is minimally invasive, has an insignificant rate of complications, and there is no retained hardware. The principles of external fixation involve longitudinal traction (ligamentotaxis) and, most importantly, palmar translation. Multiplanar ligamentotaxis is used for the treatment of fractures of the distal radius. It provides palmar translation which can restore palmar tilt, which distraction alone cannot achieve.[37]

To achieve good functional results in intra-articular comminuted fractures of the distal radius, adequate restoration of radial length, articular congruity and alignment of the radius are needed. When articular fragments are too displaced or impacted and in cases with marked cancellous defects, secondary open reduction and internal fixation with bone grafts is recommended.[9]

Disruption of the pelvic ring. In high-energy pelvic injuries the external fixator is used either acutely or as a delayed means of stabilisation. In the early management of such an injury an external fixation frame may decrease blood loss, increase patient comfort, and facilitate nursing care. It can function as a temporary, definitive or adjunctive means of fixation. When used in resuscitation, application of the external fixator can be accomplished in less than 30 minutes.

Almost all frame configurations for pelvic injury are based anteriorly and the fixator substitutes for mechanical stability which is lost principally in the anterior pelvis. It must be noted that posterior instability of the pelvis cannot be fixed reliably with an external device.

There are three sites of pin insertion: a) the iliac crest; b) between the anterior iliac spines; and c) transiliac. For pin insertion we use the percutaneous technique, but some authors suggest direct visualisation of the ilium before insertion.

Simple frames are sufficient for emergency measures and for the stabilisation of stable anterior and lateral compression injuries. More rigid configurations are needed to hold unstable compression injuries and vertical shear injuries. Various configurations of frame have been described. The simplest connection between two groups of iliac pins is a single transverse rod. Poor abdominal clearance and poor flexibility for adjustments hamper this configuration. Two

Table I. Local indications for different configurations of external fixation

Fixator configuration	Femur	Tibia	Humerus	Forearm
Monolateral	-	+	++	++ (if 1 bone)
Bilateral	-	+	-	+ (if 2 bones)
Circular	+	++	+	+
Hybrid	++	++	++	-

shorter rods forming an apex over the abdomen overcome both disadvantages.

Our ideas about the local indications for different configurations of external fixators are summarised in Table I.

REFERENCES

1. **Ilizarov GA.** *Transosseous osteosynthesis: theoretical and clinical aspects of the regeneration and growth of tissue.* Berlin: Springer-Verlag, 1991.
2. **Lammens J, Bauduin G, Driesen R, et al.** Treatment of nonunion of the humerus using the Ilizarov external fixator. *Clin Orthop* 1998;353:223-30.
3. **Paley D, Maar DC.** Ilizarov bone transport treatment for tibial defects. *J Orthop Trauma* 2000;14:76-85.
4. **O'Sullivan ME, Chao EYS, Kelly PJ.** Current concepts review: the effects of fixation on fracture-healing. *J Bone Joint Surg [Am]* 1989;71-A:306-10.
5. **Kocius M.** Lithuanian traumatology and orthopaedics 2000. *In: Lithuanian traumatology and orthopaedics 2000.* 2000:5-20.
6. **Vidal J.** External fixation: yesterday, today and tomorrow. *Clin Orthop* 1983;180:7-14.
7. **Chao EYS, Kasman RA, An KN.** Rigidity and stress analyses of external fracture fixation devices: a theoretical approach. *J Biomech* 1982;15:971-83.
8. **Caja VL, Kim W, Larsson S, Chao EYS.** Comparison of the mechanical performance of three types of external fixator: linear, circular and hybrid. *Clin Biomechanics* 1995;10;401-6.
9. **Müller ME, Allgöwer M, Schneider R, Willenegger H.** *Manual of internal fixation: techniques recommended by the AO-ASIF group.* 3rd edition, Berlin: Springer Verlag, 1991.
10. **Tencer AF, Claudi B, Pearse S, Bucholz RW, Johnson KD.** Development of a variable stiffness external fixation system for stabilization of segmental defects of the tibia. *J Orthop Res* 1984;1:395-404.
11. **Claes LE, Wilke H-J, Augat P, Rübenacker S, Margevicius KJ.** Effect of dynamization on gap healing of diaphyseal fractures under external fixation. *Clin Biomech* 1995;10:227-34.
12. **Hannu TA, Markel MD, Chao EYS.** Cortical bone reactions at the interface of external fixation half-pins under different loading conditions. *J Trauma* 1993;35:776-85.
13. **Ilizarov GA.** Basic principles of transosseous compression and distraction osteosynthesis. *Ortop Traumatol Protez* 1971;32:7-15.
14. **Lundy DW, Albert MJ, Hutton WC.** Biomechnical comparison of hybrid external fixators. *J Orthop Trauma* 1998;12:496-503.
15. **Pugh KJ, Wolinsky PR, Dawson JM, Stahlman GC.** The biomechanics of hybrid external fixation. *J Orthop Trauma* 1999;13:20-6.
16. **Schneider E, Sasse S, Schmidt HG, Schumann U.** Biomechanics of the ring fixator: contributions of individual structural elements. *Unfallchirurg* 1992;95:580-7.
17. **Catagni MA.** Upgrade of the Ilizarov method. In: Jakob RP, Fulford P, Horan F, eds. *European instructional course lectures, Vol 4.* 1999:152-8.
18. **Nork SE, Hoffinger SA.** Skeletal traction versus external fixation for pediatric femoral shaft fractures: a comparison of hospital costs and charges. *J Orthop Trauma* 1998;12:563-8.
19. **Sisk TD.** External fixation: historic review, advantages, disadvantages, complications and indications. *Clin Orthop* 1983;180:15-22.
20. **DeCoster TA, Crawford MK, Kraut MA.** Safe extracapsular placement of proximal tibial transfixation pins. *J Orthop Trauma* 1999;13:236-40.
21. **Green SA.** Complications of external skeletal fixation. *Clin Orthop* 1983;180:109-16.
22. **Hyman J, Moore T.** Anatomy of the distal knee joint and pyarthrosis following external fixation. *J Orthop Trauma* 1999;13:241-6.
23. **Kortmann H-R, Papenhagen M.** Treatment of femoral fracture with the Ilizarov fixator. *Unfallchirurg* 1992;95:534-6.
24. **Mikulak SA, Gold SM, Zinar DM.** Small wire external fixation of high energy tibial plateau fractures. *Clin Orthop* 1998;356:230-8.
25. **Rööser B, Bengtson S, Herrlin K, Önnerfält R.** External fixation of femoral fractures: experience with 15 cases. *J Orthop Trauma* 1990;4:70-4.
26. **Watson JT, Coufal C.** Treatment of complex lateral plateau fractures using Ilizarov techniques. *Clin Orthop* 1998;353:97-106.
27. **Huch K, Hünerbein M, Meeder PJ.** External fixation of intra-articular fracture of the distal radius in young and old adults. *Arch Orthop Trauma Surg* 1996;115:38-42.
28. **Olson SA.** Open fractures of the tibial shaft. *Instr Course Lect* 1997;46:293-302.
29. **Ostermann PAW, Hahn MP, Ekkernkamp A, Josten C, Muhr G.** Management of tibial shaft fractures with soft-tissue compromise: nonreamed nailing and external fixation. *Orthopaedics* 1996;4:243-50.
30. **Schatzker J.** Changes in the AO/ASIF principles and methods. *Injury* 1995;26 Suppl 2:51-6.
31. **Tile M.** Pelvic ring fractures: should they be fixed? *J Bone Joint Surg [Br]* 1988;70-B:1-12.
32. **Anglen JO, Aleto T.** Temporary transarticular external fixation of the knee and ankle. *J Orthop Trauma* 1998;12:431-4.
33. **Claes L, Heitemeyer U, Krischak G, Braun H, Hierholzer G.** Fixation technique influences osteogenesis of comminuted fractures. *Clin Orthop* 1999;365:221-9.
34. **Dendrinos GK, Kontos S, Katsenis D, Dalas A.** Treatment of high-energy tibial plateau fractures by the Ilizarov circular fixator. *J Bone Joint Surg [Br]* 1996;78-B:710-7.
35. **DiCicco JD, Ostrum RF, Martin B.** Office removal of tibial external fixators: an evaluation of cost savings and patient satisfaction. *J Orthop Trauma* 1998;12:569-71.
36. **Ring D, Jupiter JB, Toh S.** Salvage of contaminated fractures of the distal humerus with thin wire external fixation. *Clin Orthop* 1999;359:203-8.
37. **Weiland AJ.** External fixation, not ORIF, as the treatment of choice for fractures of the distal radius. *J Orthop Trauma* 1999;13:570-2.

ARTHROSCOPIC TREATMENT OF INTRA-ARTICULAR FRACTURES OF THE KNEE

P. BEAUFILS*, P. HARDY†, X. CASSARD‡, AND THE FRENCH ARTHROSCOPY SOCIETY

*From the *Centre Hospitalier de Versailles, †Hôpital Ambroise Paré, Boulogne, and ‡Clinique des Cèdres, Toulouse, France*

The objectives of surgery for intra-articular fractures of the knee are to obtain anatomical, stable reduction, to address any associated intra-articular lesions, and to minimise the risk of stiffness of the knee by allowing early mobilisation. Open surgery has a high rate of complications, produces variable functional results, and can result in post-traumatic osteoarthritis.

The arthroscope is more than just another tool; it allows a different approach to intra-articular fractures. All lesions can be identified and documented, reduction can be controlled precisely, and incisions can be kept extremely small. As with other minimally invasive procedures, arthroscopic treatment of intra-articular fractures can be expected to provide lower rates of morbidity and better functional results than open surgery. As yet, follow-up is still too short to allow an evaluation of the risk of osteoarthritis.

Fractures of the tibial plateau and spine are most readily amenable to arthroscopic reduction. Selected cases of patellar and intercondylar fractures can also be treated arthroscopically and will be mentioned briefly in this article.

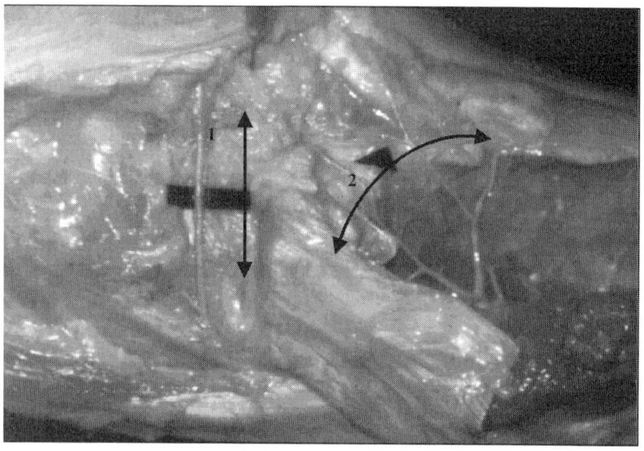

Fig. 1

Vascularisation of the lateral plateau. The vessels may be divided at open surgery when elevating the fascia lata from Gerdy's tubercle (1) and by an arthrotomy below the meniscus (2).

FRACTURES OF THE TIBIAL PLATEAU

Arthroscopic surgery is particularly well suited to the treatment of these fractures. Better preservation of the epiphyseal blood vessels is one main advantage. In a study of cadavers, Hannouche, Duparc and Beaufils[1] showed that the lateral epiphysis receives its blood supply from the branches of the lateral inferior genicular artery and the anterior tibial recurrent artery. There are consistent end-to-end anastomoses between these two networks. Injury to the extraosseous portions of the arterial branches is inevitable during open surgery (Fig. 1), but does not occur in arthroscopic surgery.

Arthroscopic surgery for split fractures or split depression fractures of the tibial plateau has been the focus of several reports of which the earliest were published in 1985.[2-4] Subsequently, a number of authors[5-11] have helped to promote arthroscopic treatment of these fractures by delineating the advantages, limitations and technical aspects of this technique. The medium-term outcome, however, has been reported in only a few studies.[12-14] The best indications for arthroscopic surgery are purely epiphyseal fractures, i.e., types I to IV of the classification of Schatzker, McBroom and Bruce[15] (Figs 2 and 3a). In our opinion, pure metaphyseal fractures and metaphyseal-diaphyseal fractures should not be treated arthroscopically, but others have advocated a combination of arthroscopic surgery and external epiphyseal-diaphyseal fixation, or even plate fixation in some complex fractures.[2,7,12]

Questions which must be addressed include the following:

1) Is arthroscopic reduction of the fracture technically possible?

2) Will sufficient stability be obtained by fixation with screws, which is the only technique feasible under arthroscopy?

3) Do the theoretical advantages of arthroscopic surgery, including better preservation of the blood supply of the tibial plateau,[1] translate into postoperative benefits such as a reduced rate of necrosis and other complications?

4) What are the medium-term functional and long-term radiological outcomes?

5) Should the defect left after elevation of a depressed

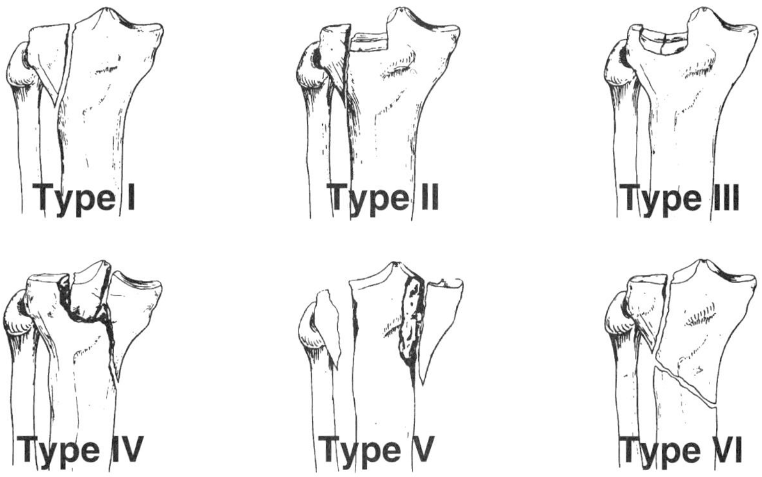

Fig. 2

The classification of Schatzker et al.[15]

fracture be filled, and if so what material should be used (autograft, allograft, bone substitute, cement)?

To answer these questions, we will refer to the literature and the results of a multicentre study (112 cases) which we performed and presented at the French Arthroscopy Society (FAS) symposium in 1999.[16]

Technique. The patient is placed supine on a simple operating table with no thigh clamp and with a tourniquet at the middle of the thigh. The knee is placed over the image intensifier to allow intraoperative fluoroscopic monitoring using Cabot's position for lateral views (Fig. 3b). Jennings,[2] Caspari et al[3] and Bobic and O'Dwyer[5] use a knee-holder with the leg hanging down.

Classic approaches are used. A 30° arthroscope is inserted through an inferolateral portal, the instruments through an inferomedial portal, and the outflow tube through a portal at the superolateral corner of the patella. The inferolateral and inferomedial portals can be alternated. Use of an inflow pump can cause compartment syndrome[5] by forcing the lavage fluid through the fracture site. Guanche and Markman[9] pointed out that using the superolateral outflow portal minimises the risk of compartment syndrome by diminishing the pressure within the joint. A case of fatal air embolism after injection of air into the joint during arthroscopic fracture surgery has been reported by Gruenwald.[17]

A shaver is useful for eliminating haematoma and intra-articular debris. Careful evaluation of the lesions is of the utmost importance. Fracture lines located under the lateral meniscus are not visible through the inferolateral portal (Fig. 3c). Perez Carro, Garera Suarez and Gomez Cimiano[18] recommended the use of a nylon loop to retract the meniscus, whereas Cassard et al[13] have advocated switching the arthroscope to the inferomedial portal after a complete evaluation of the rest of the joint. This method consistently improves visualisation of the site of the fracture. Meniscal lesions are common and usually consist of detachment of the anterior segment of the lateral meniscus. Lesions of the central pivot should be assessed. The cartilage in the unfractured femorotibial compartment should be inspected for traumatic or pre-existing lesions. In the study presented to the 1999 FAS symposium,[16] meniscal lesions were seen in 25% of patients (bucket-handle tear, 6%; rim detachment, 9%; and partial tear, 9%) and a central pivot lesion in 22.5% (anterior cruciate ligament (ACL), 20%; posterior cruciate ligament (PCL), 2.5%). A seemingly recent contusion of the condyle opposite the fracture was seen in 15% of cases and pre-existing chondropathy of the femorotibial compartment in 11%.

Small displacements can sometimes be reduced using a hook or spatula. Extensive depression must be elevated through a window in the metaphyseal cortex. If an 11 or 12 trephine is used to create the window, the piece removed can serve as a corticocancellous bone graft. To guide the trephine, we use an ACL guide (Fig. 3d).[2,7,8] All manoeuvres are performed under both arthroscopic and fluoroscopic guidance. An incision is made over the metaphysis, the aiming device is positioned in the middle of the depressed area, its angle is set to 60°, and the barrel is held in contact with the metaphysis. The trephine is used to cut out a cylinder of bone pointing toward the depression. A graft impacter is inserted into the tunnel thus created and used to lift the depressed bone under visual guidance (Fig. 3e). Because the joint cavity remains closed, spontaneous reduction is common, even with jigsaw fractures (Fig. 3f). The fluoroscope is used to check the position of the guide-pins and screws and to evaluate the quality of 'bone' reduction. In some cases, a saw-tooth forceps applied transversally to the epiphysis through the skin is used to maintain the initial reduction.

The cavity produced by lifting the depressed segment can be left[13,14] or filled partially by the cortical and cancellous bone cylinder removed by the trephine. Itokazu and Matsunaga[19] and Itokazu et al[20] recommended insertion of

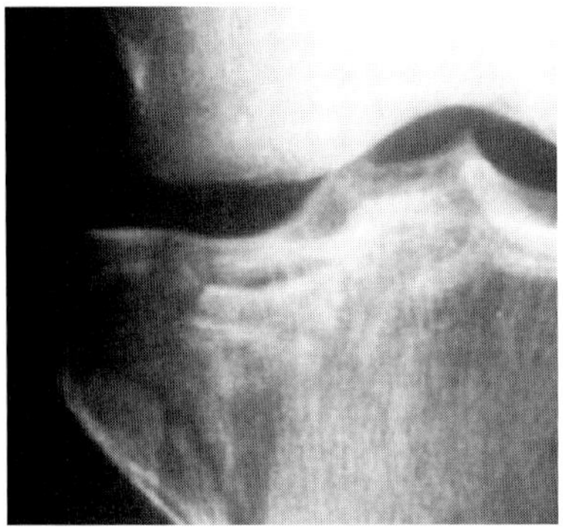

Fig. 3a

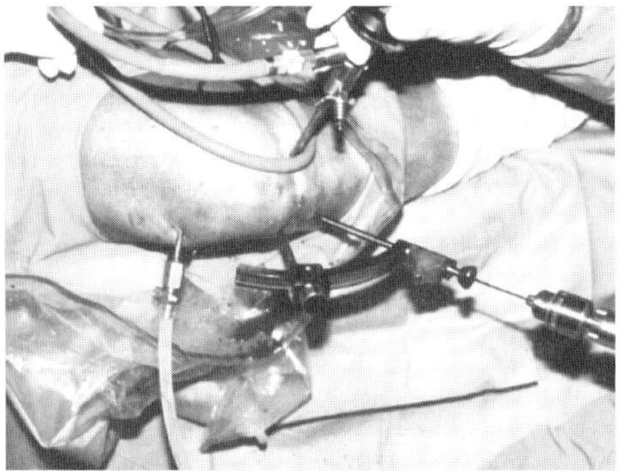

Fig. 3b

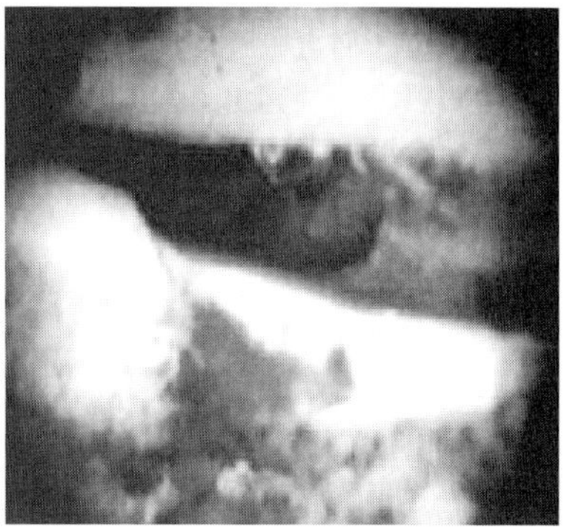

Fig. 3c

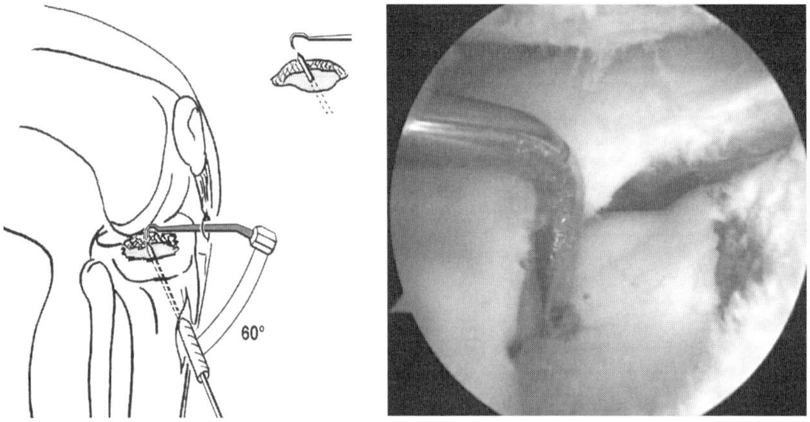

Fig. 3d

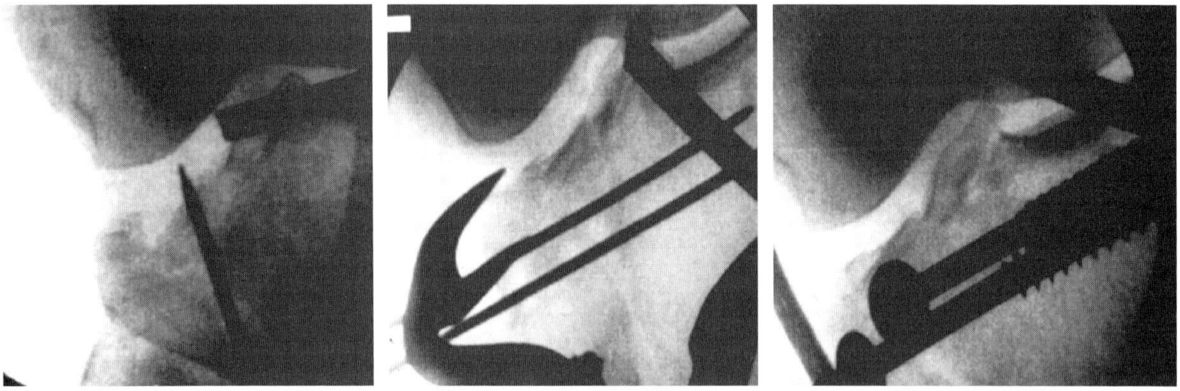

Fig. 3e

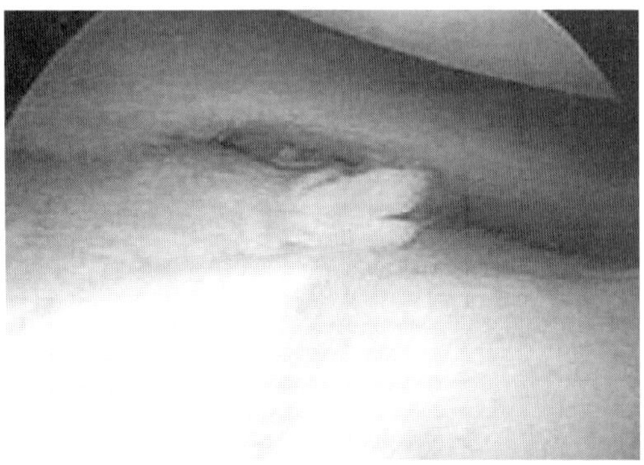

Fig. 3f

Figure 3a – Radiograph of a right knee before operation. Figure 3b – Photograph of the operative position. The knee is in Cabot's position over the image intensifier. Figure 3c – Arthroscopic view showing the depression of the lateral tibial plateau. Figure 3d – Diagram and view showing the use of the ACL guide. Figure 3e – Arthroscopic views showing the insertion of the guide-pin in the centre of the depressed area. The depression is lifted and the reduction maintained by percutaneous forceps and pins. Cannulated screws are inserted on pins. Figure 3f – Arthroscopic control of the reduction.

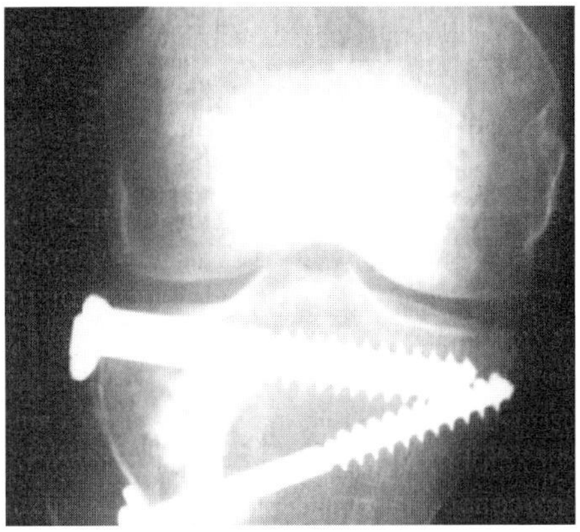

Fig. 4a

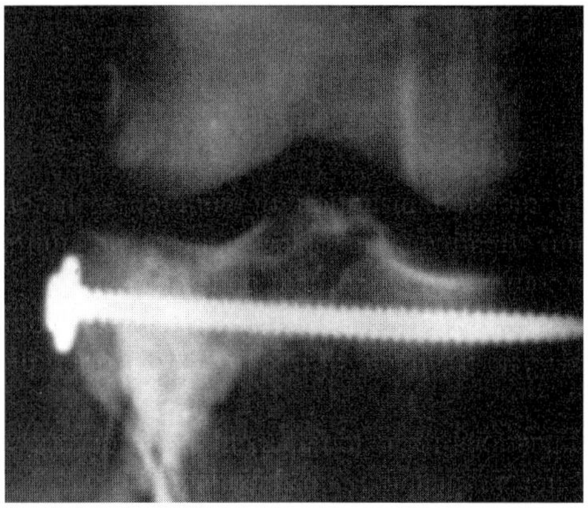

Fig. 4b

Radiographs showing filling of the bone defect by a) bone substitute and b) acrylic cement.

a cancellous bone autograft or substitute (Fig. 4a). Jennings[21] has used injections of acrylic cement, which conforms to the shape of the cavity and ensures excellent stability. The cement must be sufficiently thick. After solidification it fills the cavity and stabilises the fracture (Fig. 4b).

Fixation is usually achieved by inserting a 7 or 7.5 cm, perforated, cancellous bone screw with a short thread. Two screws (Fig. 5) are usually enough to ensure stable fixation. The use of washers is recommended[22] to increase compression at the site of the fracture. Insertion of a third, antiglide screw is unnecessary.[23]

We have used joint drainage in 15% of cases, with no specific selection criteria. There were no haematomas requiring evacuation in any of the patients who did not have a drain. Rehabilitation can be started promptly. There is general agreement that earlier mobilisation increases the chances of a favourable outcome. Jennings[2,21] suggested that early mobilisation was among the main advantages of arthroscopic management. Pain is minimal because of the small size of the incisions, and consequently rehabilitation can be started as early as the first or second postoperative day. We recommend continuous passive mobilisation with a gradual range increase to 90° within a few days. Early mobilisation is associated with a better range of movement after three months. Patients should not bear weight for two to three months, according to the type of fracture.

Results

Efficacy in reducing displacements. In the study presented at the 1999 FAS symposium,[16] reduction was both reliable and reproducible. It was considered to be excellent in 85% of cases based on arthroscopic criteria and in 78% based on postoperative radiography. Since plain radiography is the method of choice for evaluating reduction, this difference indicates that the arthroscopic findings are not sufficient to confirm that precise reduction has been obtained. Intraoperative fluoroscopic monitoring is essential.

Measurement of the overall axis of the lower limb on

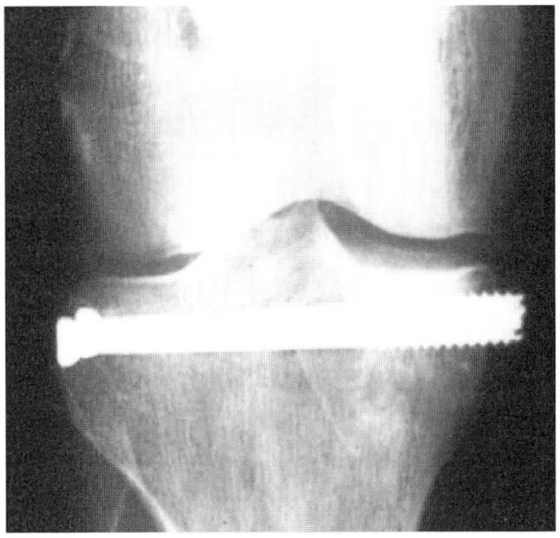

Fig. 5a

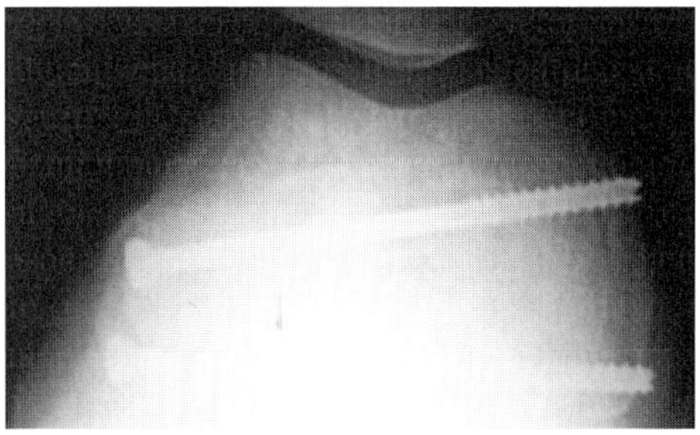

Fig. 5b

Radiographs of a right knee showing fixation by two percutaneous screws. Figure 5a – The AP view. Figure 5b – The femoropatellar projection showing the divergence of the screws.

orthopantograms of the knee showed that the residual deviation as compared with the other knee was only 1.37°, indicating excellent reduction. The absence of incisions through the fibrous sheath of the capsule, tendon, and ligament which surrounds the tibial epiphysis probably increases the likelihood of precise reduction.

Stability of fixation. This has been evaluated based on biomechanical data from cadaver studies and on the rate of secondary displacement.

Only minimal fixation can be performed during arthroscopic surgery since it is introduced percutaneously and is limited to screws in most cases. Fixation by a screw plate has long been recommended because of the stability of the fixation obtained, but it cannot be performed arthroscopically. In a study of ten pairs of cadaver knees, Boisrenoult et al[24] compared two-screw fixation and screw-plate fixation of a Schatzker type-II fracture in terms of resistance to depression in response to loading. To eliminate the possible confounding effects of osteoporosis, both knees of each subject were compared with each other. No differences were demonstrated. Koval et al[25] obtained similar results in a model of simple epiphyseal separation and Parker et al[23] showed that inserting a third screw failed to give significant advantage over two-screw fixation.

In the 1999 AS study, early or delayed disassembly occurred in only five cases, confirming the good stability of two-screw fixation.

Perioperative morbidity: early results. All 112 cases of the FAS study were included in the analysis. Data on postoperative recovery and morbidity were compared with the results of a meta-analysis[15,26-31] of 879 fractures of the tibial plateau treated by open surgery.

Of the 112 patients, only four (3.6%) had complications. There were three cases of thrombophlebitis (2.7%) and one of septic arthritis (0.9%). In the meta-analysis, the rate of septic arthritis was six times higher (6.4%) and the overall rate of complications was 17.6%. Mazoue, Guanche and Vrahas[32] reported one case of septic arthritis in a series of 14 patients. In the 1999 FAS study, there were no instances of haemarthrosis, skin necrosis (2.6% in the meta-analysis), compartment syndrome,[5,9,33] or neurological complications. The mean duration of hospital stay was only 10.2 days as compared with 13 to 22 days in other series. The range of movement was almost normal after three months (124° *v* 106°).

The minimal invasiveness of arthroscopic surgery is without doubt the main factor in the low rate of morbidity and good immediate outcome, but another crucial factor is probably the preservation of the epiphyseal blood supply.[1]

Medium-term results. In the first three years, 88% of patients were satisfied with the procedure, the knee score was 91.4, and the International Knee Society (IKS) function score was 95. Residual deviation of the axis was only 1.37°. Plain radiographs were normal in 71% of patients. Factors for poor prognosis were age over 60 years and more than 6 mm of initial depression. The type of fracture had little influence on the results, although the outcome was somewhat less favourable in Schatzker type-II fractures, but the difference was not statistically significant.

Filling the defect had no statistically significant effect on the results, perhaps because of the small number of patients. It was associated with better correction of the axis (0.5° *v* 1.9°) and a higher knee score (95.4 *v* 89.8). These improvements were most marked in the patients with Schatzker type-II fractures. The proportion of patients with normal radiographs was similar in the groups with and without filling.

Lateral meniscectomy was the main predictive factor, as shown in Table I.

The results for all clinical and radiological parameters were better in the patients who did not undergo meniscectomy, suggesting that the meniscus should be left in place whenever possible. Lesions of the lateral meniscus are extremely common and usually amenable to suturing.

Beyond the first three years, the knee score and the function score remained stable, but 40% of patients had

Table I. Influence of lateral meniscectomy on the medium-term results (FAS multicentric study[16])

	Knee score	Function score	Mean axis deviation (degrees)	% with normal radiographs
Meniscectomy	82.2	87.5	4.56	*50*
No meniscectomy	92	96	0.93	*73*

Table II. Results of filling of the defect in Schatzker type-II and type-III fractures (FAS Multicentric Study[16])

Fracture	Knee score	Function score	Number of patients with residual axis deviation	Mean axis deviation (degrees)
Type II				
Filling	94.0	88.7	2/8	0.5
No filling	85.6	91.3	9/20	2.4
Type III				
Filling	94.7	95.0	3/14	2.0
No filling	94.4	98.0	4/15	2.12

radiological abnormalities of sclerosis (20%) or narrowing of the joint space (20%). Radiographic abnormalities were more common in patients older than 45 years and in those with poorer clinical outcomes, intraoperative evidence of pre-existing chondropathy, or residual axis deviation. In patients with valgus of the knee and pre-existing chondropathy, the final axis deviation was due to a variable combination of non-reduction of the displacement and cartilage wear.

Meniscectomy had a highly significant negative influence on the results beyond three years.

Influence of filling the defect. In depression of the tibial plateau filling of the defect is usually recommended. It is believed to improve articular reduction and to diminish the risk of secondary loss of reduction. In practice, however, it is not always performed, particularly when the treatment is arthroscopic.

Fowble et al[8] and Cassard et al[13,14] did not use filling. Itokazu and Matsumaga[19] advocated filling, for which they preferred bone-graft substitutes to cancellous bone with no complications in a series of 17 cases. The use of bone-graft substitutes preserves the minimally invasive nature of the procedure by reducing the operating time and eliminating the need for a donor site. Acrylic cement with or without fixation has also been used.

In the 1999 FAS study, filling was carried out in 24 patients; autologous bone was used in four, a bone graft substitute in 16, and acrylic cement in four. The only case of septic arthritis in the series occurred after filling with a bone-graft substitute. No other complications related to the use of these materials were recorded.

No statistically significant differences in outcome were demonstrated between the patients treated with and without filling. The results, however, were better when filling was performed, particularly in patients with Schatzker type-II fractures (Table II).

Arthroscopy is technically reliable in the treatment of fractures of the tibial plateau. Screw fixation is usually adequate, except perhaps in patients with osteoporosis or with major depression of the tibial plateau. The rates of morbidity are low and substantially inferior to those seen after open surgery. The decision to fill the defect is left to the surgeon. There is some evidence, however, that filling may be preferable in Schatzker type-II fractures.

Arthroscopic treatment gives good functional results. Although the incidence of radiological abnormalities beyond three years is not negligible, it is substantially lower than that seen after open surgery.

The overall outcome after arthroscopic treatment is good or very good and substantially better than that seen after open surgery. Older age, a Schatzker type-II fracture, pre-existing chondropathy, and, particularly, lateral meniscectomy are associated with a poorer clinical and radiological outcome in the long term.

Indications. Arthroscopy can be used to treat epiphyseal separation and/or depression as defined by Duparc and Ficat[34] (Schatzker types I to IV). There is general agreement that *type-I* fractures carry a good prognosis.[15,35] Simple percutaneous screw fixation also produces excellent results.[22,36] Arthroscopy allows detection and treatment of associated intra-articular abnormalities. Joint lavage relieves pain and facilitates immediate rehabilitation.

Type-II fractures are split depression fractures of the lateral plateau (Fig. 2). We believe that arthroscopy is now the technique of choice for treating these fractures. The outcome is slightly less favourable than in other types of epiphyseal fracture, but remains substantially better than that after open surgery. Lobenhoffer et al,[36] Harper et al,[37] and Sirkin et al[38] have advocated closed reduction by traction followed by percutaneous fixation, and in their hands this technique has provided similar results to those obtained with arthroscopy. The latter, however, allows detection and treatment of any associated lesions and adds to the information on the quality of reduction provided by fluoroscopy. Trephining of the metaphysis and introduction of a graft impacter into the tunnel thus created carries no risk of further injury to the blood vessels supplying the tibial epiphysis and contributes to fast, stable and lasting healing.

The risk of disassembly deserves special attention in patients with severe depression of the tibial plateau or with osteoporosis. Filling should be performed routinely in those with severe depression and bones of good quality. Open surgery with screw-plate fixation should be considered in elderly patients with osteoporosis, but the risk of disassembly of light fixation performed arthroscopically should be weighed against the higher rates of morbidity after open surgery.

In *type-III* fractures, arthroscopy is extremely useful for checking that reduction of the depression is complete. In some cases, the depression can be elevated via the joint cavity using a spatula or hook. Palpation of the cartilage with the hook is important to detect depression of subchondral bone. Arthroscopic verification of the quality of 'bone' reduction is particularly important in type-III fractures.

Type-IV fractures are less common. Their prognosis is determined not only by the bone and cartilage lesions but also by the frequent presence of lesions of the ACL and PCL which sometimes require specific therapy.

Type-V and *type-VI* fractures require rigid fixation. The choice is between internal fixation with a plate or external fixation and is based on the condition of the skin. If external fixation is used, minimal associated percutaneous internal fixation may also be required, which is the only indication for arthroscopic treatment in type-V and type-VI fractures. In this group of fractures, arthroscopy is an ancillary tool in treatment.

FRACTURES OF THE TIBIAL SPINES

Arthroscopy allows anatomical reduction of fractures of the tibial spines under visual guidance, thus ensuring that the ACL is pulled taut.

Anecdotal cases have been reported as technical notes by Van Loon and Marti,[39] Kobayashi and Terayama,[40] Matthews and Giessler,[41] Ando and Nishihara,[42] and Kogan, Marks and Amendola.[43] Bale and Banks[44] reported eight cases in children, all of whom had an excellent outcome. Fixation can be achieved by screwing, pinning, and suturing.[45]

Screw fixation is possible only when there is a single, large fragment. A screw directed downwards and backwards so that it bites into the posterior cortex can be used. Alternatively, a screw can be inserted in a lateral-to-medial direction. This method is more difficult technically but leaves the head of the screw outside the cavity of the joint.[39,41] Fixation using a Kirschner wire[44] or a staple[40] has also been used.

Lacing techniques have been developed by Kogan et al,[43] Medler and Jansson,[46] Matthews and Giessler,[41] and Perez Carro[47] since adequate material became available. The base of the ACL is laced using a threading forceps. The laces are threaded through tibial tunnels created by an aiming device, then knotted on to the anterior cortex of the tibia. The advantages include the absence of material requiring subsequent removal, freedom from all risks of injury to the growth plate in children, and efficacy in the fixation of multiple fragments.

FRACTURES OF THE DISTAL FEMUR AND OF THE PATELLA

Only technical notes have been published on the arthroscopic treatment of these fractures. The main indications for reduction under arthroscopic guidance are unicondylar fractures,[4,48] Hoffa fractures[49] and simple, single-fragment patellar fractures.

CONCLUSIONS

Minimally invasive surgery under arthroscopic guidance is now well established for the treatment of fractures of the knee. It is technically feasible, safe and reliable in carefully selected fractures of the tibia, femur and patella.

Long-term data and comparisons with open surgery are available only for fractures of the tibial plateau, of which large series have been published.

Arthroscopic surgery not only reduces perioperative morbidity, particularly infections, but also improves the long-term functional outcome including the range of movement and the radiological outcome such as the incidence of osteoarthritis. It does not, however, eliminate the risk of osteoarthritis completely; this is dependent primarily on concomitant factors of which the most notable is meniscectomy, which should be avoided whenever possible. The respective roles of arthroscopically-assisted and strictly percutaneous techniques remain to be determined. There is sound evidence that both provide similar results when displacement is absent or minimal. In displaced fractures, however, combining fluoroscopic and arthroscopic visualisation may be the best means of ensuring anatomical reduction and therefore a good long-term outcome.

PB is grateful to Philippe Hardy, Professor of Orthopaedics at the Ambroise Paré Teaching Hospital, Boulogne, France, and Xavier Cassard. Together we prepared the study presented at the 1999 French Society for Arthroscopy Symposium. The present article draws much of its substance from that common study.

REFERENCES

1. **Hannouche D, Duparc F, Beaufils P.** Etude Anatomique de la vascularisation du plaeau tibial externe. *Ann Soc Française d'Arthroscopie.* Montpellier: Sauramps Ed, 2000.
2. **Jennings JE.** Arthroscopic management of tibial plateau fractures. *Arthroscopy* 1985;1:160-8.
3. **Caspari RB, Hutton MJ, Whipple TL, Meyers JF.** The role of arthroscopy in the management of tibial plateau fractures. *Arthroscopy* 1985;1:76-82.
4. **Lemon RA, Bartlett DH.** Arthroscopic assisted internal fixation of certain fractures about the knee. *J Trauma* 1985;25:355-8.
5. **Bobic V, O'Dwyer KJ.** Tibial plateau fracture: the arthroscopic option. *Knee Surg Sports Traumatol Arthrosc* 1993;1:239-42.
6. **Bernfeld B, Kligman F, Roffman M.** Arthroscopic assistance for unselected tibial plateau fractures. *Arthroscopy* 1996;12:598-602.
7. **Buchko GB, Johnson DH.** Arthroscopy-assisted operative management of tibial plateau fractures. *Clin Orthop* 1996;332:29-36.
8. **Fowble CD, Zimmer JW, Schepsis AS.** The role of arthroscopy in the assessment and treatment of tibial plateau fractures. *Arthroscopy* 1993;9:584-90.
9. **Guanche CA, Markman AW.** Arthroscopic management of tibial plateau fractures. *Arthroscopy* 1993;9:467-71.
10. **Handelberg F, Casteleyn PP, Deroeck P.** Arthroscopic assessment and treatment of tibial plateau fractures. *Arthroscopy* 1991;7:318.
11. **Holzach P, Matter P, Minter J.** Arthroscopically assisted treatment of lateral tibial plateau fractures in skiers: use of cannulated reduction system. *J Orthop Trauma* 1994;8:273-81.
12. **Scheerlinck T, Ng CS, Handelberg F, Casteleyn PP.** Medium-term results of percutaneous arthroscopically assisted osteosynthesis of fractures of the tibial plateau. *J Bone Joint Surg [Br]* 1998;80-B:959-64.
13. **Cassard X, Beaufils P, Blin JL, Hardy P.** Osteosynthesis under arthroscopic control of separated tibial plateau fracture: 26 case reports. *Rev Chir Orthop* 1999;85:257-66.
14. **Cassard X, Beaufils P, Hardy P.** *Fractures du plateau tibial: traitement chirurgical sous contrôle endoscopique.* In: *Arthroscopie.* Paris, Amsterdam: Elsevier, 1999:235-8.
15. **Schatzker J, McBroom R, Bruce D.** The tibial plateau fracture, the Toronto experience 1968-1975. *Clin Orthop* 1979;138:94-104.
16. **Beaufils P, Hardy P, Cassard X.** Traitement sous contrôle arthroscopique des fractures du plateau tibial: a propos de 112 cas. *Ann Soc Française d'Arthroscopie.* Montpellier: Sauramps Ed, 2000.
17. **Gruenwald JM.** Fatal air embolism during arthroscopy. *J Bone Joint Surg [Br]* 1990;72-B:929.
18. **Perez Carro L, Garcia Suarez G, Gomez Cimiano F.** The arthroscopic knot technique for fracture of the tibia in children. *Arthroscopy* 1994;10:698-9.
19. **Itokazu M, Matsunaga T.** Arthroscopic restoration of depressed tibial plateau using bone and hydroxyapatite grafts. *Arthroscopy* 1993;9:103-8.
20. **Itokazu M, Matsunaga T, Ishii M, Kusakabe H, Wyni Y.** Use of arthroscopy and interporous hydroxyapatite as a bone graft substitute in tibial plateau fractures. *Arch Orthop Trauma Surg* 1996;115:45-8.
21. **Jennings JE.** Tibial plateau fracture. In: McGinty, ed. *Operative arthroscopy.* Philadelphia: Lippincott-Raven, 1996:576-88.
22. **Keogh P, Kelly C, McGuinness AJ, O'Rourke SK.** Percutaneous screw fixation of tibial plateau fractures. *Injury* 1992;23:387-9.
23. **Parker PJ, Tepper KB, Brumback RJ, Novak VP, Belkoff SM.** Biomechanical comparison of fixation of type-I fractures of the lateral tibial plateau: is the antiglide screw effective? *J Bone Joint Surg [Br]* 1999;81-B:478-80.

24. **Boisrenoult P, Bricteux S, Beaufils P, et al.** Société Française d'arthroscopie: Vis versus plaque vissée dans les fractures séparation enforcement du plateau tibial latéral: etude biomécanique cadavérique. *Rev Chir Orthop Reparatrice Appar Mot* 2000;86:707-11.

25. **Koval KJ, Sanders R, Borrelli J, et al.** Indirect reduction and percutaneous screw fixation of displaced tibial plateau fractures. *J Orthop Trauma* 1992;6:340-6.

26. **Duwelius PJ, Connoly JF.** Closed reduction of tibial plateau fractures. *Clin Orthop* 1988;230:116-26.

27. **Honkonen SE.** Indications for surgical treatment of tibial condyle fractures. *Clin Orthop* 1994;302:199-205.

28. **Jensen DB, Rude C, Duus B, Bjerg-Nielsen A.** Tibial plateau fractures. *J Bone Joint Surg [Br]* 1990;72-B:49-52.

29. **Lachiewicz PF, Funcik T.** Factors influencing the results of open reduction and internal fixation of tibial plateau fractures. *Clin Orthop* 1990;259:210-5.

30. **Moore TM, Patzakis MJ, Harvey JP.** Tibial plateau fractures: definition, demographics, treatment rationale, and long-term results of closed traction management or operative reduction. *J Orthop Trauma* 1987;1:97-119.

31. **Young MJ, Barrack RL.** Complications of internal fixation of tibial plateau fractures. *Orthop Rev* 1994;23:149-54.

32. **Mazoue CG, Guanche CA, Vrahas MS.** Arthroscopic management of tibial plateau fractures: an unselected series. *Am J Orthop* 1999;28:508-15.

33. **Belanger M, Fadale P.** Compartment syndrome of the leg after arthroscopic examination of a tibial plateau fracture: case report and review of the literature. *Arthroscopy* 1997;13:646-51.

34. **Duparc J, Ficat P.** Fractures articulaire de l'extrémité superieure du tibia. *Rev Chir Orthop* 1960;46:339-486.

35. **Hohl M.** Tibial condylar fractures. *J Bone Joint Surg [Am]* 1967; 49-A:1455-67.

36. **Lobenhoffer P, Schulze M, Gerich T, Lattermann C, Tscherne H.** Closed reduction/percutaneous fixation of tibial plateau fractures: arthroscopic versus fluoroscopic control of reduction. *J Orthop Trauma* 1999;13:426-31.

37. **Harper MC, Henstorf JE, Vssely B, Maurizi MG, Allen WC.** Closed reduction and percutaneous stabilization of tibial plateau fractures. *Orthopaedics* 1995;18:623-6.

38. **Sirkin MS, Bono CM, Reilly MC, Behrens FF.** Percutaneous methods of tibial plateau fixation. *Clin Orthop* 2000;375:60-8.

39. **Van Loon T, Marti RK.** A fracture of the intercondylar eminence of the tibia treated by arthroscopic fixation. *Arthroscopy* 1991;7:385-8.

40. **Kobayashi S, Terayama K.** Arthroscopic reduction and fixation of a completely displaced fracture of the intercondylar eminence of the tibia. *Arthroscopy* 1994;10:231-5.

41. **Matthews D, Geissler W.** Arthroscopic suture fixation of displaced tibial eminence fractures. *Arthroscopy* 1994;10:418-23.

42. **Ando T, Nishihara K.** Arthroscopic internal fixation of fractures of the intercondylar eminence of the tibia. *Arthroscopy* 1996;12:616-22.

43. **Kogan MG, Marks P, Amendola A.** Technique for arthroscopic suture fixation of displaced tibial intercondylar eminence fractures. *Arthroscopy* 1997;13:301-6.

44. **Bale RS, Banks AJ.** Arthroscopically guided Kirschner wire fixation for fractures of the intercondylar eminence of the tibia. *J R Coll Surg Edinb* 1995;40:260-2.

45. **Lemoine J, Chassaing V.** Fracture déplacée du massif des épines tibiales: technique de réinsertion arthroscopique. In: *Arthroscopie.* Paris, Amsterdam: Elsevier, 1999:239-40.

46. **Medler RG, Jansson KA.** Arthroscopic treatment of fractures of the tibial spine. *Arthroscopy* 1994;10:292-5.

47. **Perez Carro L.** Arthroscopic management of tibial plateau fractures: special techniques. *Arthroscopy* 1997;13:265-7.

48. **McCarthy JJ, Parker RD.** Arthroscopic reduction and internal fixation of a displaced intraarticular lateral femoral condyle fracture of the knee. *Arthroscopy* 1996;12:224-7.

49. **Wallenbock F, Ledinski C.** Indications and limits of arthroscopic management of intra-articular fractures of the knee joint. *Aktuelle Traumatol* 1993;23:97-101.

DISPLACED FRACTURES OF THE PROXIMAL HUMERUS

P. HOFFMEYER

From the University Hospital, Geneva, Switzerland

Fractures of the proximal humerus may be intra-articular, involving either true articular surfaces such as the glenohumeral joint or gliding surfaces such as the subacromial joint or both. Glenohumeral motion and strength rely not only on intact articular surfaces but also on the co-ordinated interplay of the muscles and tendons around the shoulder. Contraction of the muscles of the rotator cuff creates a stabilising compressive force with a downward orientated vector which then allows smooth elevation of the humerus, in conjunction with an upwardly orientated force created by contraction of the deltoid. In pathological states, glenohumeral kinematics are disturbed. In dysfunction of the cuff as a result of poor reposition of the tuberosity, for example, after a displaced fracture, abduction will be diminished or even impossible, even although the deltoid pulls the humerus upwards,[1,2] because the cuff will not be able to produce the necessary torque for this movement to occur.

Although these fractures are probably best treated operatively, their complex pattern, comminution and displacement make secure anatomical fixation difficult. These problems may be compounded by poor bone quality because of coexisting osteoporosis. Rigid fixation and anatomical reduction are therefore not always possible and techniques must be used to restore sufficient morphology to allow painless function. Sometimes with severely comminuted and displaced fracture patterns prosthetic replacement will be the only solution.[3,4] The surgeon must therefore be aware of the technical options which will allow him to reach realistic goals, taking into account not only fracture-related components but also patient-related conditions. Techniques must be utilised which will provide sufficient stability to achieve bony union, early mobilisation and ultimately pain-free function. Depending on the osteoporosis present and the comminution of the fracture, a variety of surgical options should be considered. In some cases rigid fixation will achieve anatomical restoration while in others the anatomy will have to be sacrificed in order to achieve stability, with a predictably different outcome.

ANATOMY OF THE GLENOHUMERAL JOINT

The anatomy of the glenohumeral joint is complex and in the case of fracture the components must be reconstructed if the kinetics of the joint are to be preserved.[1,2]

The dynamics of this highly mobile joint are the consequence of its particular bony anatomy and of its soft-tissue envelope. The skeletal anatomy of the glenohumeral joint comprises two retroverted non-constrained articular surfaces. That of the glenoid is pear-shaped because of the anterior incisura acetabuli. Mallon et al[5] have made measurements of the glenoid and found a mean transverse diameter of 24 ± 3.3 mm, a mean superoinferior diameter of 35 ± 4.1 mm, a mean version of 2.0 ± 4.2° posterior (-7 to -12) and a mean radius of curvature of 36.6 ± 7.4 mm (24 to 50).

The proximal humerus has a cartilaginous surface which is tilted upwards 45° and posteriorly about 20° with reference to the distal intercondylar line.[6] Using radiological techniques, Cyprien et al[7] and Debevoise, Hyatt and Townsend[8] determined humeral retroversion. The former found a mean value of 26.9 ± 12.22° on the right and 21.2 ± 11.02° on the left and the latter group a mean value of 61.6° (47 to 65) on the right and 60.8° (47 to 85) on the left. The quasispherical surface of the humeral head occupies approximately one-third of a sphere with an angular value ranging between 120° and 150°. The radius of curvature in the axial plane is 22 ± 1.7 mm and the radius of curvature in the coronal plane is 24 ± 2.6 mm.[9]

The vascular anatomy of the humeral head plays a major role in the outcome of trauma. A devascularised humeral head will collapse and become incongruent with the development of secondary arthritis. The arteria arcuata circulates within the humeral head and receives its blood supply from four major sources: the metaphyseal artery, the branch of the anterior circumflex artery in the bicipital groove, arteries from the rotator cuff and the medial branch of the posterior circumflex artery.[10-12] Because of this arterial pattern a fracture through the anatomical neck will lead to complete devascularisation of the articular surface-bearing fragment of the head (Fig. 1).

The power link between the scapula and the humerus is ensured by the glenohumeral muscle groups which directly cross the joint: teres major, the deltoid with its three functionally independent anterior, middle and posterior segments, and the rotator cuff. The last consists of the musculotendinous units of subscapularis, supraspinatus, infraspinatus, and teres minor.[13] The biceps and its tendinous long head may also be considered as part of the rotator cuff. The biceps tendon is a valuable surgical landmark

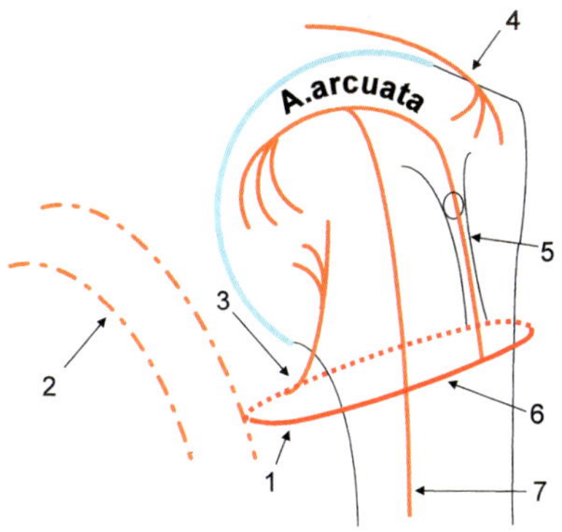

Fig. 1a

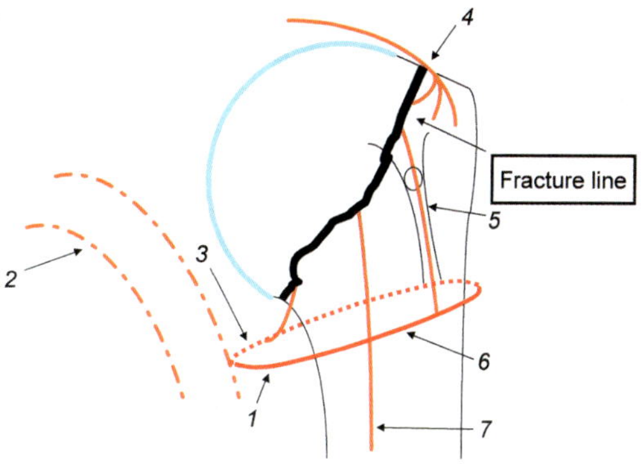

Fig. 1b

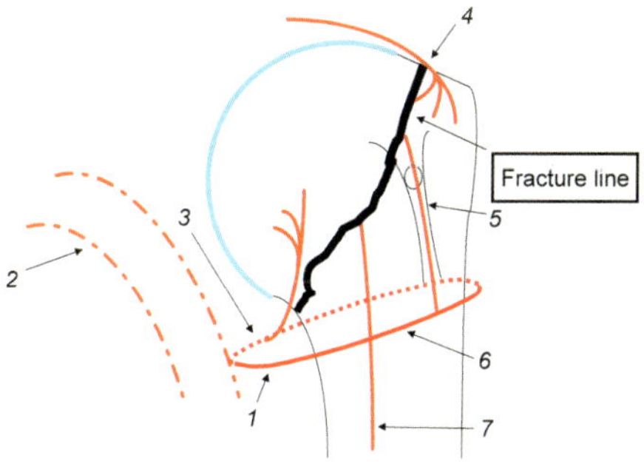

Fig. 1c

Figure 1a – Diagram of the sources of vascularisation of the humeral head. Figure 1b – Diagram showing fracture through the anatomical neck cutting off all blood supply to the head. Figure 1c – Diagram showing the line of the fracture sufficiently lateral to spare the posterior circumflex artery and preserve some blood supply to the head from that source. This may be seen in valgus-impacted fractures with good medial contact (1, circumflex artery; 2, axillary artery; 3, ascending branch of the posterior circumflex artery; 4, arterial supply of the rotator cuff from the thoracoacromial and suprascapular arteries; 5, ascending branch of the anterior circumflex artery; 6, anterior circumflex artery; 7, intraosseous metaphyseal artery).

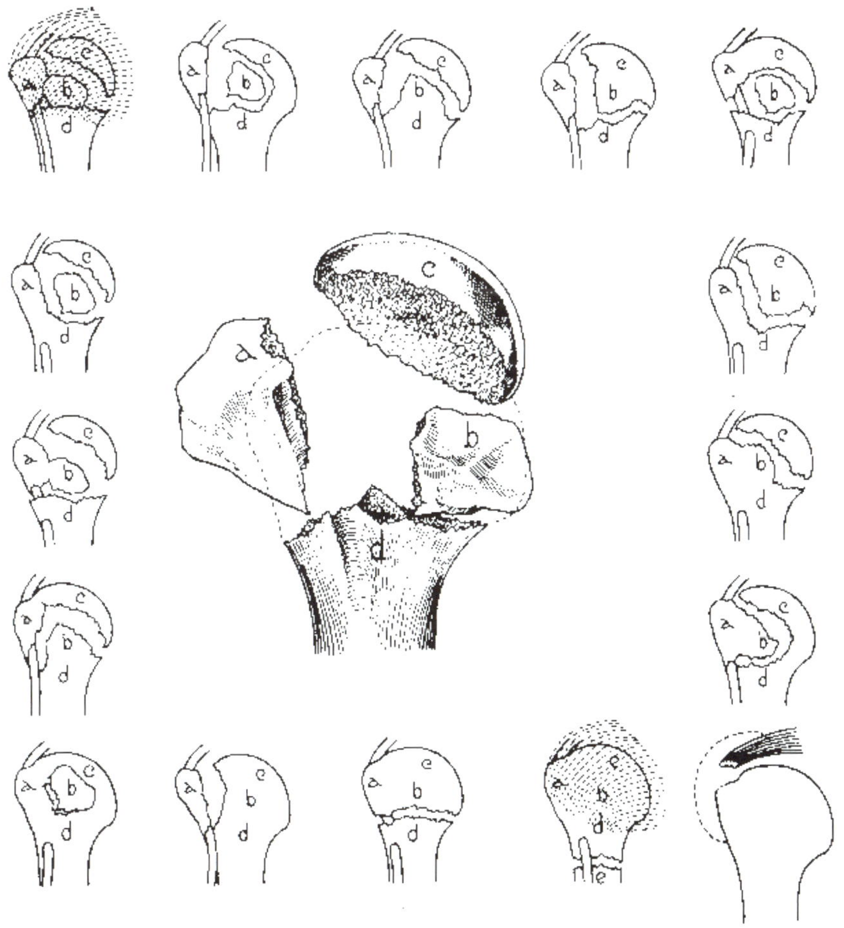

Fig. 2

Diagram of Codman's classification.[18]

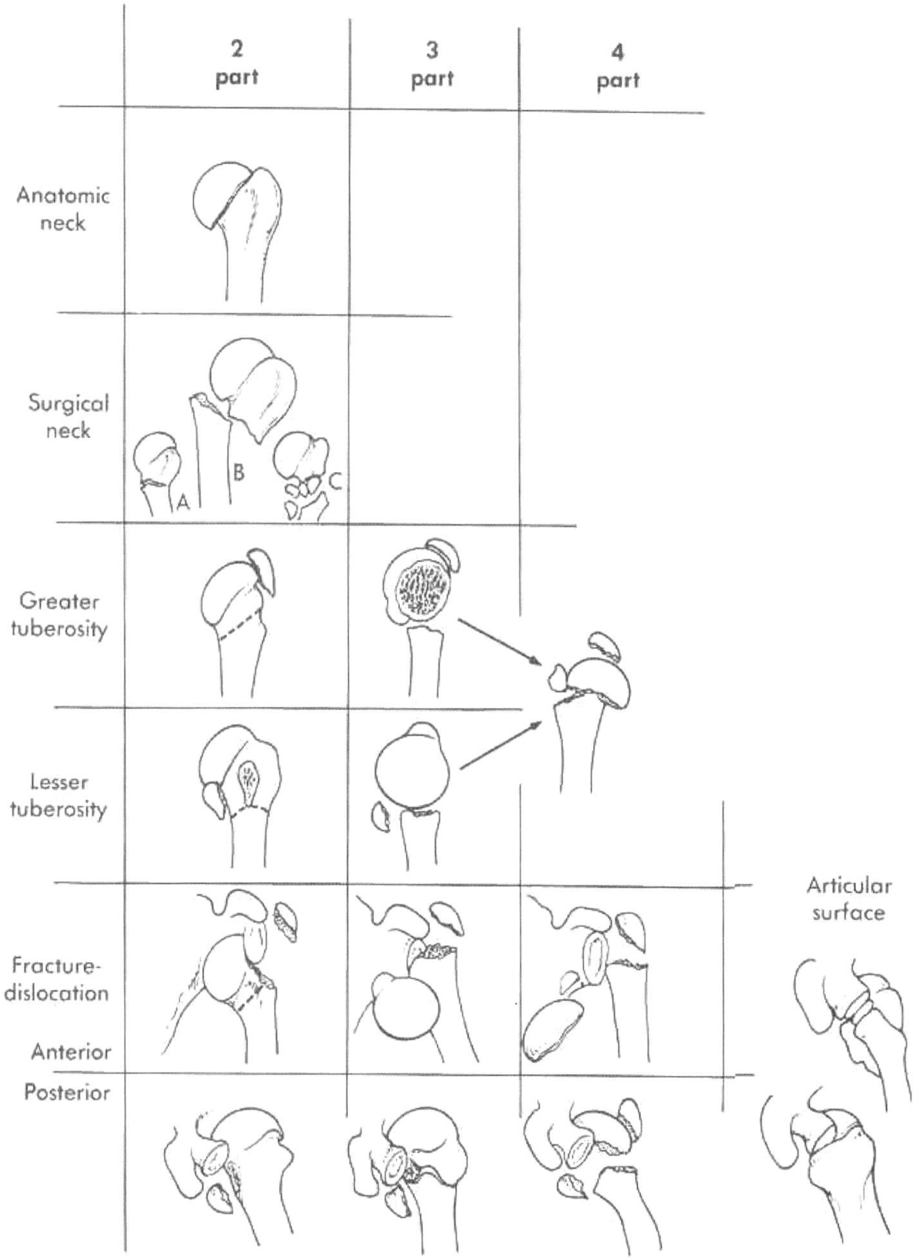

Fig. 3

Diagram of Neer's classification.[3]

separating the lesser from the greater tuberosity and therefore is of help in identifying the various fragments with their attached cuff tendons when dealing with a displaced fracture of the proximal humerus. Structures medial to the biceps tendon are subscapularis and the lesser tuberosity while those lateral to it are part of the greater tuberosity and attached tendons of supraspinatus and infraspinatus.[14]

The axillary nerve is an important structure at risk in fractures of the proximal humerus.[15] It innervates the deltoid and teres minor muscles and should be tested for motor and sensory function on the lateral aspect of the shoulder before any manoeuvre, reduction or otherwise, is attempted for fracture of the humeral head. It should be visualised at surgery, or at least palpated, as it lies anterior to subscapularis before it plunges beneath the tendon of subscapularis and the glenohumeral capsule into the quadrilateral space on its way to the deltoid and to teres minor. It must also be remembered that the axillary nerve is tensed in internal rotation and relaxed in external rotation.[15]

The musculocutaneous nerve should also be checked clinically, including its motor innervation of biceps and sensory innervation of the medial forearm. It is usually not necessary to visualise the nerve at surgery but it must be borne in mind that the nerve enters the biceps approximately 5 to 8 cm below the tip of coracoid; this distance, however, has been shown to be very variable.[16]

Vascular lesions are infrequently associated with fractures

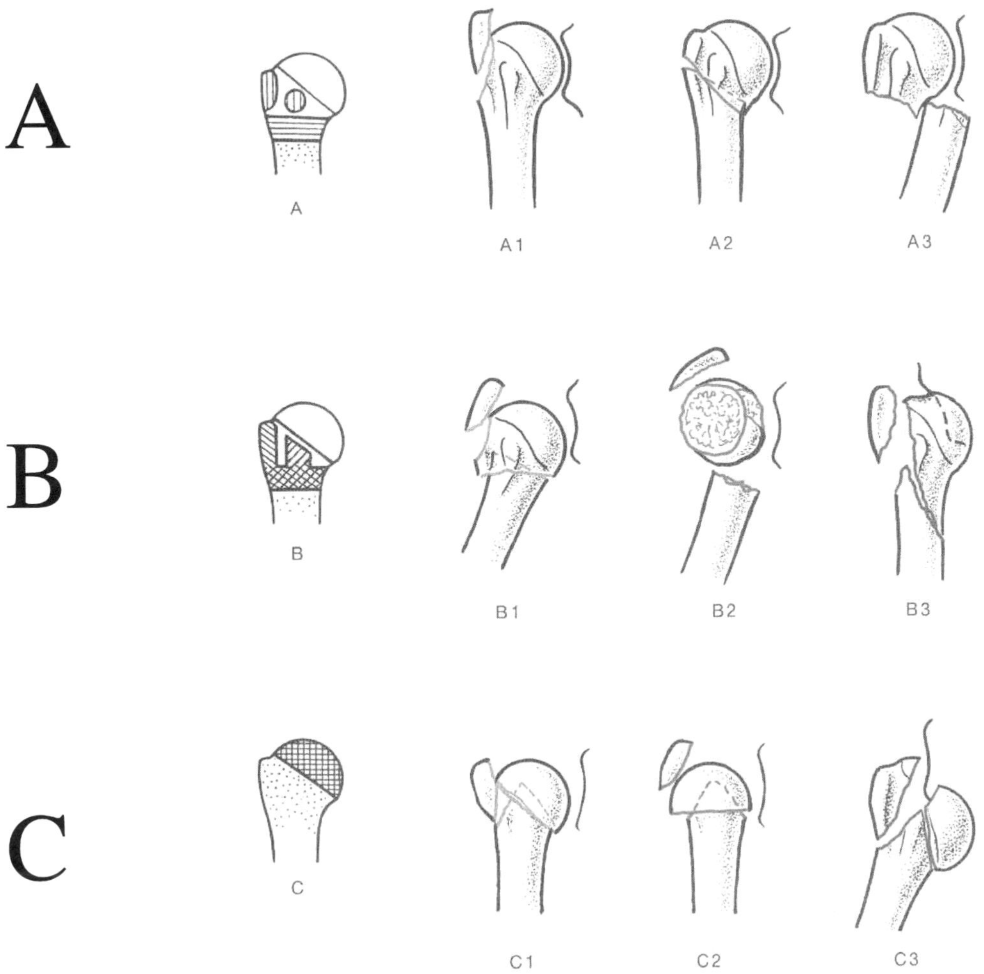

Fig. 4

Diagram of the AO-ASIF classification.[20]

of the proximal humerus.[17] In the presence of a fracture an enlarging ecchymosis or a painful tense haematoma should alert the surgeon to underlying haemorrhage either venous or, more rarely, arterial. Ideally, angiographic assessment should be considered. If this is not possible surgical exploration is mandatory.

CLASSIFICATION OF FRACTURES

Many classification schemes have evolved in order to guide treatment and to aid in determining the prognosis. Codman[18] first suggested that the number and type of fragment found in each fracture may play an important role (Fig. 2). Neer[3,4] and Brien et al[19] refined this concept into an accepted classification which takes account of the amount of displacement (of more than 1 cm linear and 45° angular) of each fragment and the number of fragments involved. The presence or absence of dislocation is also important (Fig. 3). The Association for the Study of Internal Fixation (AO-ASIF)[20] has also developed an alpha-numeric classification scheme which differentiates between articular and extra-articular fractures (Fig. 4). These classification systems have their shortcomings and do not always show inter- and intra-observer reliability.[21,22] Furthermore, none takes into account the quality of the bone or soft tissues. These difficulties may pertain more to imaging techniques than to the patterns of the fracture themselves, and future developments in imaging may improve the classification schemes. Nevertheless, although they may not always be accurate enough for reliable assessment of each individual patient, they have brought considerable understanding to the interpretation of the fracture patterns and therefore to patient care.

PREOPERATIVE ASSESSMENT

A thorough history should be taken to determine the circumstances of the fracture. Displaced fractures of the proximal humerus often occur in a population which is at risk. In eight published series between 1974 and 1995, totalling 487 cases in patients with a mean age of 65.7 years and a mean follow-up of three years (maximum of 14 years), there were

Table I. Mortality of patients with fractures of the proximal humerus from eight series reported in the literature

Author	Treatment	Reported mean age (yr)	Number of cases	Reported number of patients deceased at follow-up (number, %)	Maximum reported follow-up (yr)
Svend-Hansen[29]	Operative and closed	66	63	8 (*12*)	7
Keene et al[23]	Closed	68	92	32 (*34*)	12
Lim et al[25]	Operative and closed	62	31	7 (*22*)	6
Stableforth[28]	Hemiarthroplasty	67	81	6 (*7*)	14
Ko and Yamamoto[24]	Operative	52	17	1 (*5*)	5
Rasmussen et al[26]	Closed	77	65	15 (*23*)	4
Zyto et al[30]	Operative and closed	71	47	6 (*12*)	3
Schai et al[27]	Operative and closed	66	91	3 (*3*)	14

78 reported deaths (16% of all cases)[23-30] (Table I). It is therefore important to determine exactly the nature of the injury and to look for associated medical conditions.[31]

High-energy injuries such as occur in motor-vehicle accidents usually produce significant associated injuries such as spinal or thoracic lesions. If there is no injury a pathological fracture should be suspected and an underlying tumour whether primary or secondary should be sought. The absence of injury in a fracture-dislocation must make epilepsy a consideration and the possible causes should be considered. Moderate injury, such as a fall in the home, must raise suspicions of osteoporosis and this will call for preventive measures. Persistent pain after a fall with initially negative radiographs should alert the physician to repeat the radiography with added views; often a hidden fracture of the tuberosity will be revealed. In these cases of almost undisplaced fractures there is the risk of an underlying tear of the rotator cuff and this should be investigated by ultrasonography or MRI. Adequate neurological and vascular investigations may also be necessary.

RADIOLOGICAL INVESTIGATIONS

For a successful diagnosis of a fracture of the proximal humerus it is imperative to have two views perpendicular to each other, and the glenohumeral joint line should be completely open with no overlap of the head upon the glenoid. The most common standard views are the true AP view of the glenohumeral joint perpendicular to the plane of the scapula and the axillary view parallel to this plane and perpendicular to the acromion. These can *always* be accomplished. The axillary view necessitates only a few degrees of abduction or, if the arm is held in internal rotation by a bandage, a Velpeau view can be made in which the patient leans backwards with the x-ray beam directed supero-inferiorly from the top of the shoulder on to a cassette located at the patient's elbow. AP internal and external rotation views may be helpful but are difficult to obtain in cases of acute injury. Scapular Y views are sometimes of use but notoriously difficult to interpret and, unless perfectly performed, should not be used to exclude, for example, posterior fracture-dislocations.[14] CT is a useful adjunct and three-dimensional reconstructions can show features not readily recognisable on plain films.[32-34] MRI may accurately delineate suspected soft-tissue injury. In case of doubt angiography should be used to determine vascular integrity. Other imaging techniques such as scintigraphy may be difficult to interpret in the acute phase of a fracture of the proximal humerus and should be reserved for more chronic conditions associated with previously undiagnosed trauma.

SURGICAL APPROACHES

Deltopectoral approach. In displaced fractures of the proximal humerus the most common surgical approach is the deltopectoral approach with the patient in the 'beach-chair' or semi-sitting position.[3,4] General anaesthesia is used and sometimes a scalene block may be performed before intubation. This allows for lighter anaesthesia. In addition, the absence of pain on awakening will prevent uncontrolled movement by the patient and therefore protect the osteosynthesis. An oblique incision 15 cm long is made starting from below the clavicle and passing over the coracoid. After appropriate haemostasis of the subcutaneous tissue, the deltopectoral interval and the cephalic vein are identified. If there is difficulty in finding the interval because of swelling the search should be made more proximally near the clavicular insertion of the deltoid and pectoralis major muscles where, usually, the interval widens. The cephalic vein is left either with the deltoid muscle or with the pectoralis muscle. It may be ligated. The conjoined tendons are then retracted and a curved blunt retractor is placed under the deltoid muscle around the fragments of the humeral head in the subacromial space after blood clot and bursal tissue have been removed. The axillary nerve is identified and palpated by sliding the index finger under the conjoined tendons on to the anterior aspect of subscapularis. It is then important to identify the biceps tendon and to use it as a landmark to help to identify the fragments of the greater and lesser tuberosities with their attached tendons. With two-part fractures involving the surgical neck, the alignment of biceps may reflect the adequacy of the reduction. In a fracture in which the lesser tuberosity is not detached but where the surgeon wishes to inspect the articular surface, a small incision

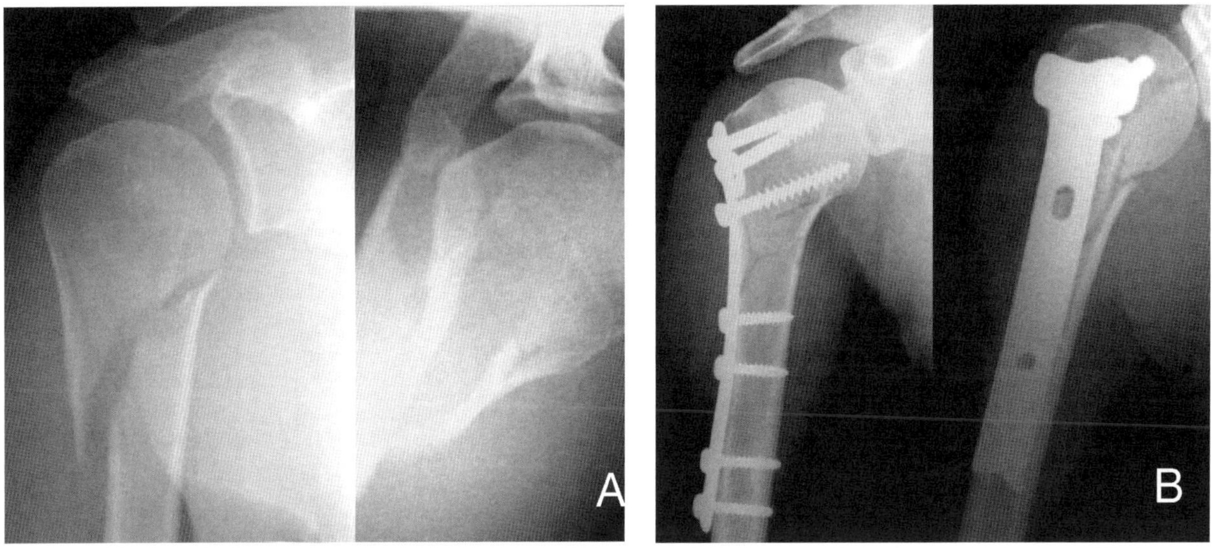

Fig. 5a Fig. 5b

Radiographs showing plate osteosynthesis. Figure 5A – A 35-year-old woman with a two-part displaced fracture (AO type A3). Figure 5B – Treatment consisted of rigid fixation with a plate osteosynthesis.

through the interval can be made and the articular surface observed. All the tendinous structures should then be identified with stay sutures. Reduction may be accomplished by various techniques from the use of plates and screws in particularly strong bone to obtain a 'rigid' fixation, to relying on osteosutures or wires to obtain a tension band construct. This last technique may be particularly indicated in the presence of osteoporosis. A control radiograph should always be obtained before closure. In order to obtain a satisfactory view the x-ray tube should be placed on the contralateral side of the patient and the cassette applied to the body of the scapula. This will give a view perpendicular to the plane of the scapula allowing interpretation of the quality of the reduction and of the position of the tuberosities.

Transdeltoid split approach. In cases of isolated fractures of the tuberosity or if an intramedullary device is used, it is sometimes sufficient to use a transdeltoid split approach. The patient is in a semi-sitting position and the skin incision may be directed following the direction of the muscle fibres along the upper deltoid at the junction of the anterior and middle thirds or as a vertical 'sabre-cut'. The deltoid is split along its fibres no more than 5 cm from the acromion in order to avoid injury to the axillary nerve. The cuff is then identified and the haemorrhagic subacromial bursa partially removed. The fragments of the fracture are then identified and reduced. Fixation may be by means of isolated screws, wiring or heavy sutures. If proximal intramedullary nailing is chosen the same transdeltoid split approach can be used. The tendon of supraspinatus is split to allow the introduction of the nail into the tuberosity. The proximal part should be buried under the level of the articular cartilage. Image-intensifier control is essential to ensure a satisfactory outcome.

OVERVIEW OF SURGICAL TECHNIQUE

Plate fixation. In a two- or three-part fracture occurring in strong bone, usually in a younger or very active individual, the goal should be anatomical reconstruction in order to achieve the best possible function.[35] As these fractures are intra-articular, the aim must be rigid fixation to avoid secondary loss of reduction. In order to obtain an optimal reduction, an open procedure using either the transdeltoid split (for an isolated fracture of the greater tuberosity) or the deltopectoral approach should be used. The fragments of the fracture must be carefully identified and tagged with stay sutures at the tendon-bone interface using the long head of biceps as a landmark. Usually, it will be possible to reposition the fragment of the head on to the metaphyseal fragment and to obtain provisional fixation with Kirschner (K-) wires. This is especially true in fractures which are aligned in varus, while in valgus-impacted fractures, if the impaction is extreme, the head may be disimpacted and held in place by an intercalated bone graft. In this situation, and when using this technique, care must be taken not to disturb the soft-tissue attachments of the medial head-neck junction (Fig. 1c). It is in this area that the medial circumflex artery penetrates the humeral head and this may be its only remaining blood supply.[36,37] The greater and/or lesser tuberosities are also reduced and a contoured T-plate (ASIF 3.5 or 4.5 mm) is applied taking care not to injure the long head of biceps. Screws are then inserted and the stay sutures may be either removed or tied into the plate holes or transosseously, if needed, for further stability (Fig. 5).

In the case of a limited head-splitting fracture, which is usually associated with a dislocation, screw fixation only may be used. In these cases, however, the vascular supply of the head is compromised and the prognosis remains guard-

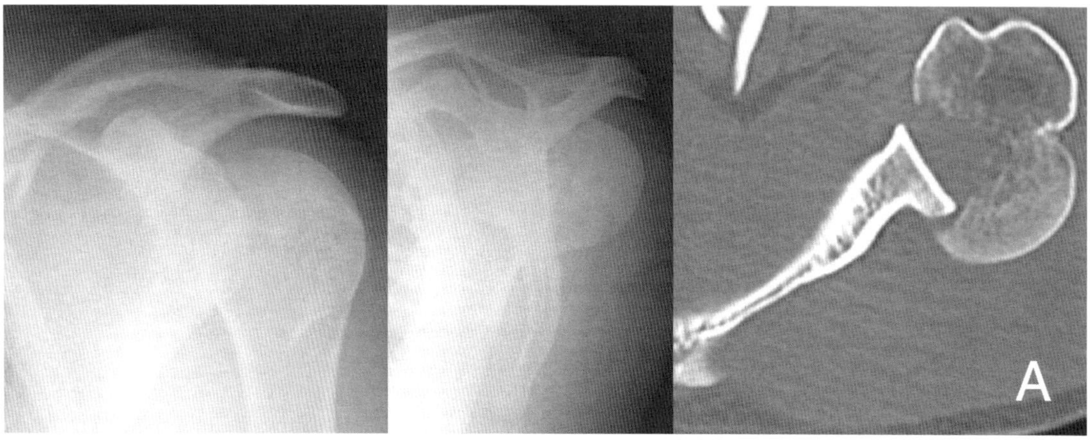

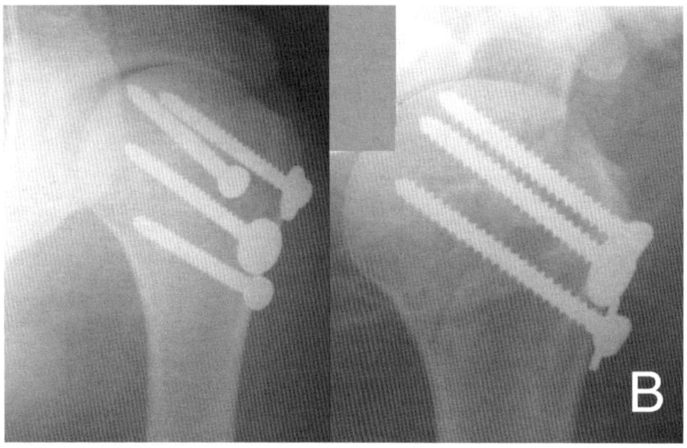

Fig. 6

Radiographs and CT showing osteosynthesis with screws. Figure 6A – A 34-year-old man with a head-splitting fracture dislocation. Figure 6B – Osteosynthesis with compression screws. The prognosis was guarded with the possibility of collapse of the head.

ed[38,39] (Fig. 6). Newer designs of implant (ASIF Locking Compression Plates) have screw heads which lock into the plates thus allowing angular stability of the screws in relation to the plate. These types of implant give improved stability and may therefore speed bony healing and functional recovery.

Osteosuture. For three- and four-part fractures occurring in older individuals or patients with fragile osteopenic bone, the goal is to obtain a reduction which is anatomical enough to allow acceptable function.[40-43] Also, in valgus-impacted three- or four-part fractures the anatomy may be restored by pulling the tuberosities below the level of the head without disturbing it or its vascularisation. Osteosuture requires the use of wire, cable or heavy sutures (Ethibond no. 6) to obtain fixation. A deltopectoral approach in a semi-sitting position will allow the surgeon to visualise the bone fragments. The head of the humerus is impacted on to the metaphysis in a stable valgus position. The greater and lesser tuberosities are identified and heavy sutures, wire or cable are passed through the fragments at the bone-tendon junction. These sutures are then fixed to the metaphysis between 1 and 2 cm below the metaphyseal fracture line either through transosseous holes or tied around a screw with washers (4.5 mm) introduced into the metaphysis. The long head of biceps will give orientation as to the reduction of the fragments. It should lie within its groove and be in a straight vertical line from its origin to the muscle belly. A radiograph should be taken before closure of the wound to ascertain the quality of the reduction (Figs 7 and 8).[37]

Extramedullary pinning. Many techniques have been described, all of which entail closed reduction and percutaneous pinning of the fragments using an image intensifier either under local, regional or general anaesthesia.[44-48] Two to three pins (K-wires) are inserted into the cephalic fragment from the distal insertion of the deltoid and another two to three into the fragment of the tuberosity from above. Care must be taken to avoid the axillary nerve and other neurovascular structures. The pins may be left protruding through the skin and can be removed six to eight weeks later. If the pins are cut beneath the surface of the skin their ends must be bent at 90° to avoid potentially fatal migration into the thorax or other cavities. This technique should be reserved for situations in which open surgery is not possible and bone quality is of sufficient strength to hold the pins which would displace in osteoporotic bone.

Intramedullary pinning. Fasciculated multiple pinning is an established technique.[49-51] This requires general, local or regional anaesthesia. The supracondylar area of the distal humerus is prepared and an oval opening is made at least 1 cm above the olecranon fossa. Using image-intensifier guidance long K-wires with bent tips are passed up the humeral shaft with two to three introduced into the head and

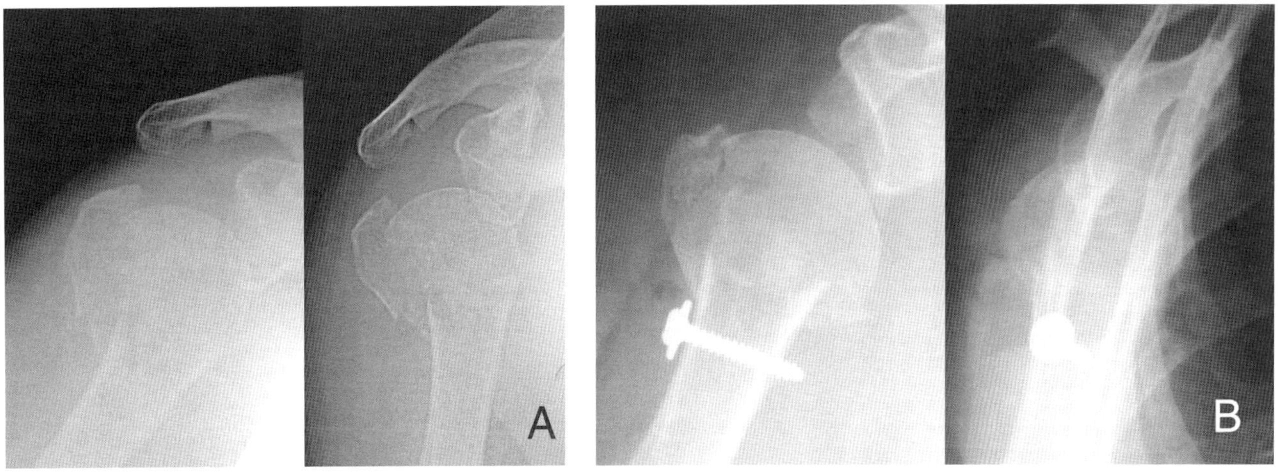

Fig. 7

Radiographs of a 69-year-old woman showing A) a four-part valgus-impacted fracture (AO type C2) and B) the technique of osteosuture because of poor bone quality. Heavy sutures (Ethibond no 6) were placed at the tendon-bone junction of the greater and lesser tuberosities and tied around a 4.5 mm cortical screw placed in the intact metaphyseal region 2 cm below the fracture.

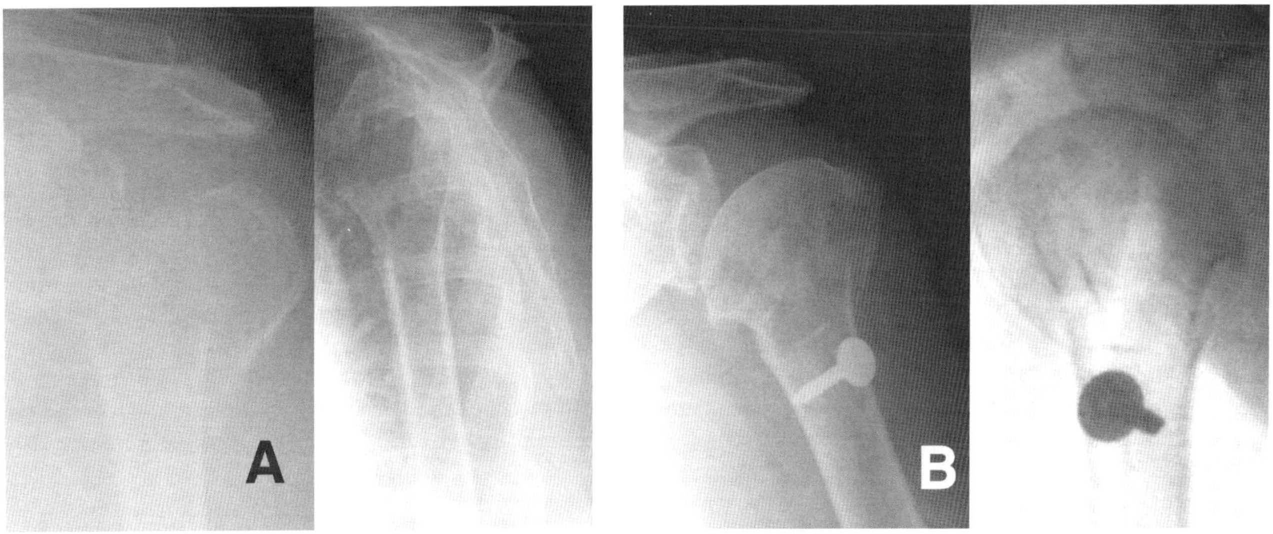

Fig. 8

Radiographs of a 69-year-old woman showing A) a four-part valgus (AO C2) fracture after a fall from a height and B) osteosuture with satisfactory function.

another two to three twisted so that they obtain purchase within the greater tuberosity. The bone must be sufficiently strong to allow fixation by the K-wires thereby avoiding protrusion into the subacromial or glenohumeral joint.

In some two-part fractures it is possible to combine intramedullary pinning with tension-band wiring. In this technique two Ender-type nails are inserted through the humeral head, using a transdeltoid split approach, and into the shaft. Wires are then passed through the eyelets, crossed and fixed transosseously into the metaphyseal region below the line of the fracture. This will have the effect of a tension band and augment the stability of the construct.[41]

Intramedullary nailing. These are used for the fixation of fractures of the proximal humerus including three- or four-part fractures.[52] The patient is usually placed in a semi-sitting position under general, local or regional anaesthesia. A transdeltoid split approach is used. The rotator cuff is exposed and incised and the nail is passed through the head, at the interface of the tendon and cartilage, into the humeral shaft. The fragments of the head are then held together with locking screws introduced with the appropriate jig. Care must be taken to avoid damage to the axillary nerve and the tendon of the long head of biceps.

Prosthetic replacement. In the case of four-part fractures in which vascularisation of the head is compromised or in the case of an intra-articular head-splitting fracture, sometimes only a prosthetic replacement can be considered.[3,4,53-55] This creates a series of inherent technical problems such as determination of the height of the prosthesis, the diameter of the head, head version, the fixation, and height of the

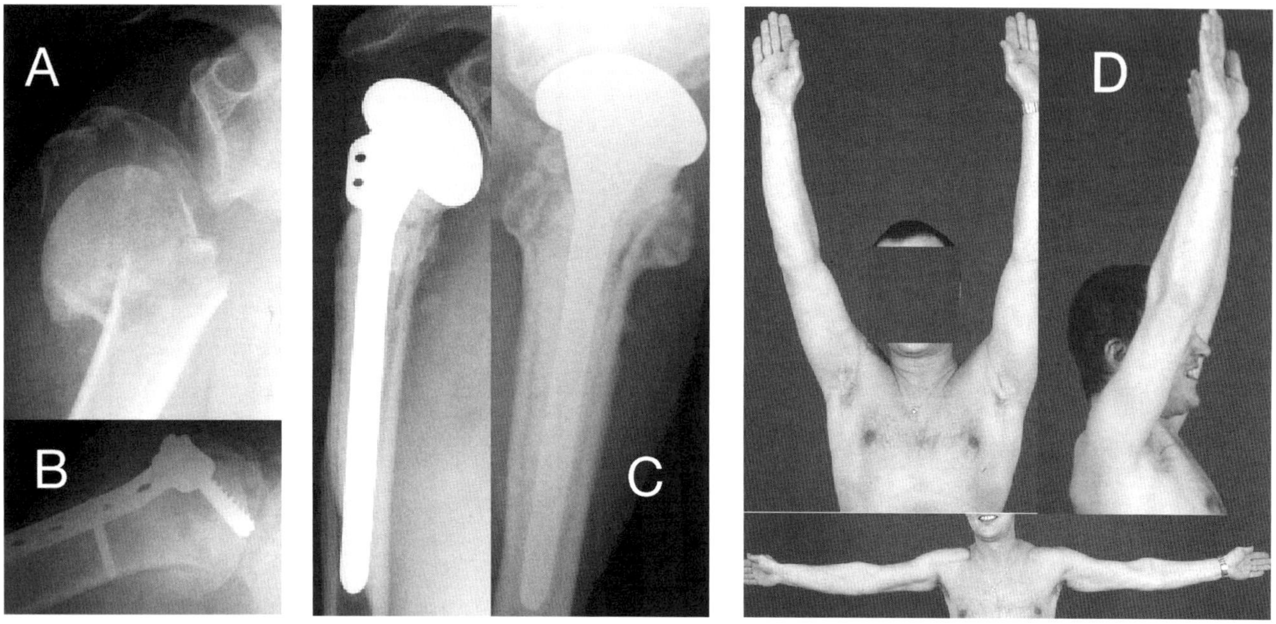

Fig. 9

Radiographs of a 35-year-old man showing A) a valgus four-part (AO C2) fracture after a fall from a height, B) a trial of plate fixation with unacceptable reduction (an intraoperative decision was made to introduce a hemiarthroplasty) and C) four years later. Figure 9D – Photographs show excellent, painless function with a full range of movement and symmetrical strength. He works full-time as a cook.

tuberosity, the type of fixation and diameter of the stem, and each must be addressed carefully. The height of the prosthesis can be determined either preoperatively by radiography of the contralateral side, allowing a preoperative plan to be made, or intraoperatively as judged by the position of the line of the fracture; there is usually a medial metaphyseal beak which is where the fracture occurs at the junction of the head and neck. Soft-tissue tension when pulling the tuberosities around the head will also give an indication as to the appropriate height and size of the head. Usually, the diameter of the head of the prosthesis should be the same or very close to the measured diameter of the retrieved head, the exception being fracture-dislocations (anterior or posterior) in which added stability may be sought by using a head of slightly larger diameter. As a rule head version should be determined with the arm at the side and the forearm on the abdomen; the centre of the head of the prosthesis should be facing the centre of the glenoid. Too much retroversion may stretch the rotator cuff and lead to pull-out of the tuberosity and too little may lead to loss of stability. In the case of posterior fracture-dislocations, less retroversion may ensure better stability, and inversely in the case of anterior fracture-dislocations more retroversion than usual may be necessary. The determination of retroversion should therefore not only rely on bony contours and fixed angles, such as 20° to the epicondyles of the distal humerus and 30° to the forearm, but should be tailored to each individual shoulder. The tuberosities should be fixed to the stem and the holes in the fins should be avoided. Sutures should pass circularly all around the stem and when tightened should compress the fragments onto it. If necessary, bone graft taken from the head of the humerus can be intercalated between the stem and the tuberosities, the goal being to have the tuberosities heal to one another. Sutures should also fix the tuberosities vertically to the shaft, thus lowering them 10 to 15 mm below the top of the head of the prosthesis. The stem should be cemented; non-cemented stems cannot ensure primary stability. The diameter of the stem should not be too tight in case it produces stress-shielding reactions resulting in loss of bone from the proximal humerus around the stem (Fig. 9).

COMPLICATIONS

The most common complications after surgical treatment of fractures of the proximal humerus are stiffness, persistent pain, postoperative infection, failure of fixation, osteonecrosis and late rupture of the rotator cuff.[14,56]

To avoid stiffness, the fixation must be stable enough to allow immediate passive movement so that adhesive scarring is limited and recovery of function is allowed. This applies to all forms of fixation and especially to patients treated by hemiarthroplasty and reattachment of the tuberosities. Persistent pain has many causes including non-union, musculotendinous damage, instability, capsulitis, osteonecrosis, migration of the implant, neurovascular damage and low-grade infection. All of these must be considered and the appropriate diagnostic procedures performed.

Postoperative infection is always a possibility and must therefore be borne in mind at all times. In the shoulder, the signs and symptoms of infection may be minor and loss of glenohumeral joint space accompanied by persistent pain and discomfort may be one of the first warnings before any other radiological or biological indicators. In case of doubt intra-articular aspiration must be performed with culture of the fluid obtained. After aspiration, and with the needle left in place, contrast medium should be injected into the joint and a radiograph taken to establish that the aspiration was from the joint. The diagnosis may show that the infection is either acute (<three weeks), intermediate (between 3 and 8 weeks) or chronic (>8 weeks). In all cases surgical revision and debridement are necessary. In acute infection, the implants may be left in place if they contribute to stability. In the intermediate situation judgement must be made as to whether to remove or leave the implants and a secondary intervention may have to be contemplated, such as fusion or reimplantation of the prostheses. In chronic infection removal of the implant is mandatory. An intravenous antibiotic regime should be started preferably with the guidance of a specialist in infectious diseases.

Secondary failure of fixation may be due to poor technique or to poor bone stock (Fig. 10). The risks of a further operation must be weighed carefully against the chances of success. In case of early avulsion of a tuberosity (less than six weeks) after insertion of a hemiarthroplasty, refixation should be attempted to avoid superior migration of the head of the prosthesis and loss of function.

Nonunion of fractures of the proximal humerus is uncommon, but when it occurs it is disabling and should be dealt with surgically. Fixation may be obtained by various methods including plates or intramedullary implants. Occasionally, it is necessary to supplement the construct with a bone graft.[57] Walch has described a technique in which a cortical graft from the fibula or iliac crest is introduced into the fragment of the humeral head and into the diaphysis. A compression plate and screws give stability to the construct and the intramedullary graft allows solid purchase for the screws.[58] Osteonecrosis cannot be avoided but a meticulous

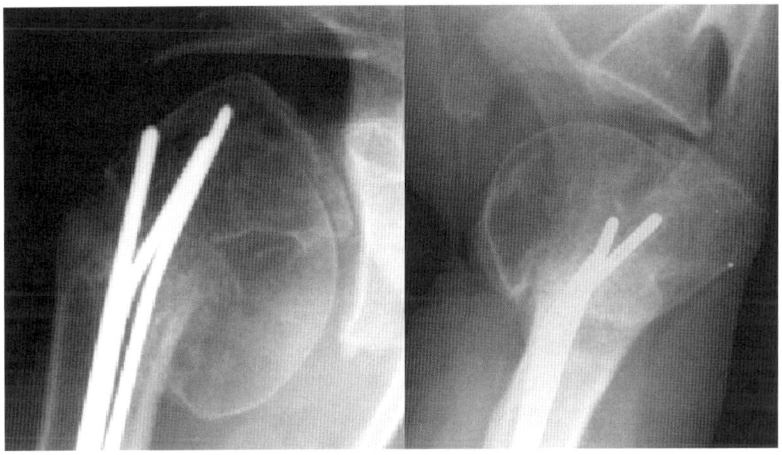

Fig. 10

Radiographs showing the complication of malunion and nail protrusion after the use of an intramedullary flexible nail for a three-part fracture.

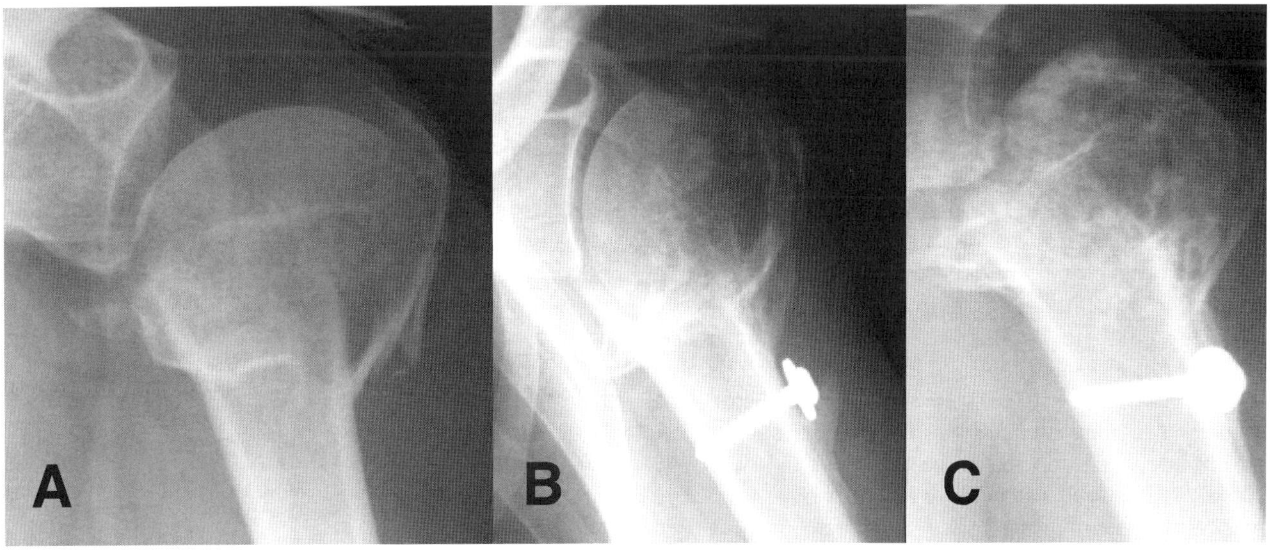

Fig. 11

Radiographs of a 52-year-old man showing A) a valgus four-part (AO C2) fracture after a fall, B) osteosuture with satisfactory union and C) at 24 months, aseptic necrosis, with collapse of the humeral head.

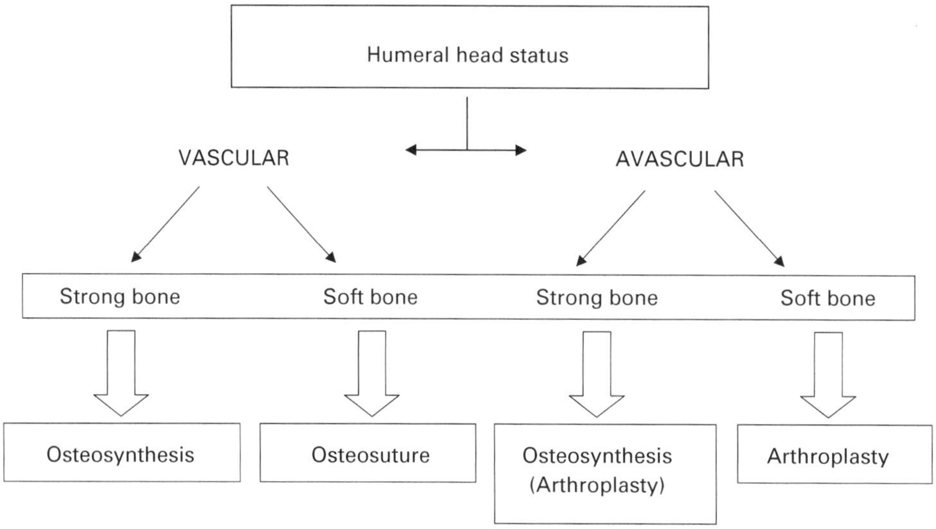

Fig. 12

Proposed algorithm for the surgical treatment of displaced fractures of the proximal humerus.

surgical technique should strive to preserve the blood supply of all fragments. Usually, however, osteonecrosis is well tolerated by the patient when the head and tuberosities have been reconstructed as closely to the normal anatomy as possible[59-61] (Fig. 11).

Late tearing of the rotator cuff may occur with hemiarthroplasty when the subacromial space narrows progressively. In case of chronic pain, reconstruction of the cuff may be the solution.

REHABILITATION

In the immediate postoperative period control of pain is a primary concern. Patients should benefit from a scalene block performed immediately before operation and, if possible, the catheter should be left in place and the pain controlled by a PCA (patient controlled anaesthesia) computerised pump.[62] After inserting a percutaneous catheter in the sheath of the interscalene plexus, 20 to 30 ml of ropivacaine 0.5% should be given before operation. Postoperatively, a PCA pump connected to the catheter allows the infusion of 5 to 10 ml/hour continuously for up to 72 hours. The patient can self-administer boluses of 10 to 15 ml every 60 to 90 minutes depending on tolerance, body-weight and other factors. During this period the arm is passively mobilised and elevated in the plane of the scapula as high as tolerated, two to three times a day. The patient is also encouraged to exercise the hand, wrist and elbow. On the third postoperative day the wound is covered with a watertight dressing and the patient is mobilised under supervision in water. Hydrotherapy is continued for six weeks at which time dry exercises are commenced with active and passive movement. Strengthening exercises are started at ten weeks depending on the fracture or consolidation of the tuberosity. It usually takes about a year to achieve a definitive level of function which may still progress for a further 12 months.

CONCLUSIONS

Fractures of the proximal humerus are complex injuries involving two articulating surfaces, the glenohumeral joint and the subacromial arch. Ideally, the principles of reconstruction of the articular fracture, including the restoration of the anatomy and stable fixation, with minimal injury to the soft tissues and to the vascularisation, should be applied. The head and tuberosities should be carefully repositioned not only to avoid weakness due to shortening of musculotendinous units and a decreased moment arm, but also stiffness and pain because of secondary subacromial impingement or excessive scarring. The options as to the surgical approach or type of implant used depend on the pattern of the fracture, the quality of the bone encountered, the patient's goals and the surgeon's familiarity with the techniques (Fig. 12). An adequate surgical technique will minimise complications and an aggressive rehabilitation regime will ensure the best possible result.

REFERENCES

1. **Poppen NK, Walker PS.** Forces at the glenohumeral joint in abduction. *Clin Orthop* 1983;135:165-70.
2. **Poppen NK, Walker PS.** Normal and abnormal motion of the shoulder. *J Bone Joint Surg [Am]* 1976;58-A:195-201.
3. **Neer CS.** Displaced proximal humeral fractures: Part I classification and evaluation. *J Bone Joint Surg [Am]* 1970;52-A:1077-89.
4. **Neer CS.** Displaced proximal humeral fractures: Part II treatment of three-part and four-part displacement. *J Bone Joint Surg [Am]* 1970;52-A:1090-103.
5. **Mallon WJ, Brown HR, Vogler JB III, Martinez S.** Radiographic and geometric anatomy of the scapula. *Clin Orthop* 1992;277:142-54.

6. **Boileau P, Walch G.** The three dimensional geometry of the proximal humerus: implications for surgical technique and prosthetic design. *J Bone Joint Surg [Br]* 1997;79-B:857-65.

7. **Cyprien JM, Vasey H, Burdet A, et al.** Humeral retrotorsion and glenohumeral relationship in the normal shoulder and in recurrent anterior dislocation (scapulometry). *Clin Orthop* 1983;175:8-17.

8. **Debevoise NT, Hyatt GW, Townsend GB.** Humeral torsion in recurrent shoulder dislocations: a technic of determination by X-ray. *Clin Orthop* 1971;76:87-93.

9. **Iannotti JP, Gabriel, Schneck SL, Evans BG, Misra S.** The normal glenohumeral relationship: an anatomical study of 140 shoulders. *J Bone Joint Surg [Am]* 1992;74-A:491-500.

10. **Gerber C, Schneeberger AG, Vinh TS.** The arterial vascularisation of the humeral head: an anatomical study. *J Bone Joint Surg [Am]* 1990;72-A:1486-96.

11. **Laing PG.** The arterial supply of the adult humerus. *J Bone Joint Surg [Am]* 1956;38-A:1105-16.

12. **Moseley HF, Goldie I.** The arterial pattern of the rotator cuff of the shoulder. *J Bone Joint Surg [Br]* 1963;45-B:780-9.

13. **Lauman V.** Kinesiology of the shoulder joint. In: Kölbel R, Helbig B, Blauth W, eds. *Shoulder replacement.* Berlin: Springer, 1987:23-31.

14. **Cofield RH.** Comminuted fractures of the proximal humerus. *Clin Orthop* 1988;230:49-57.

15. **Perlmutter GS.** Axillary nerve injury. *Clin Orthop* 1999;368:28-36.

16. **Flatow EL, Bigliani LU, April EW.** An anatomic study of the musculocutaneous nerve and its relationship to the coracoid process. *Clin Orthop* 1989;244:166-71.

17. **Pretre R, Hoffmeyer P, Bednarkiewicz M, Kursteiner K, Faidutti B.** Blunt injury to the subclavian or axillary artery. *J Am Coll Surg* 1994;179:295-8.

18. **Codman EA.** *The shoulder.* Rupture of the supraspinatus tendon and other lesions in or about the subacromial bursa. 2nd ed. Malabar: RE Krieger Publishing Company Inc, 1984:313-31.

19. **Brien H, Notfall F, MacMaster S, et al.** Neer's classification system: a critical appraisal. *J Trauma* 1995;38:257-60.

20. **Müller ME, Allgöwer M, Schneider R, Willenegger H.** *Appendix A: the comprehensive classification of fractures of long bones.* In: Manual of internal fixation: techniques recommended by the AO-ASIF group, 3rd edition. Berlin: Springer-Verlag, 1991:118-25.

21. **Sidor ML, Zuckerman JD, Lyon T, et al.** The Neer classification system for proximal humerus fractures: an assessment of interobserver reliability and intraobserver reproducibility. *J Bone Joint Surg [Am]* 1993;75-A:1745-55.

22. **Siebenrock KA, Gerber C.** The reproducibility of classification of fractures of the proximal end of the humerus. *J Bone Joint Surg [Am]* 1993;75-A:1751-5.

23. **Keene JS, Huizenga RE, Engber WD, Rogers SC.** Proximal humeral fractures: a correlation of residual deformity with long-term function. *Orthopedics* 1983;6:173-8.

24. **Ko JY, Yamamoto R.** Surgical treatment of complex fracture of the proximal humerus. *Clin Orthop* 1996;327:225-37.

25. **Lim TE, Ochsner PE, Marti RK, Holscher AA.** The results of treatment of comminuted fractures and fracture-dislocations of the proximal humerus. *Netherlands J Surg* 1983;35:139-43.

26. **Rasmussen S, Hvass I, Dalsgaard J, Christensen BS, Holstad E.** Displaced proximal humeral fractures: results of conservative treatment. *Injury* 1992;23:41-3.

27. **Schai P, Imhoff A, Preiss S.** Comminuted humeral head fractures: a multicenter analysis. *J Shoulder Elbow Surg* 1995;4:319-30.

28. **Stableforth PG.** Treatment of four-part proximal humeral fractures. *J Bone Joint Surg [Br]* 1984;66-B:104-8.

29. **Svend-Hansen H.** Displaced proximal humeral fractures. *Acta Orthop Scand* 1974;45:359-64.

30. **Zyto K, Kronberg M, Broström L-A.** Shoulder function after displaced fractures of the proximal humerus. *J Shoulder Elbow Surg* 1995;4:331-6.

31. **Lind T, Kroner K, Jensen J.** The epidemiology of fracture of the proximal humerus. *Arch Orthop Trauma Surg* 1989;108:285-7.

32. **Bernstein J, Adler LM, Blank JE, et al.** Evaluation of the Neer system of classification of proximal humeral fractures with computerized tomographic scans and plain radiographs. *J Bone Joint Surg [Am]* 1996;78-A:1371-5.

33. **Castagno AA, Shuman WP, Kilcoyne RF, et al.** Complex fractures of the proximal humerus: role of CT in treatment. *Radiology* 1987;165:759-62.

34. **Jurik AG, Albrechtsen J.** The use of computed tomography with two- and three-dimensional reconstructions in the diagnosis of three- and four-part fractures of the proximal humerus. *Clin Radiol* 1994;49:800-4.

35. **Esser RD.** Treatment of three- and four-part fractures of the proximal humerus with a modified cloverleaf plate. *J Orthop Trauma* 1994;8:15-22.

36. **Jakob RP, Miniaci A, Anson P, et al.** Four-part valgus impacted fractures of the proximal humerus. *J Bone Joint Surg [Br]* 1991;73-B:295-8.

37. **Resch H, Beck E, Bayley I.** Reconstruction of the valgus-impacted humeral head fracture. *J Shoulder Elbow Surg* 1995;4:73-80.

38. **Compito CA, Self EB, Bigliani LU.** Arthroplasty and acute shoulder trauma: reasons for success and failure. *Clin Orthop* 1994;307:27-36.

39. **Knight RA, Mayne JA.** Comminuted fractures and fracture dislocations involving the articular surface of the humeral head. *J Bone Joint Surg [Am]* 1957;39-A:1343-55.

40. **Cornell CN, Levine D, Pagnani MJ.** Internal fixation of proximal humerus fractures using the screw-tension band technique. *J Orthop Trauma* 1994;8:23-7.

41. **Cuomo F, Flatow EL, Maday MG, et al.** Open reduction and internal fixation of two- and three-part displaced surgical neck fractures of the proximal humerus. *J Shoulder Elbow Surg* 1992;1:287-95.

42. **Darder A, Darder A Jr, Sanchis V, Gastaldi E, Gomar F.** Four-part displaced proximal humeral fractures: operative treatment using Kirschner wires and a tension band. *J Orthop Trauma* 1993;7:497-505.

43. **Hawkins RJ, Bell RH, Gurr K.** The three-part fracture of the proximal part of the humerus: operative treatment. *J Bone Joint Surg [Am]* 1986;68-A:1410-4.

44. **Chen CY, Chao EK, Tu YK, Ueng SW, Shih CH.** Closed management and percutaneous fixation of unstable proximal humerus fractures. *J Trauma* 1998;45:1039-45.

45. **Herscovici D Jr, Saunders DT, Johnson MP, Sanders R, DiPasquale T.** Percutaneous fixation of proximal humeral fractures. *Clin Orthop* 2000;375:97-104.

46. **Jaberg H, Warner JJ, Jakob RP.** Percutaneous stabilization of unstable fractures of the humerus. *J Bone Joint Surg [Am]* 1992;74-A:508-15.

47. **Kocialkowski A, Wallace WA.** Closed percutaneous K-wire stabilization for displaced fractures of the surgical neck of the humerus. *Injury* 1990;21:209-12.

48. **Soete PJ, Clayson PE, Costenoble VH.** Transitory percutaneous pinning in fractures of the proximal humerus. *J Shoulder Elbow Surg* 1999;8:569-73.

49. **Gautier E, Slongo T, Jakob RP.** Treatment of subcapital humerus fracture with the Prevot nail. *Z Unfallchir Versicherungsmed* 1992;85:145-55.

50. **Habernek H, Schneider R, Popp R, et al.** Spiral bundle nailing for subcapital humeral fractures: preliminary report of the method of Henning. *J Trauma* 1999;46:400-6.

51. **Mestdagh H, Butruille Y, Tillie B, Bocquet F.** Results of the treatment of proximal humeral fractures by percutaneous nailing: à propos of 142 cases. *Ann Chir* 1984;38:5-13.

52. **Lin J, Hou S-M, Hang Y-S.** Locked nailing for displaced surgical neck fractures of the humerus. *J Trauma* 1998;45:1051-7.

53. **Bosch U, Skutek M, Fremerey RW, Tscherne H.** Outcome after primary and secondary hemiarthroplasty in elderly patients with fractures of the proximal humerus. *J Shoulder Elbow Surg* 1998;7:479-84.

54. **Frich LH, Sojbjerg JO, Sneppen O.** Shoulder arthroplasty in complex acute and chronic proximal humeral fractures. *Orthopedics* 1991;14:949-54.

55. **Tanner MW, Cofield RH.** Prosthetic arthroplasty for fractures and fracture-dislocations of the proximal humerus. *Clin Orthop* 1983;179:116-28.

56. **Movin T, Sjoden GO, Ahrengart L.** Poor function after shoulder replacement in fracture patients: a retrospective evaluation of 29 patients followed for 2-12 years. *Acta Orthop Scand* 1998;69:392-6.

57. **Healy WL, Jupiter JB, Kristiansen TK, White RR.** Nonunion of the proximal humerus: a review of 25 cases. *J Orthop Trauma* 1990;4:424-31.

58. **Walch G, Badet R, Nove-Josserand L, Levigne C.** Nonunions of the surgical neck of the humerus: surgical treatment with an intramedullary bone peg, internal fixation, and cancellous bone grafting. *J Shoulder Elbow Surg* 1996;5:161-8.

59. **Brooks CH, Revell WJ, Heatley FW.** Vascularity of the humeral head after proximal humeral fracture. *J Bone Joint Surg [Br]* 1993;75-B:132-6.

60. **Lee CK, Hansen HR.** Post-traumatic avascular necrosis of the humeral head in displaced proximal humeral fractures. *J Trauma* 1981;21:788-91.

61. **Seggl W, Weiglein A.** Die arterielle Blutversorgung des Oberamkopfes und ihre prognostische Bedeutung bei Luxationen, Frakturen und Luxations-Frakturen des Oberamkopfes. *Acta Chir Austriaca* 1991;23:1-19.

62. **Culebras X, Van Gessel E, Hoffmeyer P, Gamulin Z.** Clonidine combined with a long lasting local anesthetic does not prolong postoperative analgesia after brachial plexus block but induces hemodynamic changes. *Anesth Analg* 2001;92:199-204.

THE CERVICAL HIP FRACTURE

MARTYN J. PARKER

From Peterborough District Hospital, England

Fractures of the hip are described as constituting an orthopaedic epidemic; an estimated 1.3 million occurred worldwide in 1990.[1] These numbers are expected to increase, particularly in Asia and Africa, to about 4.5 million by 2050. Approximately half of these fractures will be cervical.

The mean age of patients with a hip fracture is about 80 years, and three-quarters are female. In comparison with patients with extracapsular fracture, those with intracapsular fractures are about two years younger, more mobile and are less likely to use walking aids or to live in residential accommodation. In addition, patients with intracapsular fractures have a shorter length of hospital stay and a lower mortality.[2,3]

TERMINOLOGY

The term 'cervical hip fracture' is synonymous with 'intracapsular hip fracture'. Other terms which have been used for this type of fracture are 'femoral neck', 'medial femoral', 'subcapital', 'transcervical' and 'mid-cervical'.

Traditionally, the term 'subcapital' referred to a fracture immediately distal to the articular surface, while 'transcervical' and 'mid-cervical' described fractures lower in the femoral neck. This differentiation between low and high fracture is imprecise and unnecessary. Most intracapsular fractures start from a fairly constant point on the superior/lateral aspect of the femoral neck, but cross the calcar at a distance of between 0 to 2.5 cm from the articular surface. The mid-cervical fracture in which the fracture line only involves the middle of the neck is rare.

Basal, basicervical or basilar fractures have been considered by different sources as either an intracapsular or an extracapsular fracture, since the fracture line may cross the capsular attachments. In clinical practice the treatment and prognosis of these fractures are more akin to those of an extracapsular fracture. Such fractures are not considered further in this article.

PATHOLOGY

The femoral head derives its blood supply from three sources, the retinacular vessels, the ligamentum teres and vessels within the medullary cavity. The main supply is the retinacular vessels which arise from an extracapsular arterial ring formed by the medial and lateral femoral circumflex arteries. The retinacular vessels from this ring pass proximally along the femoral neck in three groups. The posterior-superior retinacular arteries form the lateral epiphyseal vessels and supply most of the femoral head. The posterior-inferior retinacular arteries form the inferior metaphyseal arteries supply a small part of the femoral head in the posterior/inferior region. In addition, there are small anterior retinacular arteries. The contributions of the posterior-inferior and the anterior vessels are less important in the aetiology of avascular necrosis.[4,5]

Additional vessels pass within the medullary cavity of the femur and are transected in displaced fractures. A further source of blood supply to the femoral head is by way of the arteries of the ligamentum teres. These enter the head via the fovea capitis and supply a small area of bone around the fovea.

Revascularisation of the femoral head after a fracture occurs from three sources. Vascular ingrowth from the medullary cavity at the site of the fracture can only occur if the fixation is stable. If there is significant movement this ingrowth will be damaged. The arteries of the ligamentum teres will maintain the viability of the bone around the fovea capitis, and further vascular ingrowth to surrounding bone may occur. Finally, the epiphyseal vessels will revascularise the bone depending on the degree of damage to these vessels. This process has been described as the creeping substitution of bone, which may be seen histologically and radiographically as increased bone density. The upper segment of the femoral head tends to be the last area to become revascularised and is the portion most prone to avascular necrosis.

It is this tenuous vascular supply of the femoral head which causes the high incidence of nonunion and avascular necrosis in patients with intracapsular fractures of the femur. The greater the damage to the vascular supply the larger is the risk of these complications of fracture healing.

CLASSIFICATION

There are many different systems of radiological classification for intracapsular fractures.[6] To be of any value the classification must be able to predict outcome and be reproducible between clinicians with an acceptable degree of intra- and interobserver variation.

The degree of displacement of the fracture is the main radiological predictor of nonunion.[7-9] Unfortunately, there is no succinct method of classifying the fracture to define this displacement.

Garden classification. Described by Garden in 1961,[10] this commonly used system divided fractures into four groups depending on the appearance of the trabeculae of the femoral head as seen on the anteroposterior (AP) radiographs.

Grade I. Impacted, valgus or abduction fracture. The fracture remains essentially undisplaced although the principal trabeculae within the medial part of the femoral head are distorted at the site of the fracture by the impaction of the bone which has occurred laterally.

Grade II. The fracture remains totally undisplaced. No impaction has occurred and the trabeculae are not distorted.

Grade III. The fracture has displaced. The two fragments are in contact and have cog-wheeled together as the leg shortens. The trabeculae within the femoral head have rotated to a trabecular angle of less than 160°.

Grade IV. A displaced fracture in which separation of the fracture surfaces means that cog-wheeling has not occurred, and the trabecular angle of 160° is preserved. The trabeculae of the femoral head remain aligned with those within the pelvis.

A number of studies of the Garden classification have found an unacceptably high degree of interobserver variation.[11-13] A summary of previous reports using this classification to predict complications of fracture healing indicated that the difference between Garden grade-III and grade-IV fractures was insufficient to justify separation into the two grades.[14] A study using the degree of displacement on radiographs of intracapsular fractures related to the Garden grade found no significant difference in the degree of displacement between Garden grade-I and grade-II fractures and between grades III and IV.[15]

In summary, the Garden classification has no relevance in current practice, other than for the division into those fractures which are essentially undisplaced (Garden grades I and II) and those which are displaced (Garden grades III and IV).

Pauwels classification. First described in 1935,[16] this classification is based on the theory of greater shearing forces at the site of the fracture for those fractures with a more vertical fracture line. The three grades are determined by measuring the angle of the fracture on the AP radiograph as follows:

Type I. Pauwels angle less than 30°.

Type II. Pauwels angle 30° to 70°.

Type III. Pauwels angle more than 70°.

However, some later users of the Pauwels classification have used different angles and some use the shearing angle which is the angle of the fracture line with the vertical. Initially, the angle was measured on the postoperative radiographs with the leg in 10° of internal rotation. Clinical studies have since used this angle measured on the preoperative AP radiograph to see if it will correlate with complications of fracture healing. A summary of previous clinical studies of the Pauwels classification has indicated that other than for undisplaced fractures which are being treated conservatively, the preoperative Pauwels angle has no correlation with the subsequent incidence of complications.[17] It also has an unacceptable degree of intraobserver variation.[12] The Pauwels classification therefore has no value in current clinical practice.

AO classification. This is the most recently devised and complex system for classifying cervical fractures.[18] It divides intracapsular fractures into three broad groups, namely, undisplaced/minimally displaced, transcervical/basicervical/basal and displaced subcapital fractures. Each of these groups is then subdivided into three groups. One study of this system found it unnecessarily complicated and not useful for determining treatment[19] and a further assessment found the system to be impractical.[20] A more recent study[21] found that it had an unacceptably high degree of intra- and interobserver variation. In addition, other than for the division into displaced and undisplaced fractures, the further subdivision into the other categories was unnecessary. Therefore the AO classification for intracapsular hip fractures has no practical value and should not be used.

Classifications related to the level of the fracture. A number of clinicians have suggested that the more proximal cervical fractures will have an increased risk of complications. Most studies on this topic have failed to find a relationship between the level of the fracture and such problems.[6,22] There have, however, been studies which have reported a relationship between fracture healing and size of the femoral head.[23] At the present time further research is required before this can be used as a method of determining outcome.

Other radiological features. Posterior comminution or comminution of the calcar at the site of the fracture has a questionable influence on healing. Two studies have shown an increased rate of failure with comminution,[23,24] but a third study did not.[8] The Singh index as a measure of osteoporosis has not been found to have any clinical value in predicting union.[8,25]

Summary of radiological classifications. The earliest classification of intracapsular fractures was the simple division into those which are essentially undisplaced and those which are displaced. Undisplaced fractures equate to Garden grades I and II, while displaced fractures refer to Garden grades III and IV. This is the only classification system which has been shown to have an acceptable degree of intra- and interobserver variation and to be useful in predicting complications.[21] Because numerous other factors influence the healing of fractures the radiological appearances of the fracture cannot be used reliably to predict complications in healing.

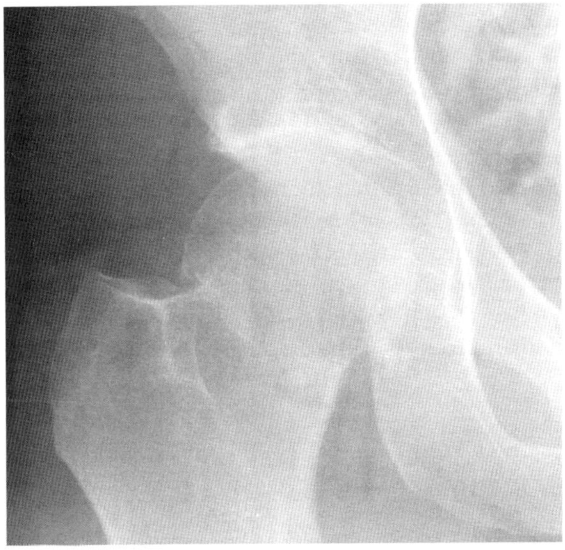

Fig. 1a

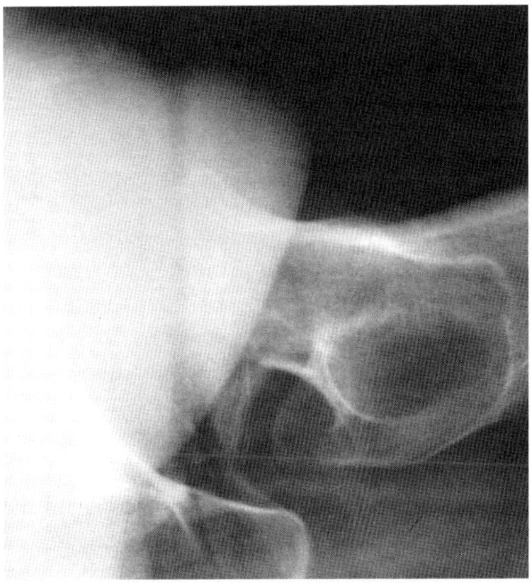

Fig. 1b

Lateral radiographs showing an impacted fracture which is partially displaced. Such a fracture is still customarily termed undisplaced.

OTHER ASSESSMENTS OF VIABILITY OF THE FEMORAL HEAD

Over the years a number of different investigative procedures have been used to determine if they will predict the viability of the femoral head and the subsequent occurrence of complications in healing. Investigations which have been used include injecting Coomassie blue,[26] measuring the oxygenation of the femoral head,[27] arteriography,[28] measurement of the intraosseous pressure,[29] intraosseous venography,[30] the Kiton fast green test,[31] tetracycline labelling,[32] bone isotope scintimetry,[33] intraosseous Doppler ultrasound and nuclear MRI.[34] None of these techniques has proved to be either reliable or practical for routine use.

THE UNDISPLACED CERVICAL FRACTURE

Other terms for this fracture are an impacted, abduction or valgus fracture. The radiological changes may be subtle, such that the initial diagnosis may be missed.[35,36] The fracture may be either completely undisplaced (as a grade-II fracture) or impacted (Garden grade-I fracture). This impaction may mean that the term undisplaced is used somewhat loosely for intracapsular fractures, and those fractures which are partially displaced or retroverted (Fig. 1).

The treatment of an undisplaced intracapsular fracture may be either operative or conservative. Conservative treatment involves a period of bed-rest while the acute pain subsides, then gentle mobilisation.[37] Weight-bearing is generally allowed. Earlier reports of this method of treatment indicated that although the rate of nonunion was increased in comparison to those cases treated by internal fixation (15% *v* 5%),[38] the failure rate was acceptable, and even if the fracture did displace internal fixation could still be undertaken. There is no evidence that the incidence of avascular necrosis, about 10%,[38,39] is influenced by the method of treatment used.

More recent reports have suggested that as the population which sustains an undisplaced intracapsular fracture became more elderly, the rate of nonunion has increased to 40% or more.[40] Comparative studies of the two methods of treatment have suggested that operative treatment is preferable because of the lower risk of complications in healing.[40,41] There is little difference in the cost of treatment between these two methods.[42]

Conservative treatment should only be used for carefully selected fractures; Raaymakers and Marti[37] suggested that it be used mainly in patients aged less than 70 years who are physically healthy. For those fractures which are partially displaced, as illustrated in Figure 1, internal fixation is recommended. At the time of surgery, the fracture should be screened using the image intensifier and may be reduced by internal rotation of the limb.

THE DISPLACED CERVICAL FRACTURE

Many authors have described the displaced cervical fracture as the unsolved fracture,[43-45] because of the continuing debate as to whether the femoral head should be preserved or replaced. Many surgeons choose their treatment according to local preference or tradition, such that in Scandinavian countries, internal fixation is conventionally used, while in much of the rest of Europe and North America, replacement of the femoral head is the technique of choice. There are numerous misconceptions about what factors influence the risk of the occurrence of complications. These are then used to support replacing the femoral head with an arthroplasty.

When presented with a displaced cervical fracture, the clinician must assess each patient individually to determine the relative risks and merits of each method of treatment in order to make the optimum choice. Besides the radiological features of the fracture, the following clinical factors will influence the choice of treatment.

The age of the patient. With increasing age there is a progressive increase in the risk of nonunion.[8,46,47] Rates of nonunion of about 5% to 15% are to be expected for younger patients but for those over 80 years of age this rises to 25% to 30%. Symptomatic avascular necrosis is less common in the elderly.

There are other factors which need to be considered with age. For example, in those aged less than 50 to 60 years, preservation of the femoral head is essential because of the long life expectancy of these patients and their higher functional demands in comparison with the elderly. If an arthroplasty is used there is a high risk of the need for a later revision. With increasing age the arguments against arthroplasty diminish since the life expectancy of the patient becomes less than that of the implant.

When considering the cervical hip fracture an 'elderly' person is one aged over 70 to 80 years. A more appropriate definition for a 'young' patient is one who is able independently to get out of his/her house, while 'elderly' relates to a patient who is housebound or lives in an institution.

Pathological fractures. For a displaced cervical fracture which is secondary to a localised area of bone abnormality and weakness, such as in Paget's disease or from metastatic tumour, the incidence of nonunion after internal fixation is markedly increased. Arthroplasty is therefore customarily preferred. A cemented hemiarthroplasty is the most appropriate type of implant. If there is evidence of acetabular damage or involvement of the acetabulum by tumour, then a total hip replacement is indicated.

Chronic renal failure/metabolic bone disease. Hyperparathyroidism and chronic renal failure have been associated with a markedly increased risk of nonunion. Thornhill and Creasman[48] presented the results of 36 patients in whom all the fractures failed to unite. There is, however, a lack of other reports in the literature to support these observations. In addition, it may be that with the advent of the use of vitamin-D analogues as part of the adjuvant treatment for chronic renal failure, the incidence of nonunion will fall. At the present time it is not possible to come to definite conclusions other than that there may be an increased risk of nonunion, making arthroplasty a more appropriate method of treatment.

Arthritis of the hip. Although an intracapsular fracture in a symptomatic arthritic hip is uncommon, when it does occur, arthroplasty is the preferred method of treatment.

Rheumatoid arthritis. A number of previous reports had indicated a marked increase in the risk of both nonunion and avascular necrosis in displaced intracapsular fractures, but not in undisplaced lesions, in patients with rheumatoid arthritis.[49-51] The results of internal fixation are worse for those hips affected with arthritis. Replacement arthroplasty is therefore appropriate for displaced cervical fractures in all but the very young. A total hip replacement may be the choice of implant if there is significant arthritis of the hip.

Factors not related to fracture-healing complications. The gender, weight, degree of osteoporosis and mental state of the patient have not been shown to have any relationship to the incidence of complications in healing,[8,46] neither has the presence of neurological impairment such as a previous stroke, Parkinson's disease or neuromuscular disorders.

INTERNAL FIXATION OR ARTHROPLASTY FOR DISPLACED CERVICAL FRACTURES IN THE ELDERLY

Comparison between these two methods of treatment is difficult outside the context of randomised trials, because of the difficulties of patient selection. The groups compared are often not well matched. Comparative series have produced conflicting results.[52,53] A meta-analysis of previous reports of the treatment of cervical hip fractures up to 1990[54] gave an incidence of nonunion of 33% and of avascular necrosis of 16% after internal fixation. Secondary operations were required in 20% to 36% of patients, typically for conversion to an arthroplasty. After an arthroplasty, the reoperation rate was from 6% to 18%. The mortality was marginally lower for internal fixation but the difference did not persist beyond three months.

The earlier randomised trials on this topic have produced contradicting results, but with a trend towards favouring arthroplasty.[55-57] All these previous randomised studies are currently being summarised into a single Cochrane review.[58] These older trials may not be so pertinent in current practice, with progressive improvements in surgical technique and implants. Three larger and more carefully controlled studies are currently in progress which should help to clarify this issue. The results to date indicate that internal fixation has a markedly increased rate of readmission and reoperation in comparison with arthroplasty of approximately 30% to 40% *versus* 5% to 10%, but there is a tendency to a slightly lower mortality with internal fixation. Both procedures produce comparable final functional outcomes.[59,60]

INTERNAL FIXATION OF CERVICAL FRACTURES

If the fracture is reduced closed the operation is shorter and the implant may be inserted percutaneously. This may result in a reduced mortality for the frail elderly patient in comparison with that of arthroplasty. This minimally traumatic surgery can even be done under local anaesthesia.

The main disadvantage of internal fixation is either redisplacement of the fracture after reduction or failure of the fracture to heal (Fig. 2). Conventionally, these compli-

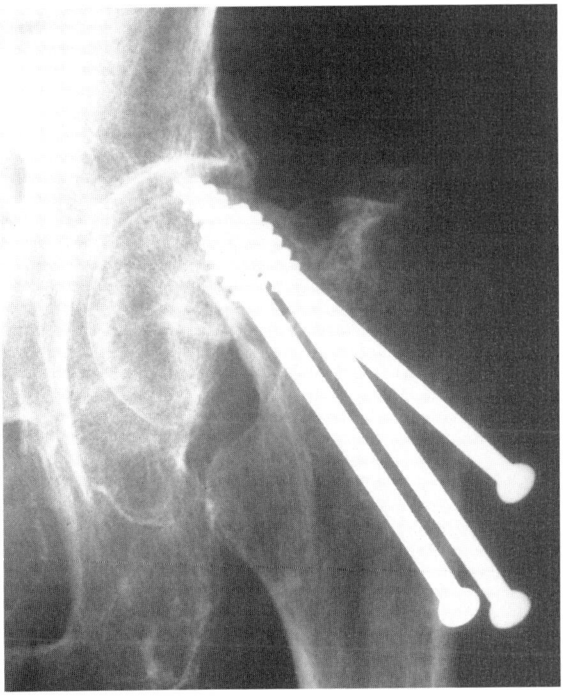

Fig. 2

Radiograph showing nonunion associated with displacement of a cervical fracture which had been reduced and fixed by three parallel screws.

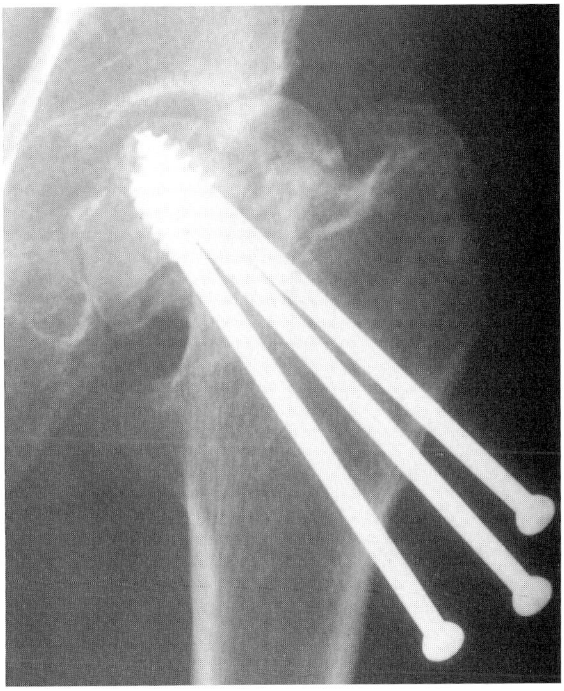

Fig. 3

Radiograph showing advanced avascular necrosis of the femoral head with fragmentation.

cations are termed nonunion. The overall risk of nonunion is between 10% and 35%.[38,54] Substantial diversities in the reported incidence of nonunion are found. This is partially explained by patient selection, differences in surgical technique, and whether the results only apply to the long-term survivors or a consecutive series of patients. Noteworthy improvements in the results of internal fixation have occurred with better radiography and understanding of the reduction of the fracture and the position of the implant.

Avascular necrosis is the second most common complication and occurs if there is damage to the blood supply of the femoral head with failure of revacularisation (Fig. 3). The incidence of this complication is 10% to 20%.[38,54] Other problems of internal fixation are fracture around the implant, backing out of the implant as the fracture collapses, and breakage of the implant which is associated with nonunion or delayed union. Overall, the risk of re-operation after internal fixation is from 20% to 36%, which is markedly greater than that after arthroplasty.

Compared with arthroplasty the advantages of internal fixation are that patients are allowed to retain their own femoral head, there is less surgical trauma, the mortality and morbidity may be marginally reduced and there is a lower risk of complications in wound healing and of sepsis. The disadvantages are the risk of nonunion and of avascular necrosis and an increased rate of reoperation.

Method of reduction of the fracture. For displaced fractures, reduction may be either closed or open. While open reduction has been recommended in a few reports, most orthopaedic opinion is in favour of closed reduction with an open procedure reserved only for those rare cases in which closed reduction proves impossible. The one randomised trial which addressed this issue[61] reported a reduced rate of nonunion for open reduction, but a markedly increased rate of mortality in the elderly.

The technique of closed reduction involves the use of a fracture table and radiographic image intensification.[62] The technique can be divided into three steps. First, the patient is positioned on the fracture table. This should be supervised by the orthopaedic surgeon to minimise excessive movement of the injured limb, which may damage the tenuous vascular supply to the femoral head. Secondly, the fracture is reduced in the AP radiograph using gentle longitudinal traction. This must be undertaken while screening the fracture with the image intensifier in the AP view. Thirdly, the fracture is reduced on the lateral view by internal rotation of the foot while screening with the image intensifier in the lateral position. Internal rotation of the limb is the key to fracture reduction. Frequently, full internal rotation of the limb is required to achieve a satisfactory position in the lateral view.

The ideal reduction is an anatomical or slight valgus position of the femoral head on the AP view. This is akin to placing a hat (the femoral head) on a coat-hook (the superior part of the femoral neck). A varus position must be avoided as this leads to a marked increase in the risk of nonunion. On the lateral radiograph, the femoral head, neck, trochanteric region and shaft should be in a straight

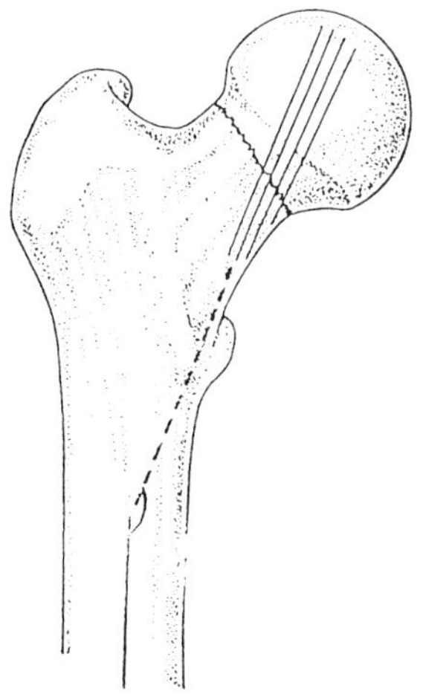

Fig. 4a

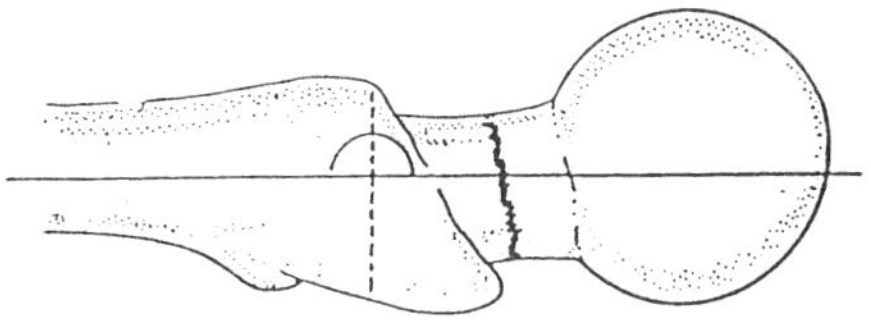

Fig. 4b

Diagram showing the method of assessing fracture reduction on AP and lateral radiographs. Figure 4a – On an AP view the trabecular angle is the angle between that of the femoral head and the shaft of the femur. An anatomical reduction angle is 160°. Figure 4b – On a lateral view the femoral head, neck, trochanteric region and shaft should be in a straight line (180°).

line. This is comparable with placing a circular ice-cream cornet back onto its cone.

The criteria for a correct reduction of the fracture are derived from the trabecular angle on the AP and lateral radiographs (Fig. 4). These have been defined as an angle of 155° to 180° on the AP and lateral views.[63] This would be considered to be too lax for current orthopaedic practice and more appropriate criteria are 165° to 175° on the AP and 170° to 190° on the lateral view.[38,62]

Failure to achieve a satisfactory reduction becomes less common with experience. When faced with a suboptimal reduction, the surgeon has to decide between fixation in this position, open reduction or proceeding to an arthroplasty. Factors which need to be considered are the fitness of the patient and the importance of preserving the femoral head. Generally, fixing the fracture in the best position possible is recommended, with an arthroplasty later should the fracture fail to heal.[55]

Choice of implant. Many different implants have been used for the internal fixation of cervical fractures. Essentially, they are either single or multiple screws or pins, in some cases attached to a side plate. A meaningful comparison between implants is only possible by randomised trials, because of the differences in the selection of patients for internal fixation within case series. A summary of all previously undertaken randomised trials[64] indicates that screws are probably better than pins, although the addition of a hook extruded from the tip of a pin may make such a modified pin similar to screws. The sliding hip screw is associated with an incidence of complications in healing comparable to that of multiple parallel screws, but requires a more protracted surgical procedure to insert. There is

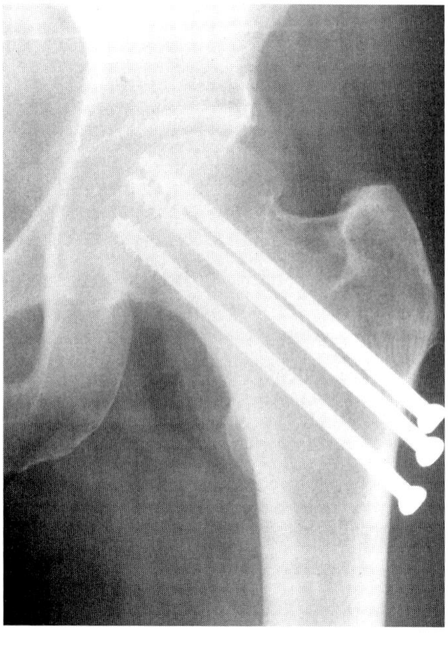

Fig. 5a

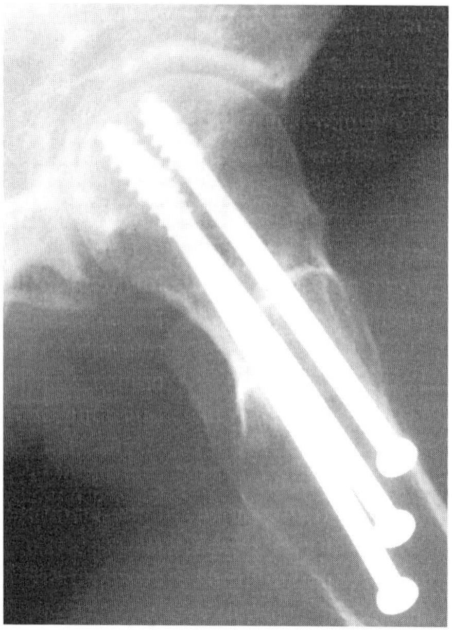

Fig. 5b

Radiographs showing the correct positioning of the screws. Figure 5a – On the AP view the lower screw is touching the calcar with two screws superior to this. The tips of the screws are close to the subchondral bone. Figure 5b – On the lateral radiograph one screw has calcar contact to give three-point fixation.

insufficient evidence to say which design of screws or pins is preferable or if two, three or more are best. A multiple parallel screw technique,[65] preferably inserted percutaneously or by minimum surgical exposure, is recommended.

Operative technique. Current opinions regarding the positioning of the implant tend to advocate that the lower screw should be just superior to the calcar on the AP radiograph, with the tip in the subchondral bone close to the joint line. This gives a three-point fixation at the femoral head, calcar and the cortical bone laterally. The second screw should be central on the AP view, touching the inferior cortical bone (calcar) on the lateral radiograph and again close to the subchondral bone to achieve a three-point fixation.[62] If a third screw is used it is possibly best placed centrally on both views. Figure 5 illustrates the correct placement of three cancellous screws.

Often it is not possible to achieve this ideal position but the surgeon should avoid placing the screws superiorly or anteriorly as these areas of the femoral head do not give good purchase. The aim of keeping the screws exactly parallel is probably not essential. It may be better to achieve a spread of the screws within the femoral head into different areas of bone.

Some surgeons have advocated compression or impaction of the fracture at the time of surgery, but clinical studies on this topic suggest that both of these techniques may be harmful.[66-68]

Aspiration or decompression of the hip. After an intracapsular fracture of the hip, bleeding from the site of the fracture may be confined within the joint capsule. This is more likely to occur with an undisplaced fracture in which the capsule is less likely to be torn. The pressure within the joint from this haematoma may rise to such an extent that it may impede the blood supply to the femoral head by a tamponade effect. Pressures as high as 320 mmHg have been reported,[69] although average pressures are normally between 30 and 140 mmHg for undisplaced fractures and 10 and 30 mmHg for those displaced.[38,70]

Drainage of this haematoma by either needle aspiration or capsulotomy may therefore increase the blood supply to the femoral head and possibly reduce the subsequent incidence of complications. Whereas aspiration of the hip has been shown to reduce intracapsular pressures and increase the blood flow in the femoral head as assessed by scintimetry,[69] it remains to be determined if removing this haematoma actually lowers the incidence of complications of healing. At the present time it would seem prudent to recommend needle aspiration of the hip at the time of surgery to remove any haematoma which may be present.

Timing of surgery. For undisplaced fractures, delay from injury until surgery will probably not influence the risk of complications of healing. There are those who state that the potentially high intracapsular pressures may damage the vascular supply to the femoral head, but this remains to be proved in clinical practice. The other potential risk of delay in surgery is that an undisplaced fracture will displace.

For displaced fractures it has been suggested that the stretching of the capsular vessels may impede the blood supply to the femoral head. Further damage may occur with time as the fracture displaces further. For those which have been displaced for more than one week, the radiograph may show characteristic changes of a blunting of the sharp margins of the fracture where the two surfaces have been moving together (Fig. 6). There may also be excessive proximal displacement of the femur. Closed reduction of such a fracture is generally impossible and nonunion is markedly increased.[46] In this situation treatment by an arthroplasty is advised, but for a young patient in whom preservation of the head is necessary, open reduction, possibly supplemented by a pedicle bone graft or osteotomy, should be planned.[38]

There is controversy about the effects of shorter delays from fracture to internal fixation. Reports from one centre have suggested that a delay of six or more hours may be detrimental.[71] Others have produced alternative results. Two large studies involving over 3000 patients reported that delays of up to six days made no difference.[46,72] A number of other smaller studies have failed to document any relationship between delay to surgery and complications of healing.[38]

Because of these conflicting reports it is not possible to give any firm advice regarding the timing of surgery for displaced cervical fractures which are to be treated by internal fixation, other than for those with a delay of more than one week. It would seem prudent to restrict delays to surgery to less than one to two days and for those in which preservation of the femoral head is essential shorter delays are preferable. Delays of more than two days from injury are associated with the problems of recumbency, namely pressure sores, pneumonia and thromboembolic complications.[73]

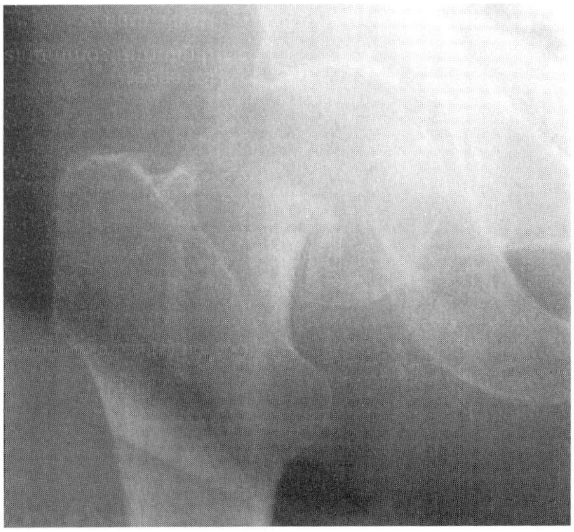

Fig. 6

Radiograph showing a displaced intracapsular fracture with delay until diagnosis. Closed reduction of such fractures is generally impossible.

Postoperative mobilisation. After internal fixation there is no need to restrict movement of the hip. The value of different strategies of physiotherapy has not been well studied.[74] Weight-bearing is a more controversial topic. Non-weight-bearing may actually increase the forces across the hip due to the muscle acting around the hip. Partial weight-bearing may reduce the forces on the hip while the fracture heals. The only clinical study to address this issue adequately found better results for those who were allowed to bear weight.[75]

In summary, after internal fixation weight-bearing should be unrestricted, but the cautious physician may advise a period of partial weight-bearing for six to eight weeks after surgery in the younger patient in whom preservation of the femoral head is paramount.

ARTHROPLASTY FOR CERVICAL HIP FRACTURES

Replacing the femoral head with a prosthesis incurs a different set of complications than those for internal fixation. Early complications are related to wound healing and include sepsis (superficial sepsis 5% to 15%, deep sepsis about 3%) and haematoma (2% to 5%), dislocation (2% to 5%), peroperative fracture of the femur (4%) and toxicity from insertion of cement (0.5% to 1%). Late complications of arthroplasty are fracture around the implant (1% to 3%), loosening of the prosthesis (2% to 10%) and acetabular erosion (4% to 20%). While the overall incidence of complications is less than that for internal fixation, when they occur they are associated with a higher mortality.[76]

The advantage of arthroplasty is a lower rate of reoperation (6% to 18%). The disadvantages include a risk of deep infection around the implant, a risk of superficial wound infection, a higher risk of wound haematoma, a risk of dislocation, toxicity from insertion of cement, a risk of fracture around the implant, a later risk of loosening of the prosthesis, a later risk of acetabular wear, and a possible higher mortality than for internal fixation.

The higher risk of complications of wound healing and sepsis may make internal fixation a more appropriate option for those patients with a source of sepsis, such as chronic leg ulcers or an indwelling urinary catheter. In addition, for those on anticoagulation medication, internal fixation may be preferable.

Unipolar hemiarthroplasty. The most common types of arthroplasty are the Moore and the Thompson (Fig. 7). Despite being implanted in vast numbers since their inception in the 1950s comparative series and randomised trials comparing the two implants are rare. Numerous reports of these implants are available but due to differences in study design, patient selection and operative technique they are of little value for comparing implants. Consequently, at the present time it is not possible to determine which is the best design of unipolar hemiarthroplasty.[77]

Bipolar hemiarthroplasty. A bipolar hemiarthroplasty incorporates a second interprosthetic joint. This gives the potential advantage of reducing acetabular wear and the degree of residual pain. Most of the randomised trials which have compared these implants with unipolar hemiarthroplasties have been too small or had too short a follow-up to

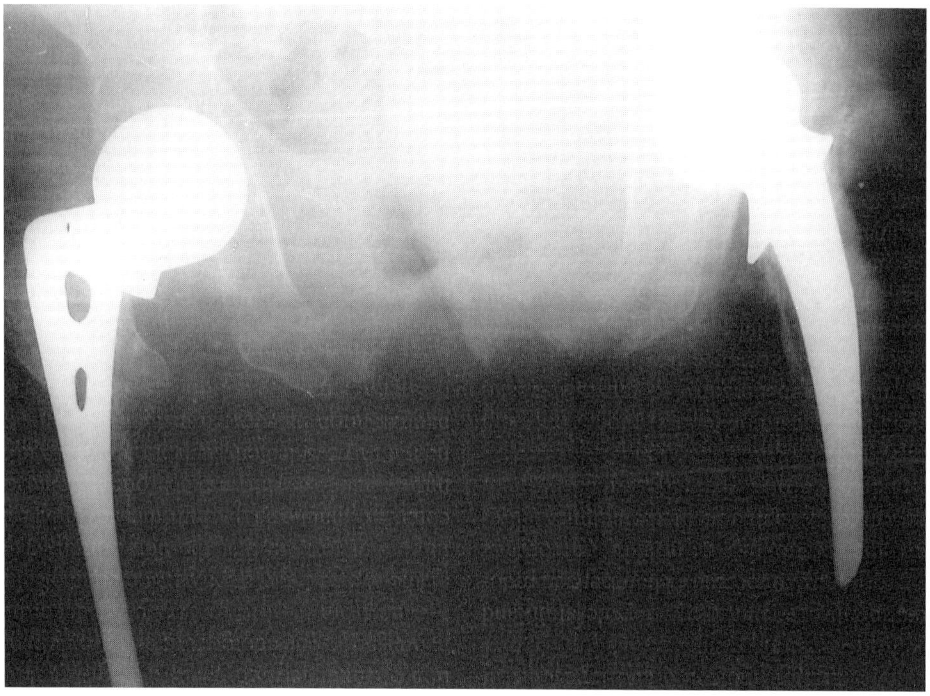

Fig. 7

Radiograph showing an uncemented Austin Moore hemiarthroplasty and a cemented Thompson prosthesis.

determine if there are any significant differences.[77] The only randomised trial to address this issue adequately[78] failed to find any significant difference between unipolar and bipolar hemiarthroplasties in patients aged over 80 years.

Summation of case reports of bipolar hemiarthroplasties indicate that there is no difference in the rate of dislocation between them and unipolar prostheses, but when dislocation occurs, a bipolar prosthesis is less likely to be reduced by closed reduction.[38] Another disadvantage of bipolar implants is the increased cost. Consequently, at the present time the use of bipolar prostheses remains open to discussion.

Total hip replacement. The use of total hip replacement for cervical fractures has been reported in a small number of case series and one randomised trial.[56] Most of these studies have restricted its use to the more healthy patients. They indicate that both the rate of dislocation (11%) and the later rate of revision were considerably increased than when this procedure is used for arthritis of the hip.[38]

Since total hip replacement is a more extensive procedure than hemiarthroplasty and at present has an undetermined place in the treatment of a hip fracture, it should be reserved only for those patients with associated arthritis of the hip or pathological fractures with acetabular involvement.

Cement or not. The use of bone cement gives a firmer fixation of the prosthesis, which probably results in less pain and a reduced long-term revision rate because of loosening.[77] Further adequately conducted studies are still required to confirm this. The disadvantages of cement are that it makes the initial surgery longer and more technically demanding. Furthermore, there is a risk of major cardiovascular collapse occurring at the time of insertion of the cement. This complication has an incidence of about 1% in the frail elderly. Another disadvantage of using cement is that revision surgery is more difficult.

Operative technique. The main decision related to the operative technique is the approach to the hip. Either an anterolateral approach through the anterior capsule or one via the posterior route may be used. A trochanteric osteotomy is not appropriate for surgery for hip fractures. The posterior approach has the advantages of being technically easier with a better exposure of the femur for reaming and of being associated with a lower operative blood loss. The anterior approach has a lower risk of dislocation (1.7% *v* 4.4%) but is more technically demanding and has a higher risk of preoperative fracture of the femur.[38,79]

Clinical studies which have compared the two approaches tend to favour the anterior approach.[54,79] Regardless of which is used, the joint capsule must be repaired to reduce the risk of dislocation.

CONCLUSIONS

The cervical fracture need not be termed the 'unsolved fracture'. There are certain patients for whom internal fixation is indicated, others for whom arthroplasty is required and in some either treatment may be used. The decision on the choice of treatment cannot be based solely on the radiological appearance of the fracture. Other factors to be considered are the facilities available, surgical expertise, delay from fracture to surgery, the age of the patient and the presence of other medical conditions. The choice of treatment can only be made on an individual patient basis. The clinician has to assess if the risk of failure of internal fixation of the fracture is high enough to justify replacing the femoral head by an arthroplasty.

If internal fixation is chosen as the method of treatment the fracture, if displaced, should be reduced closed, using the fracture table and image intensification. At the present time the implant of choice is two or more cancellous screws. The addition of a side plate is probably unnecessary. If arthroplasty is chosen, an uncemented hemiarthroplasty is acceptable for the very frail elderly since it avoids the potential hazards of cement. A cemented hemiarthroplasty, possibly incorporating a bipolar joint, should be used for the younger patient in whom internal fixation is inappropriate. At the present time total hip replacement should be reserved for those patients in whom there is damage to the hip from other causes.

Continued audit of the outcome of hip fracture should be undertaken using standardised methods.[80,81] Future research will help to clarify the importance which should be attached to the different factors that influence healing of the fracture after internal fixation. Clarification of the choice of implant for internal fixation can only be made using larger randomised trials and the choice of prosthesis and of cement still remains controversial because of the lack of adequate clinical studies.

REFERENCES

1. **Gullberg B, Johnell O, Kanis JA.** World-wide projections for hip fracture. *Osteoporosis Int* 1997;7:407-13.
2. **Keene GS, Parker MJ, Pryor GA.** Mortality and morbidity after hip fractures. *Br Med J* 1993;307:1248-50.
3. **Parker MJ, Pryor GA, Anand JK, Lodwick R, Myles JW.** A comparison of presenting characteristics of patients with intracapsular and extracapsular proximal femoral fractures. *J R Soc Med* 1992;85:152-5.
4. **Claffey TJ.** Avascular necrosis of the femoral head: an anatomical study. *J Bone Joint Surg [Br]* 1960;42-B:802-9.
5. **Sevitt S.** Avascular necrosis and revascularisation of the femoral head after intracapsular fractures: a combined arteriographic and histological necropsy study. *J Bone Joint Surg [Br]* 1964;46-B:270-96.
6. **Parker MJ.** Proximal femoral fractures. In: Pynsent PB, Fairbank JCT, Carr AJ, eds. *Classification of musculoskeletal trauma.* Oxford: Butterworth-Heinemann Publications, 1999.
7. **Alho A, Benterud JG, Rønningen H, Høiseth A.** Radiographic prediction of early failure in femoral neck fracture. *Acta Orthop Scand* 1991;62:422-6.
8. **Parker MJ.** Prediction of fracture union after internal fixation of intracapsular femoral neck fractures. *Injury* 1994;25(Suppl 2):3-6.
9. **Saito N, Miyasaka T, Toriumi H.** Radiographic factors predicting nonunion of displaced intracapsular femoral neck fractures. *Arch Orthop Trauma Surg* 1995;114:183-7.
10. **Garden RS.** Low-angle fixation in fractures of the femoral neck. *J Bone Joint Surg [Br]* 1961;43-B:647-63.
11. **Frandsen PA, Andersen E, Madsen F, Skjodt T.** Garden classification of femoral neck fractures: an assessment of inter-observer variation. *J Bone Joint Surg [Br]* 1988;70-B:588-90.

12. **McCabe J, O'Farrell D, O'Byrne J, O'Brien T.** Observer variation in the radiographic classification of femoral neck fractures. *J Bone Joint Surg [Br]* 1994;76-B:(Suppl II & III):120.

13. **Thomsen NO, Jensen CM, Skovgaard N, et al.** Observer variation in the radiographic classification of fractures of the neck of the femur using Garden's system. *Int Orthop* 1996;20:326-9.

14. **Parker MJ.** Garden grading of intracapsular fractures: meaningful or misleading? *Injury* 1993;24:241-2.

15. **Eliasson P, Hansson LI, Kärrholm J.** Displacement in femoral neck fractures. A numberical analysis of 200 fractures. *Acta Orthop Scand* 1988;59:361-4.

16. **Pauwels F.** *Der Schenkelhalsbruch: Ein mechanisches Problem.* Stuttgart: F. Enke, 1935.

17. **Parker MJ, Dynan Y.** Is Pauwels classification still valid? *Injury* 1998;29:521-3.

18. **Müller ME, Nazarian S, Koch P, Schatzker J.** *The comprehensive classification of fractures of long bones.* Berlin, etc: Springer-Verlag, 1990.

19. **Newey ML, Ricketts D, Roberts L.** The AO classification of long bone fractures: an early study of its use in clinical practice. *Injury* 1993;24:309-12.

20. **Johnstone DJ, Radford WJ, Parnell EJ.** Interobserver variation using the AO/ASIF classification of long bone fractures. *Injury* 1993;24:163-5.

21. **Blundell CM, Parker MJ, Pryor GA, et al.** Assessment of the AO classification of intracapsular fractures of the proximal femur. *J Bone Joint Surg [Br]* 1998;80-B:679-83.

22. **Rajan D, Parker MJ.** Does the level of an intracapsular femoral fracture influence fracture healing after internal fixation?: a study of 411 patients. *Injury* 2000;32:53-6.

23. **Alho A, Benterud JG, Rønningen H, Høiseth A.** Prediction of disturbed healing in femoral neck fractures: radiographic analysis of 149 cases. *Acta Orthop Scand* 1992;63:639-44.

24. **Lagerby M, Asplund S, Ringqvist I.** Cannulated screws for fixation of femoral neck fractures: no difference between Uppsala screws and Richard screws in a randomized prospective study of 268 cases. *Acta Orthop Scand* 1998;69:387-91.

25. **Unger AS, Shuster HF.** Predicting the healing of displaced subcapital hip fractures via postoperative roentgenographic factors. *Orthop Rev* 1986;15:575-80.

26. **Price ER.** Evaluation of the viability of the femoral head at operation. *J Bone Joint Surg [Br]* 1963;45-B:618.

27. **Woodhouse CF.** Dynamic influences of vascular occlusion affecting the development of avascular necrosis of the femoral head. *Clin Orthop* 1964;32:119-29.

28. **Brünner S, Christiansen J, Kristensen JK.** Arteriographic prediction of femoral head viability in medial femoral neck fractures. *Acta Chir Scand* 1967;133:449-54.

29. **Arnoldi CC, Lemperg RK.** Fracture of the femoral neck: II Relative importance of primary vascular damage and surgical procedure for the development of necrosis of the femoral head. *Clin Orthop* 1977;129:217-22.

30. **Outerbridge RE.** Perosseous venography in the diagnosis of viability in subcapital fractures of the femur. *Clin Orthop* 1978;137:132-9.

31. **Milligan GF.** The use of Kiton Fast Green to measure the viability of the head of the femur after fractures of the neck of the femur. *Injury* 1979;10:235-8.

32. **Strömqvist B.** Femoral head vitality after intracapsular hip fracture: 490 cases studied by intravital tetracycline labeling and Tc-MDP radionuclide imaging. *Acta Orthop Scand* 1983;Suppl 2001:1-71.

33. **Holmberg S, Thorngren KG.** Preoperative ^{99m}Tc-MDP scintimetry of femoral neck fractures. *Acta Orthop Scand* 1984;55:430-5.

34. **Ragnarsson JI, Ekelund L, Kärrholm J, Hietala SO.** Low field magnetic resonance imaging of femoral neck fractures. *Acta Radiol* 1989;30:247-52.

35. **Parker MJ.** Missed hip fractures. *Arch Emerg Med* 1992;9:23-7.

36. **Pathak G, Parker MJ, Pryor GA.** Delayed diagnosis of femoral neck fractures. *Injury* 1997;28:299-301.

37. **Raaymakers ELFB, Marti RK.** Nonoperative treatment of impacted femoral neck fractures. *J Bone Joint Surg [Br]* 1991;73-B:950-4.

38. **Parker MJ, Pryor GA.** *Hip fracture management.* Oxford: Blackwell Scientific Publications, 1993.

39. **Parker MJ, Pryor GA.** Treatment of undisplaced subcapital fractures. *J R Coll Surg Edinb* 1992;37:263-4.

40. **Bédat B, Rossier J, Peter R.** Garden I fractures of the femoral neck: conservative or surgical treatment? *J Bone Joint Surg [Br]* 1997;79-B (Suppl II):243.

41. **Cserháti, Kazár G, Manninger J, Fekete K, Frenyó.** Non-operative or operative treatment for undisplaced femoral neck fractures: a comparative study of 122 non-operative and 125 operatively treated cases. *Injury* 1996;27:583-8.

42. **Parker MJ, Myles JW, Anand JK, Drewett R.** Cost-benefit analysis of hip fracture treatment. *J Bone Joint Surg [Br]* 1992;74-B:261-4.

43. **Dickson JA.** The "unsolved fracture": a protest against defeatism. *J Bone Joint Surg [Am]* 1953;35-A:805-22.

44. **Nicoll EA.** Editorial. The unsolved fracture. *J Bone Joint Surg [Br]* 1963;45-B:239-41.

45. **Speed K.** Unsolved fracture. *Surg Gynecol Obstet* 1935;60:341-52.

46. **Barnes R, Brown JT, Garden RS, Nicoll EA.** Subcapital fractures of the femur: a prospective review. *J Bone Joint Surg [Br]* 1976;58-B:2-24.

47. **Gray AJ, Parker MJ.** Intracapsular fractures of the femoral neck in young patients. *Injury* 1994;25:667-9.

48. **Thornhill TS, Creasman C.** *Hip fractures in patients with renal failure.* Presentation to the AAOS 52th meeting, January 24, 1985.

49. **Bogoch E, Ouellette G, Hastings D.** Failure of internal fixation of displaced femoral neck fractures in rheumatoid patients. *J Bone Joint Surg [Br]* 1991;73-B:7-10.

50. **Strömqvist B.** Hip fracture in rheumatoid arthritis. *Acta Orthop Scand* 1984;55:624-8.

51. **Hadden WA, Abernethy PJ, Haw C.** Hip fractures in rheumatoid arthritis. *Clin Orthop* 1982;170:252-9.

52. **Johnson JTH, Crothers O.** Nailing versus prosthesis for femoral-neck fractures: a critical review of long-term results in two hundred and thirty-nine consecutive private patients. *J Bone Joint Surg [Am]* 1975;57-A:686-92.

53. **Parker MJ.** Internal fixation or arthroplasty for displaced subcapital fractures in the elderly? *Injury* 1992;23:521-4.

54. **Lu-Yao GL, Keller RB, Littenberg B, Wennberg JE.** Outcomes after displaced fractures of the femoral neck: a meta-analysis of one hundred and six published reports. *J Bone Joint Surg [Am]* 1994;76-A:15-25.

55. **Sikorski JM, Barrington R.** Internal fixation versus hemiarthroplasty for the displaced subcapital fracture of the femur: a prospective randomised study. *J Bone Joint Surg [Br]* 1981;63-B:357-61.

56. **Skinner P, Riley D, Ellery J, et al.** Displaced subcapital fractures of the femur: a prospective randomised comparison of internal fixation, hemiarthroplasty and total hip replacement. *Injury* 1989;20:291-3.

57. **Søreide O, Mölster A, Raugstad TS.** Internal fixation versus primary prosthetic replacement in acute femoral neck fractures: a prospective, randomized clinical study. *Br J Surg* 1979;66:56-60.

58. **Parker MJ, Briggs D, Fleschner S.** *Internal fixation or arthroplasty for intracapsular fractures: Cochrane review in progress: protocol on Cochrane Library.* Oxford: Update software.

59. **Parker MJ, Pryor GA.** Internal fixation or arthroplasty for displaced cervical hip fractures in the elderly: a randomised controlled trial of 208 patients. *Acta Orthop Scand* 2000;71:440-6.

60. **Rodén M, Ellene B, Fredin H.** Treatment of displaced femoral neck fracture: internal fixation versus bipolar endoprosthesis: a preliminary report of a prospective randomized study. *Acta Orthop Scand* 1996;67(Suppl 270):33.

61. **Gray DH.** The evolution of a personal philosophy for the treatment of displaced subcapital fractures. *J Bone Joint Surg [Br]* 1988;70-B:161.

62. **Parker MJ, Pryor GA, Thorngren K-G.** *Handbook of hip fracture surgery.* Oxford: Butterworth-Heinemann Publications, 1997.

63. **Garden RS.** Malreduction and avascular necrosis in subcapital fractures of the femur. *J Bone Joint Surg [Br]* 1971;53-B:183-97.

64. **Parker MJ, Blundell C.** Choice of implant for internal fixation of femoral neck fractures: meta-analysis of 25 randomised trials including 4925 patients. *Acta Orthop Scand* 1998;69:138-43.

65. **Parker MJ, Porter KM, Eastwood DM, et al.** Intracapsular fractures of the neck of the femur: parallel or crossed Garden screws? *J Bone Joint Surg [Br]* 1991;73-B:826-7.

66. **Frandsen PA, Andersen PE Jr, Christoffersen H, Thomsen PB.** Osteosynthesis of femoral neck fracture: the sliding-screw-plate with or without compression. *Acta Orthop Scand* 1984;55:620-3.

67. **Jacobsson B, Dalén N.** Femoral head vitality after peroperative impaction of hip fractures. *Acta Orthop Scand* 1985;56:312-3.

68. **Parker MJ, Dynan Y.** Surgical approaches and ancillary techniques for internal fixation of intracapsular proximal femoral fractures. *Cochrane Database Syst Rev* 2000;3:CD001705.

69. **Strömqvist B, Nilsson LT, Egund N, Thorngren K-G, Wingstrand H.** Intracapsular pressures in undisplaced fractures of the femoral neck. *J Bone Joint Surg [Br]* 1988;70-B:192-4.

70. **Wingstrand H, Strömqvist B, Egund N, Gustafson T, Nilsson LT, Thorngren KG.** Hemarthrosis in undisplaced cervical fractures. *Acta Orthop Scand* 1986;57:305-8.

71. **Manninger J, Kazar G, Fekete G, et al.** Significance of urgent (within 6 h) internal fixation in the management of fractures of the neck of the femur. *Injury* 1989;20:101-5.

72. **Holmberg S, Kalén R, Thorngren K-G.** Treatment and outcome of femoral neck fractures: an analysis of 2418 patients admitted from their own homes. *Clin Orthop* 1987:218:42-52.

73. **Parker MJ, Pryor GA.** The timing of surgery for proximal femoral fractures. *J Bone Joint Surg [Br]* 1992;74-B:203-5.

74. **Parker MJ, Handoll HHG, Dynan Y.** Mobilisation strategies after hip fracture surgery in adults. *Cochrane Database Syst Rev* 2000;3:CD001704.

75. **Graham J.** Early or delayed weight-bearing after internal fixation of transcervical fracture of the femur: a clinical trial. *J Bone Joint Surg [Br]* 1968;50-B:562-9.

76. **Palmer S, Parker MJ, Hollingworth W.** Complications and financial implications of re-operations in hip fracture surgery. *J Bone Joint Surg [Br]* 2000;82-B:864-6.

77. **Parker MJ, Rajan D.** Choice of arthroplasty (and cement) for arthroplasty for hip fractures. *Cochrane Database Syst Rev* Review expected November 2000.

78. **Calder SJ, Anderson GH, Jagger C, Harper WM, Gregg PJ.** Unipolar or bipolar prosthesis for displaced intracapsular hip fracture in octogenarians: a randomised prospective study. *J Bone Joint Surg [Br]* 1996;78-B:391-4.

79. **Keene GS, Parker MJ.** Hemiarthroplasty of the hip: the anterior or posterior approach?: a comparison of surgical approaches. *Injury* 1993;24:611-3.

80. **Parker MJ, Currie CT, Mountain JA, Thorngren K-G.** Standardised audit of hip fracture in Europe (SAHFE). *Hip Int* 1998;8:10-5.

81. **Thorngren KG.** Full treatment spectrum for hip fractures: operation and rehabilitation. *Acta Orthop Scand* 1997;68:1-2.

NERVE REPAIR IN EXTENSIVE OPEN INJURIES

JAN SKOWROŃSKI

From the Medical University of Bialystok, Poland

Extensive open injuries of the limbs present a considerable clinical problem. Their repair is not simply an exercise in reconstructing the anatomy, but also in restoring the function of the limb after healing.

In every such injury proper surgical debridement of the wound plays the key role. The requirements of debridement are the resection of non-viable tissue, the removal of foreign bodies, good haemostasis, and the elimination of dead space. These create conditions for good healing and decrease the risk of infection. After debridement, the repair of injured structures such as the skin, blood vessels, bones and nerves is carried out, in order of importance, together with re-establishment of an adequate circulation and stabilisation of the skeletal structures followed by restoration of nerves, tendon continuity and skin cover. Lacerations to vessels are the most dangerous injuries.

In major injuries, particularly if they are high-energy, restoration of the circulation guarantees the survival of the limb. A stable circulation in the limb and perfusion of local tissues around the wound promote good wound healing and regeneration of nerves. The final result is directly related to the level of reinnervation. For this reason cases of devascularising trauma associated with nerve injuries are the most difficult in which to obtain good functional results.

Devascularising injuries. This injury is not clearly defined in the literature. The surgical techniques available for restoring the circulation in these injuries fall into three categories: 1) reimplantation (complete amputation); 2) revascularisation (incomplete amputation); and 3) simple vascular repair (non-critical vascular injury).

The functional results after reconstruction of neurovascular trauma depend on the regeneration of the nerves and on the quality of motor recovery, which probably reflects the level of the muscle damage due to anoxia. In addition, the results of repair of devascularising injury can be decreased by symptoms of cold intolerance and pain. Jupiter and Kleinert[1] suggest that these symptoms are caused by poor reinnervation of the pre-existing vascular system.

Other complications occur with severe soft-tissue defects. In such cases the nerve must be repaired after local or free flap transfer (skin, skin-muscle or skin-muscle-bone). This supports the local tissue perfusion giving an adequate microenvironment for nerve regeneration. Some cases require nerve reconstruction to be delayed and secondary nerve repair may give a better chance of reinnervation.

A surgeon carrying out operative nerve repair must remember that he can only create the conditions for the regeneration process. For this he must have knowledge of the nerve structure and problems of its regeneration and be familiar with microsurgical techniques.

STRUCTURE OF THE NERVE

The nerve trunk is a unique composition of nerve fibres and connective tissues. Nerve fibres consist of motor, sensory or sympathetic neurones in various proportions. Connective-tissue elements create layers called endoneurium, perineurium and epineurium. They divide the trunk into compartments and give a scaffolding for the vascular network. The endoneurium covers single nerve fibres, and the perineurium surrounds fascicles and fascicle groups acting as diffusion barrier to the endoneural space and is resistant to mechanical trauma. The epineurium has an extended vascular network connected to an intraneural vascular system.[2-5] It also provides a secure gliding mechanism between the tissues.

DEGENERATION AND REGENERATION

Every regenerative process depends on Wallerian degeneration which occurs after injury. When the nerve trunk is severed all axons are disrupted into separate stumps. In the distal stump the initial changes consist of fragmentation of the axon, myelin sheath and Schwann cells and the phagocytosis of debris by macrophages. In the proximal stump degeneration reaches the nearest Ranvier's node.[6-9] During the process of regeneration the nerve cells do not proliferate but only undergo metabolic changes to increase the volume and transport of axoplasm.[8] The remaining cell components of the trunk present a different picture of proliferating cells (Schwann cells, fibroblasts and endothelial cells). The endothelial cells form and reconstruct intraneural vessels while Schwann cells rapidly form columns (Bünger's bands) for the reconstruction of endotubes. The sprouting proximal axonal stump embeds in the cytoplasm of Schwann cells in order to make proper connections between the axons and the peripheral target organs by endotubes.[4,8] This unique process takes time and depends on some active biomolecules such as nerve growth factor, laminin 1, neural cell adhesion molecule and tenascin, all of which are growth promoters.[6,8]

From a biological point of view injury, degeneration and regeneration are inseparably connected. The clinical implication of Wallerian degeneration is that it is the appropriate time for repair and correct coaptation of the stump.

TYPES OF INJURY AND THEIR CLASSIFICATION

Injuries to nerves involve mechanical compression and thermal, stretching or anoxic forces, but irrespective of which is involved the tissue has a limited number of morphological and clinical responses; these include neurapraxia, axonotmesis and neurotmesis as described by Seddon[7] and particularly in detail by Sunderland.[9]

Neurapraxia refers to a local conduction block, but with axonal continuity preserved. Clinically, it corresponds to the motor block seen after a compression injury, such as palsy of the radial nerve. The block disappears when restoration of myelin is complete.

Axonotmesis is a loss of axonal continuity at the site of the lesion but with the endoneural tubes intact. This injury appears after traction or crush and creates Wallerian degeneration. In most cases regeneration is satisfactory without operative intervention, but takes days, weeks or months.

Neurotmesis is a severe injury with loss of continuity of the nerve fibres and connective-tissue elements. In this type of injury operative repair is required and there is no chance of spontaneous regeneration.

DIAGNOSIS

The clinical picture after injury is a simple motor palsy, loss of sensation and sympathetic symptoms depending on which nerve is involved. Examination of sensation involves evaluation of classical cutaneous functions such as pain, vibration, heat and cold, touch and pressure. Electronmicroscopic data have allowed these functions to be ascribed to specific receptors, e.g., cold to Krause's end bulb, heat to Rupini's receptor, touch to the Messner corpuscle and pressure to Pacinian corpuscles. Practically, the most important and useful tests are the static two-point discrimination Weber test and the moving two-point test described by Dellon.[10] They allow for correct diagnosis and monitoring of reinnervation.

Motor testing involves evaluating muscle contraction. With knowledge of the anatomical details of motor branches of the nerves we can obtain fundamental diagnostic help in regard to the injury or information about the extent of reinnervation. Repeated examination may be required to give an overall picture of reinnervation.

Pseudomotor tests of sympathetic function are considered to be most reliable when performed shortly after injury and are most helpful in determining complete anaesthesia. The Ninhydrin printing test and the O'Riain wrinkle test are the most popular, and accepted especially in the detection of malingering.[11]

Sensation and motor function are defined from the S0 to S4 and from the M0 to M5 scales according to the criteria of the World Federation of Societies of Hand Surgery. It is important to note that the nerve injury is only a part of a complex diagnosis in multitissue injuries. The details of nerve diagnosis allow the proper choice of the method of repair to be selected such as 'end-to-end', nerve grafting, neurotisation or nerve transfer.

'END-TO-END' REPAIRS

Conventional 'end-to-end' nerve repair is performed in three steps as follows: 1) preparation and resection of neural stumps as far as healthy fascicles which promotes axonal regeneration; 2) approximation and coaptation of the nerve stumps without tension in order to prevent ischaemia; and 3) connection of the neural stumps with an appropriate choice of suture.

Surgeons following these procedures should bear in mind the increased risk of intraneural bleeding, fibrosis and oedema.[2,4] Despite multiple connections between the epineurium, perineurium and endoneurium, stretching the nerve by more than 15% can result in complete loss of the intraneural circulation, as was demonstrated by Lundborg and Dahlin[2] and Lundborg and Rydevic.[5] The maximal distance between stumps which allows for 'end-to-end' repair is 2 cm.[12,13] The choice of fascicular suture and epineural and group suture depends on the cross-sectional anatomy of the nerve, which was classified by Sunderland[9] into three types: mono-, oligo-, and polyfascicular. Fascicular suture should not be used for polyfascicular nerves containing many groups of fascicles which cannot be easily separated, identified or matched.[14] The few indications for fascicular suture include the partially severed nerve with few fascicles injured, a 'blow-out' injury to small nerves disrupted at different levels, and neuroma in continuity in small nerves. Practically, fascicular repair is used in the digital nerves of the hand. Epineural and group fascicular repair is used in all other cases. It should be borne in mind that a nerve may change its cross-sectional anatomy throughout its course. For example, near the brachial plexus the ulnar nerve is polyfascicular, at the elbow it is oligofascicular and at the hand monofascicular. This means that modifications have to be made to the techniques of repair.

Although sutureless repair using tissue glue and laser techniques has never become popular, good clinical results have been obtained.[6,15] The largest number of good or excellent results were achieved in repairs of the radial

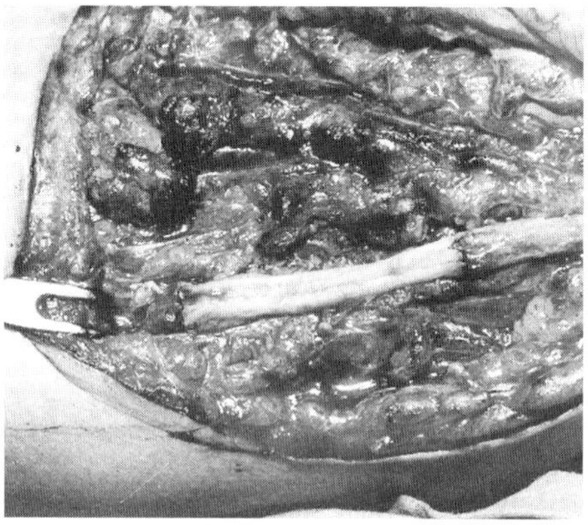

Fig. 1a

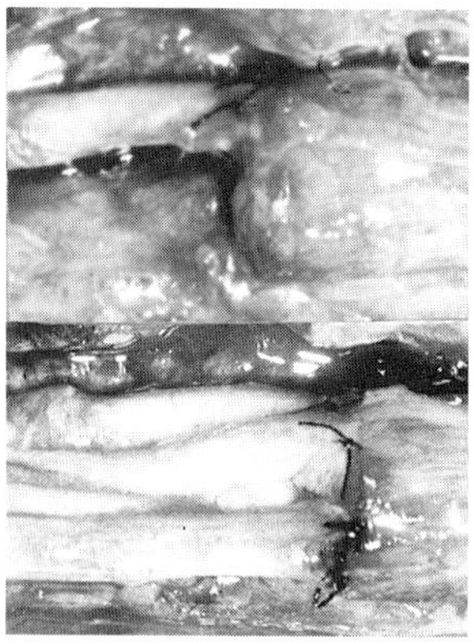

Fig. 1b

General (a) and close-up (b) views of grafting of the ulnar nerve.

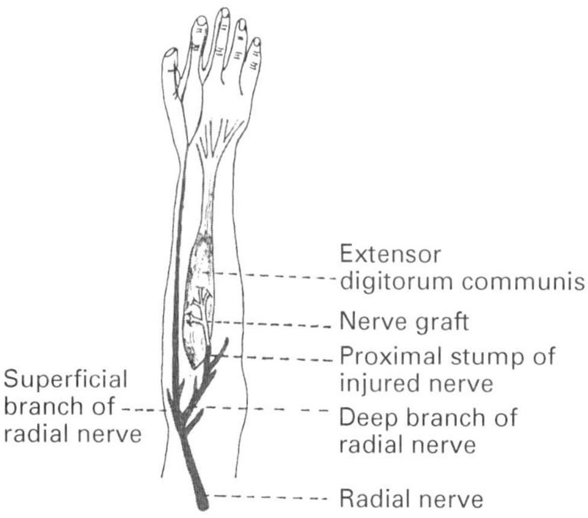

Fig. 2a

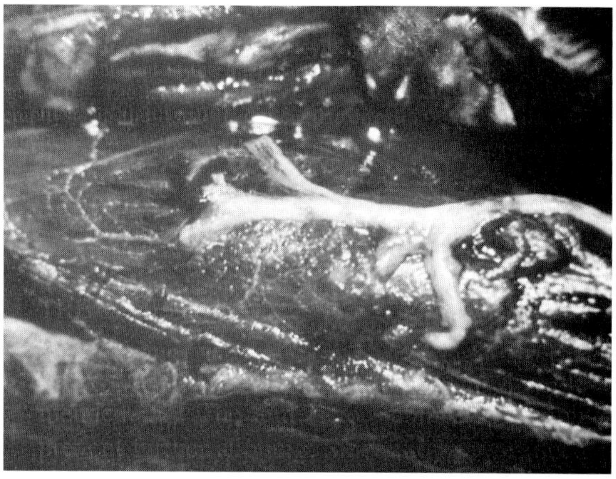

Fig. 2b

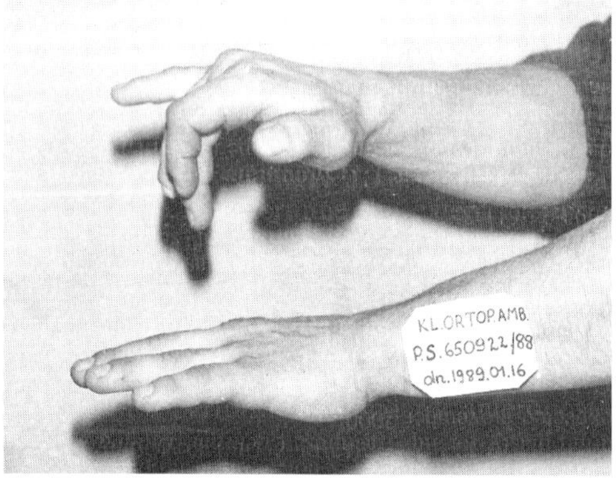

Fig. 2c

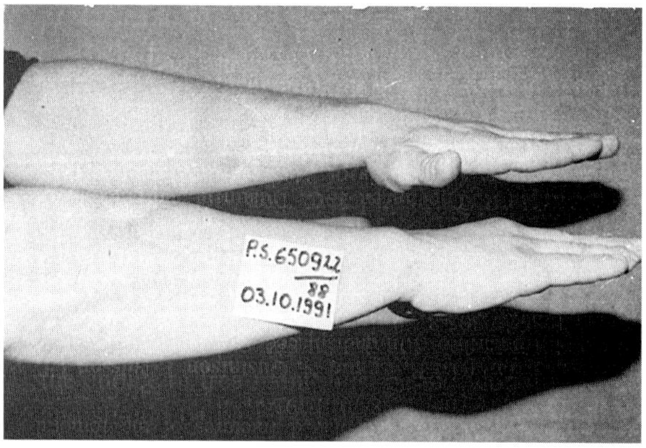

Fig. 2d

Diagram (a) and photographs (b to d) of neurotisation of extensor digitorum communis by the radial nerve extended by graft.

(80%) and musculocutaneous nerves (90%). There was good and excellent recovery of sensation in repairs of the median nerve (60%).[6]

NERVE GRAFTING

The most important indication for nerve grafting is a significant gap between nerve stumps. This occurs when there is primary loss of nerve substance, such as after a sharp laceration when the nerve is left unsutured for at least three weeks, or because of failure of recovery after primary repair requiring resection of the scar. The clinical background of nerve grafting was established by Millesi.[12] According to his experience gaps over 2.5 cm are most suitable for grafting. The main advantage is the abolition of tension at the suture line and good coaptation (Fig. 1).

Donor nerves which are used for grafting come from the upper limb and include the medial or lateral antebrachial cutaneous nerve, the posterior interosseous nerve and the dorsal cutaneous branch of the ulnar nerve. In the lower limbs the sural and lateral femoral nerves are used. Free nerve grafts are revascularised by recipient site vessels and vessels which arise from the nerve stump. In the case of a heavily scarred recipient bed vascularised nerve grafts should be used.

It is now accepted that with grafting a good functional outcome will be achieved in 70% to 80% of patients.

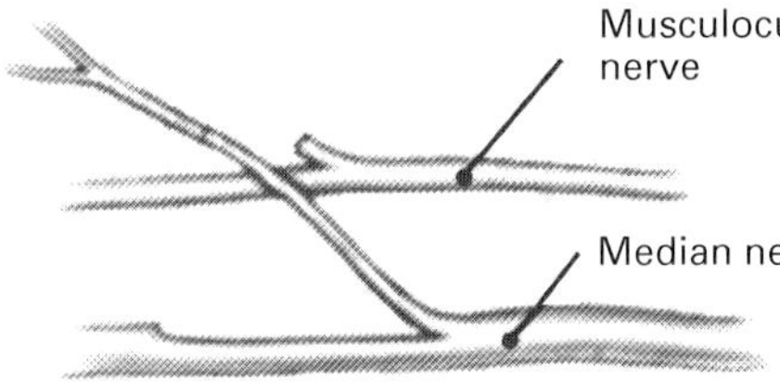

Fig. 3

Diagrammatic representation of nerve transfer.

NEUROTISATION

The classical techniques of nerve repair have no place when there is no distal stump of the damaged nerve. This is an irreparable injury and may be caused by dividing or destroying the nerve near its entrance into the muscle or by avulsion of the nerve from the muscle. In such injuries only implantation of the proximal stump of the nerve into the denervated muscle belly can give reinnervation of the muscle. The only means of restoring neuromuscular transmission is neurotisation. The first clinical experiments on direct neurotisation were performed in the 1970s. Further experimental work has shown that after reinnervation the power in a neurotised muscle is 50% to 90% of that in healthy muscle.[16-18]

It has been shown that placing nerve endings between the muscle fibres of the degenerated muscle causes the formation of new motor endplates between the nerve and previously denervated muscle fibres.[18] Brunelli[16] and Brunelli and Monini[17] improved and established the basis of the technique which involves resection of the epineurium from the proximal aspect of the stump, selection of fascicle groups and direct implantation between muscle fibres through non-bleeding small slits (Fig. 2). The only contraindication is a long reinnervation time which may mean that the reparative ability of the neurones is exhausted. Neurotisation in multitissue crush injuries requires further consideration if all of the muscle belly is fibrotic. Brunelli and Monini[17] reported 28 patients treated by the direct muscle neurotisation technique with satisfactory results from M3 to M5. Most were comparable to those obtained by conventional repair techniques. We have used neurotisation since 1990 and obtained similar results to those of Brunelli.[19]

NERVE TRANSFER

The aim is to reinnervate the target organ in the same way as in nerve repair. The main idea and philosophy of nerve transfers are to convert a proximal into a distal nerve injury.[20-22] Examples of motor transfer are: 1) musculocutaneous nerve injury at the brachial plexus (the transfer of motor fascicles of the median nerve to the musculocutaneous nerve) (Fig. 3); and 2) proximal ulnar-nerve injury (the transfer of the nerve to pronator quadratus to motor branches of the ulnar nerve). An example of the transfer of sensitivity is transfer of the fourth webspace to the first webspace in proximal median-nerve injury. The major requirement for this concept is irreversible atrophy of the target organ.[22]

The indications for nerve transfer are: 1) very proximal nerve injury or injury to the brachial plexus; 2) major limb trauma with segmental loss of the substance of the nerve trunk; and 3) partial nerve injuries in which a defined functional loss is present in one distal area with good function remaining in other areas supplied.

Nerve transfer can be used in combination with other nerve repairs. The primary repair of proximal median or ulnar nerve injuries with simultaneous tendon transfer, or tendon transfer with simultaneous neurotisation are examples of these reconstructions. The main concept is always the same: to restore function.

REFERENCES

1. **Jupiter JB, Kleinert HE.** Vascular injuries in the upper extremity. In: Tubiana R, ed. *The hand, vol. 3.* Philadelphia: WB Saunders, 1988:593-611.
2. **Lundborg G, Dahlin LB.** Structure and function of peripheral nerve. In: Gelberman R, ed. *Operative nerve repair and reconstruction.* Philadelphia: Lippincott, 1991:3-18.
3. **Lundborg G.** The intrinsic vascularization of human peripheral nerves: structural and functional aspects. *J Hand Surg [Am]* 1979;4:34-41.
4. **Lundborg G.** *Nerve injury and repair.* Edinburgh: Churchill Livingstone, 1988.
5. **Lundborg G, Rydevic B.** Effects of stretching the tibial nerve of the rabbit: a preliminary study of the intraneural circulation and the barrier function of the perineurium. *J Bone Joint Surg [Br]* 1973;55-B:390-401.
6. **Gelberman RH.** *Operative nerve repair and reconstruction.* Philadelphia: JB Lippincott, 1991.
7. **Seddon HJ.** *Surgical disorders of the peripheral nerves.* Edinburgh, etc: Churchill-Livingstone, 1972.
8. **Stoll G, Müller HW.** Nerve injury axonal degeneration and neural regeneration: basic insights. *Brain Pathol* 1999;9:313-25.
9. **Sunderland S.** *Nerves and nerve injuries.* Edinburgh, London, New York: Churchill Livingstone, 1978.
10. **Dellon AV.** *Evaluation of sensibility and re-education of sensation in the hand.* Baltimore: Williams and Wilkins, 1981:169.
11. **Lister G.** *The hand: diagnosis and indications.* 3rd ed. Edinburgh: Churchill Livingstone, 1993.
12. **Millesi H.** Techniques for grafting. *Hand Clin* 2000;16:73-91.
13. **Vanderhooft E.** Functional outcomes of nerve grafts for upper and lower extremities. *Hand Clin* 2000;16:93-104.
14. **Urbaniak JR.** Fascicular nerve suture. *Clin Orthop* 1982;163:57-64.

15. **Bora FW Jr, Bednar JM, Osterman AL, Brown MJ, Sumner AJ.** Prosthetic nerve grafts: a resorbable tube as an alternative to autogenous nerve grafting. *J Hand Surg [Am]* 1987;12:685-92.

16. **Brunelli G.** Direct neurotization of severely damaged muscles. *J Hand Surg [Am]* 1982;7:572-9.

17. **Brunelli G, Monini L.** Direct muscular neurotization. *J Hand Surg [Am]* 1985;10:993-7.

18. **Skowroński J, Bielecki M.** *Direct neurotization of muscle in irreparable nerve injuries.* SIROT/CSOS 200 China, Abstracts, Shanghaj-Beijing, 2000:118.

19. **Monach J, Skowroński J.** Direct muscular neurotization as a method of treatment of irreparable nerve injuries. *Rocz Akad Med Bialymst* 1992;37:58-63.

20. **Battiston B, Lanzetta M.** Reconstruction of high ulnar nerve lesions by distal double median to ulnar nerve transfer. *J Hand Surg [Am]* 1999;24:1185-91.

21. **Mackinnon SE, Novak CB.** Nerve transfers: new options for reconstruction following nerve injury. *Hand Clin* 1999;15:643-66.

22. **Nath RK, Mackinnon SE.** Nerve transfers in the upper extremity. *Hand Clin* 2000;16:131-9.

SLIPPED CAPITAL FEMORAL EPIPHYSIS (SCFE)

R. KRAUSPE, A. WILD, B. WESTHOFF

From the University of Düsseldorf, Germany

Slipped capital femoral epiphysis (SCFE), displacement of the epiphysis from the metaphysis, is a common disorder of the hip which affects adolescents. Patients are generally between the ages of 11 and 15 years, but it seems that this has decreased during the last part of the 20th century possibly because of a decrease in the age of puberty. Boys are affected almost twice as often as girls and usually at a later age, but approximately in the same pubertal period. The incidence is reported to be about 4 to 5/100 000 for all patients in prepuberty and puberty. SCFE occurs more often in tall and obese children. The left hip is slightly more affected than the right. The study of Hagglund, Hansson and Sandstrom[1] indicated that there was a hereditary factor in the aetiology which is still obscure.[2]

There are several pathogenic factors which lead to alteration of the cellular components and matrix at the growth plate resulting in physeal instability of the femoral head.[3,4] The angle of the epiphysis during puberty has an oblique plane which leads to higher forces at the epiphyseal-metaphyseal junction. These mechanisms are regularly enhanced by a reduced anteversion of the femoral neck[5] while the acetabulum shows normal anteversion.[6] Retroversion alone is a risk factor for osteoarthritis.[7] If the hip develops a slip the risk of developing osteoarthritis increases. Thus the cellular changes of various components, hormonal dysregulation and biomechanical factors such as oblique orientation of the growth plate or retroversion of the femoral neck are important pathogenetic factors in the displacement. The rate of late stages of SCFE in patients treated for osteoarthritis of the hip is about 10% in those coming to total hip replacement.

CLASSIFICATION

Clinically, SCFE is classified according to the type and duration of symptoms as well as the severity of the slip. Acute slips are those with sudden onset of severe symptoms which prevent walking or bearing weight on the affected leg. Radiographs show epiphyseal displacement with no evidence of bone healing or remodelling. Chronic slips are characterised by a gradual or intermittent onset and symptoms of more than three weeks' duration. Radiographs show some bone healing and remodelling of the femoral neck. The acute-on-chronic slip is defined as having a sudden onset, but radiographs show signs of remodelling of the proximal femur, and if reducible only the degree of the acute slip can be reduced by closed manipulation. The chronic form is found in about 75% of the cases, the acute slip in about 10% and the acute-on-chronic in nearly 15%[2] (Krauspe et al, unpublished data).

Loder et al[8] proposed a classification of stable and unstable SCFE by clinical parameters, mainly the ability to bear weight and walk (stable slip) or the inability to bear weight (unstable slip).

Radiologically, a slip of less than 30° is considered to be grade I, between 30° and 60° grade II, and of more than 60° grade III. Some authors prefer to differentiate between grade II and grade III at an angle of 50°. The severity of the condition may also be determined by measuring the percentage of the slip in relation to the width of the femoral neck. There are inter- and intraobserver errors as well as differences in measured angles because the radiographic technique and projection are significantly dependent on the positioning of the leg.

SYMPTOMS

The most frequently presenting complaint is a painful hip. Pain also may be referred to the knee and may be the only presenting symptom. It is usually intermittent and gradual in onset. Some patients describe episodes of trauma in the recent past. Physical examination most often reveals mild pain on movement with limited internal rotation and abduction. Flexion of the hip results in obligatory external rotation at the hip because of the slip, a positive Drehmann sign (Fig. 1). In severe slips the flexion may be limited to 60° to 70° because already at these low rates of flexion there is an impingement caused by the anterior prominence of the femoral neck (see Fig. 7b). The incidence of bilateral SCFE has been reported as 79% by Hagglund et al[1] and as 59% by Jerre et al[9] at follow-up. Both groups, however, found bilateral SCFE at the time of the first clinical presentation in only 23% and 8% to 27%, respectively. These data underline the importance of frequent follow-up examina-

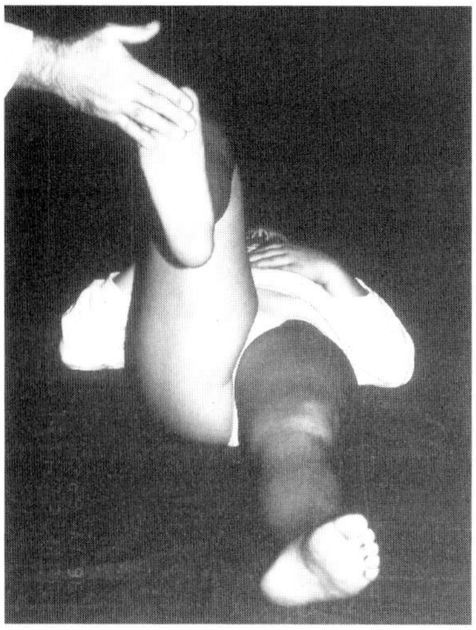

Fig. 1a

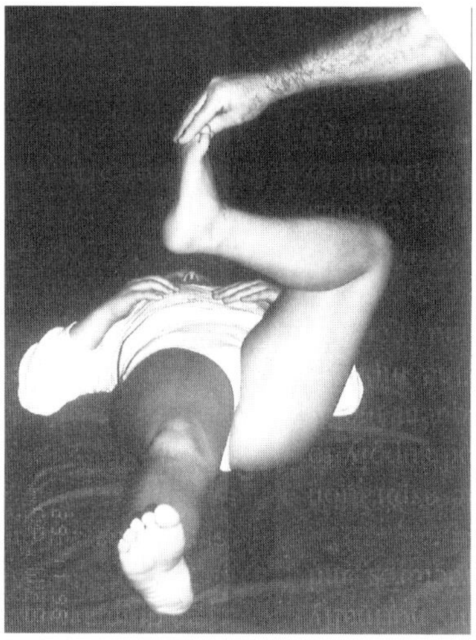

Fig. 1b

Photographs of the clinical examination of an 11-year-old girl with severe SCFE. Figure 1a – On the contralateral, non-affected side the hip can be moved into flexion without any rotation. Figure 1b – On the left side the characteristic Drehmann sign is seen. While moving the hip from extension into flexion the affected side shows external rotation because of the epiphyseal slip.

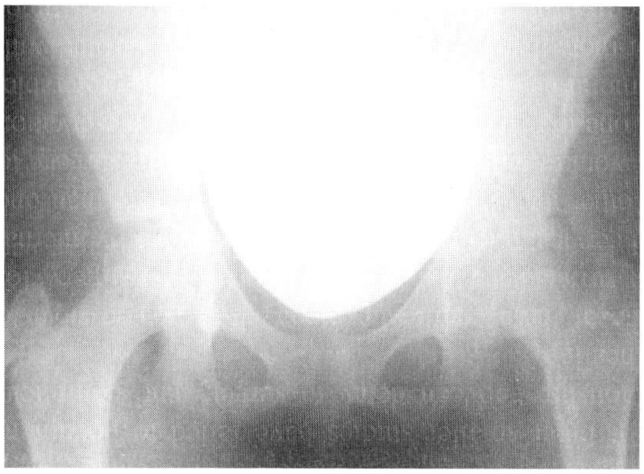

Fig. 2a

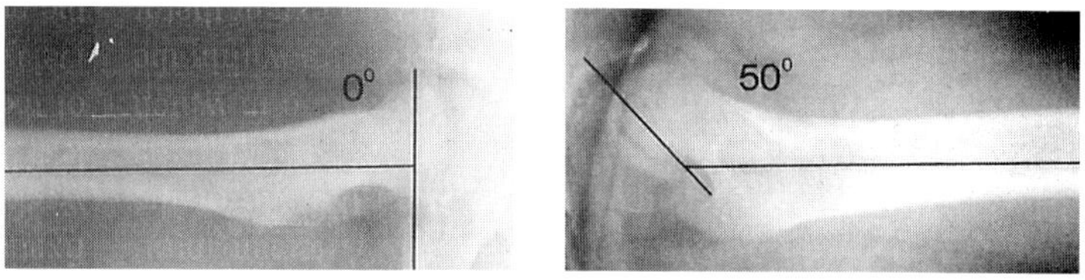

Fig. 2b

Radiographs of the pelvis of an 11-year-old girl with severe SCFE on the AP view. Figure 2a – The tangent at the lateral neck does not cross the physis on the affected side. Figure 2b – The lateral (Imhäuser) view shows the typical direction of the slip of the epiphysis in the dorso-medio-caudal direction and this projection allows for measurement of the degree of slip.

tion of the contralateral hip or simultaneous prophylactic pinning of the unaffected hip, which has been our method of treatment for more than 20 years.

RADIOLOGY

On the anteroposterior film the epiphysis is displaced posteriorly and inferiorly. A rim of new bone is found at the posterior aspect of the neck adjacent to the femoral head (see Fig. 7a). In addition, the femoral neck becomes uncovered anteriorly, producing the characteristic ‘prominence’ of its superior and anterior aspects (see Fig. 7b). A true lateral view can help to determine the extent of posterior displacement of the epiphysis, and a ‘frog-leg’ lateral view detects minor slips. The radiographic technique described by Imhäuser[10] allows for both diagnosis and measurement, and classification in a reproducible manner (Fig. 2). We therefore prefer to perform a standard anteroposterior radiograph of the pelvis and a lateral projection using this method which is performed with the hip in 90° of flexion and as much abduction as the measured result of the projected caput-collum-diaphysis angle minus 90°.

TREATMENT

Early diagnosis and surgical treatment are widely recommended.[4,9,11] The aim is to stabilise the epiphysis and to prevent further slipping. Since the best results are obtained in grade-I slips it is clear that diagnosis and treatment should be established as early as possible to prevent a progression to grade II or grade III.

There is, however, controversy regarding the appropriate surgical procedure, which may involve percutaneous or open pinning in situ, open reduction and internal fixation, epiphyseodesis, osteotomy, cheilectomy and internal fixation of the epi- and metaphysis by nails, screws or pins (Kirschner (K-) wires). The indications for prophylactic pinning of the undisplaced contralateral side are also controversial.

Each technique has its advantages and disadvantages and the choice of treatment must be individualised for each case and should be based on the experience of the surgeon with the method applied. Details of treatment are shown in Table I.

In the case of grade-I SCFE, fixation with K-wires is the

Table I. Algorithm showing details of treatment

Acute SCFE/unstable SCFE	Reduction and fixation with pins (K-wires), screws
Acute-on-chronic/unstable SCFE	Reduction of acute slippage and fixation with pins or screws. If necessary one- or two-stage surgery with a second-stage osteotomy for correction of the remaining deformity from the chronic slip
Chronic SCFE/stable SCFE	Fixation with pins (K-wires), screws and if the degree is more than 60%, osteotomy according to Imhäuser[19] (blade plate fixation) or a subcapital closing-wedge osteotomy including resection of bump and osteosynthesis with at least two screws
Degree of slip < 30°, grade I	Fixation in situ with pins (K-wires), screws
Degree of slip between 30° and 60°, grade II	Fixation in situ with pins (K-wires) or screws. If necessary osteotomy according to Imhäuser[19] (blade plate fixation) or subcapital closing wedge osteotomy including resection of bump and osteosynthesis with at least two screws
Degree of slip > 60°, grade III	Fixation with pins (K-wires) and osteotomy according to Imhäuser[19] (blade plate fixation) or subcapital closing-wedge osteotomy including resection of bump and osteosynthesis with at least two screws

method of choice (Fig. 3). König et al[12] reported that this method gave the best results in the short and long term with the lowest complication rates, compared with stabilisation by screws or Smith-Petersen nails. After fixation by K-wires significantly better long-term results were found with regard to pain and objective parameters such as the Harris hip score, the development of osteoarthritis, sphericity of the femoral head, differences in leg-length and the neck/shaft ratio of the proximal femur. Patients who needed a second or even a third operation because of withdrawal of the wires while the femoral neck grew further (see Fig. 6) were a mean of 11 years of age at the time of initial treatment, which was significantly lower compared with other series. We estimate that the advantages of fixation with K-wires are greater in these young patients despite the risk of further surgery because of the remaining growth of the proximal femur and the maintenance of the sphericity of the femoral head by this method of fixation. Careful placement and radiological intraoperative control are mandatory to detect any perforation of the joint and to place the wires or screws in a correct position (Fig. 4). De Sanctis et al[13] favoured a single percutaneous screw and argued that fixation with pins has a higher rate of complications of 18% compared with other methods, but they reported minor complications, such as superficial wound infection in the pin group and severe complications, such as avascular necrosis or chondrolysis, in the group treated with screws. In a study by Seller et al[14] no major complications occurred in hips pinned prophylactically in 109 patients treated with K-wires bilaterally at the first presentation. Rostoucher et al[15] did not advocate routine treatment of the non-affected contralateral side except in cases of severe slip before puberty; they gave no statistical data in support of their recommendation.

In the case of severe slip, after a few days in traction, if partial reduction is achieved Hansson, Hägglund and Ordeberg[16] prefer bilateral pinning without further reduction. However, reduction by a cuneiform osteotomy and internal fixation may be necessary. The reported rate of complications, such as avascular necrosis and chondrolysis, is high with this procedure.[17]

Jerre[18] recommended that chronic slips should not be reduced. A chronic slip which has united in a poor position may require intertrochanteric osteotomy according to the technique of Imhäuser[19] (Fig. 5). The rate of avascular necrosis after this procedure is lower than with a closing-wedge osteotomy of the femoral neck.[20] When performing an intertrochanteric osteotomy the remaining growth and

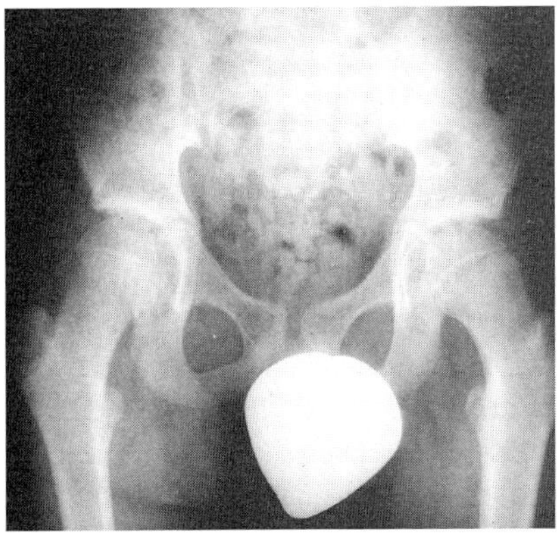

Fig. 3a

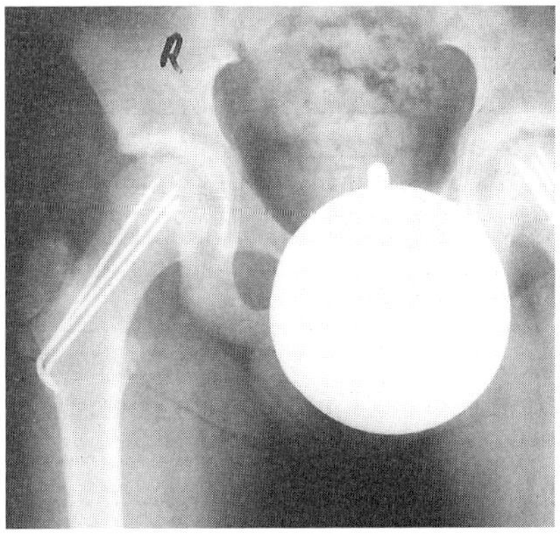

Fig. 3b

Preoperative (a) and postoperative (b) radiographs of grade-I SCFE of the left hip showing fixation of the slipped epiphysis with four K-wires and prophylactic pinning on the contralateral side with three K-wires.

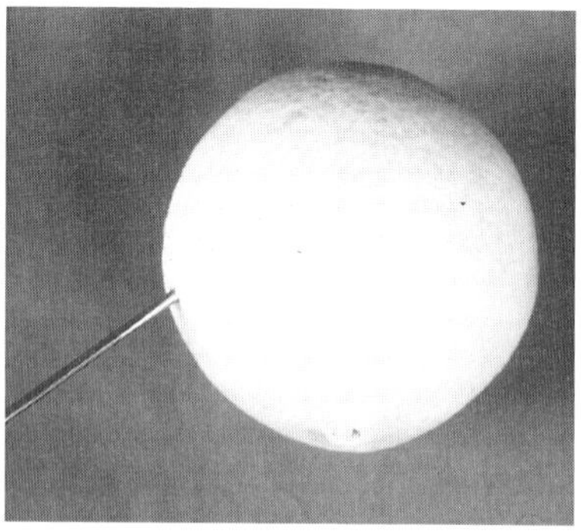

Fig. 4a

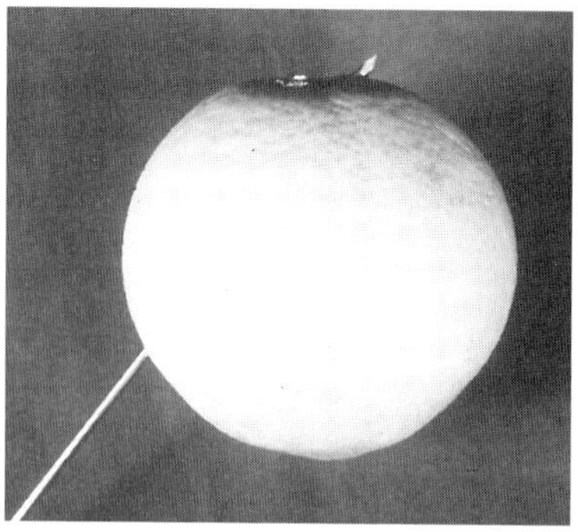

Fig. 4b

Figure 4a – Photograph of a model showing possible pin perforation of the femoral epiphysis, which may be undetected because of the projection. Figure 4b – By rotating away the bony area, either by moving the leg or by changing the direction of the x-ray beam, an incorrect position of the implant can be detected.

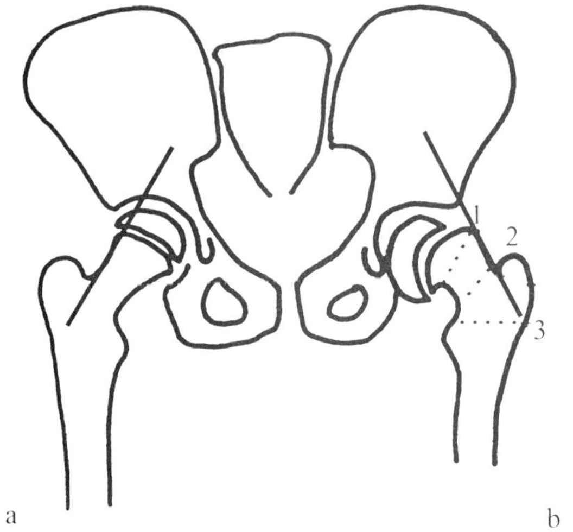

Fig. 5

Diagram of a normal proximal femur (a) compared with the typical appearance of a SCFE (b). In the normal bone the tangent at the lateral neck crosses the epiphysis (a) and in SCFE the tangent does not cross the epiphysis because of the epiphyseal slip in the dorso-medio-caudal direction (b). The dotted lines indicate the planes of: 1) intra-articular cuneiform osteotomy of the femoral neck; 2) extra-articular cuneiform osteotomy of the femoral neck; and 3) intertrochanteric osteotomy.

deformity have to be considered to determine whether additional pinning is indicated (Fig. 6). For a closing-wedge procedure it is strongly recommended that stable internal fixation be achieved with at least two screws (Fig. 7).

COMPLICATIONS

The complications of SCFE are chronic loss of range of movement and secondary degenerative arthritis, avascular necrosis of the femoral head and chondrolysis.

The risk of avascular necrosis depends on the degree of slip, whether it is acute or chronic and the treatment.[21,22] It is rare in untreated patients and probably results from interruption of the retrograde blood supply by the initial injury. In treated patients forceful repetitive manipulation, by open reduction or by osteotomy of the femoral neck, could be the cause. The risk is higher with moderate or severe displacement than with mild slips. Overall, avascular necrosis has been reported in 20% of all cases of SCFE, with boys and coloured patients having a higher risk. With repetitive manipulation the risk increases up to 47%.[8] If avascular necrosis becomes evident it may be possible to rotate the area of avascular necrosis away from the main area of loading by intertrochanteric valgus and flexion osteotomy and allow for at least some remodelling of the affected area (Figs 6 and 8). In some acute cases total necrosis of the epiphysis occurs and arthrodesis or total joint arthroplasty may be required as a salvage procedure.

Maussen, Rozing and Obermann[23] reported that in a long-term study only one of ten hips with a slip of less than 40° showed signs of osteoarthritis, compared with 15 of 16 hips with a slip of more than 40°. All patients had been treated by an intertrochanteric osteotomy. The higher the degree of slip the higher is the risk of osteoarthritis. Therefore they postulate that it is not the treatment which is the main factor for developing secondary osteoarthritis but the degree of the initial slip. This again supports the requirement for early diagnosis and treatment of the condition.

The most frequent cause of chondrolysis is penetration of the joint by the pins. The diagnosis of chondrolysis requires a joint space of less than 3 mm wide and a restricted range of movement of the hip. Treatment is bed rest, intensive physiotherapy, traction and control of pain. If a pin is left penetrating the joint it must be replaced immediately. The rate of success, however, with this type of treatment is not very high and if severe narrowing of the joint space persists with a limited range of movement and pain, salvage procedures such as arthrodesis or arthroplasty may be necessary.

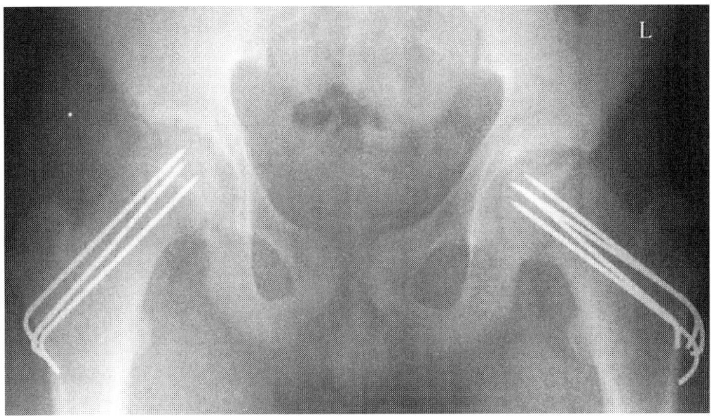

Fig. 6a

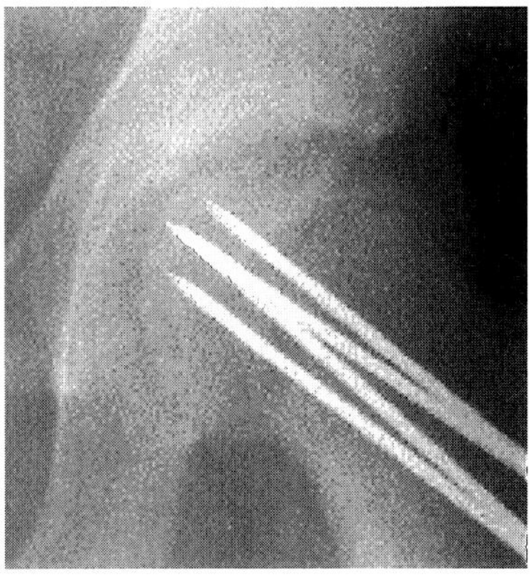

Fig. 6b

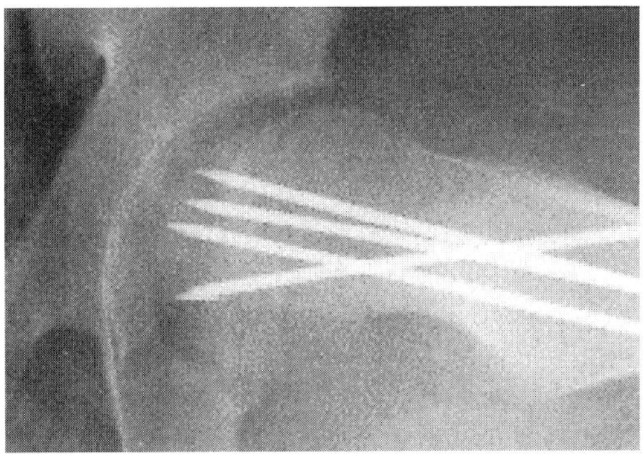

Fig. 6c

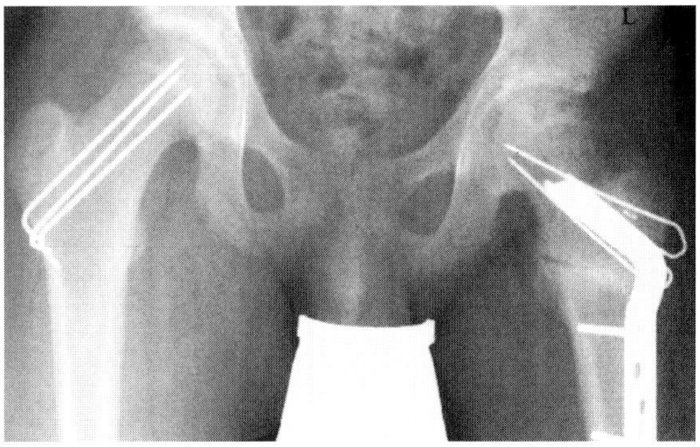

Fig. 6d

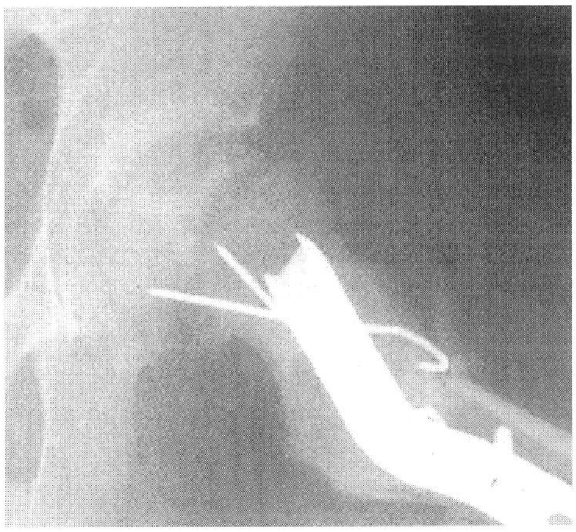

Fig. 6e

Figures 6a, 6b and 6c – SCFE of the left hip (grade II) in a 14-year-old boy four months after fixation by K-wires. There is partial avascular necrosis of the femoral head anterolaterally outside the area of the pins which do not penetrate. A valgus, flexion and rotation osteotomy gives improvement of the position of the femoral head and contributes to the remodelling capacity of the necrotic area. Figures 6d and 6e – Radiographs at six weeks after the osteotomy show signs of consolidation and there is no further collapse of the necrotic area. Clinically, the patient is free from pain.

AFTER-TREATMENT

After the operation of pinning in situ in chronic SCFE we recommend treatment by continuous passive motion and partial weight-bearing for six weeks. Physiotherapy should aim to improve the range of movement of the hip and to build up the muscle strength and co-ordination in the leg. After the wound has healed we allow partial weight-bearing of 20 kg beginning on the 15th day after operation. If the patient is free from pain and the range of movement is adequate full weight-bearing is allowed after six weeks. If there is any sign of pain or effusion in the joint, partial weight-bearing for another six weeks is recommended. Clinical and radiological follow-up is at 2, 6, 12 weeks and at 6 and 12 months after operation.

In acute SCFE we recommend bed-rest for three days after operation with continuous passive movement. The patient is then mobilised on crutches with non-weight-bearing for 14 days and 20 kg of partial weight-bearing for a total of three months after operation. The movement of the hip should be commensurate with the result of the reduction or the persistent angle of slip, and the patient should be free from pain when full weight-bearing is allowed. Any sign or symptom which may indicate AVN or chondrolysis should

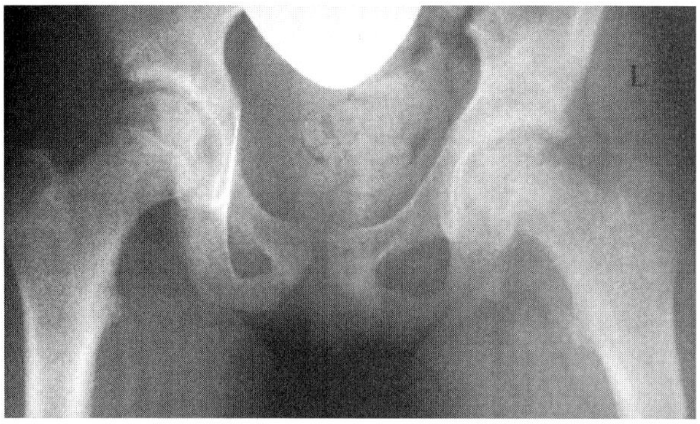

Fig. 7a

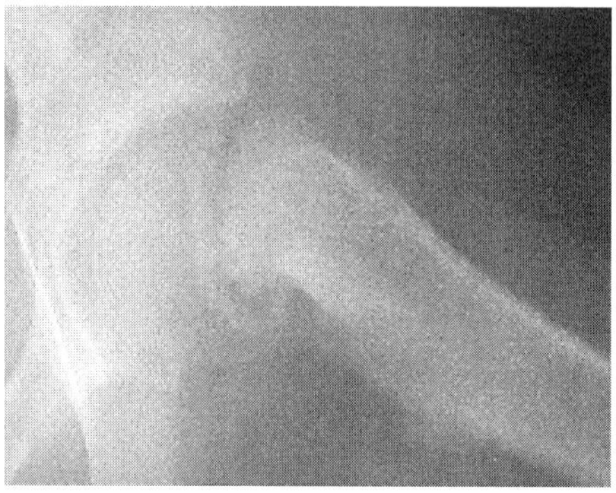

Fig. 7b

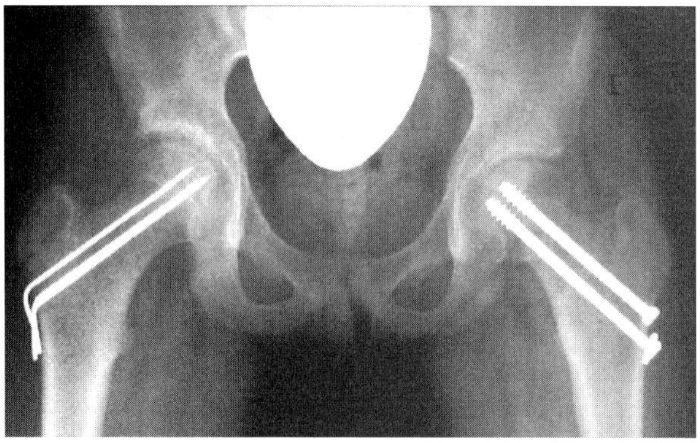

Fig. 7c

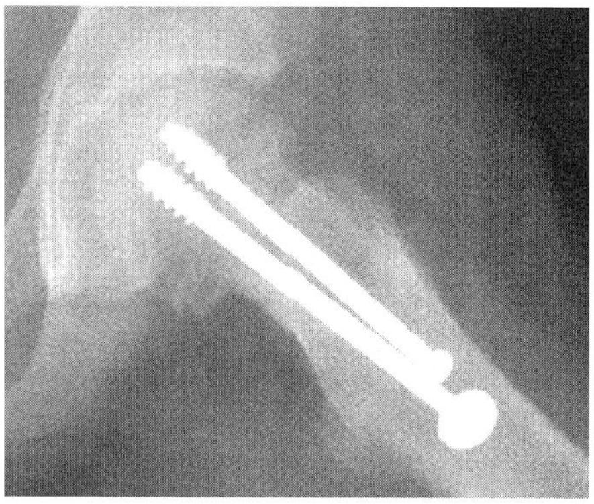

Fig. 7d

Pre- and postoperative radiographs of a 12-year-old girl with severe grade-III SCFE on the left side. Figure 7a – The AP view shows the typical appearance of SCFE compared with the unaffected contralateral side. Figure 7b – The lateral view shows the severe slip and significant bony remodelling as hip flexion was limited to 70°. Radiographic examination by the Imhäuser[16] views was not possible. Anatomical reduction was achieved after cuneiform closing-wedge osteotomy, and fixation with two screws. Prophylactic pinning of the opposite side was also performed. Figures 7c and 7d – Five months after operation there is no evidence of avascular necrosis and clinically the range of movement is normal in both hips.

influence the regimen and we then recommend further partial weight-bearing using crutches until relief of symptoms, with or without further therapy or surgery. In patients who have had an intertrochanteric osteotomy as described by Imhäuser[19] we recommend bed-rest with continuous passive movement and physiotherapy for two to three days, followed by non-weight-bearing for 14 days. The patient is then mobilised on crutches for another three months of partial weight-bearing with 20 kg. Full weight-bearing is allowed after healing of the osteotomy.

PROGNOSIS

The study of Hagglund et al[1] showed that 25% of the primarily untreated and the unaffected hips developed secondary osteoarthritis before the age of 50 years, with significant slips on the initially unaffected side. No degenerative joint disease was found in contralateral hips, which were simultaneously stabilised prophylactically. In patients with untreated SCFE the reduced range of movement results in the contraction of the external rotators with a persistent Drehmann sign which is related to the degree of the slip. Secondary osteoarthritis develops late, usually not before the fifth decade. In cases of severe slip the restriction of flexion can also lead to loss of function and secondary problems in the lumbar spine.

In more than 80% of patients with a slip of less than 40° the results are good. If the degree of slip is more than 60° osteoarthritis is likely to occur in more than 50% of the cases after 20 or 30 years.[21] If an osteotomy needs to be performed it must be considered that later in the patient's life an arthroplasty may become necessary. The risks of high-neck cuneiform and lateral osteotomies are such that these procedures are only indicated if the slip is more than 60°. The long-term results after the intertrochanteric osteotomy are good or satisfying in more than 80%.[20]

It is very important that consultation is held with the patient and his or her family as to their profession in life and the risk and benefits of the different types of treatment. If the degree of slip is more than 60° a physical job and heavy weight-lifting should not be considered.

SUMMARY

The simultaneous transfixation of the epiphysis with pins (K-wires) in SCFE is the treatment of choice for the

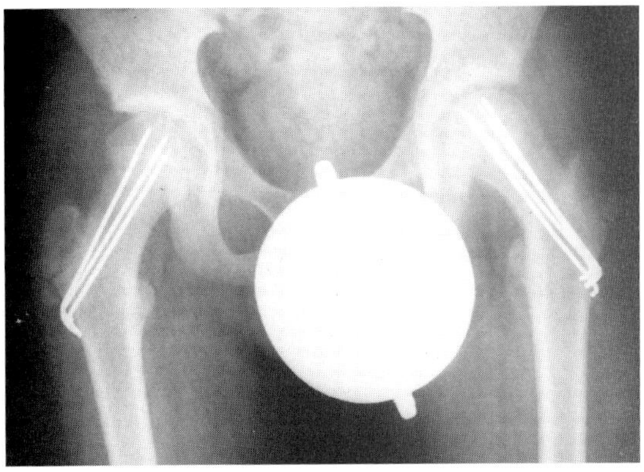
Fig. 8a

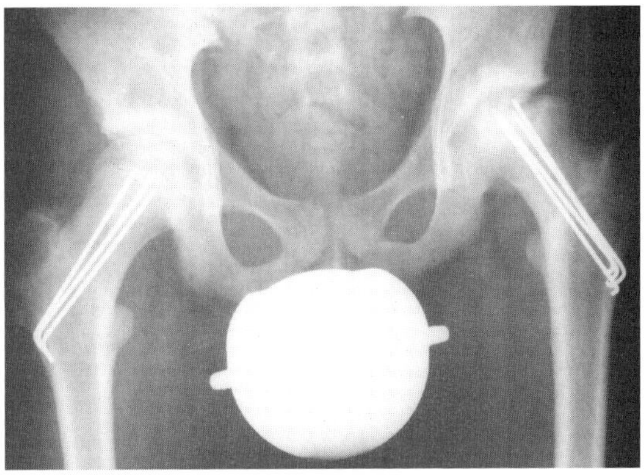
Fig. 8b

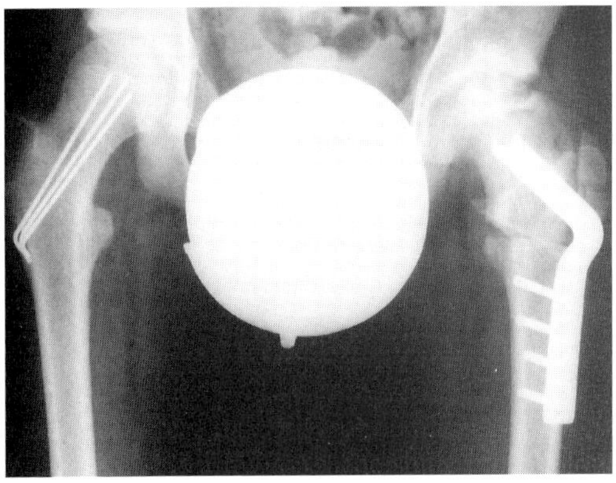
Fig. 8c

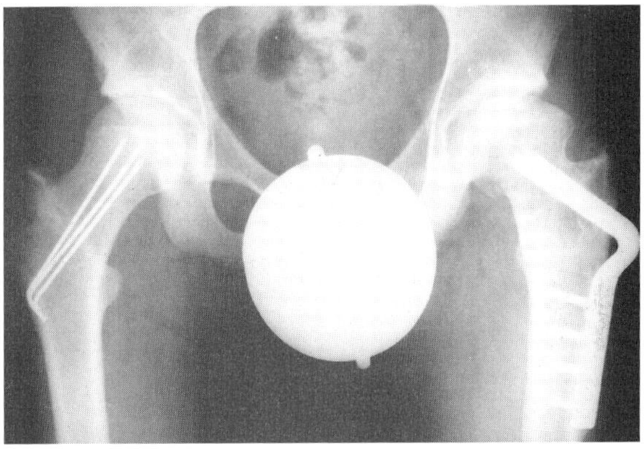
Fig. 8d

Development of avascular necrosis after operative treatment of an acute slipped capital epiphysis. Figure 8a – Postoperative radiograph after fixation by K-wires of a slipped capital epiphysis on the left side in an acute-on-chronic case and prophylactic pinning of the right side. Figure 8b – Eight months later there is development of a severe avascular necrosis without pin perforation. Figure 8c – Flexion-valgus-rotation-osteotomy of Imhäuser with a trochanteric osteotomy as a 'salvage procedure' was performed. Figure 8d – One year after the osteotomy there is clear evidence of remodelling of the femoral head and complete consolidation of the osteotomy. The patient is free from pain with good joint mobility and no limitation in walking distance. On the contralateral side further growth of the femoral neck is evident by the relation of the growth plate to the tip of the K-wires.

affected hip as well as for the contralateral undisplaced femoral epiphysis. The low rate of morbidity and the benefits of prophylactic surgical treatment of the non-affected opposite side in one stage should be appreciated. The pins should cross the growth plate until physeal closure to prevent relapses.

In the case of a severe slip, reduction by a cuneiform osteotomy and internal fixation, including resection of the anterior bump, may be necessary. The reported rate of complications such as AVN and chondrolysis with this procedure is relatively high. In a chronic slip which has united in a poor position an intertrochanteric osteotomy as advised by Imhäuser[19] may be indicated. The rate of avascular necrosis after this procedure is lower than with a closing-wedge osteotomy of the femoral neck but the degree of correction is limited and in severe slips with significant bumps a subcapital closing-wedge osteotomy allows for better correction. We will carefully follow the recently introduced technique of the surgical dislocation and corrective osteotomy in patients with severe SCFE.

REFERENCES

1. **Hagglund G, Hansson LI, Sandstrom S.** Familial slipped capital femoral epiphysis. *Acta Orthop Scand* 1986;57:510-2.
2. **Tachdjian MO.** *Pediatric orthopedics.* Philadelphia: Saunders, 1990.
3. **Krauspe R.** Epiphyseolysis capitis femoris. In: Tschauner C, ed. *Die Hüfte.* Stuttgart: Enke, 1997:135-41.
4. **Weiner D.** Pathogenesis of slipped capital femoral epiphysis: current concepts. *J Pediatr Orthop B* 1996;5:67-73.
5. **Stanitski CL, Woo R, Stanitski DF.** Femoral version in acute slipped capital femoral epiphysis. *J Pediatr Orthop B* 1996;5:74-6.
6. **Stanitski CL, Woo R, Stanitski DF.** Acetabular version in slipped capital femoral epiphysis: a prospective study. *J Pediatr Orthop B* 1996;5:77-9.
7. **Tönnis D, Heinecke A.** Decreased acetabular anteversion and femur neck anteversion cause pain and arthrosis: aetiology, diagnosis and therapy. *Z Orthop Ihre Grenzgeb* 1999;137:160-7.
8. **Loder RT, Richards BS, Shapiro PS, Reznick LR, Aronson DP.** Acute SCFE: the importance of physical stability. *J Bone Joint Surg [Am]* 1993;75-A:1134-40.
9. **Jerre R, Billing L, Hansson G, Karlsson J, Wallin J.** Bilaterality in slipped capital femoral epiphysis: importance of a reliable radiographic method. *J Pediatr Orthop B* 1996;5:80-4.
10. **Imhäuser G.** Pubertäre Hüfterkrankungen. In: Witt AN, Rettig H, Schlegel KF, eds. *Orthopädie in Praxis und Klinik 2.* Aufl, Stuttgart, New York: Thieme, 1987.
11. **Krauspe R, Eulert J.** Differentialdiagnose des Hüftschmerzes in Kindes-und Jugendalter. *Z Allg Med* 1991;67:1741-8.

12. **König A, Krauspe R, Fella E, Eulert J.** Die Entwicklung des koxalen Femurendes nach operativer Therapie der Epiphyseolysis capitis femoris. *Orthop Praxis* 1996;32:515-20.

13. **De Sanctis N, Gennaro di G, Pempinello C, Corte della S, Carannante G.** Is gentle manipulative reduction and percutaneous fixation with a single screw the best management of acute and acute on chronic slipped capital femoral epiphysis? A report of 70 patients. *J Pediatr Orthop B* 1996;5:90-5.

14. **Seller K, Raab P, Wild A, Krauspe R.** Risk-benefit analysis of prophylactic pinning in slipped capital femoral epiphysis (SCFE). *J Pediatr Orthop* 2001:in press.

15. **Rostoucher P, Bensahel H, Pennecot GF, Kaewpornsawan K, Mazda K.** Slipped capital femoral epiphysis: evaluation of different modes of treatment. *J Pediatr Orthop B* 1996;5:96-101.

16. **Hansson LI, Hägglund G, Ordeberg G.** Slipped capital femoral epiphysis in southern Sweden 1910-1982. *Acta Orthop Scand* 1987;226:58.

17. **Crawford AH.** Role of osteotomy in the treatment of slipped capital femoral epiphysis. *J Pediatr Orthop B* 1996;5:102-9.

18. **Jerre T.** A study in slipped capital femoral epiphysis. *Acta Orthop Scand* 1950:6.

19. **Imhäuser G.** Late results of Imhauser's osteotomy for slipped capital femoral epiphysis. *Z Orthop Ihre Grenzgeb* 1977;115:716-25.

20. **Schai PA, Exner GU, Hansch O.** Prevention of secondary coxarthrosis in slipped capital femoral epiphysis: a long-term follow-up study after corrective intertrochanteric osteotomy. *J Pediatr Orthop B* 1996;5:135-43.

21. **Davidson RS, Weitzel PP, Stanton RP, et al.** SCFE: a review of 432 cases: its treatment and complications. *Procs Shrine Surgeons Association Annual Meeting*, Philadelphia, 1994.

22. **Lubicky JP.** Chondrolysis and avascular necrosis: complications of slipped capital femoral epiphysis: a long-term follow-up study of 26 patients. *J Pediatr Orthop B* 1996;5:162-7.

23. **Maussen JP, Rozing PM, Obermann WR.** Intertrochanteric corrective osteotomy in slipped capital femoral epiphysis: a long-term follow-up study of 26 patients. *Clin Orthop* 1990;259:100-10.

THE FLAT FOOT DURING GROWTH

S. GIANNINI

From the University of Bologna, Bologna, Italy

Flat foot can be defined as a foot which during weight-bearing remains in persistent or prevalent pronation. The aetiology may be congenital, neuromuscular, ligamentous laxity, post-traumatic, infective, rheumatic, iatrogenic and idiopathic (flexible) (Fig. 1).

If the deformity is not carefully evaluated and treated during growth it results in chronic pronation and secondary deformities of the forefoot in the adult.[1,2] Accurate evaluation of a pronated foot during growth and proper diagnosis followed by correct treatment avoid future problems. Thus treatment during growth is prophylactic.[2-4]

NATURAL HISTORY

Flat foot is present in nearly all infants.[5-7] The arch appears after three to four years. At ten years of age 4% of children have flat feet,[6,8] a percentage which remains into adulthood. This pattern can be clearly observed on physical or radiological examination.[8,9] During growth, development of the arch occurs as a result of a combination of factors: loss of the thick subcutaneous fat present in the infant foot, an increase in muscle strength, a reduction in ligamentous laxity which normally occurs with growth and a change in bone configuration.[10]

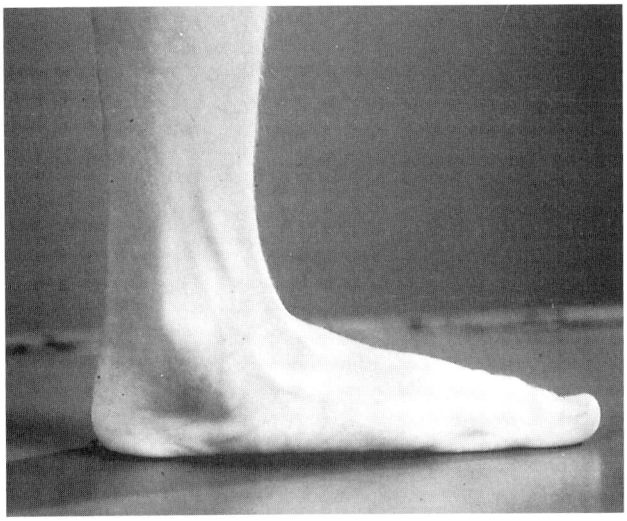

Fig. 1

Photograph showing the clinical aspect of flexible flat foot.

In our experience the flat foot which does not necessarily have a flat footprint, but which is functionally flat,[3,4] leads to chronic pronation sydrome of the foot.

Because the capsules, ligaments, tendons, vessels and nervous structures of the medial aspect of the foot are continuously stretched by the pronation of the foot, chronic pronation may lead to symptoms arising from the functional deficit and to altered working loads on the foot. Pain varies and depends on three main factors: flexibility, the extent of damage and functional deficit, and the work-load borne by the foot. This is why a juvenile flat foot, flexible and mobile, is seldom painful. Occasionally, after a long walk or run, young patients complain of tiredness and pain located on the plantar aspect or near the distal insertion of the tendon of tibialis posterior. Symptoms become more common as the child grows due to an increase in bodyweight, the start of activities which require standing for a long time or the beginning of playing sport. Usually, an associated genu valgum increases the symptoms. Sometimes, a fixed deformity develops as a consequence of the adaptation of tissues in the foot.

Pain and secondary arthritis follow and increase with the passage of time. In women the typical changes of the post-menopausal hormonal pattern aggravate the problems of flat foot. Inflammatory degenerative changes of the medial tendon, dysfunction of the tibial posterior tendon,[1] tarsal tunnel syndrome plantalgia by protrusion of the talus and degenerative changes in the spring ligament,[11] heel pain due to stretching of the plantar fascia, and lateral pain due to impingement between the talus, the calcaneus and lateral malleolus are typical consequences.

Chronic pronation of the hindfoot causes secondary metatarsalgia and deformities of the forefoot due to biomechanical imbalance. During growth these deformities are rare. A mild and flexible hallux valgus may sometimes be present. With time this becomes increasingly fixed and the functional deficit of the first ray determines the secondary deformity of the remaining forefoot.

An accurate evaluation of the flat foot during growth and a proper diagnosis followed by correct treatment will avoid the aforementioned problems. Correct assessment prevents incorrect treatment or overtreatment, but all functional flat feet which may lead to secondary painful deformities can be treated.

Clinical and radiological examination should be supported by a functional evaluation in order to make the correct diagnosis.

DIAGNOSIS

When assessing patients with flat foot, it is important to consider whether a member of the family has the same deformity and if this is, or has ever been, symptomatic.

Clinical examination. This should consist of a general assessment of the patient as well as an evaluation of the foot and footwear. The examination should determine any general disease or ligamentous laxity.[10] If present, anteversion of the femoral neck, genu varum, valgus or recurvatum and tibial malrotation can all contribute to pronation of the foot.

An assessment of the walking pattern by gait analysis should aim to determine if the normal phases take place or if there is a collapse in the hindfoot on contact with the ground, marked tibial malrotation, an early heel lift or a decrease in the push-off phase.

Some functional tests are particularly indicated. In a functional flat foot poor alignment can be observed with the heel remaining in valgus when the patient is asked to stand on tip-toe. Walking on the heel is difficult because of the limited dorsiflexion of the ankle due to secondary contracture of the triceps. Passive dorsiflexion of the hallux does not completely restore the plantar arch.[11] The patient has difficulty in balancing and standing on one leg. Manual realignment of the relationship between the talus and calcaneus with the hindfoot in a neutral position[7] causes limitation of dorsiflexion of the foot and the disappearance of the rotational secondary defects in the limb.[2,4,12-14]

Functional anlaysis. In doubtful cases gait analysis can be an important tool for validating clinical tests, and can be used for screening, diagnosis, the choice of treatment and verification.

At the Movement Analysis Laboratory of the Rizzoli Institute we have analysed a group of 24 children with flat feet. There were 16 boys and 8 girls with a mean age of 11.6 years (8 to 16).

Functional evaluation of gait was performed using the ELITE stereophotogrammetric system for the acquisition of kinematic variables of the lower limb and two dynamometric platforms for foot-ground reaction forces. Kinematic and kinetic analysis of data was made according to the Calibrated Anatomical System Technique (CAST). The activity of the muscles of the lower limb during walking was examined by means of surface electromyography. The gait pattern was recorded during three consecutive trials at self-paced velocity. The patients' data were compared with the results from a control population of healthy subjects matched for gender and age. In order to extract synthetic and discriminating features of flat foot from the data for ground reaction forces (GRF), a technique of pattern recognition was applied.[15] In this procedure only a limited number of the principal component of suitable linear combinations of the data is needed to represent and classify the GRF gait patterns, allowing classification of flat foot and its control by means of a functional score. The functional score was then correlated with the most common clinical and radiological measurements used in the diagnosis of flat foot to determine the relevance of such parameters when functionally impaired flat foot might be detected by clinical diagnosis alone.

The gait pattern of flat foot was found to be characterised by typical kinematic, kinetic and EMG abnormalities. There is a tendency for the foot to land with the ankle dorsiflexed so that plantar flexion during toe-off is decreased. An eversion joint moment is present throughout the stance phase. In most patients premature activation of gastrosoleus and peroneus longus was present at heel-strike.

The technique of pattern recognition[15] for the analysis of GRF enabled us to identify crucial parameters discriminating the flat from the normal foot. Most features determining flat with regard to the three-force components were concentrated in the loading-response phase and in the propulsive phase. On the bases of these selected features, this technique has considerable ability to distinguish flat foot with an error of misclassification of less than 7%.

The functional score obtained by means of pattern recognition analysis was significantly correlated with the following clinical measurements: heel valgus, subtalar range of pronation/supination, ankle dorsiflexion and the ability to correct the deformity during functional tests. It also correlated with talonavicular lateral radiographic alignment. A less significant correlation was found with the resting footprint.

Radiological examination. Weight-bearing anteroposterior and lateral radiographs are generally sufficient to assess flat foot, both with regard to measuring the characteristic angles of curvature and to revealing skeletal alterations, the presence of an accessory navicular bone and other congenital defects. Oblique and Harry's views can identify coalition (Figs 2 and 3) which is demonstrated better by CT. The most reproducible angle is the talometatarsal angle in the lateral view, formed by the axis passing through the neck of the talus and that of the first metatasal.[16] If the angle is zero the foot is normal. If the apex of this angle is pointing plantarwards, it means that the arch has collapsed and as the deformity increases, the angle becomes wider. The break in the line can be located in the talonavicular and navicular-cuneiform or both joints, depending on the type of flat foot (Fig. 4). In the anteroposterior view a talocalcaneal angle can be seen, formed by the talus and the calcaneal axis: in the flat foot this angle is over 35° (Fig. 5).

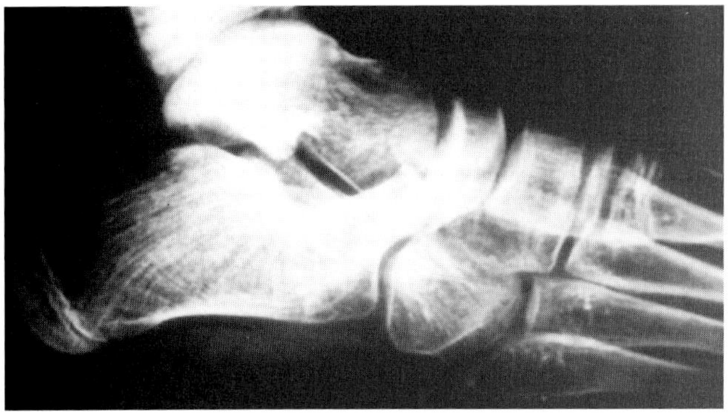

Fig. 2

An oblique radiograph showing calcaneonavicular coalition.

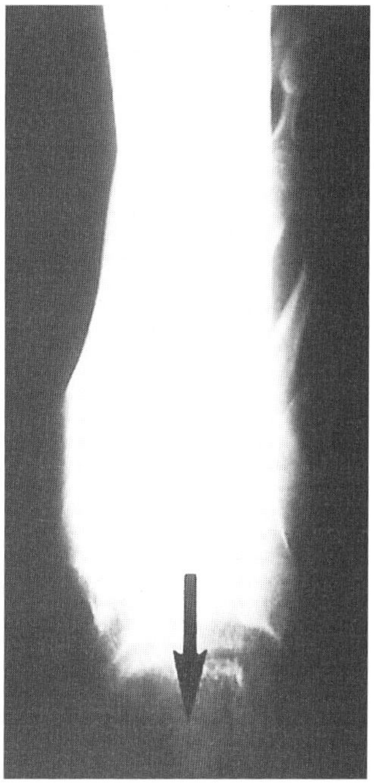

Fig. 3

Harry's view shows talocalcaneal coalition.

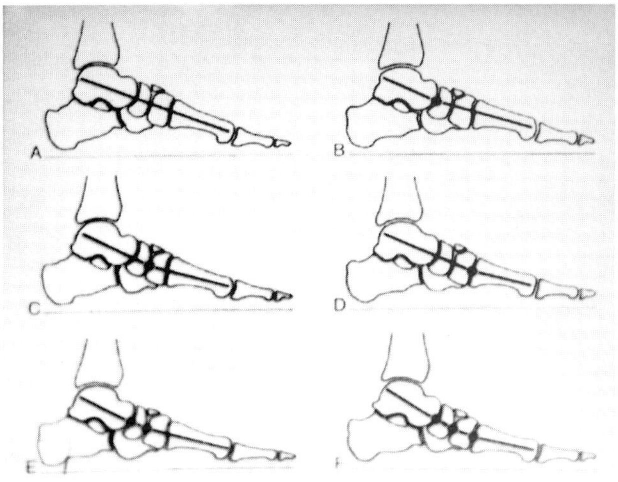

Fig. 4

Diagrams showing Meary's line (see text).

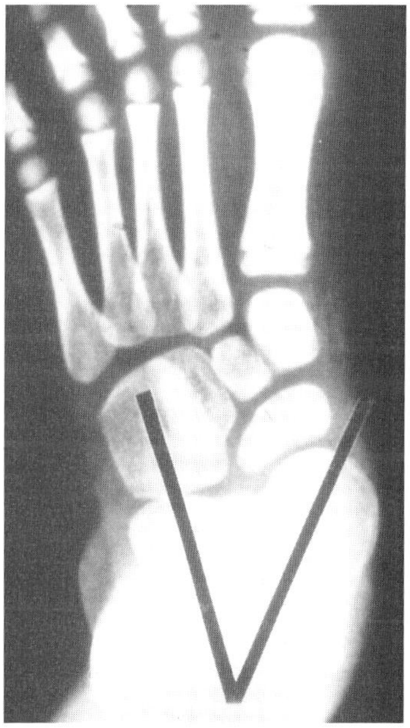

Fig. 5

Radiograph showing the talocalcaneal angle.

These measurements allow only the static morphology of the foot to be examined and do not represent an indication for surgical treatment.

TREATMENT

In agreement with most authors,[12,13,17,18-21] we think that most flat feet, being only morphologically flat, should not be treated. We do maintain, however, that about 10% of functionally flat feet, i.e. feet with excessive pronation which can be painful, or if painless may lead to future problems, should be treated. Treatment may be operative or conservative.

Conservative. This includes rehabilitation and the use of inserts and special footwear. Isolated rehabilitation, consisting of exercises for strengthening the extrinsic and intrinsic muscles, walking on tip-toe, picking up pencils with toes, electrostimulation and heelcord stretching exercises, has not proved to be very effective.

There is general scepticism concerning the use of plantar inserts and special footwear, indicated only in cases of flexible flat foot.[19-22] Bleck and Berzins,[23] and Bleck[24] and Bordelon[25] are in favour of conservative treatment with inserts. Our experience has shown that conservative treatment which is well carried out can lead to good results in 60% of cases. Treatment should not begin before four years of age.[6-8] Only then does the plantar arch start to appear. It should be aimed at restoring the normal talocalcaneal rela-

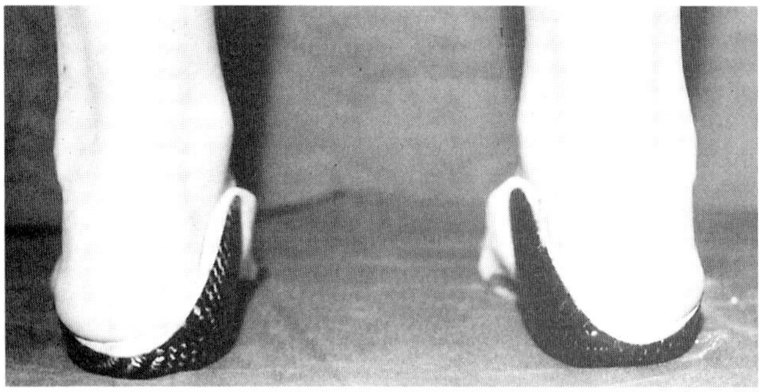

Fig. 6

Photograph showing the custom-made inserts to restore the normal talocalcaneal relationship and to hold the correct position of the hindfoot.

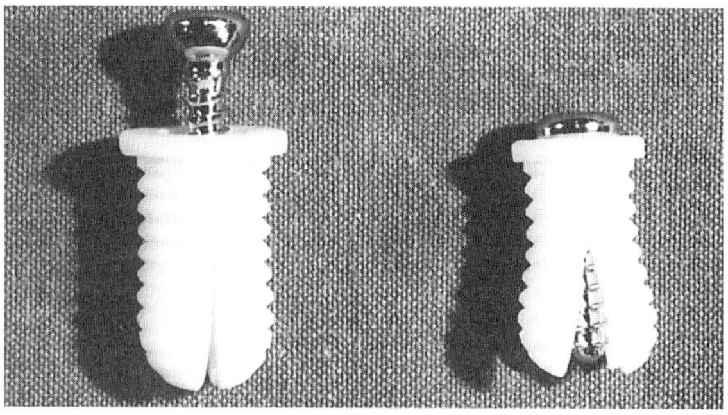

Fig. 7

Photograph showing the first type of implant designed in 1981.

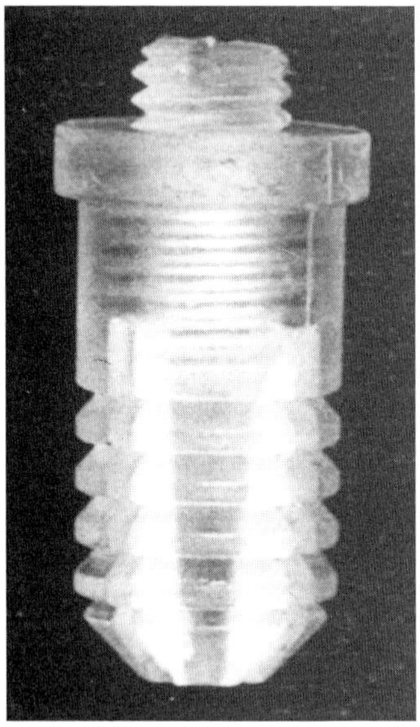

Fig. 8

Photograph showing the new type of bioresorbable implant designed in 1991.

tionship and at holding it in the correct position to avoid excessive pronation (Fig. 6). Only with a corrected stable hindfoot can remodelling of the skeletal structures take place during the subsequent period of growth. In order to achieve correction, the insert should be constructed to stabilise the hindfoot with a posterior shell made of carbon fibre or polyethylene which is light but stiff. The construction should be custom-made. The insert should be worn all day and treatment should last for at least two years since morphogenesis is a slow process.

Generally, treatment continues until the foot is functionally compensated. If there is no effect after two to three years, it can be justifiably abandoned, otherwise it should be continued up to the age of ten years. If treatment has been abandoned or if the results are not satisfactory, operative treatment will be required.

Operative. The aim of surgery is to restore the physiological alignment between the talus and calcaneus and to maintain it for the time that the bones of the foot remodel during the subsequent period of growth. Thus, definitive[26] or temporary[27,28] subtalar fusion is commonly carried out. Arthrodesis with bone graft[29-33] may be performed, but this leads to subtalar stiffness or recurrence of the deformity caused by resorption of the graft. Subtalar arthrodesis may also be carried out using a screw[34,35] but frequent overcorrection, osteolysis around the screw and particularly its breakage have made modifications to the approach[34] and design[34,36,37] necessary. A medial procedure with tightening of the tendon of tibialis posterior, combined or not with tenodesis of tibialis anterior or with retention of the calcaneonavicular ligament,[38] if performed alone, does not ensure longstanding stability of the correction. Calcaneal osteotomy with medialisation of the posterior tuberosity,[39] even if it can rebalance the load of the hindfoot, does not correct the deformity by taking into account the pathology. Lengthening of the lateral column[40] causes subluxation of the subtalar anterior articular facets and an intra-articular fracture, which, in one-third of the cases, is because the anterior and medial facets are not divided. Arthrodesis of the subtalar joint may also be performed using various types of endo-orthotic implant.[32,41]

In 1981 we designed an implant made of a hollow cylinder of Teflon with a small saddle proximally. It is partially divided longitudinally in order to provide four expansible fins. The fins are made to expand by a screw inserted into the device after its insertion into the sinus tarsi (Fig. 7). To avoid further surgery for removal of the implant, since 1991 we have been using the same device made of a bioreabsorbable material (poly-L-lactic acid)[14,42] (Fig. 8).

A 1 cm incision is made over the sinus tarsi. With a pair of curved round-headed scissors the extensor retinaculum is incised just in front of the cuboid bone. The instrumentation for the insertion of both devices is very simple and consists of a handle, three blunt rods of different diameter (6, 8, 10 mm), one positioner and one screwdriver.[2]

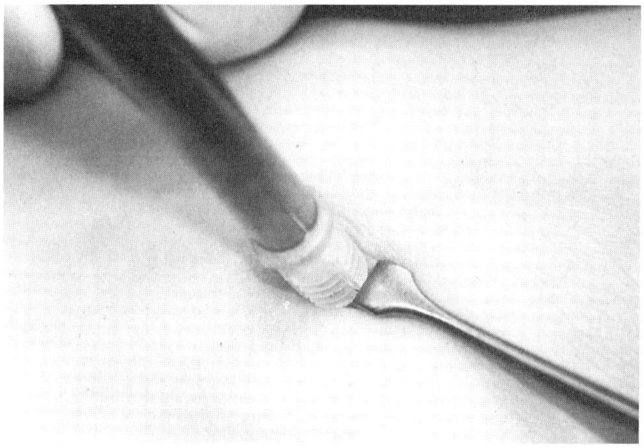

Fig. 9

Photograph showing the insertion of the implant.

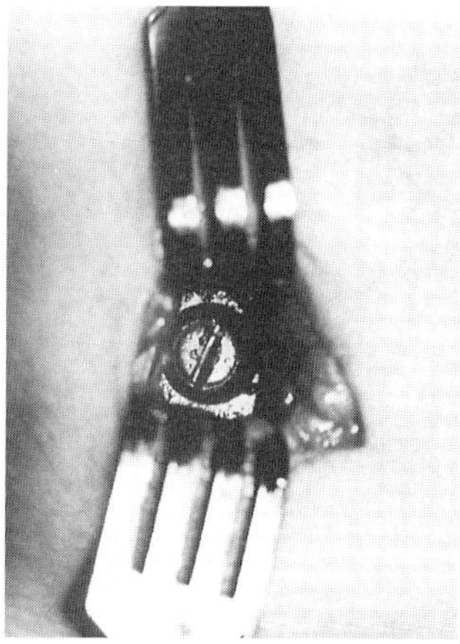

Fig. 10

Photograph showing that the inserted screw causes the fins of the implant to open.

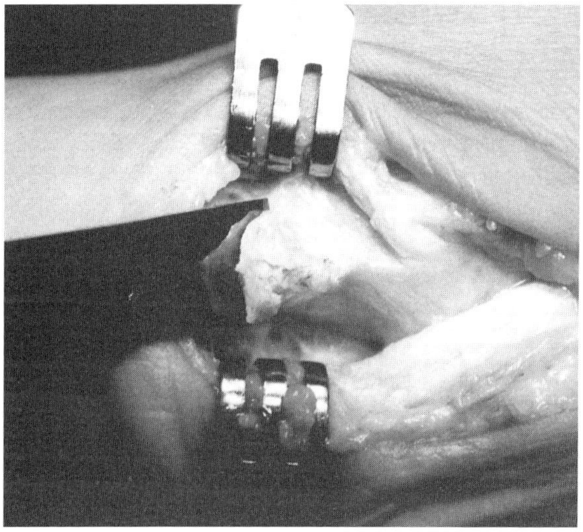

Fig. 11

Photograph showing the resection of the accessory bone or the prominence of the navicular bone.

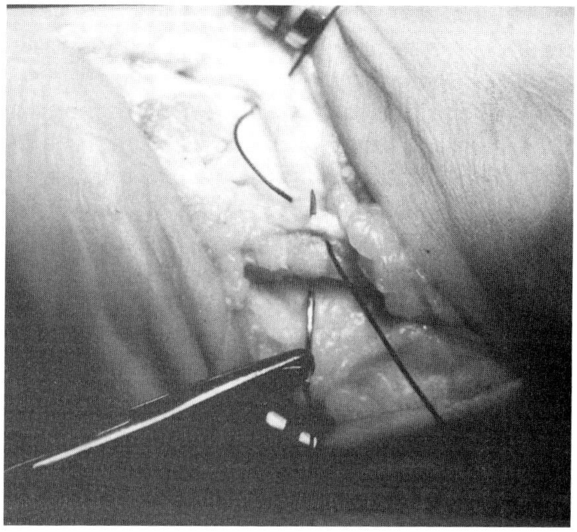

Fig. 12

Photograph showing tightening of the tendon of tibialis posterior (see text).

A number 6 blunt rod is introduced behind the cervical ligament. Blunt rods of increasing size (8, 10 mm) are inserted until correction is obtained. The diameter of the last rod used, usually 8 mm, indicates the correct size of implant required which is inserted with an appropriate positioner (Fig. 9). The screw is then introduced causing the fins of the implant to open and allowing its stable fixation in the sinus tarsi (Fig. 10). The extensor retinaculum is repaired with one 2.0 stitch, and, the skin is sutured with another single stitch.

Additional procedures. Usually the introduction of the implant is the only surgical procedure required.[2,14,42] Percutaneous lengthening of tendo Achillis with alternated hemi-incisions may be necessary only if the foot fails to reach 90° dorsiflexion after the implant has been inserted. A medial surgical procedure[34] is indicated only if a painful os tibialis is present, if there is a painful prominence of the navicular, or if the cuneonavicular joint is displaced by more than 15° to the talonavicular line. A 4 cm incision is made across the prominence of the navicular. The tendon of tibialis posterior is detached from the tubercle of the navicular and the periosteum is elevated. The tendon is then retracted plantarwards and the accessory bone, if present, or the prominence of the navicular bone is removed (Fig. 11). The plantar aspect of the navicular is decorticated. A number 2.0 resorbable suture is passed through the dorsal periosteum at the level of the talonavicular joint and a Bunnell type suture[43] is introduced through the tibialis posterior tendon, 2 cm proximal to its detached insertion, and then through the navicular bone from the proximoinferior to the distal superior edge. Thus, by tightening the suture the tendon is tightened (Fig. 12), the suture is rein-

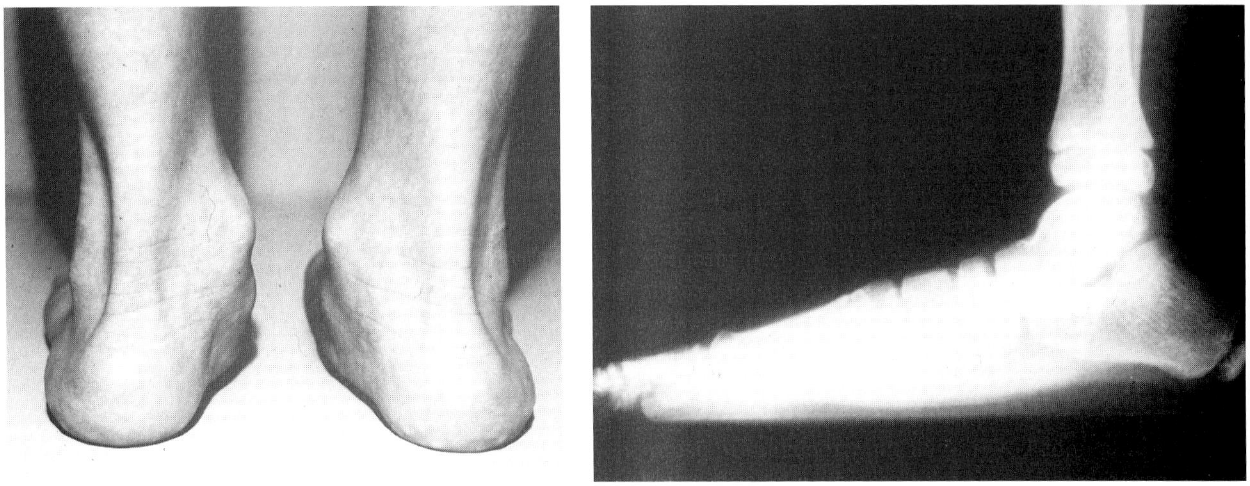

Fig. 13a

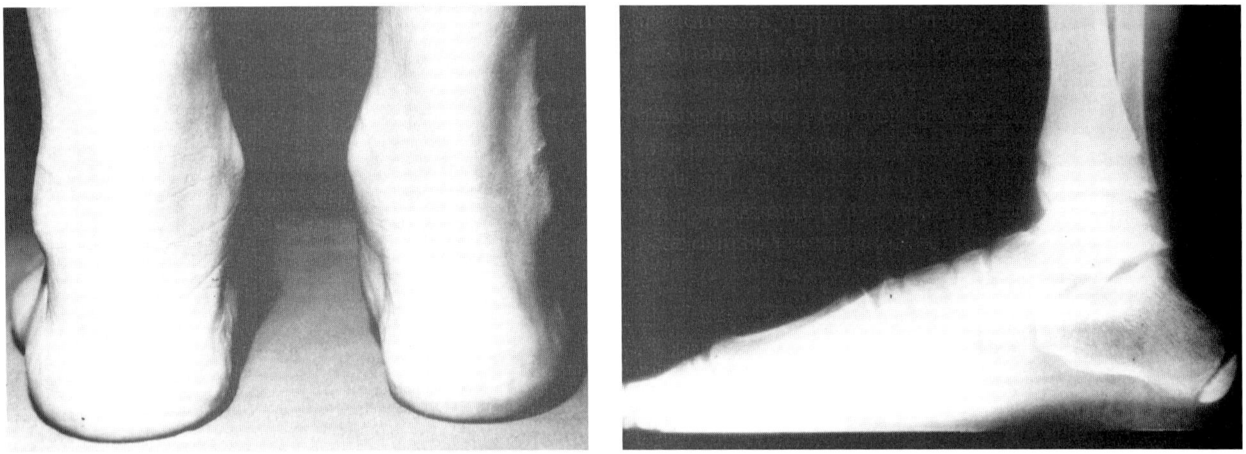

Fig. 13b

Photographs and radiographs of a flexible flat foot a) before operative treatment and b) after five years.

forced by two more stitches and the tendon sheath is closed. Finally, the skin is sutured.

Postoperative treatment. A weight-bearing short-leg cast is worn for two weeks to allow early walking without pain when only the insertion of the implant is performed. With one or both additional procedures a short-leg cast is worn for five weeks, in three without weight-bearing and in the last two with walking. After the cast has been removed, the wearing of normal shoes, swimming and bicycling are allowed.

Indications and contraindications. Surgical treatment is indicated only in functionally flat feet in patients aged between 8 and 12 years. The bioreabsorable implant is indicated in the flexible flat foot in children from 8 to 12 years of age when symptomatic or even asymptomatic if the functional deficit is well established by clinical examination or, in unclear cases, confirmed by gait analysis. Another indication for the endorthotic implant is the foot with a vertical talus. In such severe flat foot it is necessary to free all soft tissues which prevent the reduction of the talonavicular joint. The implant prevents the talus from becoming vertical again.[14] In addition, a flat foot with a calcaneonavicular or a talocalcaneal coalition can be corrected by introducing the implant after the bar has been resected.[42]

Neurological flat foot, or flat foot due to a severe ligamentous laxity, is better treated by a Grice procedure.[26] No muscular rebalance of the foot during growth should be expected in these patients. An iatrogenic flat foot with overcorrection of a club foot should be corrected by a Grice procedure or by a calcaneal osteotomy in order to obtain proper alignment of the hindfoot.[44]

RESULTS

In the first 50 cases using the non-resorbable implant we had good results in 94%.[14] In two there was slight overcorrection and in one recurrence because the patient was too young at seven years of age. The only disadvantage is that removal of the implant is recommended after one year.

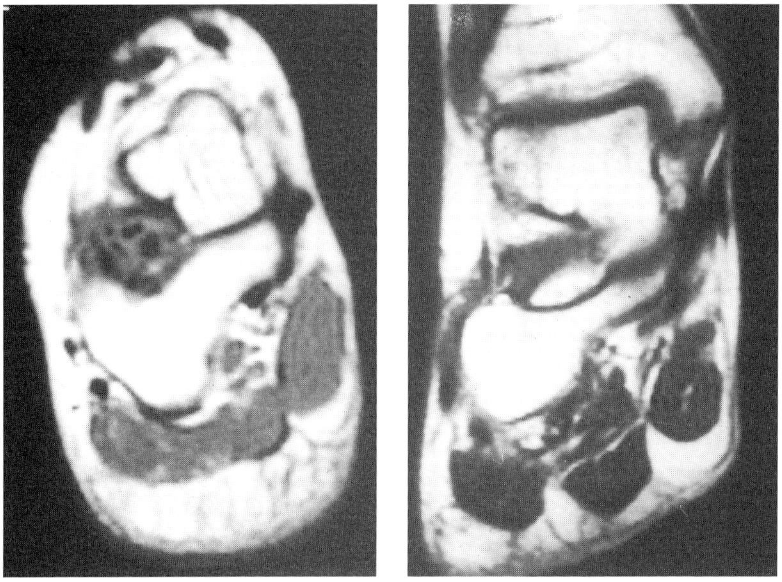

Fig. 14a Fig. 14b

MRI at a) three and b) five years after correction by a bioreabsorbable implant.

The first 20 flat feet treated by the bioresorbable implant had a minimum follow-up of 7 years and 8 months. All were evaluated taking into account the morphology, pain, function, return to sports activity and patient satisfaction (Fig. 13).

The morphological aspect of the foot was normal. There was full movement in all, except for the four patients with tarsal coalition, who had a limitation of one-third of supination. From a functional point of view, data regarding pre-treatment and post-treatment gait analyses provided evidence of the effectiveness of treatment with normalisation of the parameters of gait. All the patients returned to their previous activity including even the seven who played sports before operation.

We did not observe muscular contracture of the foot secondary to irritation of the structures of the sinus tarsi. All patients were satisfied with the results.

MRI carried out from three months to five years after surgery did not reveal sinus formation or ligamentous or bony changes within the sinus tarsi.

Modification of the implant becomes evident at six months. After three years it is almost completely resorbed and only asymptomatic oedema in the sinus tarsi can be seen. After five years it is completely resorbed (Fig. 14).

CONCLUSIONS

Flat foot is one of the most common disorders seen by the orthopaedic surgeon. The deformity is first recognised by the child's mother or by a paediatrician. The diagnosis, however, is not easy.

Flat foot does not usually cause problems if it is not associated with functional impairment. If this judgement is followed, overtreatment is avoided as is the risk of not treating flat feet which, in our experience, will prove to be the cause of chronic pronation. Because the soft tissues of the medial aspect of the foot, capsules, ligaments, tendons, vessels and nervous structures are continuously stretched, chronic pronation may lead to complaints caused by the functional deficit and to the altered working load of the foot. Clinical and radiological examination should be supported by a functional evaluation in order to make a correct diagnosis.

Gait analysis and particularly the GRF pattern, was found to give good evaluation of forefoot function. The correlations found between the functional score and clinical tests support the relevance of clinical and functional-related measurements.

Treatment can be conservative or surgical. The former is indicated in patients aged between four and eight years and the latter in older patients. A fundamental requirement of surgical treatment is to obtain a stable and complete restoration of the normal relationship between the talus and the calcaneus, which must be maintained for enough time to allow remodelling of the medial soft tissues and bone, with subsequent regrowth. Several techniques have been described but they do have their disadvantages.

We have found that the most simple and effective procedure is the introduction of the expanding implant, which in our experience has been shown to achieve stable correction and to maintain subtalar movement. It is a quick and simple technique, which respects the structures of the foot, has a very low rate of complications and avoids the need for secondary surgery for the removal of the implant.

REFERENCES

1. **Dyal CM, Feder J, Deland JT, Thompson FH.** Pes planus in patients with posterior tibial tendon insufficiency: asymptomatic versus symptomatic foot. *Foot Ankle Int* 1997;18:85-8.
2. **Giannini S.** Operative treatment of the flat foot: why and how. *Foot Ankle Int* 1998;19:52-8.

3. **Giannini S, Catani F, Ceccarelli F, Girolami M, Benedetti G.** Kinematic and isokinetic evaluation of patients with flat foot. *Ital J Orthop Traumatol* 1992;18:241-51.

4. **Rose GK, Welton EA, Marshall T.** The diagnosis of flat foot in the child. *J Bone Joint Surg [Br]* 1985;67-B:71-8.

5. **Gould N, Moreland M, Alvarez R, Trevino S, Fenwick J.** Development of the child's arch. *Foot Ankle* 1989;9:241-5.

6. **Morley AJM.** Knock-knee in children. *Br Med J* 1957;2:976-9.

7. **Staheli LT, Chew DE, Corbett M.** The longitudinal arch: a survey of eight hundred and eighty-two feet in normal children and adults. *J Bone Joint Surg [Am]* 1987;69-A:426-8.

8. **Ozonoff MB.** Anatomy and development of the foot. In: *Pediatric orthopaedic radiology.* Philadelphia: W B Saunders, 1979:300.

9. **Vanderwilde R, Staheli LT, Chew DE, Malagon V.** Measurements on radiographs of the foot in normal infants and children. *J Bone Joint Surg [Am]* 1988;70-A:407-15.

10. **Carter C, Wilkinson JA.** Persistent joint laxity and congenital dislocation of the hip. *J Bone Joint Surg [Br]* 1964;46-B:40-5.

11. **Jack EA.** Naviculo-cuneiform fusion in the treatment of flat foot. *J Bone Joint Surg [Br]* 1953;35-B:75-82.

12. **Bordelon RL.** Hypermobile flat foot in children: comprehension, evaluation and treatment. *Clin Orthop* 1983;181:7-14.

13. **DeRosa GP.** Flexible flatfoot. In: Gould. *Operative foot surgery.* Philadelphia: W B Saunders, 1994:834-57.

14. **Giannini S, Girolami M, Ceccarelli F.** The surgical treatment of infantile flat feet: a new expanding endo-orthotic implant. *Ital J Orthop Traumatol* 1985;9:315-22.

15. **Bertani A, Cappello A, Benedetti MG, Simoncini L, Catani F.** Flat foot functional evaluation using pattern recognition of ground reaction data. *Clin Biomech* 1999;14:484-93.

16. **Meary R.** On the measurement of the angle between the talus and the first metatarsal: symposium: LePid Creux Essential. *Rev Chir Orthop* 1967;53:389.

17. **Regnauld B.** *The foot.* Berlin: Springer Verlag, 1986:173-224.

18. **Viladot A.** Surgical treatment of the child's flat foot. *Clin Orthop* 1992;283:34-8.

19. **Penneau K, Lutter LD, Winter RB.** Pes planus: radiographic changes with foot orthoses and shoes. *Foot Ankle* 1982;2:299-303.

20. **Rao UB, Joseph B.** The influence of footwear on the prevalence of flatfoot: a survey of 2300 children. *J Bone Joint Surg [Br]* 1992;74-B:525-7.

21. **Sachithanandam V, Joseph B.** The influence of footwear on the prevalence of flat foot: a survey of 1846 skeletally mature persons. *J Bone Joint Surg [Br]* 1995;77-B:254-7.

22. **Sin-Fook L, Hodgson AR.** A comparison of foot forms among the non-shoe and shoe-wearing Chinese population. *J Bone Joint Surg [Am]* 1958;40-A:1058-62.

23. **Bleck EE, Berzins UJ.** Conservative management of pes valgus with plantar flexed talus, flexible. *Clin Orthop* 1977;122:85-94.

24. **Bleck EE.** The shoeing of children: sham or science? *Dev Med Child Neurol* 1971;13:188-95.

25. **Bordelon RL.** Correction of hypermobile flat foot in children by moulded insert. *Foot Ankle* 1980;1:143-50.

26. **Grice DS.** An extra-articular arthrodesis of the subastragalar joint for correction of paralytic flat feet in children. *J Bone Joint Surg [Am]* 1952;34-A:927-40.

27. **Judet J.** Indications for technics of the 'cavelier' operation. *Rev Chir Orthop Reparatrice Appar Mot* 1977;63:780-1.

28. **Lelièvre J, Lelièvre J-F.** *Manuale du patologia del piede.* Ed. Masson. Milano, 1985. Parte quink. cap 1; 425-444.

29. **Ombredanne L.** *Précis Clinique et Opératoire de chirurgie infantile.* Paris: Ed Masson, 1949.

30. **Richardson Greer E. Pesplanus** In: Crenshaw AH, ed. *Campbell's operative orthopaedics.* Vol 4. 8th ed. St Louis, etc:CV Mosby Year Book; 2693-2728.

31. **Voutey H.** *Manual de chirurgie orthopoedique et de reeducation du pied.* Paris: Ed Masson, 1978.

32. **Viladot A.** *Nouvelle technique chirurgicale de traitement du pied plat valgus.* Podologie, 1965:207-8.

33. **Dal Monte A, et al.** Risultati del trattamento chirurgico del piede piatto valgo essenziale mediante intervento di Grice, plastica del legamento glenoideo ed anteposizione del tibiale posteriore (90 osservazioni). *Giornale Italiano di Ortopedia e Traumatologia* 1979;5:23-38.

34. **Nogarin L, Bragantini A, Magnan B, Molinaroli F.** Calcaneo-stop: modifiche all'endortesi ed alla via chirurgica. *Chirurgia del Piede* 1987;11:57-60.

35. **Buruturan JM.** El calcaneo-stop para lo tratamiento del valgo de talon infantile. *Chiururgia del Piede* 1979;3:319-22.

36. **Castaman E.** L'intervento di calcaneo-stop nel piede piatto valgo. *Chirurgia del Piede* 1985;9:319-29.

37. **Pisani G.** La chirurgie du pied calcaneo valgus evolutif de l'enfant. *Chirurgia del Piede* 1979;3:169.

38. **Miller OL.** A plastic flat foot operation. *J Bone Joint Surg* 1927;9:84-91.

39. **Koutsogiannis E.** Treatment of mobile flat foot by displacement osteotomy of the calcaneus. *J Bone Joint Surg [Br]* 1971;53-B:96-100.

40. **Mosca VS.** Calcaneal lengthening for valgus deformity of the hind-foot. *J Bone Joint Surg [Am]* 1995;77-A:500-12.

41. **Valenti V.** Artrorisi sottoastragalica con protesi acrilica nel trattamento del piede piatto valgo dell'infanzia. *Minerva Ortopedica* 1976;27:309-14.

42. **Giannini S, Ceccarelli F, Mosca M.** Surgical treatment of flat foot by endo-orthotic implant. In: Epeldegui T, ed. *Flat foot and forefoot deformity.* Madrid: A Madrid Vincente Ediciones, 1995.

43. **Bunnell S.** *Atlante di chirurgia della mano.* In: Tsuge K, ed. Milano: McGraw-Hill Italia, 1988.

44. **Giannini S, Ceccarelli F, Girolami M, Marcacci M, Coppola G.** Il valgismo del retropiede dopo interventi di liberazione postero-mediale per piede torto congenito. *Chirurgia del Piede* 1988;12:5-7.

BIOLOGICAL RECONSTRUCTION AFTER TUMOUR RESECTION

W. WINKELMANN

From the University Hospital, Münster, Germany

Intralesional resection of a tumour leaves a bony defect. After a wide or radical resection both bony and soft-tissue defects remain. The defect may be reconstructed with foreign material such as bone cement, polyethylene or metal spacers or a special prosthesis, but biological reconstruction may be undertaken using parts of the extremities or other body tissue.

ADVANTAGES OF BIOLOGICAL RECONSTRUCTION

1) All the tissue used can be reattached to the local vascular supply.
2) A suitable level of circulating antibiotic can be established which increases the resistance of the graft to infection.
3) If autograft bone breaks, it will heal by the physiological formation of callus (see Fig. 13d).
4) Autograft bone may remodel to accommodate to a change of loading (see Fig. 4d).
5) Under load bone increases in density and circumference. This can be achieved better and faster with vascularised bone transplants (see Fig. 2d).
6) The transplanted bones can be lengthened or shortened using conventional methods.
7) Soft tissues (e.g. tendons, muscles) can reattach on to the transplanted bone. The physiological origin and insertion improve the function.
8) Transplantation of a physis, such as the proximal fibula, may allow further growth in length.
9) A joint may adjust in response to fresh loading stress (see Fig. 14).
10) Incorporated bones do not act as foreign bodies and are therefore not rejected.
11) Incorporated bones cannot loosen.

EXAMPLES OF BIOLOGICAL RECONSTRUCTION

Bony reconstruction is not necessary after resection of the scapula, clavicle, fibula or rib or similar expendable bones (Fig. 1).

Autologous cancellous or corticocancellous bone transplants may incorporate and remodel as described by Axhausen.[1] Homologous cancellous bone will not be converted as quickly or as completely as autologous bone, but it can be used for the reconstruction of defects which are not too large or heavily loaded.

The fibula is the most frequently used autologous cortical graft for reconstruction of defects. Bony ingrowth and load-dependent hypertrophy appear earlier and are better using the vascularised fibular graft. It is suitable by itself for the reconstruction of diaphyseal defects of the humerus (Fig. 2), radius and ulna or for substitution of the metacarpals or metatarsals.

If a vascularised transplanted fibula will not suffice as the only weight-bearing bone, an additional halfshell allograft may be used for further support. Capanna, Biagini and Casdei[2] and Capanna et al[3] found that the combined grafts healed without significant complications in the initial period.

The proximal fibula including the physis may be used as an autologous vascularised osteochondral graft. With its joint surface it can be used as a substitute for the distal radius or proximal humerus. Manfrini et al[4] have described this technique for substitution of the femoral head.

If the transplantation bed is sufficient, with an intact periosteum, a non-vascularised fibular graft may also show good incorporation and hypertrophy (Fig. 3).

Local vascular-supplied bone grafts are used for arthrodesis of the knee, wrist or ankle. A special method for replacement of the proximal humerus is the clavicula pro humero operation, described by Winkelmann.[5] The clavicle, retaining its vascular supply, is folded down around the acromioclavicular joint and fused to the remaining humerus using a special plate (Fig. 4).

Resection of pelvic tumours leads to substantial defects of both bone and soft tissue, as classified by Enneking et al[6] (Fig. 5).

After resection of tumours of the iliac bone (P1) which have invaded the lateral part of the sacrum, (P14) stabilisation of the pelvic ring can be achieved by transplantation of a double fibular graft or an allograft. For reconstruction of defects after resection of tumours of the upper part of the iliac bone and/or the lateral part up to the hemisacrum, a

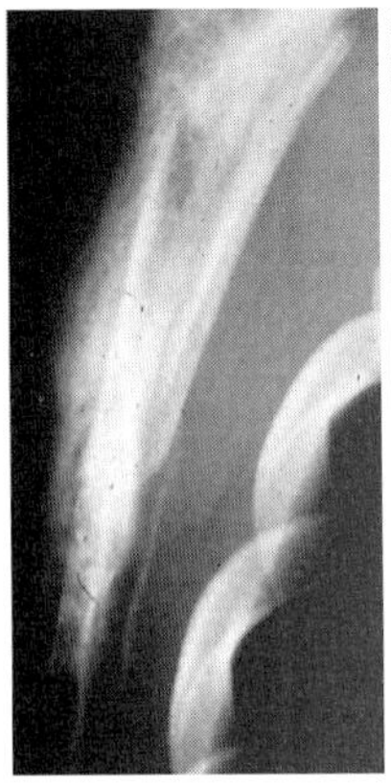

Fig. 1a

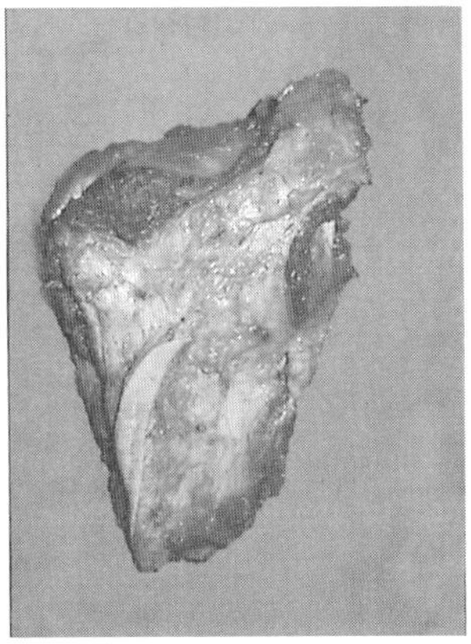

Fig. 1b

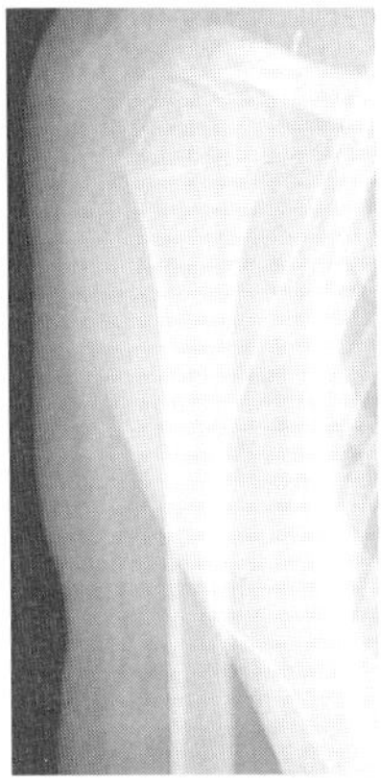

Fig. 1c

Bony reconstruction is not required after total resection of the scapula. Figure 1a – Radiograph of a seven-year-old boy with Ewing's sarcoma of the right scapula. Figure 1b – Surgical specimen. Figure 1c – Radiograph showing fixation of the humerus using Ollier's technique. Figure 1d – Photographs showing function two years after surgery.

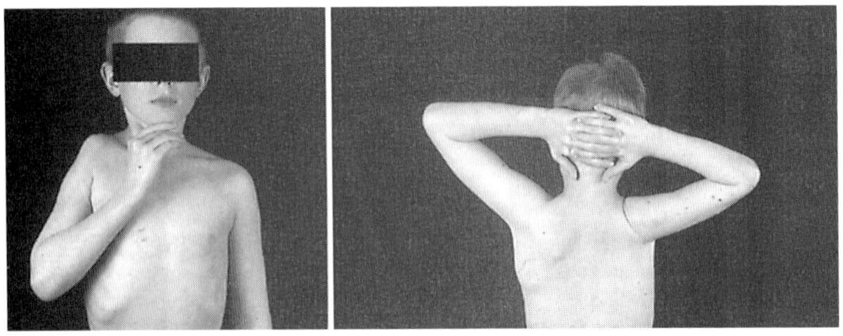

Fig. 1d

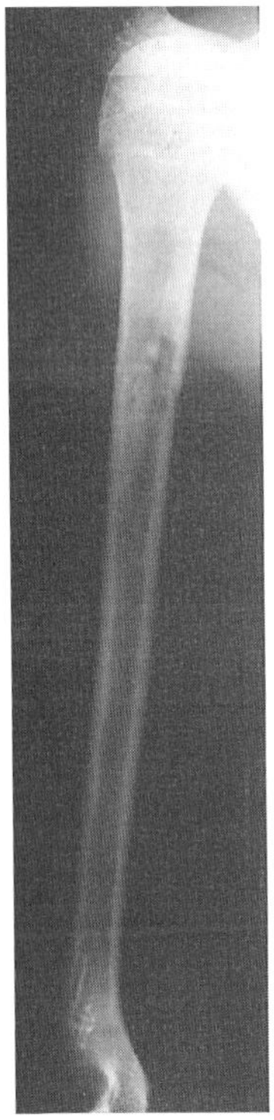

Fig. 2a

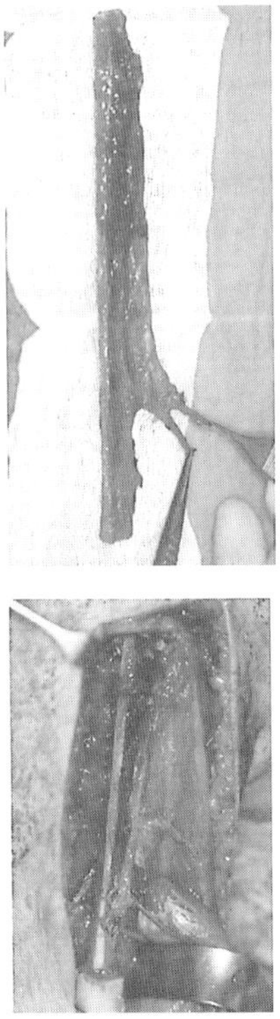

Figs. 2b, 2c

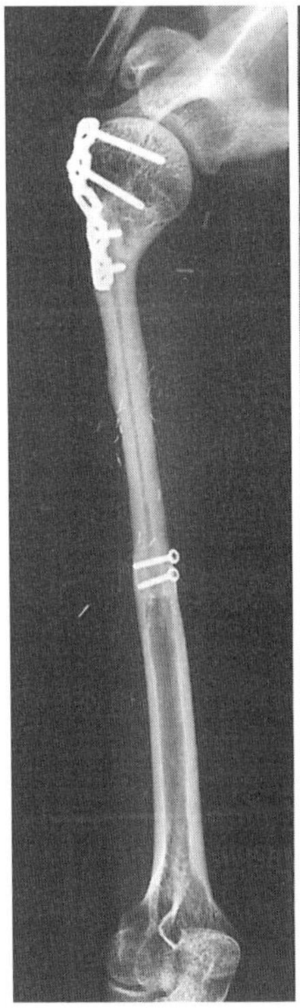

Fig. 2d

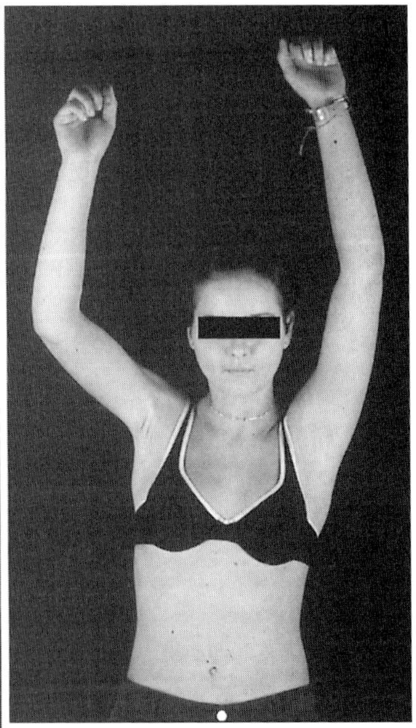

Fig. 2e

Vascularised fibular transplantation. Figure 2a – Radiograph of a 15-year-old girl with an osteosarcoma in the right proximal humerus. Figure 2b – The fibula with its vascular pedicles. Figure 2c – The fibula is transplanted with microvascular anastomosis. Figures 2d and 2e – Radiograph and photograph ten months after surgery.

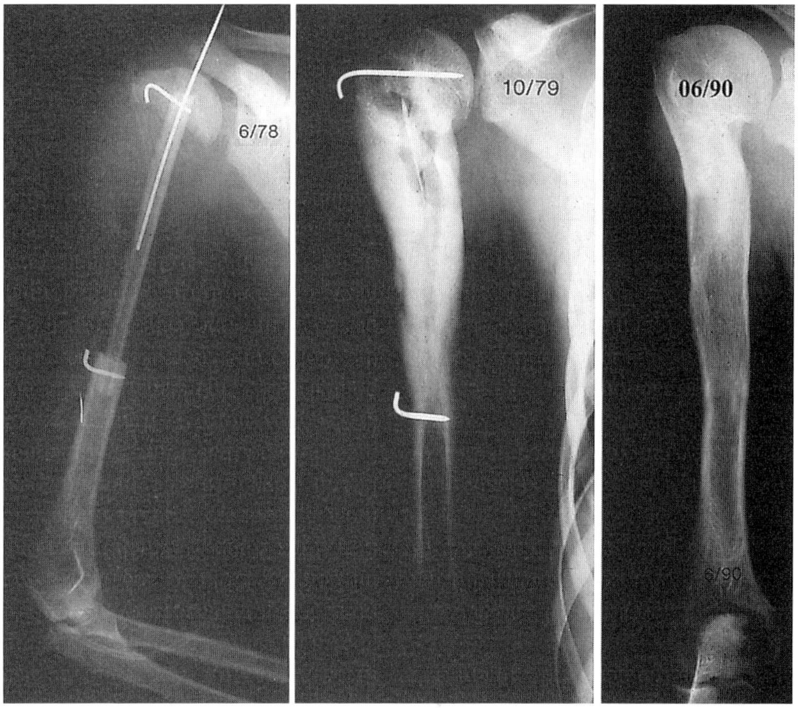

Fig. 3

Radiographs showing transplantation of a non-vascularised fibular graft after subperiosteal resection of a multiply recurrent aneurysmal bone cyst. Because of the good transplantation bed the fibula shows sound incorporation and hypertrophy.

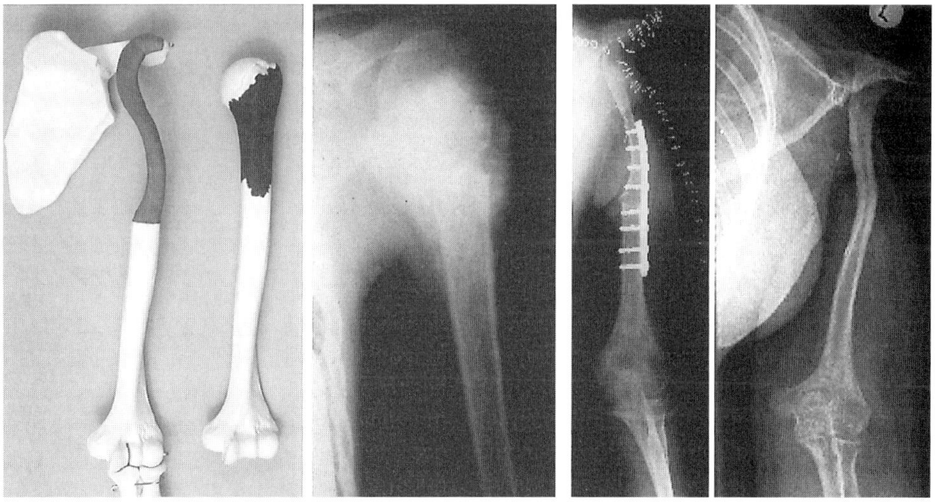

Fig. 4a Fig. 4b Fig. 4c Fig. 4d

The clavicula pro humero operation. Figure 4a – The operation is demonstrated on a model. Figure 4b – Radiograph of a ten-year-old girl with an osteosarcoma in the left proximal humerus. Figure 4c – After wide extra-articular resection of the tumour the ipsilateral clavicle with its surrounding soft tissue is downfolded on to the acromioclavicular joint and fixed to the humerus with an AO plate. Figure 4d – Radiograph six years after surgery.

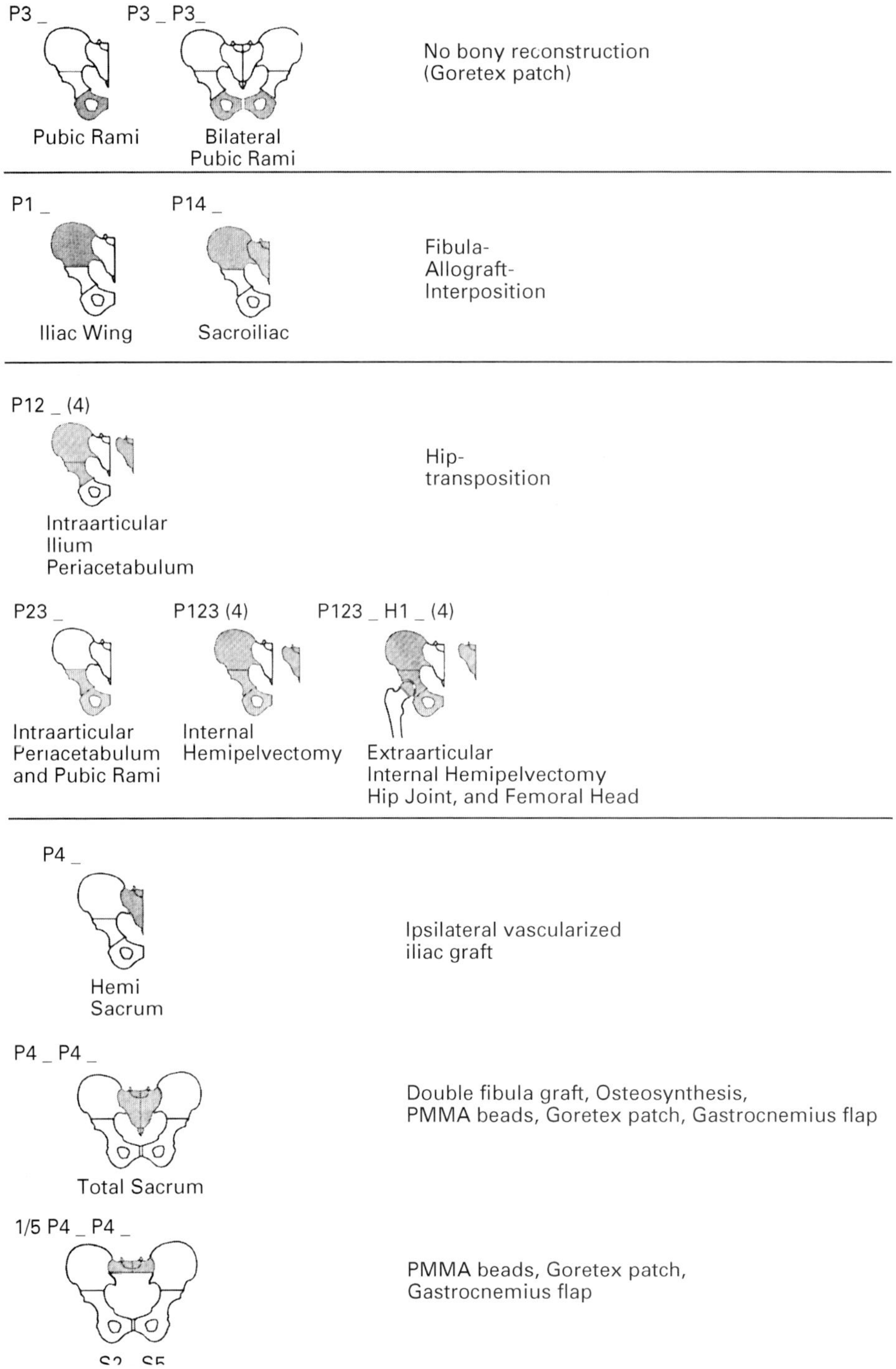

Fig. 5

Diagram of tumours in the pelvis according to Enneking et al[6] with the possible methods of biological reconstruction.

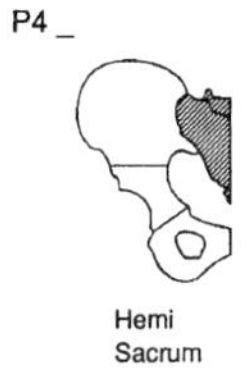

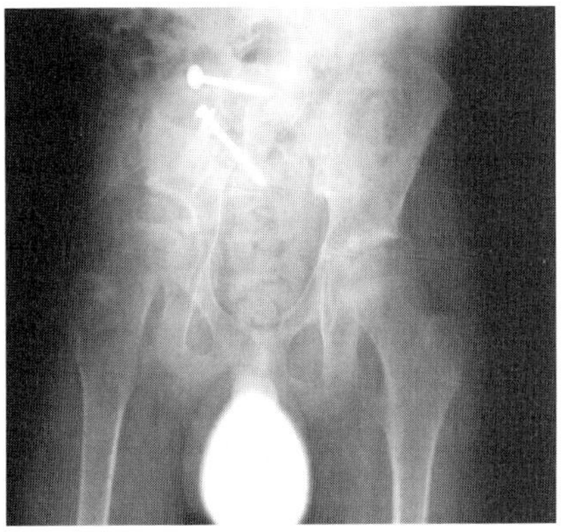

Fig. 6a

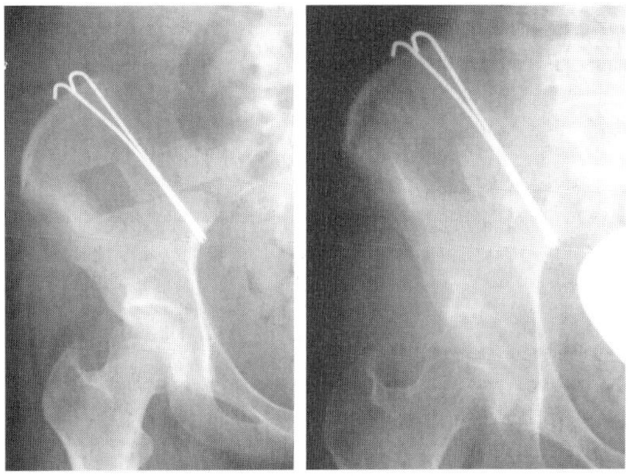

Fig. 6b

Reconstruction after resection of tumours of the lateral part of the hemisacrum (P4) and the posterior part of the iliac bone. Stabilisation of the pelvic ring can be achieved by an ipsilateral vascularised iliac graft. Two techniques are shown: a) a tilted iliac bone graft, fixed by two screws and b) a transposed iliac bone graft, fixed by two Kirschner wires.

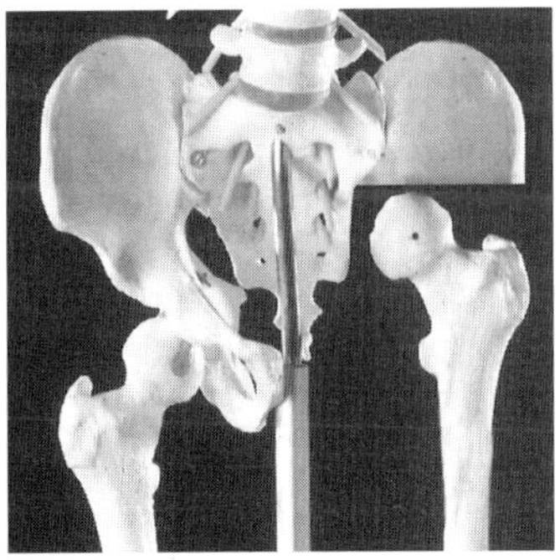

Type A

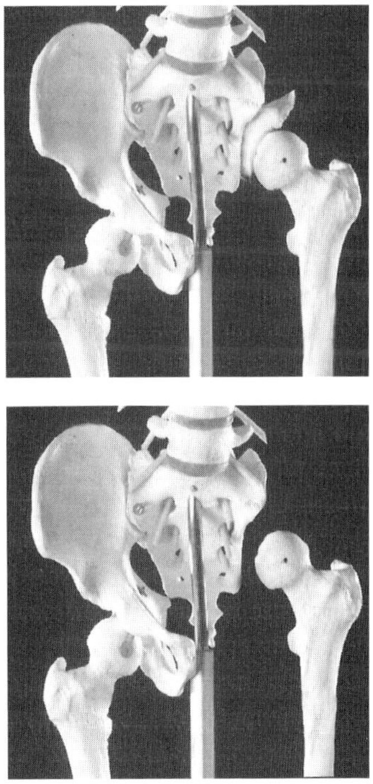

Type B

Fig. 7

Photographs of hip transposition demonstrated on models. Type A: after resection of P23 tumours. Type B: after resection of P12/4, P123/4, P123/4/H1 tumours.

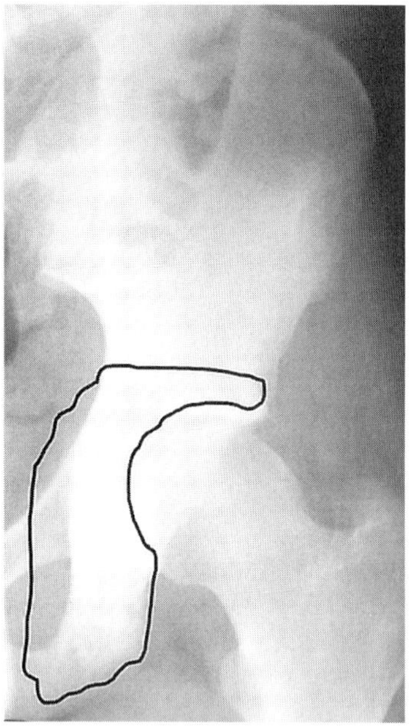

Fig. 8a

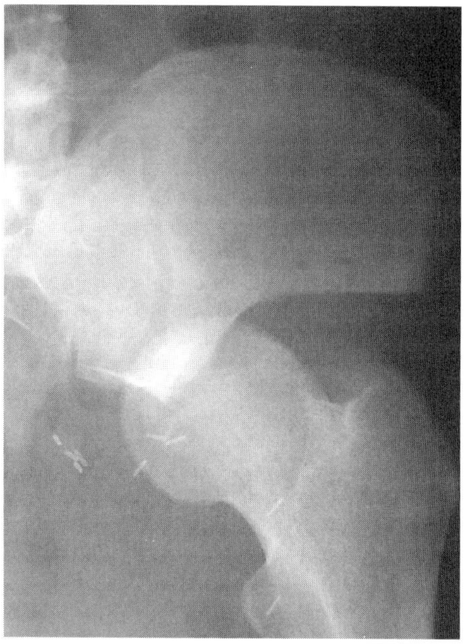

Fig. 8b

Radiographs of a 22-year-old man with a) a low-grade osteosarcoma in the left ischium and acetabulum without involvement of the hip and b) four years after surgery following type-A hip transposition.

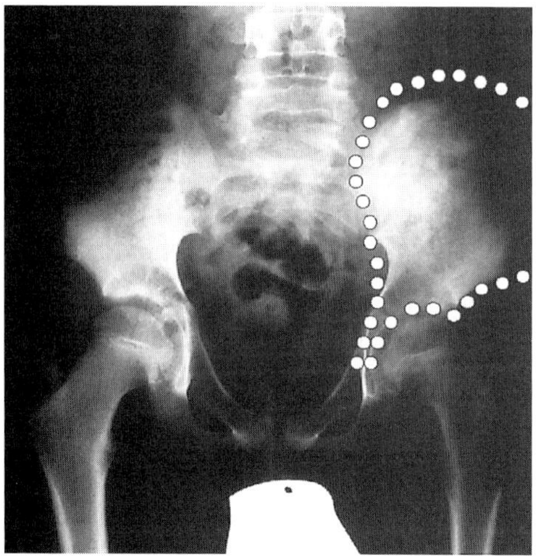

Fig. 9a

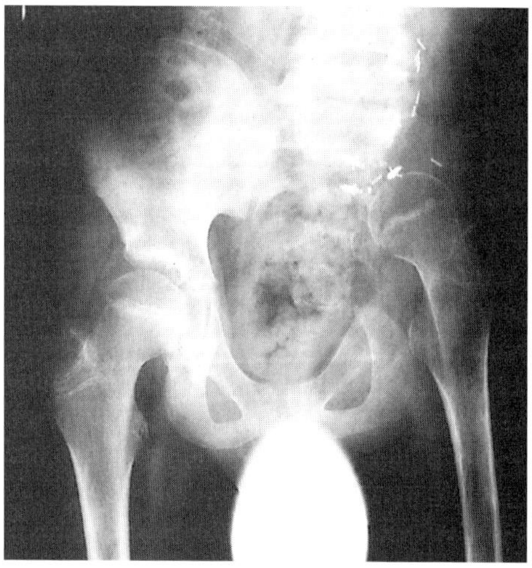

Fig. 9b

Radiographs of a 12-year-old boy with a) an osteosarcoma of the left iliac bone and acetabulum without involvement of the hip, P12/4 and b) two years after surgery following type-B hip transposition.

vascular-supplied graft of the remaining iliac bone can be moved to the sacrum (Fig. 6).

After resection of tumours in the periacetabulum and the region of the pubic rami (P23), the ilium and the peri-acetabular region (P12/4), or the whole hip region, with or without involvement of the hip (P123/4; P123/4H1), we recommend reconstruction of the defect using a hip transposition rather than employing a massive tumour prosthesis[7] (Figs 7 to 11). A mobile 'hip joint' can be produced. After resection of the tumour the femoral head can be placed against the remaining part of the iliac bone or the sacrum (Fig. 7) and a new hip capsule formed using Trevira tubes. The surrounding soft tissues grow into these tubes and under loading form a substitute joint, stabilising the femoral head which has moved cranially. The cranial shift of the soft tissue of the proximal thigh allows reconstruction of the soft tissue of the pelvis. The resulting leg-length discrepancy can be corrected later.

After resection of the pubic ramus on one or both sides (P3/P3-P3) no bony reconstruction is necessary.

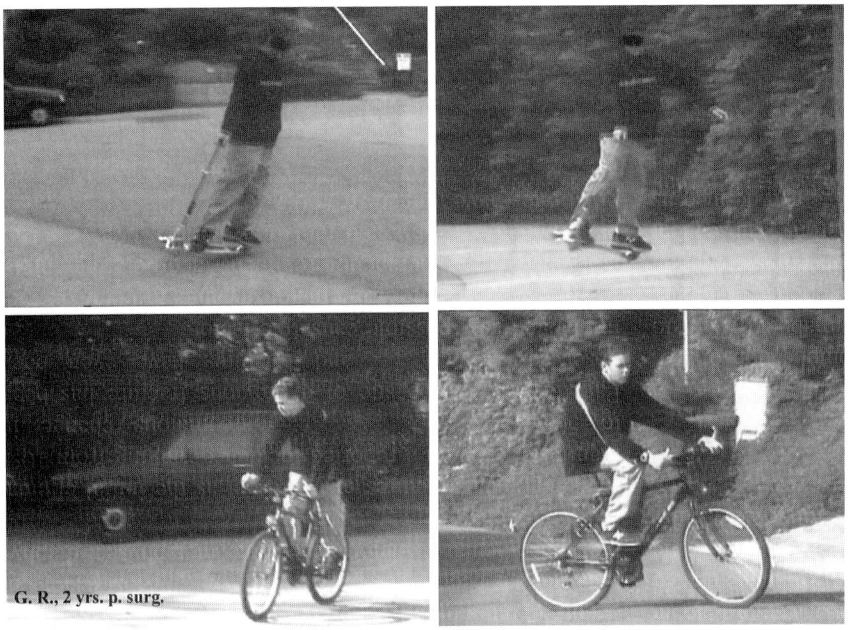

Fig. 10

Photographs of the same patient as in Figure 9 showing function two years after surgery.

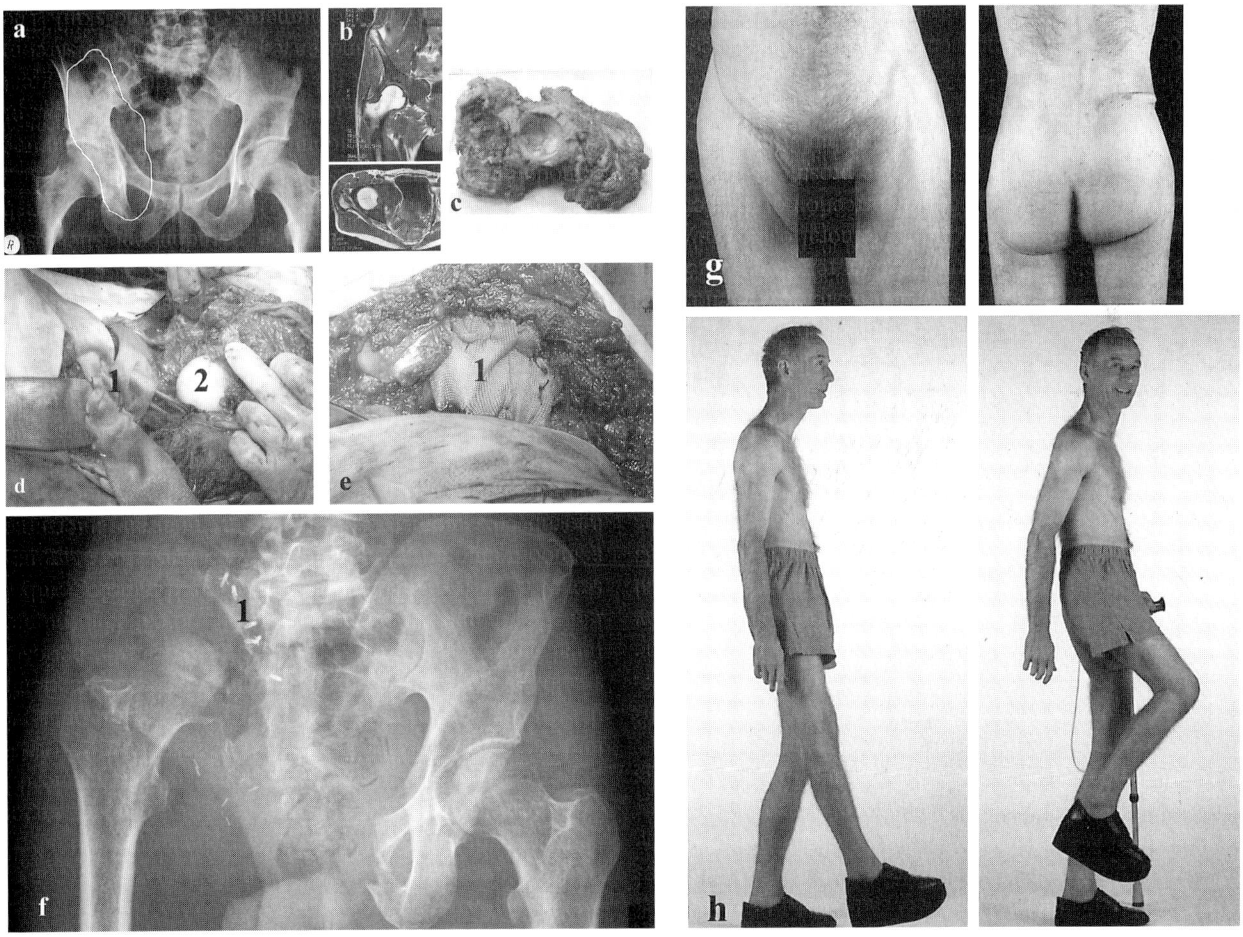

Fig. 11

Hip transposition in a 48-year-old man. A radiograph (a) and MR image (b) show a chondrosarcoma in the right iliac bone, acetabulum and pubic ramus without involvement of the hip, P123/4. Figure 11c – The surgical specimen. Figures 11d and 11e – A double Trevira tube (1) is sutured to the lateral side of the sacrum by bone anchors. The femoral head (2) is then placed into the Trevira tubes and a special capsularplasty holds the head to the sacrum. Figure 11f – A radiograph three months after surgery. Figures 11g and 11h – Photographs showing function three months after surgery.

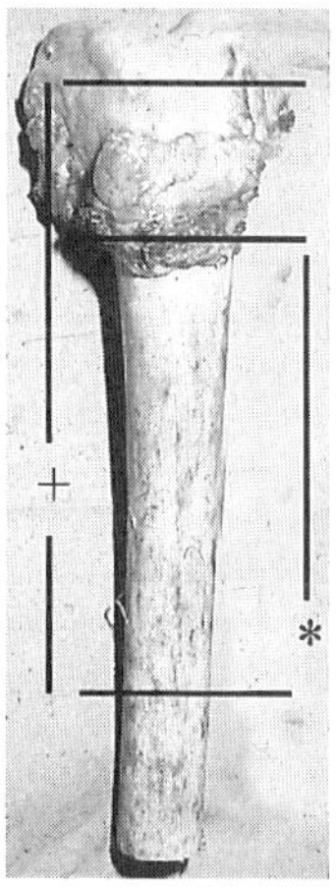

Fig. 12a

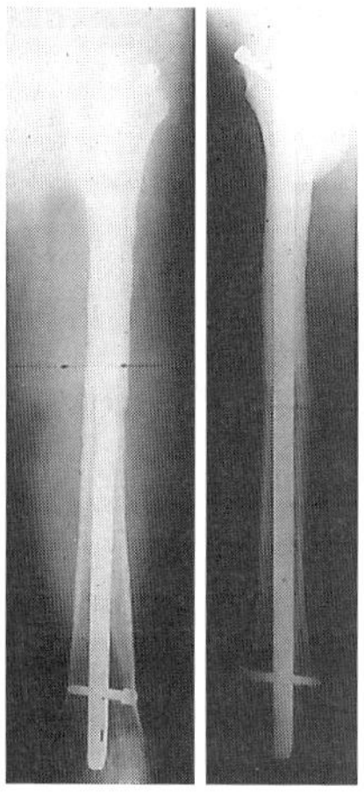

Fig. 12b

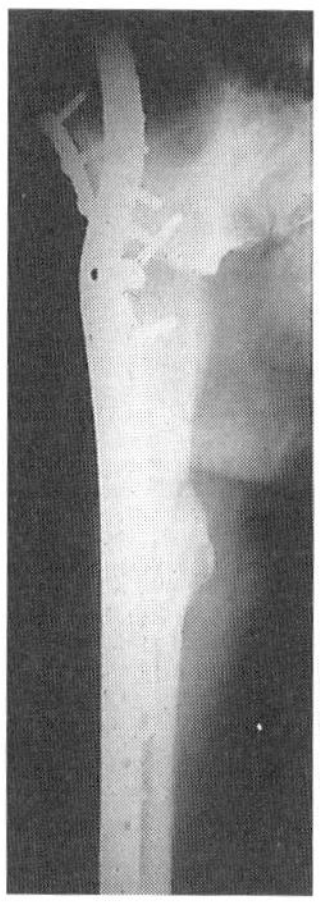

Fig. 12c

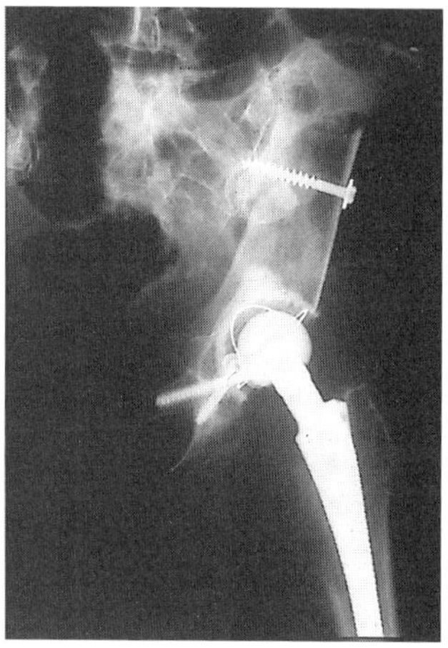

Fig. 12d

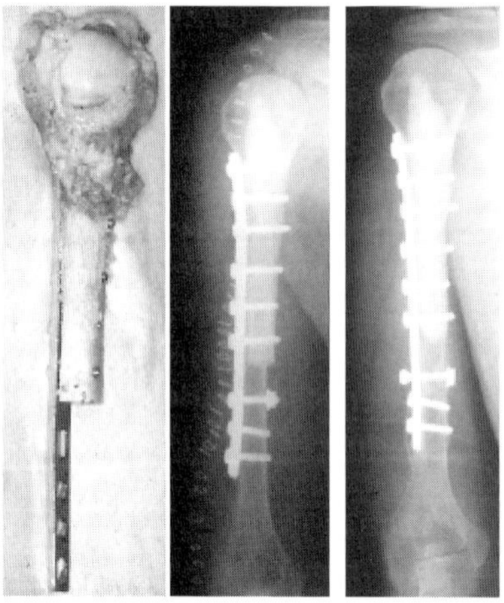

Fig. 12e

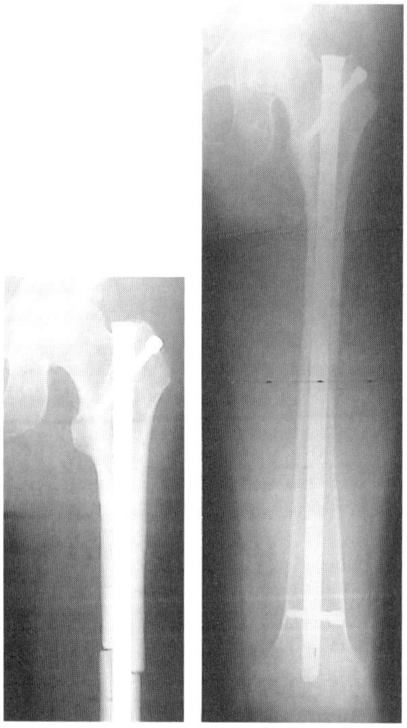

Fig. 12f

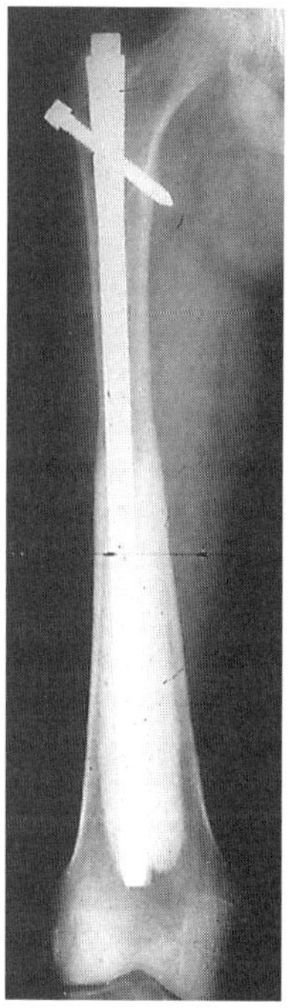

Fig. 12g

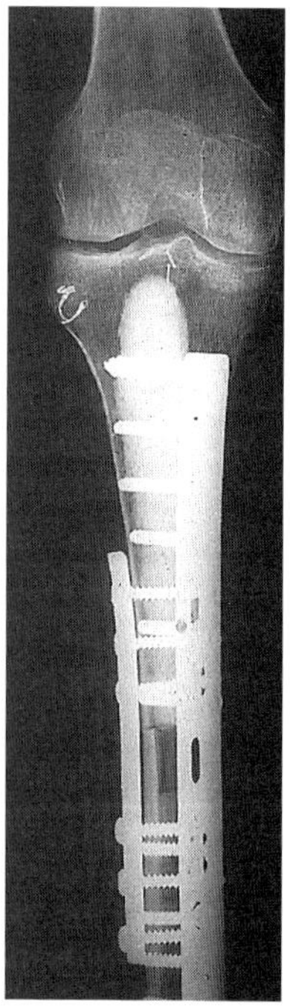

Fig. 12h

Examples of reconstruction with massive allografts. Figure 12a – Osteoarticular allograft used for an intercalary diaphyseal (*) or metadiaphyseal (+) reconstruction. Figure 12b – Radiograph showing diaphyseal intercalary allograft reconstruction in the femur fixed by an interlocking nail. Figure 12c – Radiograph showing metadiaphyseal allograft reconstruction for a hip arthrodesis with fixation by two AO plates. Figure 12d – Radiograph showing metadiaphyseal allograft reconstruction for a pelvic defect after P123/H1 resection. Figure 12e – Osteoarticular allograft for the proximal humerus and radiographs showing allograft augmentation with bone cement and fixation with an AO plate. Figure 12f – Radiographs showing osteoarticular allograft for reconstruction of the proximal femur fixed with an interlocking nail. Figure 12g – Radiograph showing osteoarticular allograft for reconstruction of the distal femur. The allograft is augmented with bone cement and fixed with an interlocking nail. Figure 12h – Radiograph showing osteoarticular allograft for reconstruction of the proximal tibia. It is augmented with bone cement and fixed with two AO plates.

SUBSTANTIAL ALLOGRAFTS FOR BIOLOGICAL RECONSTRUCTION

Massive allografts with attached tendons and ligaments may also be used for biological reconstruction. Small corticocancellous allografts are employed as onlay or inlay grafts, intercalary allografts bridge diaphyseal segmental defects, and osteoarticular allografts replace metaphyseal defects. Allografts only superficially remodel to the host bone and the centre of the allograft remains dead even after many years. Local soft tissues can grow into the allograft. Tendons and ligaments attached to it can clearly facilitate the reconstruction of joints and thus improve function (Fig. 12).

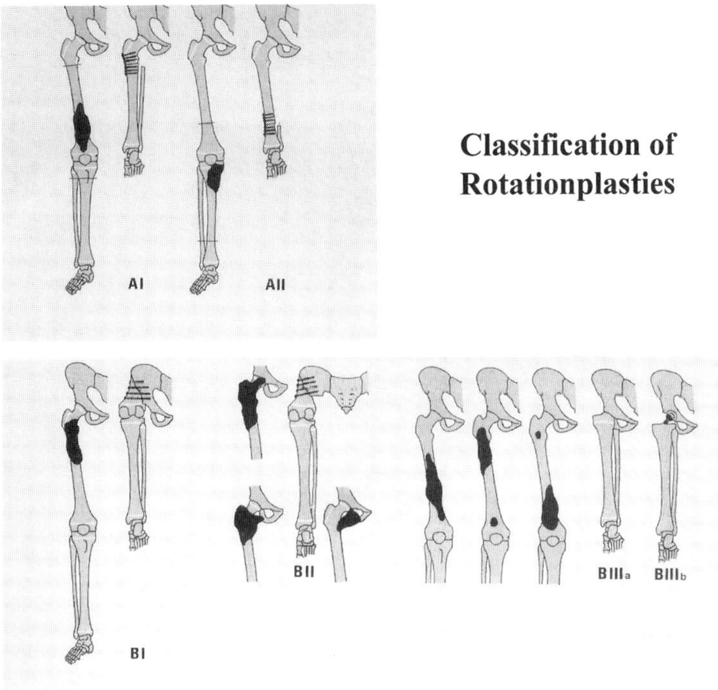

Fig. 13a

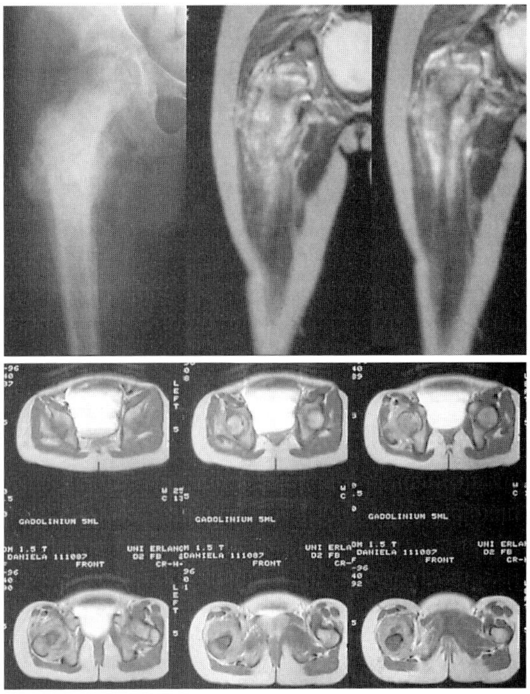
Fig. 13b

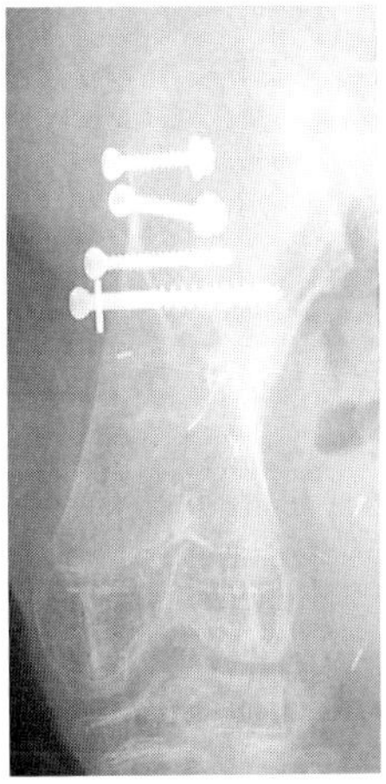
Fig. 13c

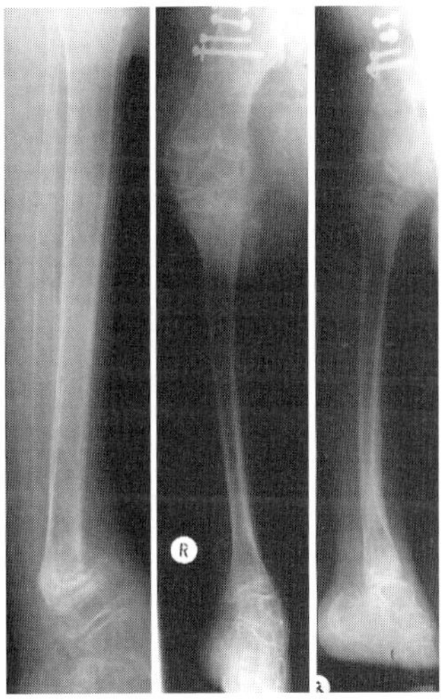
Fig. 13d

Rotationplasties for biological reconstruction. Figure 13a – Photograph showing classification of rotationplasties according to Winkelmann.[8,9] Figure 13b – Radiographs and MR images of a nine-year-old girl with an osteosarcoma in the right proximal femur with involvement of the hip. Figure 13c – Radiograph of the right pelvic region four years after hip rotationplasty type BII. Figure 13d – Radiograph showing a fracture of the distal tibia eight months after surgery which healed without axial deformation.

ROTATIONPLASTY

Rotationplasties represent a special form of biological reconstruction, since parts of whole extremities are being used.[8] In these procedures the ankle joint will become the functional knee joint, and in rotationplasty at the hip the knee joint becomes the functional hip joint (Fig. 13). An impressive example of biological reconstruction in early infancy is shown in the hip rotation plasty type BIIIa.[9] The lateral head of the tibia is transplanted into the acetabulum and is transformed into a femoral head under the new load within a few years (Fig. 14).

COMPLICATIONS

The main complications of biological reconstruction are pseudarthrosis and fatigue fracture caused by early post-operative load-bearing or relative overloading. These complications, however, almost always heal completely either by immobilisation or by an additional autologous bone transplantation. Deep infection, a common complication of tumour prostheses, also occurs in biological reconstruction but is of less significance and is substantially simpler to treat.[2,3,10-12] In allograft reconstruction the rate of major complications, such as pseudarthroses or fractures, is sig-

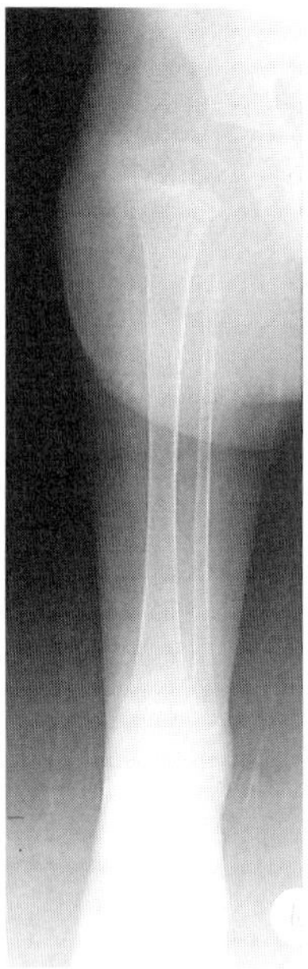

Fig. 14a

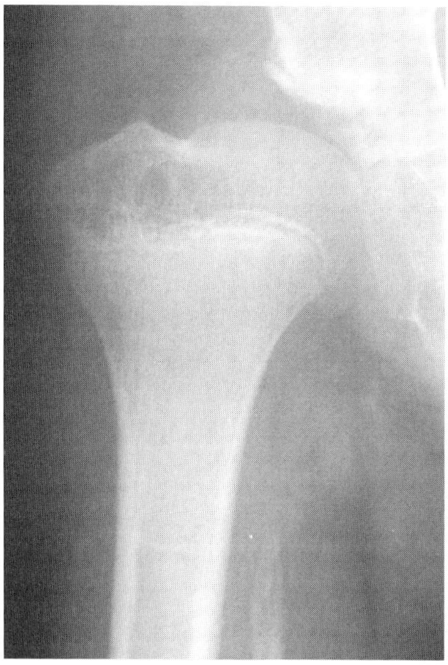

Fig. 14b

The growing bone shows enormous plasticity. In hip rotationplasty type BIIIa the tibial graft develops, due to pressure and load bearing, into a femoral head. Radiographs showing a) hip rotationplasty type BIIIa in a four-year-old girl and b) five years seven months after surgery.

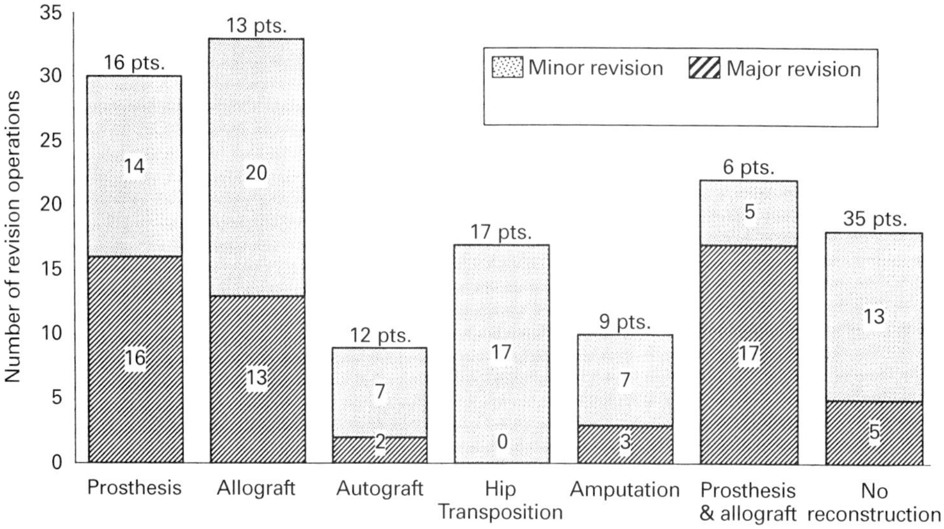

Fig. 15

The number of additional operations after resection and reconstruction of 110 tumours of the pelvis. Those with biological reconstruction have a significantly lower rate of minor or major revisions.

nificantly higher than after biological reconstruction with autologous bone material and the rate of deep infections is similar to that after implantation of tumour prostheses.[13,14] High-dose irradiation to allografts is associated with a higher rate of fracture than when similar reconstructions employ non-irradiated allografts.[15] In a series of 110 patients with pelvic tumours Hillmann et al[11] showed that after biological reconstruction the rate of additional operations for minor or major complications was significantly lower than after reconstruction with a mega-prosthesis or massive allografts (Fig. 15).

SUMMARY

Biological reconstruction is possible at all ages but the results will be better in the young. Axhausen,[1] Volkmann[16] and Hueter[17] have shown that load-dependent incorporation and remodelling are substantially better in young patients. Biological reconstruction requires a longer operation time and the postoperative rehabilitation is extended compared with the implantation of a prosthesis. Remodelling of the graft, however, may occur according to the loading required, and biological ingrowth of the surrounding soft parts, in particular muscles, tendons and ligaments, gives a better function. Late complications are significantly higher after the introduction of foreign implants.

REFERENCES

1. **Axhausen W.** The osteogenic phases of generation of bone: a historical and experimental study. *J Bone Joint Surg [Am]* 1956;38-A:593-600.
2. **Capanna R, Biagini R, Casdei R.** Autograft versus allograft reconstruction. In: Brown KL, ed. *Complication of limb salvage.* Sixth International Symposium on Limb Salvage (ISOLS). Montreal, 1990:49-52.
3. **Capanna R, Ceruso M, Innocenti M, et al.** Indication to vascularized fibula transplantation in limb salvage surgery (abstract). In: Transaction of the Ninth International Symposium on Limb Salvage (ISOLS), 1997:123.
4. **Manfrini M, Innocenti M, Ceruso M, et al.** An original biological reconstruction of the hip in a 4-year-old girl (abstract). In: Proceedings of the European Musculo-Skeletal Oncology Society Meeting, Paris 1999:38.
5. **Winkelmann WW.** Clavicula pro humero: a new surgical method for malignant tumors of the proximal humerus. *Z Orthop Ihre Grenzgeb* 1992;130:197-201.
6. **Enneking W, Dunham W, Gebhardt M, Malawar M, Pritchard D.** A system for the classification of skeletal resections. *Chir Organi Mov* 1990;75:217-40.
7. **Winkelmann W.** A new surgical approach in malignant tumors of the ilium. *Z Orthop Ihre Grenzgeb* 1988;126:671-4.
8. **Winkelmann WW.** Rotationplasty. *Orthop Clin North Am* 1996;27:503-23.
9. **Winkelmann W.** Type-B-IIIa hip rotationplasty: an alternative operation for the treatment of malignant tumors of the femur in early childhood. *J Bone Joint Surg [Am]* 2000;82-A:814-28.
10. **Delepine N, Delepine G, Desbois JC.** Update on use of expandable prostheses in limb salvage surgery for children's bone sarcomas of lower limb (abstract). In: Transaction of the Ninth International Symposium on Limb Salvage (ISOLS), 1997;9.
11. **Hillmann A, Ozaki O, Hoffmann C, Gosheger G, Winkelmann W.** Tumors of the pelvis: additional surgeries after reconstruction. *Clin Orthop* 2000 (in press).
12. **Schiller C, Windhager R, Fellinger EJ, et al.** Extendable tumour endoprostheses for the leg in children. *J Bone Joint Surg [Br]* 1995;77-B:608-14.
13. **Aho AJ, Ekfors T, Dean PB, et al.** Incorporation and clinical results of large allograft of the extremities and pelvis. *Clin Orthop* 1994;307:200-13.
14. **Mankin HJ, Doppelt SH, Sullivan TR, Tomford WW.** Osteoarticular and intercalary allograft transplantation in the management of malignant tumors of bone. *Cancer* 1982;50:613-30.
15. **Lietman SA, Tomford WW, Gebhardt MC, Springfield DS, Mankin HJ.** Complications of irradiated allografts in orthopaedic tumor surgery. *Clin Orthop* 2000;375:214-7.
16. **Volkmann R.** Chirurgische Erfahrungen über Knochenverbiegungen und Knochenwachstum. *Virch Arch Pathol Anat* 1862;24:512-40.
17. **Hueter C.** Anatomische Studien an den Extremitätengelenken Neugeborener und Erwachsener. *Virch Arch Pathol Anat* 1862;25:572-99.

PAGET'S DISEASE OF THE BONE AND ITS MANAGEMENT

ALEXANDER G. HADJIPAVLOU, IOANNIS N. GAITANIS

From the University of Crete, Greece

Paget's disease of bone (PD) is a mono-ostotic or polyostotic non-hormonal osteometabolic disorder. Over a century after the original description by Paget,[149] and despite recent intensive studies and widespread interest, its aetiology remains obscure.

The tendency to sarcomatous change, the variability of the osteoblasts (size, shape and staining), the peculiarity of the osteoclasts (size and number of nuclei up to 100, seen also in giant-cell tumours), and the control of the disease by antimitotic agents such as plicamycin (also known as mithramycin) suggest that it may be a benign neoplasm of the mesenchymal osteoprogenitor cell, as was suggested by Ramussen and Bordier.[159]

It has been postulated that the disease may be caused by a viral infection.[18,83,190] Electron microscopy of osteoclasts shows viral intranuclear inclusion structures resembling those of an RNA-type virus related to measles or subacute sclerosing panencephalitis. Immunological studies show the presence of specific viral antigens in osteoclasts and cells grown from Paget's bone.[11,39]

There is considerable evidence in support of a viral aetiology for PD.[131] A characteristic feature of paramyxoviruses is their ability to persist at very low levels, and invade the host immune system. Factors which can be activated by virally-induced ROS (e.g., IL-6, C-fos and Bcl-2) are all elevated in PD, strongly suggesting viral infection.

Some reports have indicated that PD is a zoonosis because it is associated with ownership of birds, dogs, cats or cattle.[105,120] These studies have suggested that canine distemper, a paramyxovirus closely related to measles, can contaminate human osteoclast cells, contributing to the development of PD.[96,147] Other studies, however,[167,194] found no risk factors associated with dogs or cats. In addition, it should be noted that all of the claims mentioned above are only supported by circumstantial evidence gained from electron-microscopic, immunological and epidemiological investigations.

PREVALENCE, DISTRIBUTION AND GENETIC FACTORS

PD is found more commonly in populations of Anglo-Saxon origin and is rarely encountered in China, Japan, Iran, India, Scandinavia, Africa or the Middle East.[15] Singer and Millis[190] mentioned, however, that 10% of the patients in the Los Angeles area are of African descent. A survey of PD in Johannesburg, South Africa, revealed an incidence of 1.3% among the black population and 2.4% in the white population.[76] These findings suggest that PD may not be as uncommon in Africans as was previously thought. Post-mortem reports indicate that the overall incidence of PD is 3% to 3.7%[36,185] with a tendency to increase with age. At the age of 90 years, the expected prevalence is about 10%.[185] Radiological studies revealed an incidence of 3.5%.[156] A very recent report on radiological examination of the pelvis[5] showed an estimated overall incidence in the USA of 1% to 2% with almost equal distribution between whites and blacks and between sexes.

Genetic factors play a role in the pathogenesis of PD, which is inherited as an autosomal dominant trait with high penetrance.[91,95] It often occurs in more than one member of a family.[194] A positive family history in patients or siblings was reported in 12.3% of cases compared with 2.1% of a control group. The prevalence of PD was approximately seven times higher in relatives of patients than in those of a control group.

Studies of families with PD have shown linkage to a region of chromosome 18q near the polymorphic locus D 18S42, most likely due to gene mutation.[35,91,112] Genetic heterogeneity is almost certainly present;[94,141] data from some families with PD suggest the presence of at least one additional locus, which remains to be identified.[91] Viral infection may also help to explain the genetic predisposition, by gene mutation, of PD.[131]

HISTOPATHOLOGY

The histopathology of PD is characterised by two entities: an osseous lesion and fibrosis of the bone marrow. The former is distinguished by its so-called mosaic appearance, the hallmark of a Pagetic lesion. The Pagetic cellularity consists of osteoblasts of variable size and large osteoclasts with multiple nuclei, up to 100.[159] Bone-marrow fibrosis is not associated with anaemia because the haemopoietic activity of bone marrow can expand to the appendicular skeleton;[42] uncommonly, extramedullary haemopoiesis occurs in the thoracic cavity.[166] These phenomena compensate for the extensive bone-marrow fibrosis.

PATHOMECHANICS OF BONE DEFORMITY

PD can be defined as a disturbance of remodelling, which leads to abnormal shape of the bone. Frost[61] has defined remodelling as a constant renewal or turnover of bone without changes in its size or shape. Disturbance of the bone-remodelling process, as seen in PD, changes the bone texture and gives rise to the four phases of the disease observed radiologically: the osteolytic, mixed, osteoblastic phases, and the inactive osteosclerotic phase characterised by normal or decreased activity observed on bone scans[113] (Fig. 1). Bone modelling is a process which determines the shape and geometry of bone.[72]

Modelling in PD may lead to expansion or contraction of bone by the mechanism of centrifugal or centripetal drift of cortical bone. Expansion of bone is produced by diffuse abnormal modelling and is considered to be a cardinal sign of PD.[100,136] Expansion of bone with a wide cortex is due to apposition of bone on the periosteal and endosteal envelopes. An increased external diameter of the bone with a thin cortex is caused by periosteal apposition with concomitant absorption in the endosteal envelope, leading to enlargement of the marrow cavity. Pagetic bone contraction, or centripetal cortical bone drift, is produced by apposition on the endosteal surface and absorption on the periosteal surface.

Complications include pathological fractures, delayed union, progressive skeletal deformity, chronic bone pain, neurological compromise of the peripheral and central nervous systems (compression of the ocular or facial nerves, spinal stenosis etc), Pagetic arthritis, malignant change, hearing loss, Peyronie's disease, heart disease etc.

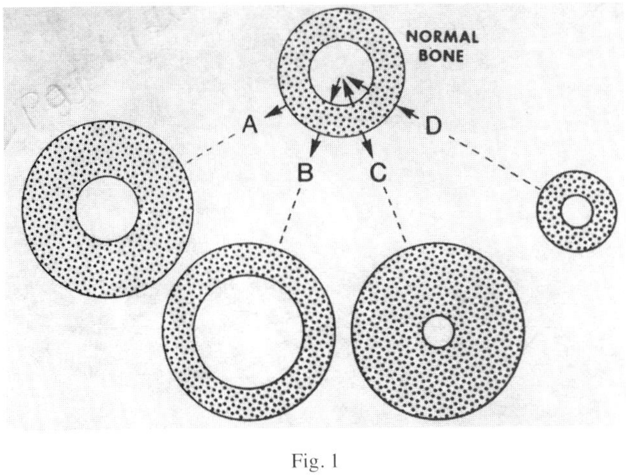

Fig. 1

Diagram of the cross-sections of a long bone to demonstrate the possible patterns of modelling in the periosteal and endosteal envelopes. The arrowheads show the direction of cortical drift due to bone apposition or absorption. Patterns A, B and C all represent bone expansion as follows: A, apposition within the periosteal envelope, endosteum unchanged; B, apposition within the periosteal envelope and absorption in the endosteal envelope resulting in a thin cortex; C, apposition in both periosteal and endosteal envelopes, resulting in a thin cortex; and D, bone contraction, periosteal absorption with endosteal apposition causing a centripetal cortical drift. (Reproduced by permission, A. Hadjipavlou, P. Lander, Paget's Disease, pp 1720–37. *Spine Care*. A. White and J. Schofferman, eds. Mosby Year Book, Inc. 1995.)

PATHOLOGICAL FRACTURES

Pathological fractures are a common complication of PD,[100,171] and may be the presenting manifestation. The reported incidence varies between 10% and 30%.[75,133] Fractures of the long bones occur in all remodelling phases, but are more common in the mixed and osteoblastic phases. Fractures in the osteolytic phase usually occur at the junction of normal bone density and the radiolucent area.[86]

There is a tendency for fractures occurring in the osteoblastic and mixed phases to be associated with delayed union,[86,109,110] whereas those in the osteolytic phase usually heal in the expected time. In the osteolytic phase, healing of the fracture can be associated with the regression phase of osteopenia.[134] Union tends to be delayed in the osteoblastic and sclerotic phases, and the incidence of nonunion increases in patients on antiPagetic therapy with disodium etidronate.[108] This drug is not recommended in the presence of fractures.[81] Predisposing factors to complete fractures are incomplete stress fractures, stress rises at the bone-plate interface and possibly treatment with etidronate disodium.[82] Incomplete stress fractures arise mostly on the tension side of long bones where they partially involve the cortex, either from the endosteal or periosteal surface. They occur mostly in blastic and sclerotic phases. Circumstantial evidence suggests that the sclerotic bone is brittle[100,122,161] and therefore may predispose to fracture.

Incomplete stress fractures associated with pain and local tenderness are suggestive of impending complete fractures. Treatment in this situation depends on the remodelling phase. In the mixed phase, walking on crutches with or without bracing may suffice. In the osteoblastic or sclerotic phases especially with associated deformity, prophylactic realignment osteotomy and intramedullary instrumental stabilisation are the most appropriate treatments. In order to avoid the stress rises associated with fixation using a plate, intramedullary nailing is preferred in cases of complete fracture. The mean time for union of femoral fractures treated by intramedullary nailing is approximately 32 weeks (26 to 42).[183]

Fractures with pronounced bone deformities are best treated surgically; this approach allows deformities, a major contributing factor to fracture, to be corrected and also improves the adjacent alignment of the joints. Patients with PD treated by electrical stimulation and bone grafting usually have exuberant formation of callus; the use of these procedures is therefore recommended for fractures occurring in the blastic or sclerotic phases.[82]

PAGET'S DISEASE AND ARTHRITIS

Arthritis in PD has been considered to be a non-specific arthropathy,[49] a coincidental finding,[78] or a specific entity.[82] Several distinct pathological processes contribute to the degeneration and destruction of articular cartilage in PD. The Pagetic process may erode the subchondral bone[100] leading to the collapse of cartilage into the underlying bones.[82] The articular cartilage can also be eroded by accelerated endochondral ossification of the subchondral bone,[68] or by the invasion of the aggressive Pagetic process.[82,168] Expansion of bone and structural deformity are other mechanisms which may produce incongruity of the articular cartilage thus contributing to arthritis.

Pain originating in the Pagetic arthritic joint may be attributed to the occurrence of microfractures or increased bone vascularity.[82] The normalisation of bone blood flow with anti-Pagetic therapy and its relationship to pain relief have been documented.[24,80] Despite the normalisation of bone blood flow, the improvement of the appearance of the bone scan and the remodelling activity of bone markers after an adequate course of antiPagetic agents, if pain persists, conservative therapy should be deemed to have failed.

In the presence of bony deformity and of joint malalignment with a relative preservation of the articular cartilage, osteotomy can correct the deformity and restore the mechanics of the joint. It can be successfully stabilised by means of either intramedullary nailing or Ilizarov external fixation.[121] Total joint arthroplasty is indicated for patients with advanced destruction of cartilage.

Osteoarthritis of the hip with a varus deformity of the femur can be successfully treated by single or multiple osteotomies of the femur, followed by implantation of a long-stemmed, fully-coated, porous ingrowth hip system.[3,142] Varus femoral deformity can also be corrected primarily by osteotomy and stabilised by a very long intramedullary nail. Later, the nail is removed and total joint reconstruction is performed. For revision surgery in the presence of a varus deformity, femoral osteotomy also facilitates removal of cement and correction of the deformity at the time of implantation of the prosthesis.[142]

The survivorship to revision for total hip arthroplasty was reported to be 98% at ten years and 91% at 15 years for the acetabular component, and 93% at ten years and 89% at 15 years for the femoral component.[198] The only increased risks identified were nonunion of the trochanteric osteotomy (13%) and the occurrence of heterotopic ossification in 29% of cases (significant in 4%). Cemented arthroplasty in PD has been reported as having slightly worse results than in non-PD patients. The long-term results of uncemented implants remain to be established.[117] Patients with sclerotic acetabular bones may be at risk of perioperative acetabular fracture when an under-reaming technique is used.[129]

MALIGNANT TRANSFORMATION

Malignant change is the most dreaded complication of PD. Fortunately, it is relatively rare, occurring in about 0.7%[87] to 0.9%[74] of patients although others have reported a higher incidence of between 5%[110] and 5.5%.[60] Since this condition was first described by Paget,[148] numerous subsequent reviews have described the malignant change and defined its clinical and radiological presentation.[14,89,99,130,153,155,197,210]

The various forms of malignant change as a complication of PD in decreasing order of frequency are as follows: (1) osteosarcoma (22% to 90%),[14,74,87,101,130,153,175,210] (2) fibrous histiocytoma (7% to 26%),[87,99,101] (3) fibrosarcoma (3% to 25%),[14,74,89,101,130,210] (4) chondrosarcoma (1% to 5%),[14,89,99,130] (5) giant-cell sarcoma (3% to 10%),[14,89,155] (6) unspecific malignant neoplasm (9%),[67,155] (7) reticulum cell sarcoma (lymphoma),[114] (8) lymphosarcoma (12%),[87] and a rare case of haemangiosarcoma.[32] Pagetic sarcomatous change constitutes between 3.3% and 14% of all osteogenic sarcomata of bone.[41,99]

The acute onset of pain or an increase in the intensity of chronic pain is usually the presenting complaint.[87,89,140] The initial radiological appearance of the primary Pagetic lesion and malignant transformation may overlap, leading to delay in diagnosis.[11,19] Swelling or associated soft-tissue masses are present in 48% to 75%.[87,89] Not all lesions with swelling, however, result from malignant change. Benign focal modelling lesions can occur in a localised periosteal Pagetic bony expansion, or a so-called 'pumice-stone'[100,112] lesion, which is characterised radiologically by a smooth uninterrupted margin. By contrast, the margins of a localised sarcomatous lesion are irregular and interrupted. Similar juxtacortical formation of soft tissue called 'pseudosarcoma' may mimic juxtacortical sarcoma.[113] CT[197] and MRI can delineate the cortical penetration and associated soft-tissue mass invariably seen with a sarcomatous lesion. Biopsy is necessary to establish a definite diagnosis. The differential radiological appearance of PD with malignant change includes the following: 1) pseudosarcomatous osteolysis secondary to medication;[173] 2) cystic degeneration of Pagetic lesions causing pseudoneoplastic lesions with central necrosis;[19] and 3) active PD with variable remodelling abnormalities.[89,112]

Some reviews have identified the pelvis as the most common site of sarcomatous change,[99,101,153] whereas others have concluded that the humerus or femur is at greater risk.[87,197] Another[9] found an equal incidence of sarcomatous change involving the humerus, femur and skull. There is no consensus in the literature regarding the most common remodelling phase at which sarcomatous change occurred, but a high frequency of osteolysis at the sarcomatous site has been reported.[87,89,99,130,153,197] Most lesions in the appendicular skeleton are in the metaphyseal-diaphyseal region.[87,89]

Pathological fractures may present as the initial clinical manifestation with a reported incidence ranging from 10% to 50%.[87,89,90,130,153,155,197,210] Sarcomatous change in Pagetic bone at the site of a previous fracture has been observed[87,130,153,155,197] and fractures have even been implicated as a possible causative factor.[153,155,197]

The prognosis after sarcomatous change in PD is dismal. Notwithstanding therapeutic regimens incorporating amputation, chemotherapy, and radiation therapy, five-year survival rates have ranged from 0% to 15% (0%,[87,153] 2%,[130] 5%,[27,89,99] 8%,[74,210] 15%[41,184]). In many series, however, most patients died from their malignant neoplasms within a few months with a rare survival of up to five years.[101] The poorer outcome of these patients compared with those with *de novo* sarcomatous lesions has been attributed to the increased vascularity of the Pagetic bone allowing unimpeded haematogenous spread of the tumour,[74] especially in older patients, who may have less resistance to malignant neoplasm. Lymphoma associated with PD has a better prognosis.[20,37,87,114,140,155,179]

Giant-cell tumours complicating PD have a good prognosis and have been described as responding very well to steroid therapy.[43,67]

PAGET'S DISEASE AND SPINAL INVOLVEMENT

Prevalence of back pain and spinal stenosis. The spine is the second most commonly affected site in PD,[7,33,102] predisposing patients to low back pain and spinal stenosis.[6,86,92,213] Hartman and Dohn[92] have shown that 15.2% of patients with PD had involvement of the vertebrae, and 26% of these patients had symptoms of spinal stenosis. The reported incidence of back pain in PD ranges from 11%[58] to 43%,[174] and a more recent paper reports 34%.[8] The causal relationship between vertebral PD and back pain has been disputed by Altman and Colins,[8] who attributed the low back pain in PD to coexisting osteoarthritis of the spine in 88% of patients and to PD alone in only 12%. Others[62] consider PD to cause back pain even more rarely. In our series,[86] however, 33% of patients with PD showed Pagetic involvement of the spine; 54% of these patients had back pain and 30% had clinical symptoms of spinal stenosis.

Pathomechanics of structural spinal stenosis and facet arthropathy. In PD disturbed modelling contributes to bone expansion which leads to spinal stenosis[112] (Fig. 2). More specifically, Pagetic spinal stenosis can be caused either by posterior expansion of the vertebral body alone (least common), by the expansion of the neural arch and the facet joints, or a combination of these[86,213] (Fig. 3).

Facet arthropathy can be produced by abnormal Pagetic remodelling and modelling changes, causing the joint to become hypertrophic and incongruous with destruction of articular cartilage, as may occur in other Pagetic joints.[79,132]

Spinal stenosis. About one-third of patients with spinal involvement have symptoms of spinal stenosis[86] which can be characterised as lateral or central. The former manifests itself as constant or intermittent leg pain of variable intensity with specific radicular distribution associated with paraesthesiae. This pain is exacerbated by walking, may improve with rest, and may be associated with motor weakness and reflex and sensory changes. Central stenosis has a bizarre symptomatology which includes leg weakness and cramps with variable pain which is provoked by walking and improves with rest. Objective clinical signs are usually absent. A combination of central and lateral stenosis may also be present. Central stenosis with myelopathy is associated with upper motor neurone manifestations.

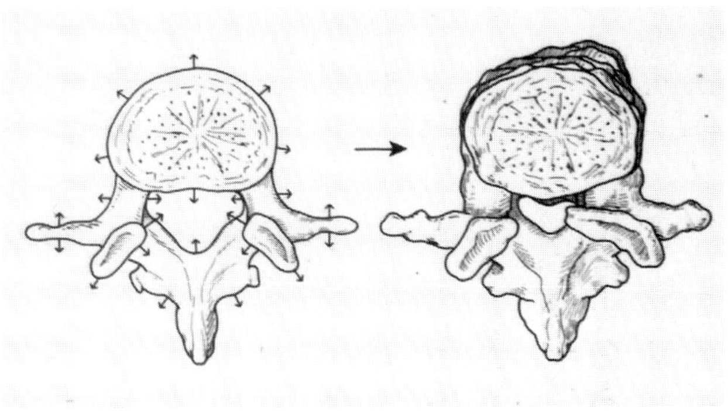

Fig. 2

Diagram of bone remodelling of the vertebra to show the tendency of bone expansion in all directions, leading to hypertrophic facet osteoarthropathy and spinal stenosis (Reproduced by permission, P. Lander, A. Hadjipavlou. A dynamic classification of Paget's disease. J Bone Joint Surg [Br] 1986; 68-B: 431–8.)

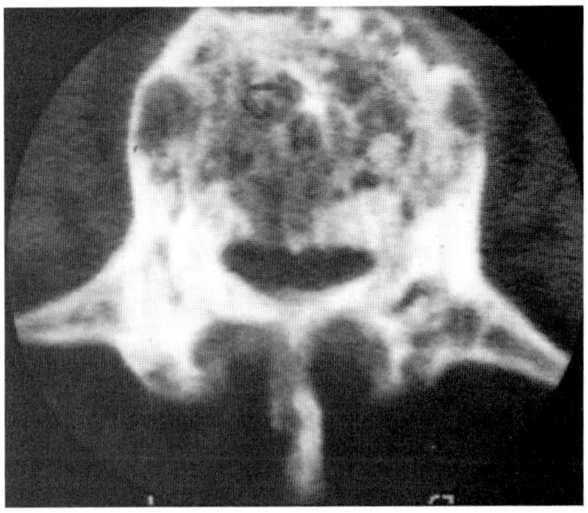

Fig. 3

CT showing mixed-phase Paget's disease of the L4 vertebra with a thickened cortex and trabeculae. There is a wide marrow space of fat density and expansion of the body and neural arch.

Several authors have mentioned that neural involvement is more commonly associated with PD of the thoracic[92,107,186] or the cervical spine,[128] rather than the lumbar spine. This is attributed to the large size of the thoracic and cervical region of the spinal cord relative to the capacity of the vertebral canal. Hence the same proliferation of bone in all vertebrae would result in compression of the cervical and thoracic thecal sacs sooner than it would in the lumbar spine.[185] Involvement of the cervical spine tends to predispose to spinal stenosis with myelopathy.[86]

Ten distinct mechanisms have been implicated as producing dysfunction of neural elements in the spine of patients affected with PD. They are as follows: 1) compression of the neural element by Pagetic bone overgrowth;[47,86,107] 2) compression by Pagetic intraspinal soft tissue;[85,86] 3) ossification of the epidural fat similar to ankylosing spondylitis;[34] 4) neural ischaemia produced by diversion of the blood supply, causing the so-called 'arterial steal phenomenon';[33,92,93,154] 5) interference with the blood supply to the cord because of arterial compression by the expanding Pagetic bone,[185] or other factors not well defined;[126] 6) vertebral fracture or atlantoaxial subluxation;[186,209] 7) platybasia with impingement on the medulla;[40] 8) compression of the spinal cord by epidural haematoma from spontaneous bleeding;[116,169] 9) the development of syringomyelia as a complication of PD of the spine, especially after cranial settling (basilar invagination);[52,169] and 10) rarely, neurocompression from Pagetic sarcomatous change.[98] Bone compression by the expanding Pagetic vertebrae is by far the most common cause of neural dysfunction;[86] it was first reported by Wyllie.[212] Severe stenosis, as seen by CT, however, may remain asymptomatic, suggesting adaptability of the thecal sac and its neural elements to severe spinal stenosis without significant loss of function.[186]

The mechanism of neural ischaemia is, however, still theoretical and supported only by circumstantial evidence. For example, patients with spinal cord symptomatology respond to calcitonin treatment better than patients with lesions of the spinal nerve roots.[40] Some patients experience progressive deterioration of neurological function without evidence of myelographic block which is not easily explained by a mechanical effect alone,[181] neurological signs do not always correlate with the site of skeletal involvement and rapid clinical improvement occurs in some patients with medical treatment alone. These observations suggest that neurological dysfunction in PD may also result from mechanisms other than simple bone encroachment on the neural elements,[50,80,93,103,154,204,212] such as reduction of local blood supply by the rapidly remodelling hypervascular Pagetic bone, the 'arterial steal phenomenon'.

Spinal pain (back and neck pain). Pagetic back pain is characterised by a deep, dull, relatively constant ache which is unrelated to activity, and is not relieved by rest or non-steroidal anti-inflammatory agents. By contrast, so-called mechanical back pain improves with rest and worsens with activity or any sustained position, and arthritic back pain is a variable aching and stiffness during inactivity which improves with walking.[69]

Pagetic facet arthropathy is a major contributing factor to both back pain and spinal stenosis, and the more severe the facet arthropathy, the greater the likelihood of spinal stenosis and/or back pain.[86] This, however, does not necessarily preclude that, although present, severe facet arthropathy may remain asymptomatic.[86] Back pain in PD may also be attributed to blood engorgement of the vertebral body caused by vascular and disorganised, hyperactive remodelling processes.[111] Other factors implicated in spinal pain may include invasion of the vertebral disc space by the Pagetic process,[111] and spinal stenosis.[213] Microfractures of the Pagetic vertebral bodies, especially in the osteolytic or mixed phase, can also lead to back pain. The most common type of spinal pain in our series[86] was mechanical or arthritic, accounting for 27% of patients Constant spinal pain attributed to PD alone was present in 13%, in a combination of mechanical or arthritic back pain in association with Pagetic pain in 14%. In the remaining 46% no spinal pain was reported.

In summary, the altered remodelling unit in PD results in abnormal bone remodelling, producing structural changes precipitating or leading to facet osteoarthropathy and spinal stenosis (Fig. 2). In most cases, the clinical picture of Pagetic spinal stenosis and facet osteoarthropathy is not expected to differ from that of degenerative spondylosis of the spine. A few patients, however, have constant spinal pain attributed to the Pagetic pathological remodelling process. Because the natural history of PD affecting the spine is progressive with bone proliferation, vertebral expansion, and structural changes (Fig. 2), preventive therapy is required.

Treatment of back pain. In most patients with PD, back pain is either mechanical or arthritic in origin, or a combination of these; only 12% of patients experience pain which is clearly due to PD.[81] Care must be taken in attributing back pain to PD, otherwise the results of antiPagetic treatment may be disappointing.[6] In one report suppressive therapy with EHDP (disodium etidronate) was beneficial in 36% of patients with low back pain and PD.[7] This suggests that unless a well-defined lesion is related to low back pain, antiPagetic therapy will not be beneficial. If antiPagetic medical therapy is ineffective within three months, a concomitant non-steroidal anti-inflammatory agent and other treatment methods for back pain should be prescribed, especially when the presenting pain is mechanical or arthritic in nature.[196]

Treatment of spinal stenosis. Treatment of the symptoms of Pagetic spinal stenosis should start with medical anti-Pagetic therapy. Calcitonin, mithramycin, sodium etidronate, pamidronate disodium and chlodronate have been reported either to improve or to completely reverse the symptoms of spinal stenosis,[4,33,53,160,206] but relapse after medical antiPagetic treatment is common.[48,49] Therefore patients should be closely monitored and cyclical therapy should be continued if necessary until the biochemical bone indices become normal. If the symptoms persist in spite of normalisation of bone remodelling markers, surgery may be an alternative treatment. The results of surgery have shown variable improvement in 85% of patients,[181] with frequent relapses or failures that may improve with subsequent medical antiPagetic therapy.[4,33,160] In our series[81] patients who showed either partial or temporary improvement after laminectomy and were treated by further antiPagetic medical treatment had marked improvement of their symptoms. From our experience and from other reports, spinal surgery for Pagetic spinal stenosis may fail to reverse the neurological deficit completely[29] and may be associated with serious complications with a mortality rate of 11%[181] and the possibility of dangerous profuse bleeding.[178] Therefore we advocate radionucleide determination of the bone blood flow to the affected spinal region before operation to assess the vascularity of bone. We have found this test to be reliable and reproducible.[24] In order to decrease bleeding during surgery[81] if there is increased vascularity, we strongly recommend a course of medical antiPagetic treatment until bone blood flow becomes normal. In our experience, this may take two to three months with calcitonin therapy, or two to three weeks with treatment with mithramycin. The new generation of intravenous bisphosphonates can also be used effectively. In an emergency embolisation of the region may be indicated. Because of the expected considerable haemorrhage during laminectomy, the use of a cell saver is strongly recommended.[11,80]

Surgery for spinal stenosis, when indicated, should be tailored to the pathology responsible for neural compression. If this is caused by posterior expansion of vertebral bodies, an anterior approach with corpectomy and fusion is indicated. If neural compression is caused by posterior vertebral elements, posterior decompression should be the operation of choice.[81] An acute onset of spinal compression seems to have a more serious prognosis than the more gradual development of symptoms, which tend to respond better to decompression.[187]

AntiPagetic medical therapy is rewarding when treating Pagetic spinal stenosis syndrome. Severe spinal stenosis of the lytic type may successfully respond to antiPagetic treatment with chlodronate.[53] It has been suggested that, for Pagetic spinal stenosis in the lytic phase, administration of vitamin D and calcium supplements to improve mineralisation of the Pagetic spinal canal may enhance the effectiveness of bisphosphonate therapy.[53] Decompression for spinal stenosis should be undertaken promptly after failure of antiPagetic therapy. In these circumstances, delaying decompression may result in irreversible myelopathy or radiculopathy.[111] In addition, surgery is indicated as primary treatment when neural compression is secondary to pathological fracture, dislocation, epidural haematoma, syringomyelia, platybasia, or sarcomatous transformation.

Other associated conditions

Malignant transformation. In our series of patients with PD,[87,88] we have not seen any cases of sarcomatous change in the spine. In that of Schajowicz et al,[182] of 62 cases of sarcomatous change, five occurred in the spine. The clinical presentation of Paget's sarcomatous change is characterised by severe and persistent pain with rapid deterioration, neurocompression and death.[98] Surgical decompression offers little, if any, true relief of pain, with the longest survival reported at just over five months.[98]

Rheumatic and arthritic conditions. Forestier's disease, or disseminated idiopathic hyperostosis (DISH) can frequently affect patients with PD. Care should be taken, however, not to confuse DISH with Paget's extraosseous bone formation.[29] The incidence of DISH in PD is reported to range from 14%[82] to 30%.[7] Pagetic tissue may invade the hyperostotic lesions produced by DISH and transform them into Pagetic exostoses,[86] which may progress to vertebral ankylosis.[125] Other rheumatic and arthritic conditions such as psoriatic or ankylosing spondylitis may coexist and may be responsible for the clinical presentation.[8,58] PD has also been noted to be associated with an increased incidence of gout[58] and pseudogout.[157] These conditions, however, are not clearly implicated in the production of back pain.[86] It should be borne in mind that treatment with sodium etidronate may be responsible for the accumulation of pyrophosphate crystals in synovial joints, producing pseudogout.[65]

PHARMACOLOGICAL TREATMENT

An important issue regarding treatment is whether physicians should treat asymptomatic patients. The progressive nature of PD, the severity of its associated complications, the potential negative impact on the quality of life of the patient, and the availability of effective antiPagetic drugs have led many experts to recommend treatment for asymptomatic patients who have active disease.[81,202] There are, however, no data to support the view that complications can be prevented by controlling bone remodelling with drug therapy.[202]

Five classes of drug are available for the treatment of PD: bisphosphonates, calcitonin, mithramycin (plicamycin), gallium nitrate, and imprіflavone. Some of these are still in experimental use and can be obtained only through clinical trials. Patients who are asymptomatic and inactive by biochemical and imaging parameters do not require treatment. Those, however, who are clinically asymptomatic but have increased disease activity as shown by the measurement of biochemical markers, bone scanning or radionucleide investigation should be treated until these indices become normal.[196]

Bisphosphonates

Bisphosphonates are chemically stable analogues of inorganic pyrophosphate. These compounds are characterised by two carbon-phosphorus (P-C-P) bonds which, in the past, were erroneously called 'disphosphonates'.[57]

According to Fleisch,[57] the mechanism of action of bisphosphonates on bone was originally ascribed to their physiochemical effect on hydroxyapatite crystals. This action consists of the inhibition of normal calcification by interfering with the growth of calcium phosphate crystals. They bind strongly to hydroxyapatite crystals and inhibit both their formation and dissolution in vitro. Although such an effect is characteristic of their overall action, their influence on cells is probably of greater importance. The bisphosphonates inhibit bone resorption at a cellular level, and after a time, formation of bone also decreases, probably because of the well-known coupling effect between the formation and resorption of bone. The mechanism of action appears to be complex[56] involving several components: a) a direct effect on osteoclastic activity; b) a direct effect on osteoclast recruitment; c) an indirect effect on osteoclast recruitment mediated by cells of osteoclastic lineage capable of stimulating or inhibiting osteoclastic recruitment; and d) a shorter osteoclast life-span because of apoptosis.

Bisphosphonates can be grouped into two pharmacological classes with a distinct molecular mechanism of action. Nitrogen-containing bisphosphonates, which are the most potent, act by inhibiting the mevalonate pathway in osteoclasts, thereby preventing prenylation of small GTPase signalling proteins required for osteoclast function. Bisphosphonates which lack a nitrogen ion in their chemical structure do not inhibit protein prenylation and have a different mode of action which may involve the formation of cytotoxic metabolites in osteoclasts or the inhibition of protein tyrosine phosphatase.[172] Dichloromethylene bisphosphonate or chlodronate (Cl_2MBP) and 1-hydroxymethylene-1,1-bisphosphoric acid (HEBP) inhibit the synthesis of prostaglandin in bone cells. These are powerful bone resorbers. Numerous other cellular effects of bisphosphonates have been described, such as an increase in the production of alkaline phosphatase, an increase or decrease in the synthesis of proteoglycans, inhibition of multiplication of bone macrophages which are osteoclast precursors and a decrease in the production of lactic acid which plays an important role in the dissolution of the crystal. The quality of newly-formed bone is lamellar in appearance without significant mineralisation defects. Large amounts of bisphosphonates, however, can also inhibit mineralisation by a physicochemical inhibition of crystal growth.[56] In addition to its direct inhibition of osteoclastic bone resorption, etidronate can directly induce apoptosis and disruption of actin rings in osteoclasts.[94] A sufficient dose of etidronate inhibits bone mineralisation and may result in osteomalacia.

Cl_2MBP displays relatively little inhibiting activity on bone mineralisation. Intravenous administration of either 4-amino-1-hydroxybuthilidene-1, 1-bisphosphonate (AHButBP), 3-amino-1-hydroxypropylidene-1, 1-bisphosphonate (AHPrBP), or 6-amino-1hydroxyhexylidene-1, 1-bisphosphonate (AHHexBP) induces an acute-phase response (APR) which, irrespective of the underlying disease, manifests as a fall in the number of circulating lymphocytes and serum zinc concentration, and a rise in the level of C-reactive protein (CRP); a febrile reaction occurs in 39% of patients. This APR occurs within 28 to 30 hours of intravenous administration of bisphosphonates and disappears two to three days later, despite continuous treatment. Bisphosphonates seem to interact with macrophage-like cells resident in the skeleton and stimulate the release of interleukin-1 which is responsible for the appearance of APR. At the same time, these cells are rendered insensitive to further stimulation for several months.[1] From these reports bisphosphonates appear to be more effective than calcitonin in suppressing the histological and biochemical activity of PD. Therefore calcitonin is no longer considered the treatment of choice for this condition.

Several bisphosphonates have been investigated, but only the following have been approved for clinical use: disodium etidronate, chlodronate, pamidronate, aledronate, risedronate aminohexane bisphosphonate, tiludronate, ibadronate, chloro-4-phenylthiomethylene bisphosphonate, aminohydroxybutylene bisphosphonate, olpadronate and zoledronate.

Disodium etidronate. The usual dose of disodium etidronate (EHDP) is either 5 mg/kg per day for six months, 10 mg/kg per day for three months, or 20 mg/kg per day for one month. Etidronate is effective in most patients. The drug should be taken on an empty stomach, at least two hours before eating; dairy products should be avoided for five to six hours to improve absorption. Higher doses or more prolonged therapy may result in osteomalacia and pathological fractures.[72,82,195] Combination treatment of 1α-hydroxyvitamin D3 with disodium etidronate, used to prevent the mineralisation defect caused by the bisphosphonate, was not successful in the treatment of PD.[158] Treatment with disodium etidronate should aim at reducing the serum levels of alkaline phosphatase by 40% to 50% at three months with subsequent adjustment of dosage,[54] and it should be repeated cyclically every six months until normalisation of bone-remodelling markers is observed. If EHDP is ineffective after six months of treatment, or if it becomes resistant after a few treatments, other agents such as Cl_2MBP, APD, or calcitonin are recommended. A study comparing oral chlodronate (Cl_2MBP) 600 mg daily and etidronate 5 to 10 mg/kg per day for six months showed that the proportion of patients responding to etidronate was less than the chlodronate group, which had a more sustained response.[73]

Chlodronate. Chlodronate, or dichloromethylene bisphosphonate, is a very potent bisphosphonate; its action on the skeleton consists of the inhibition of bone resorption without the demineralisation.[50,165] The inhibitory effect of bone resorption is mediated mainly by a cytotoxic effect on osteoclasts.[165] The clinical response seems to be better than that achieved with EHDP or calcitonin.[50] The recommended dose is 800 to 1600 mg per day orally for six months,[45,50,73] with a prolonged remission expected to last for about one to two years after withdrawal of the drug.[21,31,45] The recommended intravenous dose which can substantially suppress the activity of the disease is 300 mg daily for five consecutive days (1500 mg total).[104] Chlodronate has also been shown to reverse progression of Pagetic deformity.[21] Unfortunately, leukaemia has been associated with its treatment in three patients and this observation has halted its release for clinical practice except for investigation.[73]

Pamidronate. This is also known as 3-amino-1-hydroxypropylidene-1, 1 bisphosphonate or ADP and is a very effective drug, usually given for severe forms of PD, or if the disease becomes refractory to other medications. Pamidronate binds with crystals of hydroxyapatite in the bone matrix inhibiting osteoclastic activity by preventing attachment of osteoclast precursor cells to bone. This drug has a prolonged biochemical response and can reverse the activity of alkaline phosphatase to normal or nearly normal values in severely symptomatic patients. Transient febrile reactions which are sometimes accompanied by myalgia and lymphopenia commonly occur after the first infusion. Other reported adverse events include transient hypocalcaemia,[28] neutropenia, mild thrombophlebitis and, rarely, ocular complications (uveitis, scleritis).[38] Bone loss in the appendicular skeleton after intravenous treatment has recently been described[199] and attributed to secondary hyperparathyroidism. This effect can be prevented by the administration of calcium and calcitriol. Otherwise no major side-effects have been reported.[28,51,124] APD is available in intravenous and oral forms. Because of its profound effects on mineral and bone metabolism, close monitoring is required during intravenous treatment[51] which is given at a dose ranging from 15 to 25 mg from five to seven consecutive days, a single dose of 60 mg in a 0.9% saline infusion over two hours,[28,200,205] or a dose of 180 mg per course usually given over three days.[203] The suppression period of bone turnover after intravenous administration of this bisphosphonate has not been established with certainty. The estimated ranges are from two to 12 months.[48,200,201,205] The oral form given at a high dose of 1200 mg per day over five consecutive days induces a rapid decline of biochemical indices. As opposed to EHDP-treated patients who showed considerable deterioration in bone texture in 50% of the lytic lesions,[48] ADP was effective in healing such lesions,[48,123] The clinical and biological effects of pamidronate may vary as the number of courses increases.[203] Although APD is a useful means of rapidly suppressing bone turnover, further studies are needed to determine the optimal dosage, the length of treatment and whether oral intravenous treatments when combined would allow for prolonged remission.[205]

Aledronate. Aledronate is a potent amino-bisphosphonate which has been rigorously shown to heal lytic bone lesions[164] and to restore levels of alkaline phosphate to normal by six months in most patients. This drug is capable of producing long-term biochemical remission and is safe and well-tolerated at a daily oral dose of 40 mg for three months[104,119,164,192] or intravenously at a dose of 10 mg daily for five consecutive days.[144] Gastrointestinal[8] side-effects occur in 25% of patients. Histomorphometric assessment failed to show any evidence of impaired mineralisation.[104,164.]

Risedronate. This is a pyridinyl bisphosphonate which can be administered orally in lower dosages than other anti-resorptive bisphosphonates. The recommended dose is 30 mg per day for two to three months or less.[26,97,190] In general, it is well tolerated and has a good safety profile. Treatment for two to three months can significantly reduce or normalise the bone markers of disease activity with long-lasting remission, reduce the associated Pagetic pain[97,137] and provide additional remission in subjects who had an incomplete response to previous treatment with etidronate.[190] This drug is highly effective in osteolytic lesions after six months of treatment.[26]

Aminohexane bisphosphonate (AHBP). This has been tried successfully in PD with no adverse effects on mineralisation or significant side-effects. The oral dose is 400mg daily for one to three months and the intravenous dose is 15 to 50 mg daily for five days or 200 mg in one single dose or in two separate doses on consecutive days. It gives a suppression of biomechanical indices in most patients for up to 18 months with normalisation of specific alkaline phosphatase in more than 60%. AHBP has also been used successfully in patients in whom resistance developed after treatment with disodium etidronate[13,45] or chlodronate.[55]

Tiludronate. This is a potent oral bisphosphonate. At a dose of 400 mg/day for three months it is more effective and is as equally well tolerated as etidronate at 400 mg/day. It is a safe drug[162] with a sustained antiPagetic effect for more than 18 months[59] and can normalise bone turnover without impairing mineralisation.[176]

Ibandronate. This is another bisphosphonate for intravenous use (usual dose 2 mg).[206]

Chloro-4-phenylthiomethylene bisphosphonate. This has a relatively rapid action and gives marked clinical improvement which was observed from the first month of treatment. The drug can be given orally at a dose of 200 to 400 mg daily for six months. The mean decrease in the levels of alkaline phosphatase at six months after the onset of treatment is reported as 43 ± 4% ($p < 0.01$) for a dose of 200 mg and 48 ± 9% ($p < 0.01$) for 400 mg.[163]

Aminohydroxybutylidene bisphosphonate. This is a new bisphosphonate[151] which can be administered intravenously at a dose of 5 mg per day for four to five days and has a profound inhibition of bone resorption. A significant decrease of bone biochemical markers has been observed.[144]

Olpadronate (OPD). This is one of the latest bisphosphonates and it is characterised by dimethylation of the amino group. Its potency is similar to aledronate, but it is more soluble in the digestive system than other aminobisphosphonates. A 12-day course of 200 mg/day has been shown to be very effective and well tolerated.[69]

Zoledronate. This is a third-generation imidazole-ring-containing bisphosphonate. In animal studies it has been shown to be 850 times more potent than pamidronate. A single infusion of a dose of 400 μg inhibited bone resorption without observable clinical or biochemical toxicity.[12] It appears to be a promising drug but merits further study to determine its optimal dose and safety.

Calcitonin

Three forms of calcitonin are available, porcine, salmon and human synthetic, for intramuscular or subcutaneous administration. Salmon is also available in suppositories and as an intranasal spray and in oral form. The potency of salmon and porcine calcitonin is expressed in MRC (Medical Research Council) units. The dose for porcine calcitonin is 1 to 22 MRC units per kg of body-weight, whereas that of salmon calcitonin is 50 to 160 MRC units,[14] given either daily or three times a week in a single or divided dose for a prolonged period of six to 12 months. The dose of human synthetic calcitonin is 0.25 to 0.5 mg per day by subcutaneous injection.[194] Human calcitonin can be used when salmon becomes ineffective because of the formation of antibodies.

Salmon calcitonin has been introduced as a nasal spray or as suppository at doses of 200 to 400 units or 300 units, respectively. Injection of salmon (100 IU) calcitonin is more effective than the use of a nasal spray (200 IU). The latter was ineffective in three patients with severe PD as compared with the injectable form.[70] The decrease in serum alkaline phosphatase after three months of nasal calcitonin is expected to average 24% to 33% of pretreatment values.[63] The ease of administration and patients' acceptance make this form a suitable alternative for geriatric patients.[63] The exposure to intranasal synthetic salmon calcitonin by patients previously treated with parenteral calcitonin may cause a secondary antibody response and clinical resistance.[119]

Calcitonin acts directly on osteoclasts with immediate inhibition of their activity and a marked reduction in their number.[30] It enhances the production of 1,25-dihydroxy-vitamin D3.[65] It also promotes renal excretion of phosphate, calcium, sodium and water.[79] The responses to salmon calcitonin (100 MRC units thrice weekly) and disodium etidronate (EHDP, 400 mg daily) given for six months were similar.[145,170] The reduction in alkaline phosphatase was 53% and 56%, respectively. Combination therapy produced a reduction of 71% in alkaline phosphatase, which is significantly greater than in the non-combined treatment. More sustained control of the activity of the disease was achieved with EHDP given either alone or in combination with calcitonin.

Mithramycin-plicamycin

Mithramycin acts on bone resorption by its osteoclastic toxicity. This inhibits the DNA-directed RNA synthesis of osteoclasts.[180] It has a quick effect on bone remodelling with dramatic normalisation of bone scan activity.[80,180] It is indicated for severe compression of the cord especially when the disease is in the osteolytic phase.[73,80] The recommended dose is 15 μg/kg per day, administered in an intravenous glucose injection over six to eight hours, for five days. The same regimen should be repeated after a seven-day interval. It is toxic to the liver, kidneys and platelets. Monitoring of patients receiving mithramycin should include a platelet count, haematocrit, measurement of blood urea nitrogen, and liver-function tests every second day. We did not encounter permanent kidney, liver or bone-marrow complications in the regimen described. It may predispose to hypokalaemia which may result in death, especially in patients with predisposing cardiac disease who are receiving diuretics.[17] Patients may die of a bleeding diathesis if large doses (37.5 to 50 μg/kg) are given for cancer therapy.[103]

Gallium nitrate

This is a new drug in the treatment of PD. The duration of the response is variable lasting from 6 to 42 weeks. It is administered either intravenously at a dose of 2.5 μg/kg of body-weight per day in 5% glucose for seven consecutive days or by subcutaneous injection at a dose of 0.25 to 0.5 mg/kg body-weight per day for 14 days followed by a two-week interval free from medication, in a monthly cyclical fashion.[22,207] The effectiveness of treatment is proportional to the dose of the drug administered. The response to intravenous treatment was more marked than that to subcutaneous administration.[208] Treatment with gallium nitrate significantly reduces the serum levels of alkaline phosphatase and urinary excretion of hydroxyproline. A fall in hydroxyproline precedes the suppression of alkaline phosphatase, suggesting that suppression of osteoclastic bone resorption precedes that of bone reformation by osteoblasts. The uptake of gallium is dependent on the cellular function. The exact mechanism of action is unknown but may be related to a similar inhibitory effect of calcitonin on osteoclasts.[138] Transient hyperparathyroidism has also been recorded secondary to the decrease in the serum calcium levels during treatment. The effects of gallium nitrate seem to be long-lasting[127] and safe.[22] The treatment is still experimental, and larger trials are required to evaluate its safety and effectiveness.

Impriflavone

This is an isoflavone (7-isoproxy-3-phenyl-4h-1-bonzopyran-4-1) which has been found to have a beneficial effect on PD.[138] At a dose of 600 mg daily for 30 days, there was significant alleviation of Pagetic bone pain and improvement of biochemical bone markers. The drug was well tolerated, and only some mild gastrointestinal intolerance was reported.[150] It apparently acts indirectly on bone, inhibiting bone resorption by stimulating the release of calcitonin,[141] but it is still experimental and is available only in Europe.

METHODS FOR CLINICAL ASSESSMENT AND MONITORING ANTIPAGETIC DRUG TREATMENT

Imaging resources. The effects of treatment are monitored by the patient's clinical response, imaging parameters and the measurement of markers of bone remodelling. Radionucleide scanning can be used to monitor vascularity and therefore to assess the potential bleeding of relevant regions before proceeding with surgery, and also to monitor the effectiveness of emergency intravenous treatment with anti-Pagetic agents. Conventional bone scanning is recommended before and six months after treatment and at 12 months thereafter depending on the behaviour of the Pagetic lesion. A 24-hour retention scan, a more quantitative radionucleide assessment, can be used as an adjunct to bone scanning.[24] Quantitative bone scan scintigraphy allows early and objective assessment of PD when evaluating the effects of therapy.[152] Radiological images should be obtained before treatment and every one to two years thereafter to monitor the changes in modelling and remodelling. Although PD can be diagnosed by conventional radiography, MRI is well suited for showing the specific characteristics of certain complications, including basilar invagination, spinal stenosis and secondary neoplasm.[25]

Biochemical bone markers. Recently, the assessment and effectiveness of the treatment of patients with PD have been improved by emerging and prompt application of biochemical markers for remodelling of new bone. In serum the common bone markers used for the evaluation of bone turnover in PD are levels of total alkaline phosphatase, bone alkaline phosphatase, procollagen type I N-terminal polypeptide (PINP), beta-carboxyterminal telopeptide of type-I collagen (SCTx), osteocalcin and bone sialoprotein. In urine they are the levels of hydroxyproline (Hyp) and amino (NTX) and beta-carboxyterminal (CTX) telopeptides of collagen type I, total pyridinoline (PYD) and deoxypyrinoline (DPD). Markers of bone resorption representing degradation of type-I collagen are N-telopeptides, C-telopeptides, hydroxyproline, and collagen cross-links pyridinoline and dexopyridinoline. The urinary calcium level is also an indication of bone resorption. The serum tartrate-resistant acid phosphatase is a marker for osteoclastic activity. Bone formation markers include bone-specific alkaline phosphatase and N terminal and C terminal extension peptides of procollagen. Osteocalcin, produced by osteoblasts or released during degradation of bone matrix by osteoclasts, may indicate either formation when resorption and formation are coupled or turnover when they are uncoupled. Resorption markers respond approximately one to three months after treatment, whereas markers of formation respond much later, usually after six to nine months.[40]

The serum markers of bone turnover show lower biological variability than urinary markers, and are therefore more sensitive indices of the activity of disease.

Bone alkaline phosphatase and PINP seem most accurately to reflect Pagetic activity.[9,23,152] Total alkaline phosphatase can also be considered as a sensitive marker for the therapeutic monitoring of Paget's disease. More specific markers, however, may improve the usefulness of the biochemical assessment of PD in certain situations.[211]

Urinary N-telopeptide (NTX) has also emerged as a sensitive marker for bone resorption in the management of Pagetic patients.[44,152] Serum levels of pyridinium cross-links correlate well with its urinary excretion (a sensitive index of bone resorption)[10] in patients with PD. The determination of serum levels of pyridinium crosslinks therefore avoids the usual problems related to the collection of urinary specimens.[188] Urinary excretion of β-isomers of type-I collagen (CTX) reflects lamellar bone turnover which is impaired in PD, whereas α-CTX is an index of the structure of woven bone present in active PD.

An abnormal α/β-CTX ratio, which becomes normal after therapy, probably indicates the formation of lamellar structures in the newly-formed bone.[44,66]

Patients should be followed by measuring bone markers every three to six months depending on the activity of the Pagetic lesions and the drug used.[8] Further treatment is suggested when the remodelling indices rise above the upper limits of normal or by 25% above the previous lowest level.[177]

Other tests. The haematological profile, serum level of electrolytes, and kidney- and liver-function tests are helpful in assessing the overall medical condition of elderly patients with PD,[86] especially when administering anti-Pagetic drugs such as mithramycin or the new-generation bisphosphonates.

REFERENCES

1. **Adami S, Bhalla AK, Dorizzi R, et al.** The acute-phase response after bioshphosphonate administration. *Calcif Tissue Int* 1987;41:326-31.
2. **Agnusdei D, Cemporeale A, Conneli S, et al.** Short treatment of Paget's disease of bone with impriflavore. *Bone Miner* 1992;19 Suppl:35.
3. **Alexakis PG, Brown BA, Hohl WM.** Porous hip replacement in Paget's disease: an 8-2/3-year follow-up. *Clin Orthop* 1998;350:138-42.
4. **Alexandre C, Trillet M, Meunier P, et al.** Traitement des paraplegics pagetiques par les disphosphonates. *Rev Neurol (Paris)* 1979;135:625.
5. **Altman RD, Bloch DA, Hochberg MC, Murphy WA.** Prevalence of pelvic Paget's disease of bone in the United States. *J Bone Miner Res* 2000;15:461-5.
6. **Altman RD.** Paget's disease of bone: rheumatologic complications. *Bone* 1999;24Suppl 5:47-8.
7. **Altman RD, Brown M, Gargano F.** Low back pain in Paget's disease of bone. *Clin Orthop* 1987;217:152-61.
8. **Altman RD, Colins B.** Musculoskeletal manifestation of Paget's disease of bone. *Arthritis Rheum* 1980;23:1121.
9. **Alvarez L, Ricos C, Peris P, et al.** Components of biological variation of biochemical markers of bone turnover in Paget's bone disease. *Bone* 2000;26:571-6.
10. **Alvarez L, Guanabens N, Peris P, et al.** Discriminative value of biochemical markers of bone turnover in assessing the activity of Paget's disease. *J Bone Miner Res* 1995;10:458-65.
11. **Anderson JT, Dehner LP.** Osteolytic form of Paget's disease: differential diagnosis and pathogenesis. *J Bone Joint Surg [Am]* 1976;58-A:994-9.
12. **Arden-Cordone M, Siris ES, Lyles KW, et al.** Antiresorptive effect of a single fusion of microgram quantities of zoledronate in Paget's disease of bone. *Calcif Tissue Int* 1997;60:415-8.
13. **Atkins RM, Yates AJ, Gray RE, et al.** Aminohexane disphosphonate in the treatment of Paget's disease of bone. *J Bone Miner Res* 1987;2:273-9.
14. **Avramides A.** Salmon and porcine calcitonin treatment of Paget's disease of bone. *Clin Orthop* 1977;127:78-85.
15. **Barry HC.** *Paget's disease of bone.* Edinburgh: Churchill Livingstone, 1969.
16. **Barry HC.** Sarcoma in Paget's disease of bone in Australia. *J Bone Joint Surg [Am}* 1961;43-A:1122-34.
17. **Bashiz Y, Tomson LR.** Cardiac arrest associated with hypocalcemia in a patient receiving mithromycin. *Postgrad Med J* 1988;64:289.
18. **Basle MF, Rebel A, Fournier JG, Russell WC, Malkani K.** On the trail of paramyxoviruses in Paget's disease of bone. *Clin Orthop* 1987;217:9-15.
19. **Bawerman LW, Altman J, Hughes JL, Zadek RE.** Pseudo-malignant lesion in Paget's disease of bone. *Am J Roentgenol Radium Ther Nucl Med* 1975;124:57-61.
20. **Betoulieres PP, Romieu C, Guilbert HL.** La degenerescence maligne de la maladie osseuse de Paget. *Bull Assoc Fr Cancer* 1948;35:47-64.
21. **Bickerstaff DR, Douglas DL, Burke PH, O'Doherty DP, Kanis JA.** Improvement the deformity of the face in Paget's disease treated with disphosphonates. *J Bone Joint Surg [Br]* 1990;72-B:132-6.

22. **Bockman RS, Wilhelm F, Siris E, et al.** A multicenter trial of low dose gallium nitrate in patients with advanced Paget's disease of bone. *J Clin Endocrinol Metab* 1995;80:595-602.

23. **Bonnin MR, Moragues C, Nolla JM, et al.** Evaluation of circulating type I procollagen propeptides in patients with Paget's disease of bone. *Clin Chem Lab Med* 1998;36:53-5.

24. **Boudreau RJ, Lisbona R, Hadjipavlou A.** Observations on serial radionuclide blood-flow studies in Paget's disease. *J Nucl Med* 1983;24:880-5.

25. **Boutin RD, Spitz DJ, Newman JS, Lenchik L, Steinbach LS.** Complications in Paget disease at MR imaging. *Radiology* 1998;209:641-51.

26. **Brown JP, Chines AA, Myers WR, et al.** Improvement of pagetic bone lesions with risedronate treatment: a radiologic study. *Bone* 2000;26:263-7.

27. **Burgener FA, Perry PE.** Pitfalls in the radiographic diagnosis of Paget's disease of the pelvis. *Skeletal Radiol* 1978;2:231-8.

28. **Cantrill JA, Buckler HM, Anderson DC.** Low dose intravenous 3-amino-hydroxy-prohylidene-1, Ibisphosphonate (APD) for the treatment of Paget's disease of bone. *Ann Rheum Dis* 1986;45:1012.

29. **Cartlidge N, McCollum JPK, Ayyar RDA.** Spinal cord compression in Paget's disease. *J Neurol Neurosurg Phyhiatry* 1970;35:825.

30. **Chambers TJ, McSheehy PMJ, Thomson BM, Fuller K.** The effect of calcium regulation hormones and prostaglandins on bone resorption by osteoclasts desaggregated from neonatal rabbit bones. *Endocrinology* 1985;116:234-9.

31. **Chapuy MC, Charhon SA, Meunier PJ.** Sustained biochemical effects of short treatment of Paget's disease of bone with dichloromethylene disphosphonate. *Metab Bone Dis Relat Res* 1983;4:325-8.

32. **Chen KTK.** Hemangiosarcoma complicating Paget's disease of the bonc. *J Surg Oncol* 1985;28:187-9.

33. **Chen JR, Richard SCR, Wallach S, et al.** Neurologic disturbances in Paget's disease of bone: response to calcitonin. *Neurology* 1979;29:448.

34. **Clarke PR, Williams HI.** Ossification in extradural fat in Paget's disease of the spine. *Br J Surg* 1975;62:571-2.

35. **Cody JD, Singer FR, Roodman GD, et al.** Genetic linkage of Paget disease of the bone to chromosome 18q. *Am J Hum Genet* 1997;61:1117-22.

36. **Collins DH.** Paget's disease of bone: incidence and subclinical forms. *Lancet* 1956;2:51.

37. **Cornil L, Paoli J, Gasten H, Spitelier H.** Les tumeurs osseoses de Paget *Semaine Hop Paris* 1950;26:2357-61.

38. **Coukell AJ, Markham A.** Pamidronate: a review of its use in the management of osteolytic bone metastases, tumour-induced hypercalcaemia and Paget's disease of bone. *Drugs Aging* 1998;12:149-68.

39. **Christenson BH.** Biochemical markers of bone metabolism: an overview. *Clin Biochem* 1997;30:573-93.

40. **Curran JE.** Neurological sequelae of Paget's disease of the vertebral column and skull bone. *Austral Radiol* 1975;19:15.

41. **Dahlin HC, Coventry MB.** Osteogenic sarcoma. *J Bone Joint Surg [Am]* 1967;49-A:101-10.

42. **Danais S, Hadjipavlou A.** Etude scinntighaphique comparative des lesions osseuses et de la moelle osseuse dans la maiadie de Paget. *Union Med Can* 1977;106:1100.

43. **De Chiara A, Apice G, Fazioli F, et al.** Multicentric giant cell tumour with viral-like inclusions associated with Paget's disease of bone: a case treated by steroid therapy. *Oncol Rep* 1998;5:317-20.

44. **Delmas PD.** Biochemical markers of bone turnover in Paget's disease of bone. *J Bone Miner Res* 1999;14Suppl 2:66-9.

45. **Delmas PD, Chapuy MC, Edouard C, Meunier PJ.** Beneficial effects of aminohexane disphosphonate in patients with Paget's disease of bone resistant to sodium etidronate. *Am J Med* 1987;83:276-82.

46. **Delmas PD, Chapuy MC, Vignon E.** Effects of dichloromethylene disphosphonate in Paget's disease of bone. *J Clin Endocrinol Metab* 1982;54:837-44.

47. **Direkze M, Milnes JN.** Spinal cord compression in Paget's disease. *Br J Surg* 1970;57:239.

48. **Dodd GW, Ibbertson HK, Fraser TR, Holdaway IM, Wattie D.** Radiological assessment of Paget's disease of bone after treatment with bisphosphonate EHDP and APD. *Br J Radiol* 1987;60:849-60.

49. **Douglas DL, Duckworth T, Kanis JA, et al.** Spinal cord dysfunction in Paget's disease of bone: has medical treatment a vascular basis? *J Bone Joint Surg [Br]* 1981;63-B:495-503.

50. **Douglas DL, Duckworth T, Kanis JA, et al.** Biochemical and clinical responses to dichloromethylene disphosphonate (CI2MDP) in Paget's disease of bone. *Arthritis Rheum* 1980;23:1185.

51. **Drake S, Massie JD, Postlethwaite AE, Palmieri GM.** Pamidronate sodium and calcitonin-resistant Paget's disease: immediate response in a patient. *Arch Intern Med* 1989;149:401-3.

52. **Elisevich K, Fontaine S, Bertrand C.** Syringomyelia as a complication of Paget's disease. *J Neurosurg* 1987;67:611.

53. **Eulry F, Poirer JM, Perard D, et al.** Cauda equina syndrome with pagetic vertebral fusion: clinical recovery under calcium-vitamin D supplementation plus clodronate after apparent failure of pamidronate and acquired resistance to etidronate. *Rev Rhum Engl Ed* 1997;64:495-9.

54. **Evans RA.** Paget's disease of bone: comments by eight specialists. *Excerpta Medica* Princeton, NJ, 1988.

55. **Filipponi P, Cristallini S, Policani G, Casciari C, Gregorio F.** Paget's disease of bone: benefits of neridonate as a first treatment and in cases of relapse after clodronate. *Bone* 1998;23:543-8.

56. **Fleisch H.** Mechanisms of action of the bisphosphonates in Paget's disease of bone. *Medicina (B Aires)* 1997;57 Suppl 1:65-75.

57. **Fleisch H.** Experimental basis for the use of bisphosphonates in Paget's disease of bone. *Clin Orthop* 1987;217:72-8.

58. **Franck WA, Bress NM, Singer FR, etal.** Rheumatic manifestations of Paget's disease of bone. *Am J Med* 1974;56:592.

59. **Fraser WD, Stamp TC, Creek RA, Sawyer JP, Picot C.** A double-blind, multicentre, placebo-controlled study of tiludronate in Paget's disease of bone. *Postgrad Med J* 1997;73:496-502.

60. **Freydinger JE, Duhig JT, McDonald LW.** Sarcoma complicating Paget's disease of bone: a study of 7 cases with report of one long survival after surgery. *Arch Pathol* 1963;75:496-500.

61. **Frost HM.** Bone modelling and skeletal modeling errors. In: *Orthopedic lectures.* Vol. 4. Springfield, IL, Charles C. Thomas, 1973.

62. **Frost HM.** Bone remodelling and its relationship to metabolic bone diseases. In: *Orthopedic lectures.* Vol. 3. Springfield, IL, Charles C. Thomas, 1973.

63. **Gagel RF, Logan C, Mallette LE.** Treatment of Paget's disease of bone with salmon calcitonin nasal spray. *J Am Geriatr Soc* 1988;30:1010-4.

64. **Galante L, Colston KW, MacAuley SJ, et al.** Effect of calcitonin on vitamin D metabolism. *Nature* 1972;238:271.

65. **Gallagher SJ, Boyle IT, Capell HA.** Pseudogout associated with the use of cyclical etidronate therapy. *Scott Med J* 1991;36:49.

66. **Garnero P, Fledelius C, Gineyts E, Serre CM, Vignot E, Delmas PD.** Decreased beta-isomerization of the C-terminal telopeptide of type I collagen alpha 1 chain in Paget's disease of bone. *Bone Miner Res* 1997;12:1407-15.

67. **Gebhart M, Vandeweyer E, Nemec E.** Paget's disease of bone complicated by giant cell tumour. *Clin Orthop* 1998;352:187-93.

68. **Goldman AB, Bullough P, Kammeron S, Ambos M.** Osteitis deformans of the hip joint. *Am J Radiol* 1977;128:601.

69. **Gonzalez DC, Mautalen CA.** Short-term therapy with oral olpadronate in active Paget's disease of bone. *J Bone Miner Res* 1999;14:2042-7.

70. **Gonzales D, Vega E, Ghiringhelli G, Mantalan E.** Comparison of the acute effect of the intranasal and intramuscular administration of salmon calcitonin in Paget's disease. *Calcif Tissue Int* 1987;41:313-5.

71. **Goodman SJ.** Syringomeglia in Paget's disease. *J Neurosurg* 1987;67:790.

72. **Gray RE.** *Paget's disease of bone: comments by eight specialists.* Princeton, NJ, Excerpt Medica, 1988.

73. **Gray RE, Yates JP, Preston CJ, et al.** Duration of effect of oral disphosphonate therapy in Paget's disease of bone. *Q J Med* 1987;64:755-67.

74. **Greditzer HG, McLeod RA, Unni KK, Beabout JW.** Bone sarcomas in Paget's disease. *Radiology* 1983;146:327-33.

75. **Grundy M.** Fractures of the femur in Paget's disease of bone: their etiology and treatment. *J Bone Joint Surg [Br]* 1970;52-B:252-63.

76. **Guyer PB, Chamberlain AT.** Paget's disease of bone in South Africa. *Clin Radiol* 1988;39:51-2.

77. **Guyer PB, Shepherd DFC.** Paget's disease of lumbar spine. *Br J Radiol* 1980;53:286.

78. **Guyer PB, Dewbury KC.** The hip joint in Paget's disease (Paget's coxopathy). *Br J Radiol* 1978;52:574.

79. **Hadjipavlou A, Brooks EE.** Etude de l'action de la calcitonin sur le rein. *Union Med Can* 1976;105:915.

80. **Hadjipavlou AG, Tsoukas GM, Siller TN, et al.** Combination drug therapy in treatment of Paget's disease of bone: clinical and metabolic response. *J Bone Joint Surg [Am]* 1977;59-A:1045-51.

81. **Hadjipavlou AG, Lander PH, Enker.** Paget's disease of bone: orthopedic management in arthritis pathology and management. In: Uttof, ed. *Current concepts of bone fragility.* Berlin, etc: Uttof Springer-Verlag, 1986.

82. **Hadjipavlou A, Lander P, Srolovitz H.** Pagetic arthritis: pathophysiology and management. *Clin Orthop* 1986;208:15.

83. **Hadjipavlou A, Begin LR, Abitbol JJ.** Observations morfologiques, histochimiques et ultrastructulares de culture cellulaires in vitro d'os pagetique et normal. *Union Med Can* 1986;115:746.

84. **Hadjipavlou A.** Paget's disease of bone: comments by eight specialists. In: *Excerpta Medica* Princeton, NJ, 1988.

85. **Hadjipavlou A, Shaffer N, Lander P, Srolovitz H.** Pagetic spinal stenosis with extradural pagetoid ossification: a case report. *Spine* 1988;13:128-30.

86. **Hadjipavlou A, Lander P.** Paget's disease of the spine. *J Bone Joint Surg [Am]* 1991;73-A:1376-81.

87. **Hadjipavlou A, Lander P, Srolovitz H, Enker P.** Malignant transformation in Paget's disease of bone. *Cancer* 1992;70:802-8.

88. **Hadjipavlou AG, Lander PH.** Paget's disease. In: White AH, Schofferman JA, eds. *Spinal care.* Mosby, 1995:1720-37.

89. **Haibach H, Farrell C, Dittrich FJ.** Neoplasm arising in Paget's disease of bone: a study of 89 cases. *Am J Clin Pathol* 1985;83:594-600.

90. **Harrington KD.** Surgical management of neoplastic complications of Paget's disease. *J Bone Miner Res* 1999;14Suppl 2:45-8.

91. **Hartman JT, Dohn DF.** Paget's disease of the spine with cord or nerve-root compression: report of six cases. *J Bone Joint Surg [Am]* 1966;48-A:1079-4.

92. **Haslam SI, Van Hul W, Morales-Piga A, et al.** Paget's disease of bone: evidence for a susceptibility locus on chromosome 18q and for genetic heterogeneity. *J Bone Miner Res* 1998;13:911-7.

93. **Herzberg L, Bayllis E.** Spinal cord syndrome due to compressive Paget's disease of bone: a spinal artery steal phenomena reversible with calcitonin. *Lancet* 1980;2:13.

94. **Hiroi-Furuya E, Kameda T, Hiura K, et al.** Etidronate (EHDP) inhibits osteoclastic-bone resorption, promotes apoptosis and disrupts actin rings in isolate-mature osteoclasts. *Calcif Tissue Int* 1999;64:219-23.

95. **Hocking L, Slee F, Haslam SI, et al.** Familial Paget's disease of bone: patterns of inheritance and frequency of linkage to chromosome 18q. *Bone* 2000;26:577-80.

96. **Holdaway IM, Ibberston HK, Wattie D, et al.** Previous pet ownership and Paget's disease. *Bone Miner* 1990;8:53.

97. **Hosking DJ, Eusebio RA, Chines AA.** Paget's disease of bone: reduction of disease activity with oral risedronate. *Bone* 1998;22:51-5.

98. **Huang TL, Cohen NJ, Sahgal SA, et al.** Osteosarcoma complicating in Paget's disease of the spine with neurologic complication. *Clin Orthop* 1979;14:260.

99. **Huvos AG, Butler A, Bretsky SS.** Osteogenic sarcoma associated with Paget's disease of bone: a clinicopathologic study of 65 patients. *Cancer* 1984;52:1489-95.

100. **Jaffe HC.** Paget's disease of bone. *Arch Pathol* 1933;15:81-131.

101. **Jattiot F, Goupille P, Azais I, et al.** Fourteen cases of sarcomatous degeneration in Paget's disease. *J Rheumatol* 1999;26:150-5.

102. **Kay HD, Levy-Simpson S, Riddoch G, et al.** Osteitis deformans with roentgenologic section. *Arch Intern Med* 1934;53:208.

103. **Kennedy BJ.** Metabolic and toxic effects of mithromycin during tumour therapy. *Am J Med* 1970;48:494.

104. **Khan SA, Vasikaran S, McCloskey EV, et al.** Alendronate in the treatment of Paget's disease of bone. *Bone* 1997;20:263-71.

105. **Khan SA, Brennan P, Newman J, et al.** Paget's disease of bone and unvaccinated dogs. *Bone* 1996;19:47-50.

106. **Khan SA, McCloskey EV, Eyres KS, et al.** Comparison of three intravenous regimens of clodronate in Paget's disease of bone. *J Bone Miner Res* 1996;11:178-82.

107. **Klenerman L.** Cauda equina and spinal cord compression in Paget's disease. *J Bone Joint Surg [Br]* 1966;48-B:365-70.

108. **Krane SM.** Etidronate disodium in the treatment of Paget's disease of bone. *Ann Intern Med* 1982;96:619-25.

109. **Lake M.** The pathology of fractures in Paget's disease. *Aust NZ J Surg* 1957;27:307.

110. **Lake M.** Studies of Paget's disease (osteitis deformans). *J Bone Joint Surg [Br]* 1951;33-B:323-5.

111. **Lamovec J, Rener M, Spiler M.** Pseudosarcoma in Paget's disease of bone. *Ann Diagn Pathol* 1999;3;99-103.

112. **Lander P, Hadjipavlou A.** Intradiscal invasion of Paget's disease of the spine. *Spine* 1991;16:46-51.

113. **Lander PH, Hadjipavlou AC.** A dynamic classification in Paget's. *J Bone Joint Surg [Br]* 1986;68-B:431-8.

114. **Lauchlan SC, Walsh MJ.** Reticulum cell carcinoma complicating Paget's disease. *Can Med Assoc J* 1963;88:891-2.

115. **Leach RJ, Singer FR, Cody JD, Roodman GD.** Variable disease severity associated with a Paget's disease predisposition gene. *J Bone Miner Res* 1999;14 Suppl 2:17-20.

116. **Lee KS, McWhorter JM, Angelo JN.** Spinal epidural hematoma associated with Paget's disease. *Surg Neurol* 1988;30:131-4.

117. **Lewallen DG.** Hip arthroplasty in patients with Paget's disease. *Clin Orthop* 1999;369:243-50.

118. **Levy F, Muff R, Dotti-Sigrist S, et al** Formation of neutralizing antibodies during intranasal synthetic salmon calcitonin treatment of Paget's disease. *J Clin Endocrinol Metabo* 1988;17:541.

119. **Lombardi A.** Treatment of Paget's disease of bone with alendronate. *Bone* 1999;24Suppl 5;59-61.

120. **Lopez-Abente G, Morales-Piga A, Elena-Ibanez A, Rey-Rey JS, Corres-Gonzalez J.** Cattle pets, and Paget's disease of bone. *Epidemiology* 1997;8:247-51.

121. **Louette L, Lammens J, Fabry G.** The Ilizarov external fixator for treatment of deformities in Paget's disease. *Clin Orthop* 1996;323:298-303.

122. **Lowry AM, Rutherford JL.** Osteitis deformans (Paget's disease) fissure fractures: their etiology and clinical significance. *Am J Radiol* 1937;38:109.

123. **Maldaque B, Malghem J.** Dynamic radiologic patterns of Paget's disease of bone. *Clin Orthop* 1987;217:125.

124. **Mallete LE.** Successful treatment of resistant Paget's disease of bone with pamidronate. *Arch Intern Med* 1989;149:2765-7.

125. **Marcelli C, Yates AJ, Barjon MC, et al.** Pagetic vertebral ankylosis and diffuse idiopathic skeletal hyperostosis. *Spine* 1995;15;20:454-9.

126. **Mathe JF, Delobel R, Resche F, et al.** Syndromes medullaire au cours de la maladie De Paget: Role du facteur vasculaire. *Nouv Presse Med* 1976;5:2619.

127. **Matkovic V, Apseloff G, Shepard DR, Gerber N.** Use of gallium nitrate on bone: a pilot study. *Lancet* 1990;335:72-5.

128. **Mawhinney R, Jones R, Worthington BJ.** Spinal cord compression secondary to Paget's disease of the axis. *Br J Radiol* 1985;58:1203-6.

129. **McGrory BJ.** Periprosthetic fracture of the acetabulum during total hip arthroplasty in a patient with Paget's disease. *Am J Orthop* 1999;28:248-50.

130. **McKenna RJ, Schwinn CP, Soongy KY, Higinbotham NL.** Osteogenic sarcoma arising in Paget's disease. *Cancer* 1964;17:42-66.

131. **Mee AP.** Paramyxoviruses and Paget's disease: the affirmative view. *Bone* 1999;24 Suppl 5:19-21.

132. **Merkow RL, Lane JM.** Current concepts of Paget's disease of bone. *Orthop Clin North Am* 1984;15:747.

133. **Merkow RL, Lane JM.** Paget's disease of bone. *Orthop Clin North Am* 1990;21:171.

134. **Meyers MH, Singer FR.** Osteotomy of tibia vara in Paget's disease under cover of calcitonin. *J Bone Joint Surg [Am]* 1977;68-A:810.

135. **Meunier PJ, Salson C, Mathieu L, et al.** Skeletal distribution and biochemical parameters of Paget's disease. *Clin Orthop* 1987;217:37.

136. **Milgram JW.** Orthopaedic management of Paget's disease of bone. *Clin Orthop* 1977;127:63.

137. **Miller PD, Brown JP, Siris ES, et al.** A randomized, double-blind comparison of risedronate and etidronate in the treatment of Paget's disease of bone: Paget's risedronate/etidronate study group. *Am J Med* 1999;106:513-20.

138. **Mills BG, Singer FR.** Critical evaluation of viral antigen data in Paget's disease of bone. *Clin Orthop* 1987;217:16.

139. **Mills BG, Masuka LS, Graham CC Jr, et al.** Gallium-67 citrate localization in osteoclast nuclei of Paget's disease of bone. *J Nucl Med* 1988;29:1083-7.

140. **Molle D, Bard H, Kuntz D, et al.** Osteolyse relatrice d'un lymphome developpe sur un os pagetique. *Rev Rhum Mal Osteartic* 1983;50:217-21.

141. **Nakamura S, Mozimoto S, Takamoto S, et al.** Effect of ipriflavore on bone mineral density and calcium related factors in elderly females. *Calcif Tissue Int Suppl* 1992;1:30.

142. **Namba RS, Brick GW, Murray WR.** Revision total hip arthroplasty with correctional femoral osteotomy in Paget's disease. *J Arthroplasty* 1997;12:591-5.

143. **Nance MA, Nuttall FQ, Econs MJ, et al.** Heterogeneity in Paget disease of the bone. *Am J Med Genet* 2000;19 92:303-7.

144. **O'Doherty DP, Bickerstaff DR, McCloskey EV, et al.** Treatment of Paget's disease of bone with aminohydroxybutylidene bisphosphonate. *J Bone Miner Res* 1990;5:483-91.

145. **O'Doherty DP, McCloskey EV, Vasikaran S, Khan S, Kanis JA.** The effects of intravenous alendronate in Paget's disease of bone. *J Bone Miner Res* 1995;10:1094-100.

146. **O'Donoghue DJ, Hoskins DJ.** Biochemical response to combination of disodium etidronate with calcitonin in Paget's disease. *Bone* 1987;8:219.

147. **O'Driscoll JB, Buckler HM, Jeakurk J, et al.** Dogs distemper, and osteitis deformans: a further epidemiological study. *Bone Miner* 1990;11:204.

148. **Paget J.** On a form of chronic inflammation of bone (osteitis deformans). *Trans R Med Chir Soc Lond* 1877;60:36.

149. **Paget J.** Remarks on osteitis deformans. *Illus Med News* 1889;2:181.

150. **Passeri M, Biudi M, Costi D, et al.** Effect of ipriflavone on bone mass in elderly osteoporotic women. *Bone Miner Suppl* 1992;19:57.

151. **Pedrazzoni M, Palummeri E, Ciotti G, et al.** Short term effects on bone and mineral metabolism of 4-amini-1-hydroxybutylidene-1, 1-disphosphonate (ABDP) in Paget's disease of bone. *Bone Miner* 1989;7:301-7.

152. **Pons F, Alvarez L, Peris P, et al.** Quantitative evaluation of bone scintigraphy in the assessment of Paget's disease activity. *Nucl Med Commun* 1999;20:525-8.

153. **Porretta CA, Dahlin DC, Janes JM.** Sarcoma in Paget's disease of bone. *J Bone Joint Surg [Am]* 1957;39-A:1314-29.

154. **Porrini AA, Maldonado-Cocco JA, Morteo GO.** Spinal artery steal syndrome in Paget's disease of bone. *Clin Exp Rheumatol* 1987;5:337.

155. **Price CCHG, Goldie W.** Paget's sarcoma of bone: a study of eighty cases from the Bristol and the Leeds Bone Tumour Register. *J Bone Joint Surg [Br]* 1969;51-B:205-24.

156. **Pygott F.** Paget's disease of bone: the radiological incidence. *Lancet* 1957;1:1170.

157. **Radi I, Epiney J, Reiner M.** Chondrocalcinose et maladie asseuse de Paget. *Rev Rheum* 1970;37:387.

158. **Ralston SH, Boyce BF, Cowan RA, et al.** The effect of 1-alpha-hydroxyvitamin D3 on the mineralization defect in disodium etidronate treated Paget's disease: a double-blind randomized clinical study. *J Bone Miner Res* 1987;2:5-12.

159. **Ramussen H, Bordier P.** The physiological cellular basis of metabolic bone disease. *N Engl Med* 1973;184:25.

160. **Ravichandran G.** Neurologic recovery of paraplegia following use of salmon calcitonin in a patient with Paget's disease of the spine. *Spine* 1979;4:37.

161. **Redden JF, Dixon J, Vennart W, Hoskins DJ.** Management of fissure fracture in Paget's disease. *Int Orthop* 1981;5:103.

162. **Reginster JY, Treves R, Renier JC, et al.** Efficacy and tolerability of a new formulation of oral tiludronate (tablet) in the treatment of Paget's disease of bone. *J Bone Miner Res* 1994;9:615-9.

163. **Reginster JY, Dezoisy R, Lecart MP, Franchimont P.** (Chloro-4 phenyl) thiomethyne bisphosphonate in Paget's bone disease. *Acta Belg Med Phys* 1989;12:47-52.

164. **Reid IR, Nicholson GC, Weinstein RS, et al.** Biochemical and radiologic improvement in Paget's disease of bone treated with alendronate: a randomized placebo-controlled trial. *Am J Med* 1966;101:341-8.

165. **Reisma PH, Teitelbaum SL, Bijvoet OLM, Kahn AJ.** Differential action of bisphosphonates (3-amino-1-hydroxypropylidene)-1,1-bisphosphonate (ADP) and disodium dichloromethylidene bisphosphonate (C12MDP) on rat macrophage-mediated bone resorption in vitro. *J Clin Invest* 1982;70:927-33.

166. **Relea A, Garcia-Urbon MV, Arboleya L, Zamora T.** Extramedullary hematopoiesis related to Paget's disease. *Eur Radiol* 1999;9:205-7.

167. **Renier JC, Fanello S, Bos C, Audran M.** An etiologic study of Paget's disease. *Rev Rhum Engl Ed* 1996;63:606-11.

168. **Resnick D, Niwayama G.** *Diagnostic of bone and joint disorders with ephasis on articular abnormalities.* Philadelphia: W. B. Saunders, 1981:1738.

169. **Richter RL, Semble EL, Turner RA, Challen VR.** An unusual manifestation of Paget's disease of bone: spinal epidural hematoma presenting as acute cauda equina syndrome. *J Rheumatol* 1990;17:975-8.

170. **Rico H, Hernandez ER, Younes M, et al.** Biochemical assessment of acute and chronic treatment of Paget's bone disease with calcitonin and calcium with or without bisphosphonate. *Bone* 1988;9:63-6.

171. **Roberts RE, Cohen MJ.** Osteitis deformans (Paget's disease of bone). *Proc Soc R Lond* 1926;19:13.

172. **Rogers MJ, Gordon S, Benford HL, et al.** Cellular and molecular mechanisms of action of bisphosphonates. *Cancer* 2000;88:2961-78.

173. **Rondier J, Huchet B, Calya J.** Osteolyse pseudo-sarcomateuse chez un Pagetique traite par l'etidronate disodique (EHDP). *Rev Rhum Mal Osteoartic* 1984;51:49-54.

174. **Rosenkrantz JA, Wolf J, Kaicher JJ.** Paget's disease (osteitis deformans). *Arch Intern Med* 1952;90:610.

175. **Rosenthal L, Lisbona R.** *Current practice in nuclear medicine: skeletal imaging.* Norwalk (CT): Appleton-Century-Crofts, 1984:43-7.

176. **Roux C.** The methodology of clinical trials of oral tiludronate in Paget's disease of bone. *Bone* 1995;17Suppl 5:497-9.

177. **Russell RG, Rogers MJ, Frith JC, et al.** The pharmacology of bisphosphonates and new insights into their mechanisms of action. *J Bone Miner Res* 1999;14Suppl 2:53-65.

178. **Ryan WC, Schwartz TB.** Mithramycin and malignancy (letter). *Ann Intern Med* 1981;94:279.

179. **Ryan MD, Taylor TKF.** Spinal manifestations of Paget's disease. *Aust N Z J Surg* 1992;62:33.

180. **Ryan WG.** Treatment of Paget's disease of bone with mithramycin. *Clin Orthop* 1977;127:106.

181. **Sadar SE, Walton RJ, Grossman HH.** Neurological dysfunction in Paget's disease of the vertebral column. *J Neurosurg* 1972;37:661.

182. **Schajowicz F,Araujo ES, Berestein M.** Sarcoma complicating Paget's disease of bone: a clinicopathology study of 62 cases. *J Bone Joint Surg [Br]* 1983;65-B:299-307.

183. **Shardlow DL, Giannoudis PV, Matthews SJ, Smith RM.** Stabilisation of acute femoral fractures in Paget's disease. *Int Orthop* 1999;23:283-5.

184. **Schatzki SC, Dudley HR.** Bone sarcoma complicating Paget's disease: a report of 3 cases with long survival. *Cancer* 1961;14:518-23.

185. **Schmorl G.** Uber osteitis deformans Paget. *Virchows Arch Anat Physiol* 1932;183:694.

186. **Schwarz GA, Reback S.** Compression of the spinal cord in osteitis deformans (Paget's disease of the vertebrae). *Am Roentgenol Radi Ther* 1939;42:345.

187. **Siegelman SS, Levine SA, Walpin L.** Paget's disease with spinal cord compression. *Clin Radiol* 1968;19:421.

188. **Sinigaglia L, Varenna M, Binelli L, et al.** Serum levels of pyridinium crosslinks in postmenopausal women and in Paget's disease of bone. *Calcif Tissue Int* 1997;61:279-84.

189. **Singer RF.** *Paget's disease of bone.* New York: Plenum Medical Books Co, 1977.

190. **Singer RF, Millis BG.** The etiology of Paget's disease of bone. *Clin Orthop* 1977;127:37.

191. **Siris E, Chines AA, Altman RD, et al.** Risedronate in the treatment of Paget's disease of bone: an open label, multicenter study. *J Bone Miner Res* 1998;13:1032-8.

192. **Siris E, Weinstein RS, Altman R, et al.** Comparative study of alendronate versus etidronate for the treatment of Paget's disease of bone. *J Clin Endocrinol Metab* 1996;81:961-7.

193. **Siris ES, Kelsey JL, Flasher E, Parker S.** Familial aggregation of Paget's disease of bone. *J Bone Miner Res* 1991;6:495.

194. **Siris ES, Kelsey JL, Flasher E, Parker S.** Paget's disease of bone and previous pet ownership in the United States: dogs exonerated. *Int J Epidemol* 1990;19:455-8.

195. **Siris ES.** Paget's disease of bone: comments by eight specialists. *Excerpta Medica* Princeton, NJ, 1988.

196. **Smidt WR, Hadjipavlou AG, Lander P, Dzioba RB.** An algorithmic approach to the treatment of Paget's disease of the spine. *Orthop Rev* 1994;9:715-24.

197. **Smith J, Botet JF, Yeh SDJ.** Bone sarcoma in Paget's disease: a study of 85 patients. *Radiology* 1984;152:583-90.

198. **Sochart DH, Porter ML.** Charley low-friction arthroplasty for Paget's disease of the hip. *J Arthroplasty* 2000;15:210-9.

199. **Stewart GO, Gutteridge DH, Price RI, et al.** Prevention of appendicular bone loss in Paget's disease following treatment with intravenous pamidronate disodium. *Bone* 1999;24:139-44.

200. **Thiebaud D, Jaeger P, Gobelet C, et al.** A single infusion of the bisphosphonate AHPrBP (ADP) as treatment of Paget's disease of bone. *Am J Med* 1988;85:207-12.

201. **Thiebaud D, Jaeger P, Burchardt P.** Paget's disease of bone treated in five days with AHPrBp (ADP) per OS. *J Bone Miner Res* 1987;2:45.

202. **Tiegs RD.** Paget's disease of bone: indications for treatment and goals of therapy. *Clin Ther* 1997;19:1309-29.

203. **Trombetti A, Arlot M, Thevenon J, Uebelhart B, Meunier PJ.** Effect of multiple intravenous pamidronate courses in Paget's disease of bone. *Rev Rhum Engl Ed* 1999;66:467-76.

204. **Turner JWA.** Spinal complications of Paget's disease (osteiti deformans). *Brain* 1940;63:321.

205. **Vega E, Gonzales D, Chiringelli G, Montalen C.** Intravenous aminopropylidene bisphosphonate (ADP) in the treatment of Paget's bone disease. *J Bone Miner Res* 1987;2:267-71.

206. **Wallace E, Wong J, Reid IR.** Pamidronate treatment of the neurologic sequelae of pagetic spinal stenosis. *Arch Intern Med* 1995.

207. **Warrell RP Jr.** Gallium nitrate for the treatment of bone metastases. *Cancer* 1997;15:80Suppl 8:1680-5.

208. **Warrell RP Jr, Bosco B, Weinerman S, et al.** Gallium nitrate for advanced Paget's disease of bone, effectiveness and dose-response analysis. *Ann Intern Med* 1990;113:847-51.

209. **Whalley N.** Paget's disease of the atlas and axis. *J Neurol Neurosurg Psychiat* 1946;9:84-51.

210. **Wick MR, Siegal GP, Unni KK, et al.** Sarcomas of bone complicating osteitis deformas (Paget's disease): fifty years' experience. *Am J Surg Pathol* 1981;5:47-59.

211. **Woitge HW, Oberwittler H, Heichel S, et al.** Short- and long-term effeccts of ibandronate treatment on bone turnover in Paget disease of bone. *Clin Chem* 2000;46:684-90.

212. **Wyllie WG.** The occurrence in osteiti deformans of lesion of the central nervous system with a report of four cases. *Brain* 1923;46:336.

213. **Zlatkin MB, Lander PH, Hadjipavlou AC, Levine JS.** Paget's disease of the spine: CT with clinical correlation. *Radiology* 1986;160:155-9.

INDICATIONS FOR LUMBAR SPINAL FUSION

MARTIN KRISMER

From the University of Innsbruck, Austria

Low back pain (LBP) is a common complaint. Walker[1] has published a systematic review of the literature analysing 56 population prevalence studies of LBP. The point prevalence ranged from 12% to 33%, the one-year prevalence from 22% to 65%, and lifetime prevalence from 11% to 84%. A few studies have dealt with the prevalence of LBP in developing countries and reported much lower rates than in Western industrialised nations.

Most Western adults complaining of low back pain can cope with it and do not seek professional treatment, but a few do require help. Patients with chronic spinal disorders have worse scores for physical functional status than those with most other conditions.[2] Some of these patients are considered to be candidates for lumbar spinal fusion. The rates for both are not well known, and the regional variation of the incidence of lumbar spinal fusion is high. Although there is some evidence about the efficacy of lumbar spinal fusion, there are different opinions about the indications, which is also reflected by the considerable regional variation. A recent publication[3] has shown that in surgery for hip fracture the regional variation is low (1.9- to 2.09-fold), in total hip replacement it is intermediate (3.5- to 4.7-fold), and in back surgery it is high (6.5- to 10.1-fold). International variation in the rates of back surgery is also high. Countries with high rates of back surgery also have high rates of other discretionary procedures such as tonsillectomy and hysterectomy.[4] In an Australian investigation, the rates of lumbar spinal surgery varied fourfold from 25/100 000 to 92/100 000. In a regression model, only the rate of unemployment was negatively correlated with the variation in the rate of lumbar spinal surgery and accounted for 11% of this.[5] In another study on lumbar disc herniation, outcomes for patients who had been operated on by surgeons in areas with low rates of surgery were better than those for patients in areas with high rates. The latter generally had less severe preoperative symptoms.[6] The conclusion of this study was that the outcome of back surgery is related to rigid indications.

In this article a systematic analysis will be made of existing studies in order to arrive at clear recommendations with a proposal concerning further studies to obtain better guidelines.

We do not know to what extent factors such as genetics, occupation, access to health care, and the opinions of the general population about spinal fusion explain regional variation. The differing opinion of surgeons concerning the indications, however, is believed to play an important role and the complexity of this process is high. The following analysis therefore focuses on the most common problems and indications, and does not claim completeness. Particularly, conditions such as tumours, infections, trauma, lumbar Scheuermann's disease, kyphosis, severe lordosis, and degenerative scoliosis are not included.

THE INDICATIONS FOR FUSION

Some indications for treatment in medicine are simply related to the diagnosis and others to the severity of the disease. Acute appendicitis is an indication for appendicectomy, but osteoarthritis of the hip is not necessarily an indication for hip arthroplasty. The severity of the osteoarthritis on radiographs and the disability should reach a certain level, otherwise the intervention may be considered to be too early. Classifications are often used to establish guidelines for indications. The AO classification for vertebral fractures was created to serve as such. None of these examples is exactly in keeping with indications for lumbar spinal fusion.

The decision-making process involving surgeons and their patients is also poorly understood. The behaviour of the physician and the expectations of the patient have not been systematically studied. In the following paragraphs a personal opinion is given which cannot be based on empirical data.

Patient. There is almost no knowledge about the patient's opinion of lumbar spinal fusion. Why does the patient want to undergo this procedure? Does he perhaps want less care and less risk than surgeons offer? What does the general population think about this procedure and how does this knowledge affect the indications for surgery? In different countries there are different answers to these questions. It is astonishing that no firm guidelines have been published in the orthopaedic literature, although this is mandatory to meet the patient's needs. Recently, Weinstein[7] has pointed out that patients have a preference for avoiding risk and for non-surgical treatment rather than operation.

Doctor-patient relationship. The legal concept assumes that the doctor informs the patient about his disease, the different options for treatment, with the possible benefits and adverse events, empowering the patient to make the decision himself. The everyday experience is that patients behave differently in this relationship. Many of them simply trust the doctor, do not wish to know anything about adverse events, and hope that a good outcome will occur without their own contribution. Such behaviour may be adequate for a perforated gastric ulcer, when the simple decision to be made is between dying or undergoing surgery. It is, however, not the usual way in which a customer decides to buy a car, and it is probably not the best way to focus on the customer's needs. In other conditions there is some evidence that shared decision-making based on a fully-informed patient, perhaps helped by a video tape, can help to address the patient's requirements.[7]

Doctor. Today the doctor is the most important influence in the decision-making process and passes on his knowledge and beliefs to the patient. Carey, Garrett and Jackman[8] followed 1246 patients with acute LBP; 96 (7.7%) had had chronic continuous symptoms for three months, with unremitting pain for 22 months in 59 (4.7%) and 46 underwent various surgical procedures. Patients initially seen by an orthopaedic surgeon were more likely to undergo surgery (5.2%) than those seen in an HMO (1.8%), by a chiropracter (2.8%), or by a primary-care physician (4.4%). The decision to operate is also influenced by the financial and personal interests of the doctor. It has been shown in hip arthroplasty that a long waiting list is associated with a worse outcome. Volinn et al[9] found a nearly 15-fold variation of spinal surgery, which was weakly related to explanatory variables. They proposed to investigate surgeon-related variables such as: 1) variable diffusion of medical innovations (willingness to apply promising new *versus* well-established methods of treatment); 2) preconceptualisation (knowledge learned during residency training, later acquired knowledge may be assimilated into a preconceived knowledge base); 3) tolerance of uncertainty (surgeons are inclined towards action and resolving of uncertainty); and 4) reaction to patient expectations (pressures exerted by the patient vary by ethnic group, class, and also locally).

These variables have not been studied with regard to lumbar spinal fusion. Much more data are required for the better understanding of this process of indication.

THE GOAL

The goal of spinal lumbar fusion is not to achieve fusion between two vertebrae but to improve pain, disability, quality of life and the working capacity of the patient or to alter an unfavourable natural course. The patient's main problem is pain and the disability due to it. Most patients undergoing lumbar spinal fusion are not threatened by a progressing deformity. Fusion is carried out to relieve pain, and to improve the patient's functional status. The rates of fusion are therefore not an adequate measure of the success of the procedure.

Outcome measures. It is confusing and frustrating to compare the results of studies using different outcome measures. Penta and Fraser[10] followed 125 patients who had had anterior lumbar interbody fusions for a minimum of ten years. Of these, 78% rated themselves as having complete or considerable relief of pain, but only 34% had a good or excellent outcome as judged by a low back outcome score. Hence these outcome measures are not comparable.

Pain. This is best measured by a visual analogue scale for current and habitual pain.[11,12] A short written explanation to the patient is sufficient; an oral explanation is not necessary.

Disability. Restricted function or "the limitation of a patient's performance compared to that of a fit person of the same age and sex"[13] is measured by a disability scale. The Roland and Morris scale[14] includes 24 items and an indication of pain. The patient is asked to tick each sentence which describes his present status and the score ranges from 0 (no disability) to 24 (severe disability). It can be completed in five minutes. The Oswestry disability scale which includes ten items[15] is also often used. It offers six answers for each item ranging from 0 to 5. A percentage of the total score divided by the total possible score is calculated. It ranges from 0 (no disability) to 100 (severe disability). The Waddell and Main disability index[13] is a short nine-item scale requiring answers with high reliability ranging from 0 (no disability) to 9 (severe disability). All these disability scores are condition-specific for LBP. Kopec and Esdaile[16] have compiled a list of more than 40 scales, most of which have been developed for a single study and have not been properly validated. The Roland and Morris scale has been the most frequently cited back pain scale in the medical literature, followed by the Oswestry questionnaire and the Waddell disability index. It is also validated for the German language.[17]

Quality of life. This is most often measured by the SF-36[18-20] questionnaire. It contains 36 items and generates a profile of eight dimensional scores (physical functioning, social functioning, role limitations (physical), role limitations (emotional), pain, mental health, vitality, and general health perception ranging from 0 to 100, in which high scores indicate good health. It can be completed by most patients within ten minutes. The Euroqol[21] is also increasingly in use. It is a brief two-page questionnaire; the first page contains five items describing health status across five dimensions (mobility, self-care, usual activity, pain/distress and depression/anxiety: EQ-5D) and the second displays a 20 cm visual analogue rating scale on which the respondent marks an assessment of their overall health ranging from 100 (best imaginable health state) to 0 (worst imaginable health state) (EQ-VAS). The Euroqol therefore provides two single-index measures of health, the EQ-5D and the EQ-VAS.

Work loss. This is the hardest objective measure of outcome, but it has some limitations. It may be less important to the individual patient and is only applicable to the working population. It addresses only one specific aspect of functional disability and is a dichotomous variable with limited statistical power in comparison with continuous measures. Work loss and return to work are very dependent on non-health-related socio-economic variables such as general economic conditions and the labour market.[22]

Outcome scores. These were developed by Greenough and Fraser[23] and the North American Spine Society (NASS).[24] The Greenough low back outcome score ranges from 0 (worst) to 75 (best) and includes four items scoring nine points (current pain, employment, domestic chores, sport), four items scoring six points (resting, treatment, analgesia, sex life), and five items scoring three points (sleeping, walking, sitting, travelling, dressing). The NASS outcome instrument can be completed in 20 minutes and includes six subscales: pain and disability (11 items), neurogenic symptoms (6 items), job dissatisfaction (3 items), job exertion (5 items), expectations (6 items), and satisfaction (3 items). The NASS instrument is also validated for the German language.[25]

Natural course and alternatives to lumbar spinal fusion. In a prospective study patients who were seeking treatment in a primary-care office for the first time for a period of LBP were followed up. It was found that half who had a self-defined poor outcome at seven weeks also had a poor outcome at one year.[26]

The efficacy of our commonly used methods of conservative treatment is strongly related to disability. In a prospective trial patients with LBP were invited by advertisement in the press to undergo one of three methods of conservative treatment: physiotherapy, isoinertial training devices, and aerobic exercises. The result was a long-lasting reduction of pain from 6.5 to 5 on a 10 cm visual analogue scale, and from 8 to 6 on the Roland and Morris disability scale.[27,28] In patients undergoing lumbar spinal fusion, the Roland and Morris disability score is usually about 16, decreasing to 9 at the follow-up at two years.[8] This illustrates that disability is important in characterising a study population. Most papers on conservative treatment deal with a totally different study population compared with those on lumbar spinal fusion and are therefore difficult to compare.

Lumbar spinal fusion. In a meta-analysis of 47 articles published on lumbar spinal fusion from 1966 to 1991,[29,30] no randomised trials were found. On average, 68% of patients had a satisfactory outcome after fusion, but the range was wide (16% to 95%). The rate of satisfactory outcome was lower in prospective than in retrospective studies. The most frequently reported problems were pseudarthrosis (14%) and chronic pain at the donor site of the bone graft (9%). Clinical outcome did not differ by diagnosis or fusion technique, but anterior interbody fusions had lower rates of solid arthrodesis. Reoperations had a worse outcome. Different methods of spinal fusion will have a different outcome. There is some evidence that discogenic pain may persist after solid posterior fusion[31,32] and therefore an unfavourable result in a study on posterior fusion for the treatment of discogenic pain should be interpreted with caution. A bad outcome can be related to the wrong indication as well as the choice of the wrong technique.

Complications of fusion are relatively common.[29,30] In the studies reporting specific complications, an average of 3.7% of patients had deep-vein thrombosis, 2.8% had neurological injury, and 8.7% developed chronic pain at the donor site. Pseudarthrosis averaged 14% overall. Deyo et al[33] studied 27 111 Medicare patients who had had spinal surgery, of whom 5.6% had fusions. The rate of blood transfusion was 5.8 times greater than in surgery without fusion; the six-week mortality was 2.0 times greater and hospital charges were 1.5 times greater. Rates of reoperation at four years were not lower for patients who had undergone fusion. The authors concluded that there was an urgent need for a uniform definition of spinal instability and the indications for fusion. In a comparison of 1041 fusions and 5335 other surgical procedures of the lumbar spine, Malter et al[34] have shown that lumbar fusion is associated with a higher rate of reoperation (18% *v* 15%) and a much higher complication rate (18% in fused *v* 7% in unfused patients).

Comparison of outcomes. In a prospective cohort study[8] of 1246 patients with acute back pain, 46 had surgery. The operated patients had more initial disability (Roland score 16 *v* 11) and at 22 months (9 *v* 5). The rates of satisfaction with care (57% *v* 51%) and employment rate (72% *v* 79%) were comparable. In another study of 507 patients, 133 were receiving workers' compensation.[35] Of the latter, 65 had been treated surgically and 68 non-surgically. The patients treated surgically were more likely to have preoperative imaging, worse leg pain and decreased physical function than the non-surgically-treated patients. At six months disability was less in patients treated surgically than in those treated non-surgically. Return to work was also greater (60% *v* 40%). All of these studies, however, did not differentiate between different surgical procedures, and included many more cases of decompression of a herniated disc than lumbar spinal fusion. It is not known whether the more favourable result of surgical treatment is caused exclusively by decompression of a herniated disc.

Möller and Hedlund[36] carried out a prospective, randomised study on lumbar spinal fusion *versus* non-surgical treatment in 111 adults with isthmic spondylolisthesis. The surgical group had a better outcome than the non-surgical group, as assessed by a VAS and a disability index. In the exercise group, the disability rating index did not change at all.

NON-ORGANIC PREDICTORS OF OUTCOME

In chronic LBP, and especially in patients who have been on sick leave for more than a month, resumption of work can be predicted almost exclusively by psychosocial factors, disability, and comorbidity.[37] In a recent Swedish study,[38] quality of life was found to be the best predictor of return to work in patients with LBP. In another study[8] high disability and sciatica, defined as radiation of pain to the level of the knee or below, were the most powerful predictors of developing a chronic back problem. Unfortunately, a Roland and Morris disability score of 11 was 86% sensitive, but only 50% specific in predicting a patient's ability to perform activities of daily living at three months, resulting in a positive predictive value of only 13%. Even when a Roland and Morris score of 19 was used as a cut-off point for predicting chronicity, this resulted in a positive predictive value of only 22%.

In severely disabled patients on sick leave there is no proven efficacy of most conservative methods of treatment. Hansson and coworkers[39] investigated 2080 subjects in six countries who had been on sick leave for a minimum of 90 days because of LBP. All had been treated in a relatively uniform way. Almost none of the most frequently practised procedures had a positive effect on recorded health measures or on resumption of work. The only exception was back surgery, which had some beneficial effect on return to work in some of these countries.

Psychological and social predictors of the outcome of operative treatment are better evaluated in disc herniation than in degenerative disc disease. Hasenbring et al[40] found that persistent pain six months after discectomy was best predicted by a combination of somatic (the degree of disc displacement), psychological (depression, pain-coping strategies, endurance strategies, non-verbal pain behaviour, search for social support) and social parameters (social status, sitting position).

Tandon, Campbell and Ross[41] performed posterior lumbar interbody fusion in 55 patients. They used the DRAM (see under **Short screening tools**) and the Oswestry disability score before surgery and after a mean follow-up of 2.7 years. The Oswestry score was reduced from a mean of 51 preoperatively to a mean of 39 at follow-up. In the DRAM groups 'normal' and 'at risk' disability was reduced from 48 to 37, and in the DRAM groups 'distressed depressive' and 'distressed somatic' from 56 to 42. There was a strong association between psychological distress and Oswestry disability. There is no clear opinion as to how to treat a patient with a marked organic as well as a psychological disorder. The strong relation between both, and the possibility that psychosocial distress can also be ameliorated by organic treatment as in the study of Tandon et al,[41] suggests that both organic and psychological disorders should be treated independently. The sequence of treatment will depend on the underlying condition.

Psychosocial comorbidity. The intention of lumbar spinal fusion is to treat an organic disease. There are certainly better methods than surgery to treat a psychological or social problem. Severe psychosocial problems should therefore be actively sought before lumbar spinal fusion is undertaken. Psychological factors are strongly related to disability and outcome. Disability is associated with coping strategies, depression and belief in avoidance of fear.[28,40] In herniation of a lumbar disc it was shown that psychosocial and work-related factors played a much more important role than morphology (MRI findings) in predicting outcome.[42]

Childhood psychological trauma is reported to be associated with a worse outcome in spinal fusion. Physical abuse, sexual abuse, alcohol or drug abuse in a primary care-giver, abandonment (not uncomplicated divorce) and emotional neglect with abuse were identified. In a retrospective study of 86 patients, those with poor surgical outcome had an incidence of such trauma of 75%.[43]

Occupation. Several studies showed that LBP is strongly associated with occupation. Machine driving with whole-body vibration[44] and prolonged sitting were notable factors. The outcome of lumbar fusion is worse in a workers' compensation population. Franklin et al[45] performed a population-based study on 388 patients; 68% reported that back pain was worse and 23% required further lumbar spinal surgery two years after fusion.

Short screening tools

Pain drawings. These can demonstrate radicular pain but they are not suitable as a screening method to detect psychosocial distress.

DRAM (Distress and Risk Assessment Method). This was developed by Main et al[46] and is based on the Modified Somatic Perception Questionnaire (22 items) and the Modified Zung Depression Index (23 items). Threshold values of both questionnaires are used to define four types of patient: normal, at risk, distressed depressive and distressed somatic. The method is not time-consuming and can be applied by an orthopaedic surgeon.

Behavioural responses to examination. These are often recognised by orthopaedic surgeons. Signs like overreaction or a better performance of the straight-leg raising test when the patient is distracted are often overinterpreted. The non-organic signs are not a test of credibility or faking.[47] Waddell et al[48] developed a standardised assessment of inappropriate non-organic signs, but their interpretation is difficult. Multiple signs suggest that the patient does not have just a physical problem, but that psychological factors also need to be considered.[49]

ORGANIC INDICATIONS, GENERAL CONSIDERATIONS

In the case of a fracture of the femur the goal of treatment is simply to restore the original situation. This is definitely not the goal of lumbar spinal fusion and we are forced to consider what we aim to achieve.

The indications for lumbar spinal fusion should be based on an organic condition. In clinical practice there are sometimes different methods of verifying a particular condition. It is helpful therefore to consider which conditions can be helped by lumbar spinal fusion and which methods can confirm the condition.

Which conditions can be altered by lumbar spinal fusion in order to achieve a defined goal? A recent study has shown that positive discographic pain was found in 50% of discs with a high-intensity zone (HIZ) as an MRI sign of a tear of the annulus. In patients with abnormal testing and/or chronic pain, however, 100% of discs with an HIZ were positive on discography.[50] A tear of the annulus is a particular condition, and we shall therefore focus on the question as to whether lumbar fusion for the treatment of such a tear has a desirable outcome. This is only valid under the premise that an organic painful condition can be treated efficiently by lumbar spinal fusion. This statement is too general to be used as a premise. On the other hand, the argument is valid in the opposite direction. Many studies have compared a series of individuals with and without low back pain and tried to demonstrate that a particular condition causes pain or is not likely to be painful. These studies are often interpreted by the way in which a condition common in patients with LBP and rarely found in normal individuals can successfully be treated by lumbar spinal fusion. This is not conclusive. On the other hand, a condition occurring with the same frequency in patients with and without pain is likely not to be the cause of pain, and should therefore not be treated by fusion.

This approach is very common in medicine and orthopaedics. It is meaningful to ask whether a torn anterior cruciate ligament should be treated by a ligament repair, and to deal separately with the questions on diagnostic methods, indications, and surgical methods. The indications for most surgical procedures are based on a diagnosis and side conditions. Osteoarthritis of the hip should be treated if pain or disability exceed a certain level. Disability seems to play a role in the assessment by most surgeons, as preoperative disability in patients treated operatively is much greater than in those treated conservatively.[8] Therefore it seems necessary also to use a grading system to include other conditions so that the primary condition to be treated can be clearly defined.

The question raised above can best be answered by prospective, randomised trials evaluating whether lumbar spinal fusion compares favourably with conservative treatment or surgical treatment without fusion in a defined particular condition and with regard to a defined outcome measure.

Which diagnostic method is the best to find a particular condition? It is better to separate this question from the previous one. In most of the following studies (in INDICATIONS) this difference was not considered. Several surgeons feel that a 'black disc' in MRI is a good indication for lumbar spinal fusion by a cage. Such an approach causes considerable confusion by not clearly defining the three different problems of diagnosis, indications and choice of the surgical procedure.

There are many studies on the accuracy and reliability of diagnostic methods and on confounding variables which influence the results of a diagnostic test. The diagnostic method should be reliable so that several repetitions will give the same result. Much more important, however, is the accuracy, that is the capability of the method to find the real condition. Investigations on accuracy are much more difficult to perform than those on repeatability, and can often only be determined by comparison with a much more accurate method. The diagnostic method should be as least invasive and expensive as possible.

Diagnostic methods are used to find or define a particular condition (diagnosis, severity), to determine whether this condition is painful or relevant to the patient's symptoms (e.g., by provocative discography) and as an outcome measure.

INDICATIONS

Slosar et al[51] found a strong correlation between diagnosis and outcome (Table I). In this study, there were no statistical differences in outcome between primary or revision procedures, and between workers' compensation and non-workers' compensation groups. Remarkably, 'instability' did not occur in the list of indications.

Disc degeneration

The disc is a source of pain. Even referred pain distally below the knee can originate from the disc. In a study of 33 patients with LBP a heating coil was placed intradiscally. When the coil was heated, 66% of the patients had an exact reproduction of their presenting symptoms. Since normal temperatures were recorded adjacent to the disc, it was assumed that the provoked pain was produced by stimulation of annular nociceptors.[52]

Degeneration of the disc is assumed to cause discogenic pain. There is a sequence in degeneration of the disc which is described in various grading systems. The most important step in defining a clinically relevant lesion is the occurrence of a radiating annular tear. These were first described by Schmorl and Junghanns, and investigated in more detail by an Australian research group.[53] They can be classified as peripheral lesions, circumferential tears and radiating clefts. Experiments on sheep showed that a stab

Table I. Successful outcome as estimated by the patient

	Number	Successful outcomes (%)
Painful degenerative disc disease	89	*56*
Internal disc disruption	8	*50*
Pseudarthrosis	17	*82*
Spondylolisthesis	15	*80*
Stenosis	4	*50*

Table II. Incidence of MRI findings in individuals who had never had LBP according to Boden et al[62]

Age (yrs)	Number	Herniated disc (%)	Spinal stenosis (%)	Bulging disc (%)	Disc degeneration (%)
20 to 39	35	*21*	*1*	*56*	*34*
40 to 59	18	*22*	*0*	*50*	*59*
60 to 80	14	*36*	*21*	*79*	*93*

Table III. Degeneration patterns according to Buirski[65]

Pattern type	Intranuclear cleft	Prolapse/ bulge	Disc intensity	Disc height	Asymptomatic (n = 63) (%)	Symptomatic (n = 115) (%)
1	Thick	-	No	No	*0*	*0*
2	Thick	-	Reduced	No	*5*	*4*
3	No	Yes	No	No	*4*	*4*
4	Thick	Yes	Reduced	Reduced	*42*	*29*
5	Thick/ incomplete	Yes	Focal signal voids (HIZ)*	More reduced	*31*	*47*
6	Not seen	Yes	Severely reduced	Severely reduced	*18*	*16*

* HIZ - author's comment

wound produced in order to simulate a peripheral tear lesion does not heal, but slowly develops to a radiating cleft.[54] Degenerated discs with a radiating cleft behave differently. Axial rotation is considerably increased.[55,56] As soon as the cleft has reached the surface of the annulus (grading Adams V, Thompson V), the height of the disc decreases and flexion/extension and sidebending are reduced. Signs of tears of the annulus on MRI such as the HIZ correlate with provoked discographic pain. Nevertheless, not all discs with a radiating tear are painful.

Radiography and CT. These are not always indicative of disc degeneration. Degenerative changes are often found in radiographs[57] and CT scans[58] of symptom-free individuals. CT is not able to elucidate disc pathology adequately.

MRI. This does correspond well to the underlying pathology. Unenhanced T2-weighted MRI is usually sufficient. Gadolinium contrast-enhanced examination may give useful additional information for the differentiation of formation of a scar and disc herniation.[59] In MRI, the Thompson grading of disc degeneration[60] can be done reproducibly, but special coils are necessary. There is currently no technique which has enough quality to categorise disc degeneration other than MRI.[55] In conventional MRI, the first sign of degeneration is inhomogeneity of the intranuclear cleft followed by bulging of the disc. Late signs are decreased signal intensity and reduced disc height. In a Finnish study of 151 men aged from 40 to 45 years in whom MRI was performed twice with a four-year interval, a clear sequence of these signs was shown.[61]

Boden et al[62] have shown that degenerative changes in the disc are common in normal individuals (Table II).

Jensen et al[63] also found in their MRI study of 98 asymptomatic individuals and 27 patients with back pain that there is a high prevalence of bulges (52%) and protrusions (27%) in asymptomatic subjects. Only 36% of the asymptomatic individuals with an age range of 20 to 80 years had normal discs at all levels. Buirski and Silberstein[64] have classified patterns in the disc with increasing pathology from 1 (normal) to 6 (severely reduced disc height).

The pattern of distribution was not significantly different between 115 symptomatic patients and 63 control subjects (Table III).[65] None of these studies have separately addressed Modic changes (see **Bone-marrow changes**).

Boos et al[66] have shown in 46 asymptomatic individuals followed for a mean of five years that herniations of the disc and neural compromise did not become significantly worse at follow-up, whereas degeneration of the disc progressed in 19 individuals (41%), six of whom had to seek medical treatment with another five having to stop work temporarily. Nevertheless, LBP-related medical consultation was predicted with higher accuracy by listlessness, job satisfaction, and working in shifts. Work incapacity was best predicted by physical job characteristics, job disaffection, and working in shifts. Another study[44] has found an association of LBP with MRI signs of degeneration of the disc and of sciatic pain with posterior bulges of the disc. The adjusted odds ratios for the 12-month prevalence of LBP were 2.7 for a posterior bulge, 3.4 for an anterior bulge, and 2.0 for a dark nucleus. The adjusted odds ratios for a four-year prevalence were 1.7 for a posterior bulge, 1.9 for an anterior bulge, and 2.1 for a dark nucleus.

There is no strong correlation between MRI changes of the intervertebral disc and LBP. In most studies, however, disability was not assessed. Perhaps the incidence of degenerative lesions is much higher in a severely disabled population. Further studies are required to evaluate whether there is a correlation between degeneration of the disc and the degree of disability.

High intensity zone (HIZ). This was first described in the lumbar spine by Aprill and Bogduk[67] and is a high-intensity signal on MR scans in the substance of the posterior nucleus pulposus. It is surrounded by a low-intensity black signal of the annulus, and it is appreciably brighter than the signal of the nucleus. Provocative discography revealed that the HIZ represented painful internal disruption of the disc with a positive predictive value of 86%. Schellhas et al[68] and Lam, Carlin and Mulholland[69] confirmed these findings, whereas Ricketson, Simmons and Hauser[70] found that the HIZ is not necessarily associated with a painful disc. Carragee, Pragioudakis and Khurana[71] performed provocative discography and MRI in 42 symptomatic patients and 54 asymptomatic individuals. The prevalence of an HIZ was 59% in the symptomatic and 24% in the asymptomatic group. Provocation discography was done. In the asymptomatic group, 73% of the discs with an HIZ were positive on discography compared with 38% of the discs without an HIZ. In the symptomatic group, the respective values were 69% and 10%. The nature of the HIZ is unclear. It may represent an area of secondary inflammation as a result of a tear in the annulus.

Discography. This has also been used for grading degeneration of the disc. It is, however, more invasive than MRI. Buirski[65] has shown that the signal characteristics of MRI can accurately depict the early stages of nuclear degeneration as revealed by discography. Once protrusion of the disc occurs, MRI and discography do not correspond so well. With the current trend to perform more provocative discography, grading of disc degeneration can be done additionally, using, for example, the classification of Adams, Dolan and Hutton[72] (Figs 1 and 2).

Provocation discography. This is an attempt to reproduce symptoms. Since damage to the intervertebral disc can be seen in asymptomatic as well as symptomatic individuals, the intention is to distinguish painful from painless disc disease, and also to localise the painful disc. Colhoun et al[73] followed 137 patients in whom discography had provoked symptoms; in 25 the discs showed morphological abnormality but had no provocation of symptoms. Patients underwent anterior or posterior fusions and occasionally a laminectomy. Of the 137 with provoked symptoms 89% derived significant and sustained clinical benefit from operation, measured by subjective improvement, resumption of work and/or normal duties and no intake of analgesics, compared with 52% of patients in whom symptoms had not been provoked by discography. Carragee et al[50] performed provocation discography of the lumbar spine in 26 individuals with no history of LBP. Significant positive pain responses were found in 10% of pain-free individuals, 40% of those with chronic cervical pain and in 83% of those with a somatisation disorder. False-positive discography therefore may be low in subjects with a normal

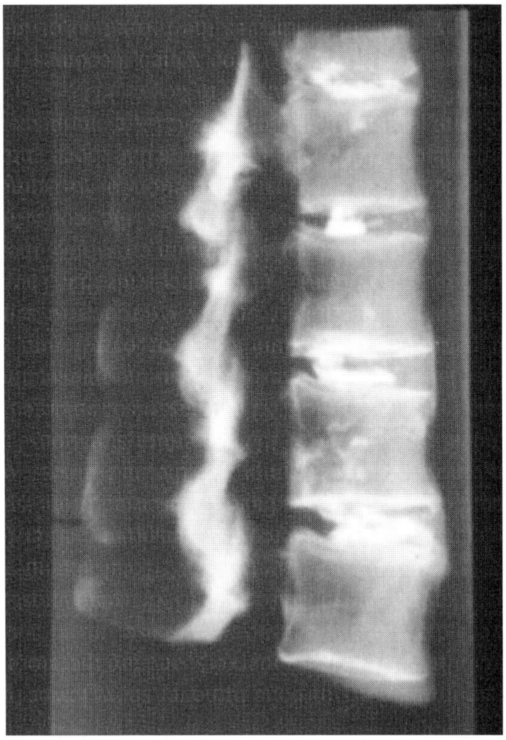

Fig. 1

Morphological categories of disc degeneration in discography according to Adams et al.[72] From top to bottom the grades 4, 2, 3 and 4 are revealed.

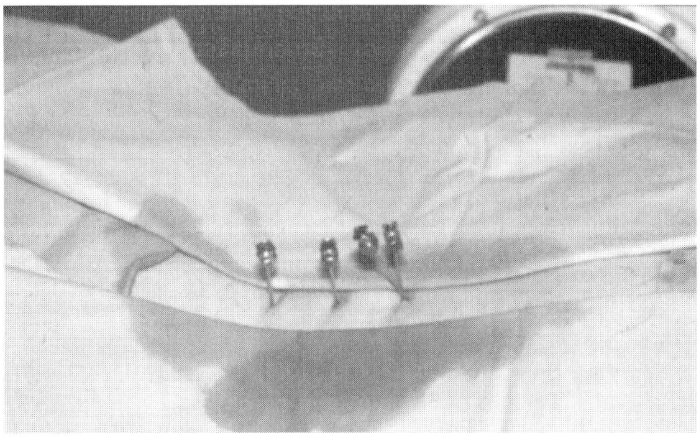

Fig. 2

The technique of discography. Needles are placed in four discs. Repeatedly, small amounts of saline and an antibiotic are injected into the disc. The patient is not aware which of the discs is provoked at any time.

psychometric profile. This may also explain the high rate of 65% of fair and poor results of single-level fusions in a workers' compensation group.[74] Carragee et al[71] also found in patients with normal psychometric testing that provocation discography in discs demonstrating an HIZ was positive in only 50%, compared with 100% in patients with abnormal psychometric testing. Although provocation discography is an instrument for assessing discogenic pain, Leufven and Nordwall[75] reported excellent and good

Table IV. Types of Modic changes as defined by signal intensity (SI) patterns in T1- and T2-weighted MR sequences, underlying pathology according to de Roos et al[78] and Modic et al[79], and their relation to reproduction of pain at provocative discography in the series of Braithwaite et al[80]

	MRI				
Type	**T1-weighted**	**T2-weighted**	**Pathology**	**No pain***	**Pain***
I	SI reduced	SI increased	Fissures of the cartilaginous endplate, increased vascularity within the subchondral bone	0	5
II	SI increased	SI increased or isotense	Fatty replacement of the marrow, perhaps a result of marrow ischaemia	2	16
III	SI reduced	SI reduced	Subchondral sclerosis	0	3
None				60	69

* numbers of patients

results in 52% of patients with a positive provocation test who had only posterior fusion.

Derby et al[76] investigated 96 patients in a retrospective study. They categorised provocative discographic pain according to the pressure required to trigger the pain: chemical, <100 kPa; mechanical, 100 to 350 kPa; and indeterminate, normal, 350 to 600 kPa. Chemical pain was associated with a better outcome after interbody or combined fusion. Hanley, Phillips and Kostuik[77] recommend diagnosis of discogenic LBP by discography reproducing the patient's symptoms, and showing advanced degeneration especially dye extravasation to the side of the leg symptoms.

Provocation discography is perhaps one of the rare techniques which is helpful in indicating the need for lumbar spinal fusion in patients with degenerative discs. It is, however, invasive, and a small amount of antibiotics should be added to the dye to protect against iatrogenic discitis. Provocation discography should be combined with psychometric testing. The painful disc should be fused and a 360° fusion is perhaps better than a posterior fusion in patients with positive provocation discography.

Vertebral bone-marrow changes. These changes, sometimes called vertebral endplate or Modic changes, were first described by de Roos et al[78] and Modic et al[79] (Table IV, Fig. 3).

Type-I changes often progress to type-II changes, but they can also resolve. Marrow oedema may also be seen in discitis, penetrating Schmorl's nodes, and following chemonucleolysis. The prevalence of Modic changes in asymptomatic individuals has not been investigated.[62-64] Braithwaite et al[80] found an additional HIZ in 7 of 23 discs with Modic changes, and Modic changes in 7 of 27 discs with an HIZ. Toyone et al[81] studied 500 MRI scans and identified 74 patients with bone-marrow changes, 37 with increased (type A, Modic II) and 37 with decreased (type B, Modic I and III) signal intensity; 73% of those with type-A changes and 11% of those with type-B changes had pain.

Lang et al[82] evaluated 33 patients who had had lumbar spinal fusion, in 30 by posterolateral fusion, in whom segmental instability was suspected at the site of the fusion; 16 of 19 patients with a solid fusion had bone-marrow changes comparable with Modic II changes. In ten of the 14 patients with segmental instability subchondral bands of low intensity in T1-weighted and increased signal intensity in T2-weighted MRI were found. It remains unclear whether the bone-marrow changes in solid fusion were also present before surgery, and whether a 360° fusion should be undertaken in all patients with bone-marrow changes, if surgical treatment is considered. In the author's opinion this is the correct procedure.

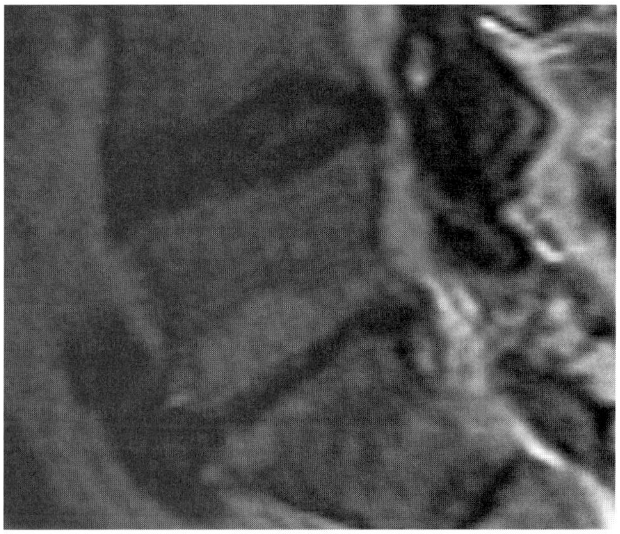

Fig. 3

Increased signal intensity in T2-weighted MRI in a Modic type-I lesion of the presacral disc.

The specificity of Modic changes for identification of a painful disc at discography is high, but sensitivity, however, is low.[80] The presence of Modic changes is therefore perhaps an indication for lumbar spinal fusion, although the literature is not very conclusive. Both T1- and T2-weighted MR scans are necessary to distinguish between the different types of Modic changes.

Facet joint degeneration. The facet joint usually degenerates later than the disc. Butler et al[83] performed CT and MRI of 330 discs; in 108 there was degeneration without changes in the facet joint, in 40 both the disc and the facet

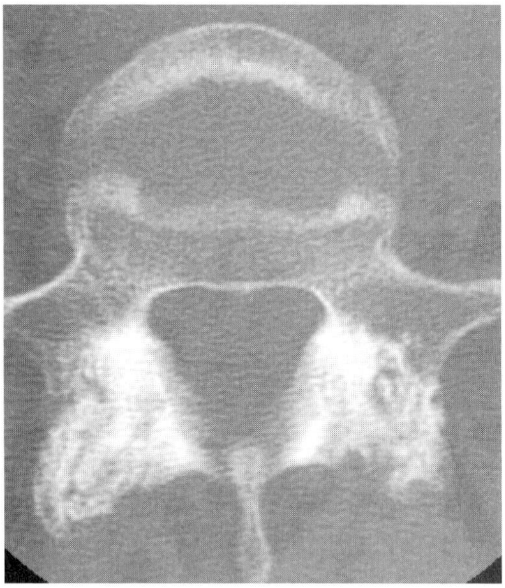

Fig. 4

Degeneration of a facet joint in the presence of a relatively intact disc in a 59-year-old woman. The patient had almost no pain at the one-year follow-up after fusion.

joints were degenerated, and in only one was there isolated facet joint degeneration without degenerative changes in the disc. Fujiwara et al[84] have confirmed this finding recently, whereas Videman et al[85] showed that osteoarthritis of the facet joint preceded degeneration of the disc in 20% (Fig. 4).

Facet joint blocks. Several studies have shown that these are not predictive in the selection of patients for lumbar fusion. In 126 patients Esses and Moro[86] failed to find any significant correlation between the outcome of fusion and the result of facet blocks.

Lovely and Rastogi[87] studied facet blocks prospectively; 28 of 91 patients had pain relief of more than 70% for more than six hours on three separate occasions. These patients underwent fusion and 19 of 23 described pain relief of 90% at follow-up. The authors applied 3 to 5 ml of a combination of 1% xylocaine, 40 mg of Depo-Medrol, and 0.5% marcaine. The facet blocks were not selective because of the amount of local anaesthetic.

In my opinion, facet blocks may determine the location of posterior facet pain; 0.5 ml of local anaesthetic per facet is adequate, otherwise the block will not be sufficiently selective.

Instability. Segmental instability has been recognised as a cause of LBP for some time. Knutsson[88] was the first to discuss the significance of instability or abnormal mobility between two lumbar vertebrae. He introduced flexion-extension radiographs to determine instability. Morgan and King[89] drew attention to the association between annular tears, radiographic instability, and LBP. Kirkaldy-Willis and Farfan[90] focused on anteroposterior lateral bending radiographs, from which rotational deformity and lateral translation were interpreted to be indicators of instability.

Flexion-extension radiographs. These were often found to be inconsistent. Shaffer et al[91] found in experiments that only relatively large translations (±5 mm) could be observed in flexion-extension radiographs in a reproducible way, when obliquity was small on radiographs, and when concomitant movements were minimal. Leivseth et al[47] compared roentgen stereophotogrammetry and distortion-compensated sagittal plane radiographs and came to a similar conclusion, recommending a threshold value of ±5 mm.

Hayes et al[92] examined 59 flexion-extension radiographs obtained from asymptomatic individuals undergoing routine pre-employment examination. Angulatory motion was 7° to 14° and translational motion 2 mm to 3 mm at each intervertebral level. Of the asymptomatic individuals in the study 20% had 4 mm or more of translational movement at the L4-L5 interspace. Boden and Wiesel[93] studied 40 normal individuals using special x-ray equipment. They found that only 5% had a dynamic AP translation of 4 mm or more. Mayer et al[94] found that the test-retest reliability of flexion-extension radiographs of 14 examiners and 18 healthy volunteers was 4.9°.

In conclusion, there is some evidence that instability can be assumed when dynamic AP translation is 5 mm or more.

Lateral bending films. Their use is not as well documented as that of flexion-extension films. Haas et al[95] found that the inter-rater reliability was poor at L5, but acceptable at levels above. Jayaraman et al[96] found that the range of lateral bending was reduced by 43% for symptomatic patients when compared with painfree individuals. Dvorak et al[97] examined healthy volunteers and found a large variation in rotation, which may limit the clinical usefulness of functional lumbar analysis. There are no reports in the English medical literature after 1990 which show a predictive value of lateral bending radiographs with regard to the outcome of lumbar fusion.

Lumbar orthosis. This restricts gross movement of the trunk rather than intervertebral mobility as has been demonstrated by roentgen stereophotogrammetry.[98] A corset test was carried out in 50 patients; 31 experienced significant pain relief of more than 50%. The clinical outcome after solid fusion did not correlate with the preoperative results of the corset test.[99] A lumbar orthosis is not of value when selecting patients for lumbar fusion.

External transpedicular fixation test. This is an invasive method in which 5 mm Schantz screws are driven into the pedicles by a closed technique and using an image intensifier. The screws are connected by bars. Pain is then assessed using visual analogue scales with locked and unlocked bars. Roentgen stereophotogrammetric analysis gave a significant reduction in sagittal intervertebral translations, in half of the cases below the accuracy of the measuring method.[100]

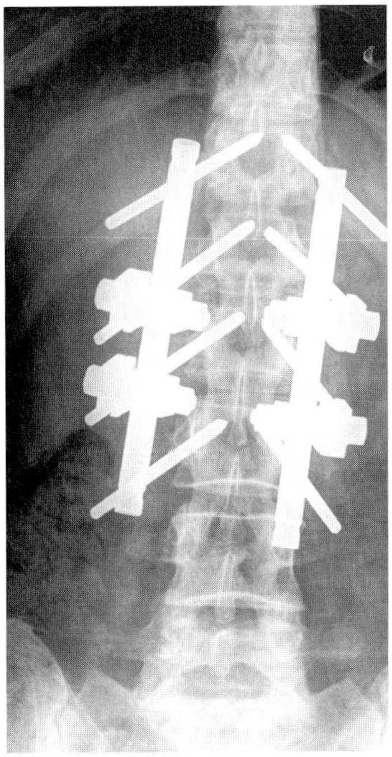

Fig. 5a

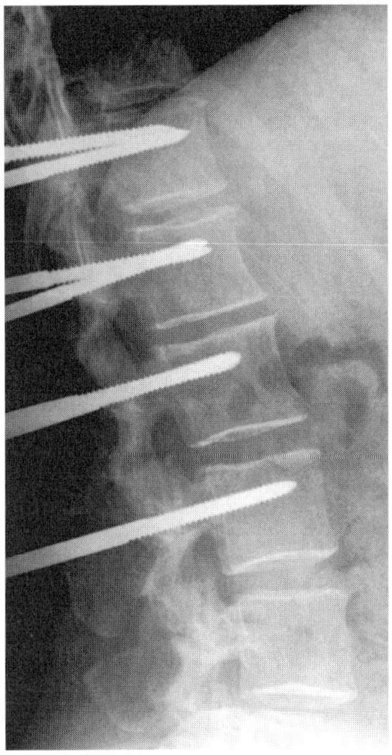

Fig. 5b

External transpedicular fixation test in a 38-year-old woman with several inappropriate signs, but severe pain at L1/L2. At intervals of two days other movement segments are fixed. At this stage only L1/L2 is fixed.

Soini et al[101] carried out a prospective study on 42 patients with chronic LBP; 29 had relief of pain in the external fixation test. At one and two years, they had significantly better pain and performance scores than the other patients. Van der Schaaf, van Limbeck and Pavlov[102] followed 133 patients, all of whom had had an external fixation test in three positions: neutral, slight distraction, and non-fixation. After two to three days for each position, pain was assessed by means of a visual analogue scale. Those patients who experienced adequate pain relief in fixation and considerably less pain relief in non-fixation were considered to be suitable candidates for fusion and of these 55 had fusion and 78 were treated conservatively. The subjective end result was good in 35 of the 55 fused patients (64%) and in 10 of 78 control subjects (13%), fair in 16 of the fused patients (29%) and in 23 of the conservatively-treated patients (29%), and poor in 4 (7%) of the fused and 45 (58%) of the conservatively treated patients. The VAS of the fusion group was 77 before operation, 26 during test fixation, 69 in non-fixation, and 40 at follow-up. The corresponding figures for the control group were 75, 53, 44 and 71.

There are no reports of a higher rate of infection in lumbar spinal fusion after the external fixation test, possibly because of the small numbers of patients in the studies. The method requires an additional operation. In difficult cases, however, the external fixation test seems suitable for proper selection of patients and segments (Fig. 5).

Other methods. Steffen et al[103] have developed a three-dimensional method based on the use of Kirschner wires inserted into the spinous processes to assess flexion-extension, lateral bending and axial rotation. Studies using videofluoroscopy[104] and cinéradiography[105] showed a stepwise occurrence of segmental movement and different patterns of movement in the lumbar spine. It remains unclear whether a thorough analysis by these methods will lead to reliable techniques for the assessment of instability.

Spondylolisthesis. In 111 patients with painful adult spondylolisthesis (Fig. 6), 62% reported LBP and sciatica, 31% low back pain only and 7% sciatic only.[106] In a study on 936 asymptomatic soldiers and 662 with LBP the incidence of spondylolisthesis was 5.3% in the symptomatic group, and 2.2% in the asymptomatic group.[107] Spondylolisthesis seems therefore to be associated with a higher incidence of LBP.

In a Swedish study, 111 patients with adult spondylolisthesis were compared with 39 with unspecific chronic LBP. The functional profile was strikingly similar for both groups.[28] Adult spondylolisthesis of minor degrees is therefore perhaps not very different from pure degenerative disc disease. Fusion in high grades of spondylolisthesis (Fig. 7) and of spondylolisthesis in children usually has a good outcome. Buttermann et al[108] used the Oswestry disability score to follow 165 patients after a mean period of five years. Children and patients with a high degree of slip (3 and more) had mean preoperative Oswestry scores of 50 and at follow-up of about 10. Those with low slips, degenerative disc disease and after discectomy had Oswestry scores of about 50 before operation and about 20 (low slips) and 30 (degenerative disc disease and post-discectomy) at follow-up. Patient satisfaction was 100% in the children and in patients with high slips and 84%, 76% and 69% in the low slip, degenerative disc disease, and post-

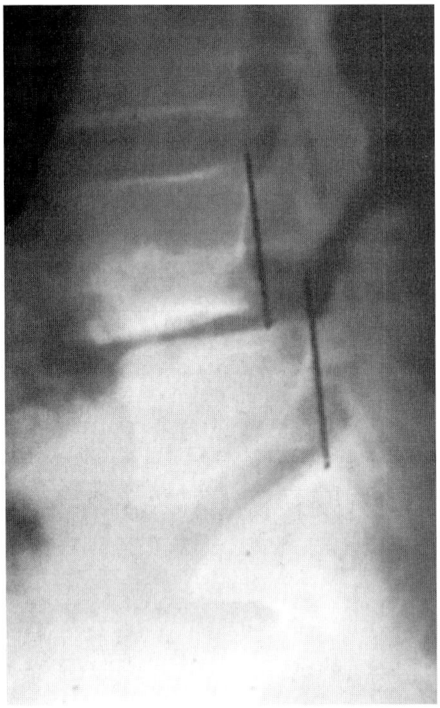

Fig. 6

Adult isthmic spondylolisthesis with severe degeneration of the disc and sclerosis of the endplates.

discectomy groups, respectively. The outcome did not differ between degenerative and isthmic spondylolisthesis, but was significantly worse in cases of pseudarthrosis.

Painful spondylolisthesis in children and in patients with high degrees of spondylolisthesis are the most accepted indications for lumbar spinal fusion.

Post-discectomy. Patients with psychosocial comorbidity have a less favourable result after operative treatment of lumbar disc herniation (see NON-ORGANIC PREDICTORS OF OUTCOME). Nevertheless, some studies report promising results of lumbar fusion in patients who had residual symptoms after discectomy,[109-111] with the same return to work rates when compared with a group after primary fusion, and rates of improvement of up to 82%. Tandon et al[41] have shown that distressed patients had the same functional benefit from lumbar spinal fusion as normal patients. Nevertheless, there is a need for more studies to establish clear guidelines for the selection of patients in those with failed back surgery.

Spinal stenosis. Spinal stenosis is outside the scope of this review. Therefore, the indication for decompression should not be considered. Some authors have recommended spinal fusion when decompression is done for spinal stenosis. Most agree that fusion should be performed when more than two-thirds of one facet joint is removed, or more than 50% of a facet pair, or more than 50% of successive facets. These general guidelines are based on biomechanical studies, but their scientific basis is inadequate.[112] When a facet-joint-preserving technique is utilised, postoperative slipping does not occur in patients without a preoperative slip. Patients with a degenerative spondylolisthesis have a 30% risk of progressive slip after a four-year follow-up, but without associated clinical problems.[113]

Spinal stenosis associated with degenerative spondylolisthesis. This condition is often seen. Fischgrund et al[114] studied prospectively 76 patients with this combination who were decompressed and fused by posterolateral intertransverse non-instrumented or instrumented fusion. The outcome was the same in both groups. Successful arthrodesis occurred in 82%. Successful fusion did not influence patient outcome. The disadvantages of this study, however, were the small statistical power and that it was not the primary intention to compare patients with successful and unsuccessful fusion.

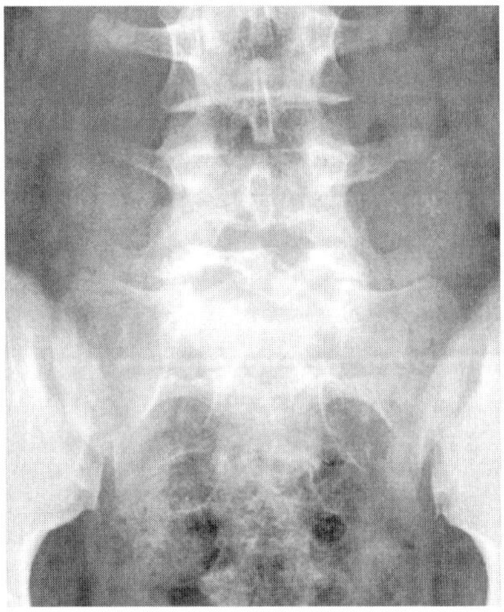

Fig. 7a

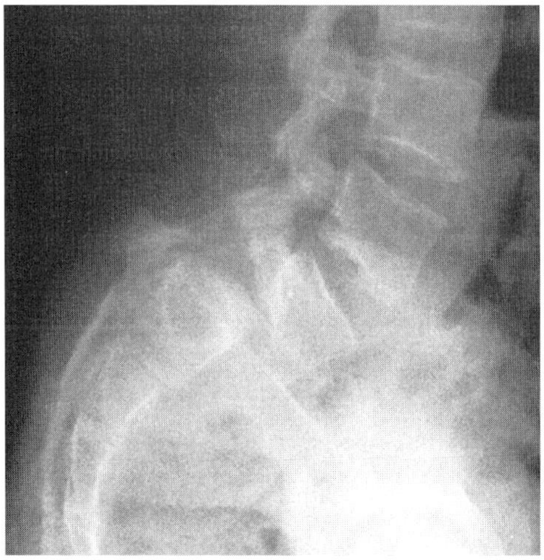

Fig. 7b

Spondylolisthesis in a 13-year-old boy.

CONCLUSIONS

The indications for lumbar spinal fusion are not well understood and there is not enough evidence for sound recommendations. A Cochrane review[115] recently came to the following conclusions:

1) There is no acceptable evidence (strength D) of the efficacy of any form of fusion for degenerative lumbar spondylosis, back pain, or 'instability'.

2) There is limited evidence (strength C) that adjunct fusion to supplement decompression for degenerative spondylolisthesis produces less progressive slip and better clinical outcomes than decompression alone.

3) There is limited evidence (strength C) that fusion alone may be as effective as combined decompression and fusion for patients with grade-I or grade-II isthmic spondylolisthesis and no significant neurology.

4) There is strong evidence that instrumented fusion may produce a higher rate of fusion (strength A), but does not improve clinical outcome (strength A).

Lumbar spinal fusion should therefore be undertaken with caution. It should be borne in mind that there is little evidence to suggest that it has a beneficial effect on patients.

Psychosocial screening should be performed and if psychosocial distress is shown a thorough evaluation should follow. If both a psychosocial and organic disorder are found, both should be treated, with discussion between the psychiatrist and the surgeon as regards the sequence of treatment.

A high-grade spondylolisthesis, a progressive slip in an adult, and iatrogenic removal of the facet joints during decompression are good indications for lumbar spinal fusion. AP translation of 5 mm in a painful motion segment may also be a good indication, if the level of disability is high.

When a highly disabled patient has localised pain and no slip and imaging techniques show bone-marrow changes or an HIZ, provocative discography or a fixation test should be considered for further evaluation. When a highly disabled patient has localised pain, and when imaging techniques show severe degeneration of the facet joints, facet blocks should be performed to determine the location of pain. In a psychosocially distressed patient provocation tests should be interpreted with caution. If provocation or pain relief tests clearly indicate that pain is related to a localised disorder, then lumbar fusion may be also indicated.

REFERENCES

1. **Walker BF.** The prevalence of low back pain: a systematic review of the literature from 1966 to 1998. *J Spinal Disord* 2000;13:205-17.
2. **Fanuele JC, Birkmeyer NJ, Abdu WA, Tosteson TD, Weinstein JN.** The impact of spinal problems on the health status of patients: have we underestimated the effect? *Spine* 2000;25:1509-14.
3. **Birkmeyer JD, Sharp SM, Finlayson SR, Fisher ES, Wennberg JE.** Variation profiles of common surgical procedures. *Surgery* 1998;124:917-23.
4. **Cherkin DC, Deyo RA, Loeser JD, Bush T, Waddell G.** An international comparison of back surgery rates. *Spine* 1994;19:1201-6.
5. **Loeser JD, Van Konkelenberg R, Volinn E, Cousins MJ.** Small area analysis of lumbar spine surgery in South Australia. *Aust N Z J Surg* 1993;63:14-9.
6. **Keller RB, Atlas SJ, Soule DN, Singer DE, Deyo RA.** Relationship between rates and outcomes of operative treatment for lumbar disc herniation and spinal stenosis. *J Bone Joint Surg [Am]* 1999;81-A:752-62.
7. **Weinstein JN.** Editorial. The missing piece: embracing shared decision making to reform health care. *Spine* 2000;25:1-4.
8. **Carey TS, Garrett JM, Jackman AM.** Beyond good prognosis: examination of an inception cohort of patients with chronic low back pain. *Spine* 2000;25:115-20.
9. **Volinn E, Mayer J, Diehr P, et al.** Small area analysis of surgery for low-back pain. *Spine* 1992;17:575-9.
10. **Penta M, Fraser RD.** Anterior lumbar interbody fusion: a minimum 10-year follow-up. *Spine* 1997;22:2429-34.
11. **Huskisson EC.** Measurement of pain. *Lancet* 1974;9:1127-31.
12. **Ogon M, Krismer M, Söllner W, Kantner-Rumplmair W, Lampe A.** Chronic low back pain measurement with visual analogue scales in different settings. *Pain* 1996;64:425-8.
13. **Waddell G, Main CJ.** Assessment of severity in low back pain disorders. *Spine* 1984;9:204-8.
14. **Roland M, Morris R.** A study of the natural history of back pain. Part I: development of a reliable and sensitive measure of disability in low back pain. *Spine* 1983;8:141-4.
15. **Fairbank JC, Couper J, Davies JB, O'Brien JP.** The Oswestry low back pain disability questionnaire. *Physiotherapy* 1980;66:271-3.
16. **Kopec JA, Esdaile JM.** Spine update: functional disability scales. *Spine* 1995;20:1943-9.
17. **Wiesinger GF, Nuhr M, Quittan M, et al.** Cross-cultural adaptation of the Roland-Morris questionnaire for German-speaking patients with low back pain. *Spine* 1999;24:1099-103.
18. **Brazier JE, Harper R, Jones NMB, et al.** Validating the SF-36 health survey questionnaire: new outcome measure for primary care. *Br Med J* 1992;305:160-4.
19. **Garrat AM, Ruta DA, Abdalla I.** The SF-36 health survey questionnaire: an outcome measure suitable for routine use within the NHS. *Br Med J* 1992;306:1440-4.
20. **Ware J, Sherbourne D.** The MOS 36-item Short-Form Health Survey (SF-36): I. conceptual framework and item selection. *Med Care* 1992;30:473-83.
21. **The Euroqol Group.** Euroqol: a facility for the measurement of health-related quality of life. *Health Policy* 1990;16:199-208.
22. **Waddell G.** Evaluation of results in lumbar spine surgery: clinical outcome measures: assessment of severity. *Acta Orthop Scand* 1993;64:134-7.
23. **Greenough CG, Fraser RD.** Assessment of outcome in patients with low back pain. *Spine* 1992;17:36-41.
24. **Daltroy LH, Cats-Baril WL, Katz JN, Fossel AH, Liang MH.** The North American Spine Society lumbar spine outcome assessment instrument: reliability and validity tests. *Spine* 1996;21:741-9.
25. **Pose B, Sangha O, Peters A, Wildner M.** Validierung des North American Spine Society Instruments zur Erfassung des Gesundheitsstatus bei Patienten mit chronischen Rückenbeschwerden. *Z Orthop Ihre Grenzgeb* 1999;137:437-41.
26. **Cherkin DC, Deyo RA, Street JH, Barlow W.** Predicting poor outcomes for back pain seen in primary care using patient's own criteria. *Spine* 1996;21:2900-7.
27. **Mannion AF, Muntener M, Taimela S, Dvorak J.** A randomised clinical trial of three active therapies for chronic low back pain. *Spine* 1999;24:2435-48.
28. **Mannion AF, Taimela S, Müntener M, et al.** Factors influencing self-rated disability scores in chronic low back pain patients. *Int Soc Study Lumbar Spine* Adelaide, 2000:3.
29. **Turner JA, Ersek M, Herron L, et al.** Patient outcomes after lumbar spinal fusions. *JAMA* 1992;268:907-11.
30. **Turner JA, Herron L, Deyo RA.** Meta-analysis of the results of lumbar spine fusion. *Acta Orthop Scand* 1993;64:Suppl 251:120-2.
31. **Barrick WT, Schofferman JA, Reynolds JB, et al.** Anterior lumbar fusion improves discogenic pain at levels of prior posterolateral fusion. *Spine* 2000;25:853-7.

32. **Weatherly CR, Prickett CF, O'Brien JP.** Discogenic pain persisting despite solid posterior fusion. *J Bone Joint Surg [Br]* 1986;68-B:142-3.

33. **Deyo RA, Ciol MA, Cherkin DC, Loeser JD, Bigos SJ.** Lumbar spinal fusion: a cohort study of complications, reoperations, and resource use in the Medicare population. *Spine* 1993;18:1463-70.

34. **Malter AD, McNeney B, Loeser JD, Deyo RA.** 5-year reoperation rates after different types of lumbar spine surgery. *Spine* 1998;23:814-20.

35. **Atlas SJ, Singer DE, Keller RB, Patrick DL, Deyo RA.** Application of outcomes research in occupational low back pain: the Maine lumbar spine study. *Am J Ind Med* 1996;29:584-9.

36. **Möller H, Hedlund R.** Surgery versus conservative management in adult isthmic spondylolisthesis: a prospective randomized study: part 1. *Spine* 2000;25:1711-5.

37. **Hiebert R, Pietrek M, Crane M, Nordin M.** The association of comorbidity and outcome in episodes of non-specific low back pain. *Int Soc Study Lumbar Spine* Adelaide, 2000:6.

38. **Hansson T, Jonsson R, Hansson E, Bergendorff S, Palmer E.** Instruments for predicting work resumption or not for low back pain and neck pain patients. *Int Soc Study Lumbar Spine* Adelaide, 2000:75.

39. **Hansson T, Hansson E, Bergendorff S, Palmer E.** Returning back patients to work in six countries: the effect of commonly used medical interventions. *Int Soc Study Lumbar Spine* Adelaide, 2000:1.

40. **Hasenbring M, Marienfeld G, Kuhlendahl D, Soyka D.** Risk factors of chronicity in lumbar disc patients: a prospective investigation of biologic, psychologic, and social predictors of therapy outcome. *Spine* 1994;19:2759-65.

41. **Tandon V, Campbell F, Ross ER.** Posterior lumbar interbody fusion: association between disability and psychological disturbance in non-compensated patients. *Spine* 1999;24:1833-8.

42. **Schade V, Semmer N, Main CJ, Hora J, Boos N.** The impact of clinical, morphological, psychosocial and work-related factors on the outcome of lumbar discectomy. *Pain* 1999;80:239-49.

43. **Schofferman J, Anderson D, Hines R, Smith G, White A.** Childhood psychological trauma correlates with unsuccessful lumbar spine surgery. *Spine* 1992;17:S138-44.

44. **Luoma K, Riihimäki H, Luukkonen R, et al.** Low back pain in relation to lumbar disc degeneration. *Spine* 2000;25:487-92.

45. **Franklin GM, Haug J, Heyer NJ, McKeefrey SP, Picciano JF.** Outcome of lumbar fusion in Washington State workers' compensation. *Spine* 1994;19:1897-903.

46. **Main C, Wood PL, Hollis S, Spanswick CC, Waddell G.** The distress and risk assessment method: a simple patient classification to identify distress and evaluate the risk of poor outcome. *Spine* 1992;17:42-52.

47. **Leivseth G, Brinckmann P, Frobin W, Johnsson R, Stromqvist B.** Assessment of sagittal plane segmental motion in the lumbar spine: a comparison between distortion-compensated and stereophotogrammetric roentgen analysis. *Spine* 1998;23:2648-55.

48. **Waddell G, McCulloch JA, Kummel E, Venner RM.** Nonorganic physical signs in low back pain. *Spine* 1980;5:117-25.

49. **Main CJ, Waddell G.** Spine update: behavioral responses to examination: a reappraisal of the interpretation of 'nonorganic signs'. *Spine* 1998;23:2367-71.

50. **Carragee EJ, Tanner CM, Khurana S, et al.** The rates of false positive lumbar discography in select patients without low back symptoms. *Spine* 2000;25:13733-80.

51. **Slosar PJ, Reynolds JB, Schofferman J, et al.** Patient satisfaction after circumferential lumbar fusion. *Spine* 2000;25:722-6.

52. **Derby R, O'Neill C, Berquam JA, Vaughan P.** Mechanisms of leg pain in patients with intervertebral disc disorders. *Inter Soc Study Lumbar Spine* Adelaide, 2000:80.

53. **Osti OL, Vernon-Roberts B, Fraser RD.** Annular tears and disc degeneration in the lumbar spine: a post-mortem study of 135 discs. *J Bone Joint Surg [Br]* 1992;74-B:678-82.

54. **Osti OL, Vernon-Roberts B, Fraser RD.** Annulus tears and intervertebral disc degeneration: an experimental study using an animal model. *Spine* 1990;15:762-7.

55. **Fujiwara A, An HS, Lim TH, Jeon CH, Andersson GBJ.** Lumbar segmental motion characteristics vary with degenerative changes in the disc and facet joints. *Int Soc Study Lumbar Spine* Adelaide, 2000:30.

56. **Krismer M, Haid C, Behensky H, et al.** Motion in lumbar functional spine units during side bending and axial rotation moments depending on the degree of degeneration. *Spine* 2000;25:2020-7.

57. **Torgerson WR, Dotter WE.** Comparative roentgenographic study of asymptomatic and symptomatic lumbar spine. *J Bone Joint Surg [Am]* 1976;58-A:850-3.

58. **Wiesel SW, Tsourmas N, Feffer HL, Citrin CM, Patronas N.** A study of computer-assisted tomography. 1. The incidence of positive CAT scans in an asymptomatic group of patients. *Spine* 1984;9:549-51.

59. **Mullin WJ, Heithoff KB, Gilbert TJ Jr, Renfrew DL.** Magnetic resonance evaluation of recurrent disc herniation: is gadolinium necessary? *Spine* 2000;25:1493-9.

60. **Thompson JP, Pearce RH, Schechter MT, et al.** Preliminary evaluation of a scheme for grading the gross morphology of the human intervertebral disc. *Spine* 1990;15:411-5.

61. **Riihimäki H, Like M, Paakkulainen H, Lamminen A, Leino-Arjas P.** Sequence of appearance of MRI signs of disc degeneration. *Int Soc Study Lumbar Spine* Adelaide, 2000;23.

62. **Boden SD, Davis DO, Dina TS, Patronas NJ, Wiesel SW.** Abnormal magnetic resonance scans of the lumbar spine in asymptomatic subjects. *J Bone Joint Surg [Am]* 1990;72-A:403-8.

63. **Jensen MC, Brant-Zawadzki MN, Obuchowski N, et al.** Magnetic resonance imaging of the lumbar spine in people without back pain. *N Engl J Med* 1994;331:69-73.

64. **Buirski G, Silberstein M.** The symptomatic lumbar disc in patients with low-back pain: magnetic resonance imaging appearances in both symptomatic and control population. *Spine* 1993;18:1808-11.

65. **Buirski G.** Magnetic resonance signal patterns of lumbar discs in patients with low back pain: a prospective study with discographic correlation. *Spine* 1992;17:1199-204.

66. **Boos N, Semmer N, Elfering A, et al.** Natural history of individuals with asymptomatic disc abnormalities in magnetic resonance imaging: predictors of low back pain: related medical consultation and work incapacity. *Spine* 2000;25:1484-92.

67. **Aprill C, Bogduk N.** High intensity zone: a diagnostic sign of painful lumbar disc on magnetic resonance imaging. *Br J Radiol* 1992;65:361-9.

68. **Schellhas KP, Pollei SR, Gundry CR, Heithoff KB.** Lumbar disc high-intensity zone: correlation of magnetic resonance imaging and discography. *Spine* 1996;21:79-86.

69. **Lam KS, Carlin D, Mulholland RC.** Lumbar disc high-intensity zone: the value and significance of provocative discography in the determination of the discogenic pain source. *Eur Spine J* 2000;9:36-41.

70. **Ricketson R, Simmons JW, Hauser BO.** The prolapsed intervertebral disc: the high intensity zone with discographic correlation. *Spine* 1996;21:2758-62.

71. **Carragee EJ, Pragioudakis SJ, Khurana S.** Lumbar high intensity zone and discography in subjects without low back complaints. *Int Soc Study Lumbar Spine* Adelaide, 2000:61.

72. **Adams MA, Dolan P, Hutton WC.** The stages of disc degeneration as revealed by discograms. *J Bone Joint Surg [Br]* 1986;68-B:36-41.

73. **Colhoun E, McCall IW, Williams L, Cassar Pollicino VN.** Provocation discography as a guide to planning operations on the spine. *J Bone Joint Surg [Br]* 1988;70-B:267-71.

74. **Knox BD, Chapman TM.** Anterior lumbar interbody fusion for discogram concordant pain. *J Spinal Disord* 1993;6:242-4.

75. **Leufven C, Nordwall A.** Management of chronic disabling low back pain with 360° fusion, posterolateral fusion, and pedicle screw instrumentation in patients with chronic disabling low back pain. *Spine* 1999;24:2042-5.

76. **Derby R, Howard MW, Grant JM, et al.** The ability of pressure-controlled discography to predict surgical and nonsurgical outcomes. *Spine* 1999;24:364-72.

77. **Hanley EN, Phillips ED, Kostuik JP.** Who should be fused? In: Frymoyer JW, ed. *The adult spine: principles and practice.* New York: Raven Press, 1991;1893-917.

78. **De Roos A, Kressel K, Spritzer C, Dalinka M.** MR imaging of marrow changes adjacent to endplates in degenerative lumbar disc disease. *AJR* 1987;149:531-4.

79. **Modic MT, Steinberg PM, Ross JS, Masaryk TJ, Carter JR.** Degenerative disc disease: assessment of changes in vertebral body marrow with MR imaging. *Radiology* 1988;166:193-9.

80. **Braithwaite I, White J, Saifuddin A, Renton P, Taylor BA.** Vertebral end-plate (Modic) changes on lumbar spine MRI: correlation with pain reproduction at lumbar discography. *Eur Spine J* 1998;7:363-8.

81. **Toyone T, Takahashi K, Kitahara H, et al.** Vertebral bone-marrow changes in degenerative lumbar disc disease: an MRI study of 74 patients with low back pain. *J Bone Joint Surg [Br]* 1994;76-B:757-64.

82. **Lang P, Chafetz N, Genant HK, Morris JM.** Lumbar spinal fusion: assessment of functional stability with magnetic resonance imaging. *Spine* 1990;15:581-8.

83. **Butler D, Trafimow JH, Andersson GBJ, McNeill TW, Huckman MS.** Discs degenerative before facets. *Spine* 1990;15:111-3.

84. **Fujiwara A, Tamai K, Yamato M, et al.** The relationship between facet joint osteoarthritis and disc degeneration of the lumbar spine: an MRI study. *Eur Spine J* 1999;8:396-401.

85. **Videman T, Battié MC, Gill K, et al.** Magnetic resonance imaging findings and their relationship in the thoracic and lumbar spine: insights into the etiopathogenesis of spinal degeneration. *Spine* 1995;20:928-35.

86. **Esses SI, Moro JK.** The value of facet joint blocks in patient selection for lumbar fusion. *Spine* 1993;18:185-90.

87. **Lovely TJ, Rastogi P.** The value of provocative facet blocking as a predictor of success in lumbar spine fusion. *J Spinal Disord* 1997;10:512-7.

88. **Knutsson F.** The instability associated with disc degeneration in the lumbar spine. *Acta Radiol* 1944;25:593-608.

89. **Morgan FP, King T.** Primary instability of lumbar vertebrae as a common cause of low back pain. *J Bone Joint Surg [Br]* 1957;39-B:6-22.

90. **Kirkaldy-Willis WH, Farfan HF.** Instability of the lumbar spine. *Clin Orthop* 1982;165:110-23.

91. **Shaffer WO, Spratt KF, Weinstein J, Lehmann TR, Goel V.** The consistency and accuracy of roentgenograms for measuring sagittal translation in the lumbar vertebral motion segment: an experimental model. *Spine* 1990;15:741-50.

92. **Hayes MA, Howard TC, Gruel CR, Kopta JA.** Roentgenographic evaluation of lumbar spine flexion-extension in asymptomatic individuals. *Spine* 1989;14:327-31.

93. **Boden SD, Wiesel SW.** Lumbosacral segmental motion in normal individuals: have we been measuring instability properly? *Spine* 1990;15:571-6.

94. **Mayer RS, Chen IH, Lavender SA, Trafimow JH, Andersson GB.** Variance in the measurement of sagittal lumbar spine range of motion among examiners, subjects and instruments. *Spine* 1995;20:1489-93.

95. **Haas M, Nyiendo J, Peterson C, et al.** Interrater reliability of roentgenological evaluation of the lumbar spine in lateral bending. *J Manipulative Physiol Ther* 1999;13:179-89.

96. **Jayaraman G, Nazre AA, McCann V, Redford JB.** A computerized technique for analyzing lateral bending behavior of subjects with normal and impaired lumbar spine: a pilot study. *Spine* 1994;19:824-32.

97. **Dvorak J, Panjabi MM, Chang DG, Theiler R, Grob D.** Functional radiographic diagnosis of the lumbar spine: flexion-extension and lateral bending. *Spine* 1991;16:562-71.

98. **Axelsson P, Johnsson R, Stromqvist B.** Effect of lumbar orthosis on intervertebral mobility: a roentgen stereophotogrammetric analysis. *Spine* 1992;17:678-81.

99. **Axelsson P, Johnsson R, Stromqvist B, Nilsson LT, Akesson M.** Orthosis as prognostic instrument in lumbar fusion: no predictive value in 50 cases followed prospectively. *J Spinal Disord* 1995;8:284-8.

100. **Axelsson P, Johnsson R, Stromqvist B.** Mechanics of the external fixation test in the lumbar spine: a roentgen stereophotogrammetric analysis. *Spine* 1996;21:330-3.

101. **Soini J, Slatis P, Kannisto M, Sandelin J.** External transpedicular fixation test of the lumbar spine correlates with the outcome of subsequent lumbar fusion. *Clin Orthop* 1993;293:89-96.

102. **Van der Schaaf DB, van Limbeck J, Pavlov PW.** Temporary external transpedicular fixation of the lumbosacral spine. *Spine* 1999;24:481-5.

103. **Steffen T, Rubin RK, Baramki HG, et al.** A new technique for measuring lumbar segmental motion in vivo: method, accuracy and preliminary results. *Spine* 1997;15:156-66.

104. **Okawa A, Shinomiya K, Komori H, et al.** Dynamic motion study of the whole lumbar spine by videofluoroscopy. *Spine* 1998;23:1743-9.

105. **Kanayama M, Abumi K, Kaneda K, Tadano S, Ukai T.** Phase lag of the intersegmental motion in flexion-extension of the lumbar and lumbosacral spine: an in vivo study. *Spine* 1996;21:1416-22.

106. **Möller H, Sundin A, Hedlund R.** Symptoms, signs and functional disability in adult spondylolisthesis. *Spine* 2000;25:683-9.

107. **Libson E, Bloom RA, Dinari G.** Symptomatic and asymptomatic spondylolysis and spondylolisthesis in young adults. *Int Orthop* 1982;6:259-61.

108. **Buttermann GR, Garvey TA, Hunt AF, et al.** Lumbar fusion results related to diagnosis. *Spine* 1998;23:116-27.

109. **Bernard TN Jr.** Repeat lumbar spine surgery: factors influencing outcome. *Spine* 1993;18:2196-200.

110. **Christensen FB, Thomsen K, Eiskjaer SP, Gelinick J, Bunger CE.** Functional outcome after posterolateral spinal fusion using pedicle screws: comparison between primary and salvage procedure. *Eur Spine J* 1998;7:321-7.

111. **Glassman SD, Minkow RE, Dimar JR, et al.** Effect of prior lumbar discectomy on outcome of lumbar fusion: a prospective analysis using the SF-36 measure. *J Spinal Disord* 1998;11:383-8.

112. **Andersson GBJ.** Surgical aspects on lateral spinal stenosis: indications and principles. *Acta Orthop Scand* 1993;64Suppl 251:74-5.

113. **Jönsson B.** Vertebral slipping after decompression for spinal stenosis. *Acta Orthop Scand* 1993;64Suppl 251:76-7.

114. **Fischgrund JS, Mackay M, Herkowitz HN, et al.** 1997 Volvo Award winner in clinical studies: degenerative lumbar spondylolisthesis with spinal stenosis: a prospective, randomized study comparing decompressive laminectomy and arthrodesis with and without spinal instrumentation. *Spine* 1997;22:2807-12.

115. **Gibson JN, Grant IC, Waddell G.** The Cochrane review of surgery for lumbar disc prolapse and degenerative lumbar spondylosis. *Spine* 1999;24:1820-32.

THE TREATMENT OF SPONDYLOLYSIS WITH OR WITHOUT SPONDYLOLISTHESIS

P. GILLET

From the Centre Hospitalier Universitaire, Liège, Belgium

Spondylolysis is a common lesion of the pars or isthmus of the posterior arch of the lower lumbar vertebrae and is often well tolerated. However, the excess of vertebral mobility that is associated with spondylolysis can lead to pain in the back which may be referred to the leg, true sciatica or even a neurological deficit, and progressive deformity of the spine in the sagittal plane. Anteroposterior displacement of the pathological vertebra in relation to the adjacent lower vertebrae is called spondylolisthesis. This can occur in degenerative disorders of the spine because of dysplasia of the posterior facet joints, or after major trauma.[1,2] This review deals only with spondylolysis and spondylolisthesis resulting from a defect of the pars.

AETIOLOGY

Spondylolysis is a fatigue fracture thought to be the result of repetitive microtrauma. In some cases, the pars interarticularis can fracture and heal several times, leading to an elongated pars. It usually occurs in youth (7 to 11 years of age); its incidence increases slightly in adulthood. The male-to-female ratio is about 2:1. Spondylolysis is not a congenital disease. Although it has occasionally been reported in newborn infants the conclusions of these reports are debatable.[3] Genetic factors can influence the incidence of isthmic spondylolisthesis but to a much less degree than in dysplastic types. The genetic influence is illustrated by a varying prevalence of the disease in different races, e.g. in white Caucasians it is 5% to 6%, in Africans 1% to 3% and in Eskimos up to 50%.[4-6] These differences, however, may be at least partially due to behavioural habits. Repetitive stress on the pars, especially in extension, and hyperlordosis, which causes impingement by the distal aspect of the lower articular facet of the upper vertebrae on the affected pars, clearly favour the occurrence of isthmic spondylolysis.[7-12] Adolescents practising sports involving hyperextension are at risk[13,14] Micheli and Wood[15] found that 47% of paediatric patients involved in sports developed spondylolysis compared with the general adult population. The occurrence of spondylolysis is probably multifactorial; radiological peculiarities such as dysplasia of the vertebral body show that there can be a predisposition which weakens the pars, which is probably of a genetic origin, and local repetitive microtrauma may lead to fracture.

CLINICAL FINDINGS

Spondylolysis and spondylolisthesis are often diagnosed incidentally since they may be asymptomatic. The patient, either child, adolescent or adult, may present, however, with acute pain in the back, thigh or leg which can be mechanical with radiation into the lower limb or true radicular pain, lumbar scoliosis, paravertebral muscle spasm, or abnormal stance or gait. If the symptoms are significant, other pathological conditions of the spine should be excluded since spondylolysis is often only mildly symptomatic. The symptoms are not proportional to the extent of the pathological condition; spondylolysis without slip can be more painful than spondylolysis with obvious spondylolisthesis. Figure 1 shows an MR scan of a 55-year-old patient who presented with moderate back pain. She was referred by her general practitioner because he was concerned about a grade-IV spondylolisthesis. She had

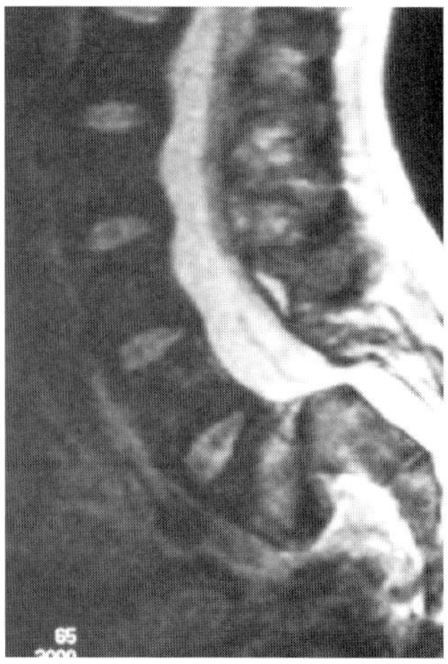

Fig. 1

MRI of a 55-year-old patient complaining of recent moderate back pain. Grade-IV spondylolisthesis is present. She worked for 30 years as a nurse in a geriatric department.

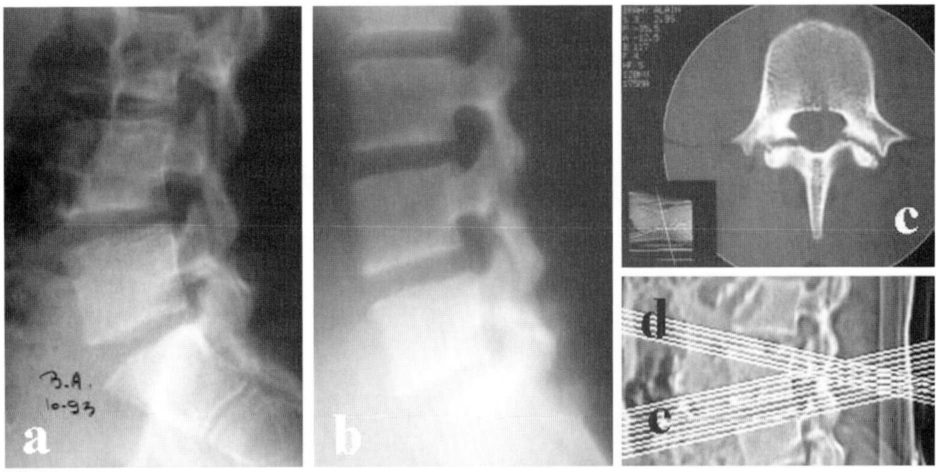

Fig. 2

Radiographs (a) may be doubtful, and conventional tomography (b) can display spondylolysis. With CT, the reversed gantry technique (d) will show spondylolysis better (c) than the standard technique (e) used for the study of the discs.

worked for 30 years as a nurse in a geriatric department. Möller and co-workers[16-18] found that symptoms were similar in adult patients with spondylolisthesis and in patients with chronic non-specific low back pain probably related to degenerative conditions. In their study the group with chronic low back pain reported greater functional disability.

RADIOLOGICAL FINDINGS

Plain lateral radiographs are useful in the evaluation of spondylolisthesis. Ideally, standing films should be obtained, centred on the lumbosacral area and not the lumbar spine. The degree of spondylolisthesis, the translational displacement in the sagittal plane, is usually defined by the classification of Mayerding: grade 0, no slip; grade 1, 1% to 25% slip; grade 2, 26% to 50% slip; grade 3, 51% to 75% slip; grade 4, 76% to 100% slip. If the slip exceeds 100%, it is grade 5 or a spondyloptosis. In practice, it can be difficult to place a particular patient in a specific category. The angle of slip is the measurement used to determine the amount of lumbosacral kyphosis. This is done by drawing a line along the posterior cortex of the sacrum and measuring the angle between its perpendicular and a line drawn along the inferior border of L5. The normal angle ranges between 0° and 10°. If deformity of the inferior border of the L5 vertebral body is significant, the superior border can be used. The angle of sacral inclination is formed by a line perpendicular to the floor and a line along the posterior margin of the sacrum. Nazarian[19] has made a complete review of the sagittal parameters related to spondylolisthesis and their measurements.

Spondylolysis can be missed on lateral views and therefore oblique views centred on the pathological vertebra must be obtained when the abnormality is suspected. Even with plain radiographs of very good quality spondylolysis can be missed, especially in the early stage. Conventional tomography can be useful (Fig. 2) and dynamic lateral views can be helpful to evaluate the mobility of the abnormal vertebra. They should be obtained in a lateral decubitus position.[20]

CT, particularly using the reversed gantry technique, may be needed to demonstrate the defect (Fig. 2).

Bone scans are also helpful in diagnosing the pars defect at an early stage; in chronic cases bone scans may be normal[21] (see Fig. 6).

Radiological peculiarities. In unilateral spondylolysis, hypertrophy of the opposite pars or pedicle may occur (Fig. 3) because of bypass of the load through these structures.[22,23]

The possibility of an osteoid osteoma must be considered, especially if the patient has persistent pain. A unilateral defect of the pars with lysis of the contralateral pedicle may be observed.

A false L5/S1 spondylolisthesis may be described because of dysplasia of the vertebral body of L5. Some patients show a trapezoidal-shaped vertebral body with a reduced anteroposterior diameter. This leads to the appearance of a spondylolisthesis because the posterior walls of L4, L5 and S1 are not aligned; it has been noticed in such cases that the anterior borders of the vertebral bodies are in perfect regular sagittal alignment. The term spondylolisthesis should not be used in these circumstances because it can lead to misinterpretation of the stability at the lumbosacral junction. Such patients illustrate the role of genetic factors in the occurrence of isthmic spondylolysis since the changes in the vertebral body are not due to secondary remodelling as demonstrated by its normal positioning in regard to the adjacent vertebrae.

Myelography. This has been and is still used by some physicians to evaluate possible root compromise. It can give false-negative results since the posterior arch remains

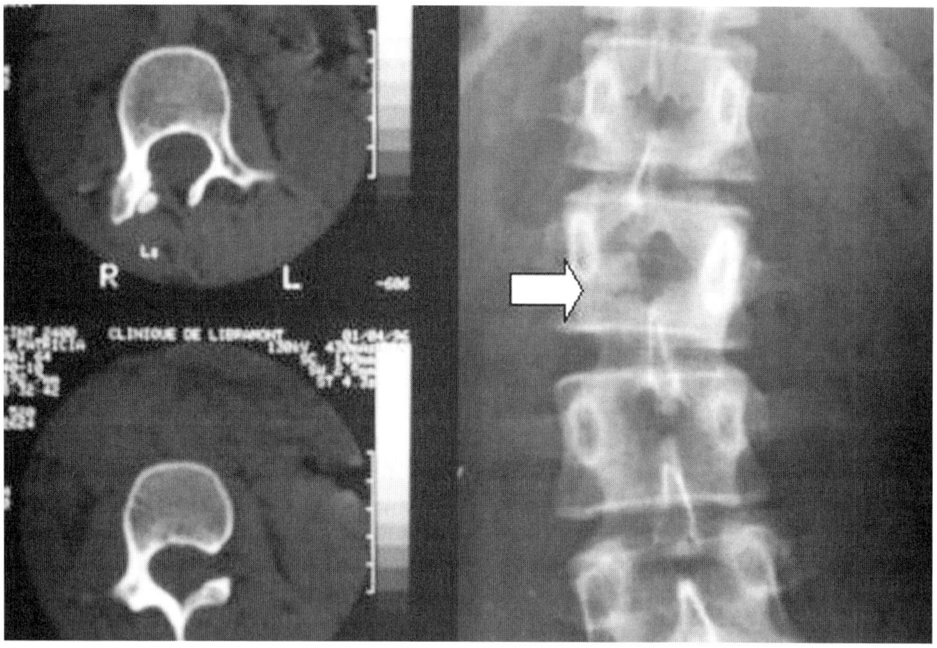

Fig. 3

In unilateral spondylolysis (arrow), the mechanical stress shunted through the opposite half of the posterior arch can lead to hyperdensity of the opposite pedicle. The differential diagnosis of an osteoid osteoma must be considered, especially if scoliosis is present, as in this case.

in place in spondylolisthesis due to spondylolysis and there is an increase in the anteroposterior diameter of the spinal canal (Fig. 4). The possible root impingement is much more lateral, in an area where the contrast material normally does not reach.[24]

CT. This is widely available and its usefulness in assessing spondylolysis and spondylolisthesis has been reported. It shows the increase in fibrocartilaginous tissue and hypertrophy of the stumps of the pars. Sagittal reconstructions may show root encroachment between remnants of the proximal pars and the underlying vertebral body.[24]

CT is useful if the diagnosis of spondylolysis cannot be made on plain radiographs, but its use in evaluating the existence of an associated herniated disc and the study of the foramina by sagittal reconstructions have been superseded by MRI in the sagittal plane. False images of herniated discs may be seen in the transverse plane if the axial slices are not perfectly parallel to the disc space, especially if spondylolisthesis is present (Fig. 4).

MRI. If there is an indication for surgical treatment, MRI in spondylolysis and spondylolisthesis is mandatory. T2-weighted images demonstrate if there are degenerative changes in the discs[25] and this information is important in deciding which type of operation to perform (Fig. 5). Associated herniated discs responsible for neurological compromise, especially at the level of the foramina, and impingement by a pincer effect of the stump of the pars and the adjacent disc and vertebral body, can be easily recognised on sagittal cuts.[26,27]

AUTHOR'S IMAGING STRATEGY

If spondylolysis is suspected, plain radiographs with AP, lateral and oblique views should be obtained and if necessary, adequate CT performed. Bone scanning should be considered if the diagnosis is not confirmed by radiological imaging (Fig. 6).

If surgery is anticipated, regular imaging investigations should include plain radiography and MRI. The latter will give the necessary information on the presence of a herniated disc which may require removal, on the choice between a reconstructive procedure of the pars if there is no degenerative disc disease at the level of the spondylolysis or some type of intervertebral fusion if degenerative disc disease is present, and on the necessary length of such a fusion to reach the level of an intact disc space. If MRI gives doubtful results, a discogram should be performed. CT and myelography should be used in exceptional cases. If they have already been obtained by the referring physician, they usually rarely influence the surgical indication or procedure.

NATURAL HISTORY OF SPONDYLOLYSIS

The natural history of spondylolysis and spondylolisthesis is difficult to assess. In most studies spondylolysis with and without initial slip are studied together. Some authors have studied symptomatic and asymptomatic patients, some symptomatic patients only and others have compared operated and non-operated patients.[28-37]

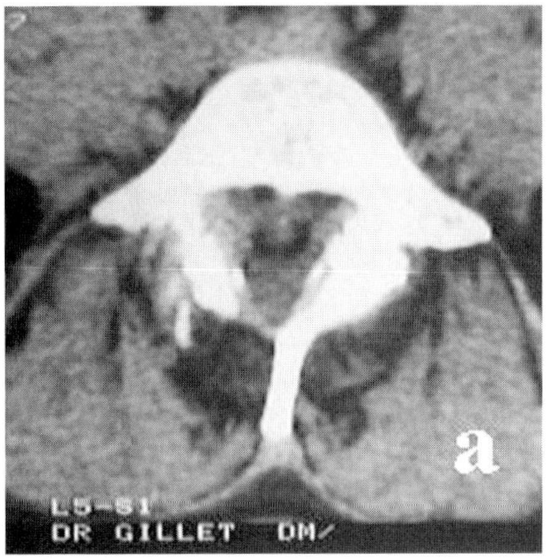

Fig. 4a

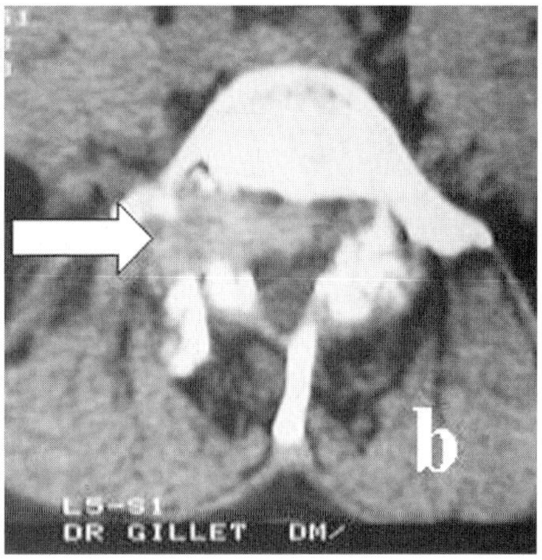

Fig. 4b

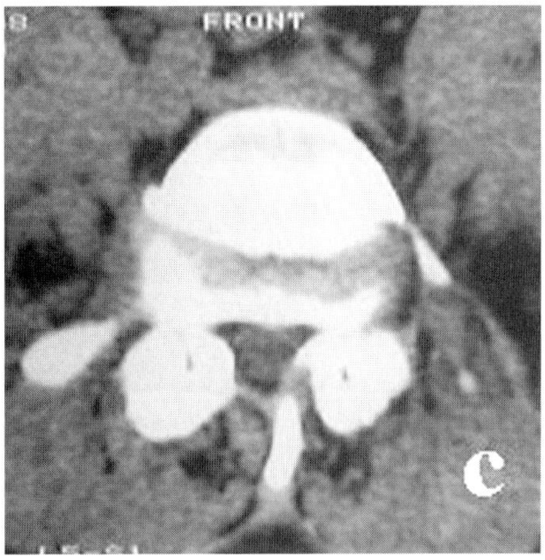

Fig. 4c

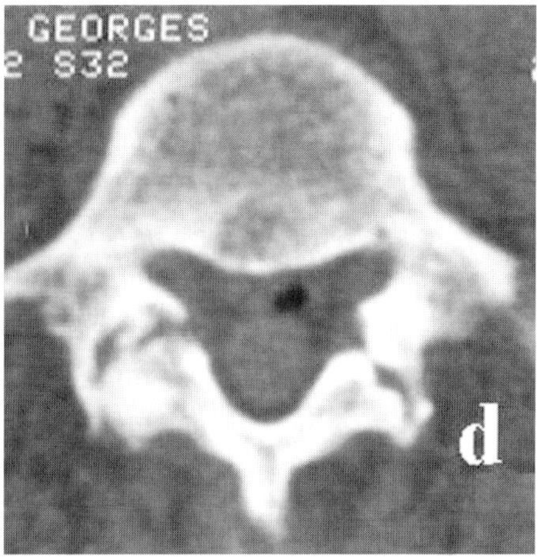

Fig. 4d

CT may show confusing images, such as false herniated discs (b, arrow) if the cuts are not parallel to the motion segment. In spondylolisthesis due to spondylolysis, the anteroposterior diameter is widened at the level of the slip (compare a with c), which accounts for possible false absence of nerve-root compromise on myelograms since the compression is more likely to occur at the level of the foramina where the isthmic stumps are hypertrophic (d), an area the contrast medium does not usually reach during myelography.

Spondylolysis can heal without sequelae, but it can also persist until adulthood, with progressive pain presenting after decades of an asymptomatic presence. Secondary symptoms can occur as the result of stress imposed on the various ligamentous structures because of instability of the motion segment induced by the pars fracture. Potential intervertebral instability is theoretically greater for L4 or L3 spondylolysis than for L5 spondylolysis because of the absence of anatomical links such as the iliolumbar ligaments. Most of the slips are less than 30% to 50%. Progressive slip is more often associated with local anatomical peculiarities but this remains debatable: these may include a vertical sacrum, a dome-shaped sacrum, or a trapezoidal-shaped L5 vertebral body.[4,11,36,38] Local kyphosis seems to be more troublesome than the degree of slip.[1,2,39] Progressive slip is unusual in adulthood but can be the result of degenerative disc disease with collapse of the disc leading to a slight amount of spondylolisthesis.[40,41] Significant slips presenting in adult patients have generally been present since adolescence. The early onset of a fracture of the pars can increase the risk of progressive spondylolisthesis. Progression of the slip usually occurs during the growth spurt.[4] The more the slip is significant during the growth period (more than grade 2), the more the patient is at risk for further displacement until skeletal maturity. An angle of slip greater than 55% is also associated with a risk of progression. Therefore, even in asymptomatic patients, there may be an occasional indication for fusion in severe spondylolisthesis.[36] Lonstein[6] has shown that spondylolisthesis occurs twice as often in males but the risk of increasing spondylolisthesis is four times greater in female than in male patients.

If not the cause of spondylolysis, trauma can increase symptoms related to the anomaly and lead to an increase in the slip.[10]

Frennered[42] studied the incidence of spondylolysis and

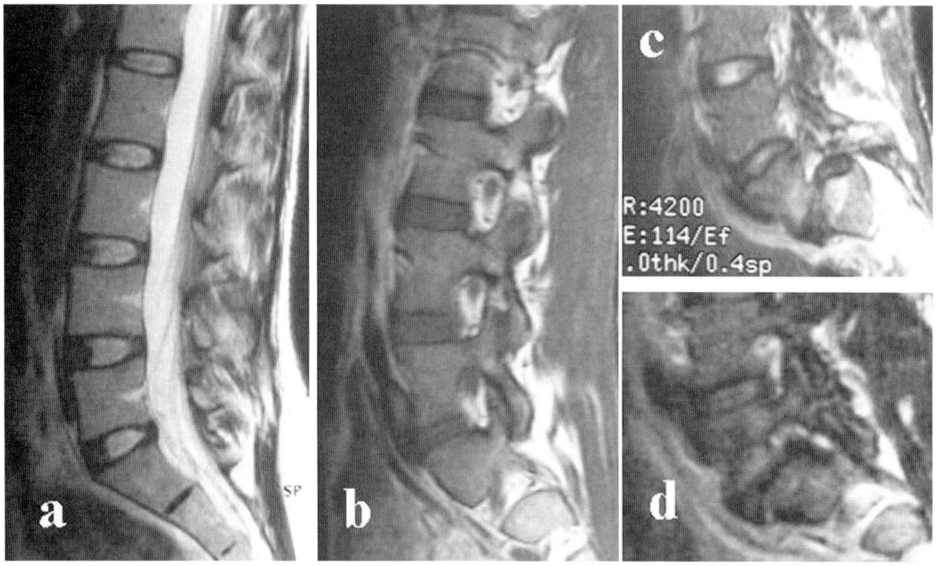

Fig. 5

T2-weighted MRI assesses the trophicity of the motion segments (a), which is important when considering what type of surgery (fusion or isthmic reconstruction) is required. Lateral parasagittal slices through the foramina show normal landmarks (b) or stenosis due to prolapse or herniation of the disc linked to the slip and possible bony compromise leading to nerve-root compression (c and d), which is important when considering whether a decompression by realignment of the spondylolisthesis or a Gill procedure should be performed.

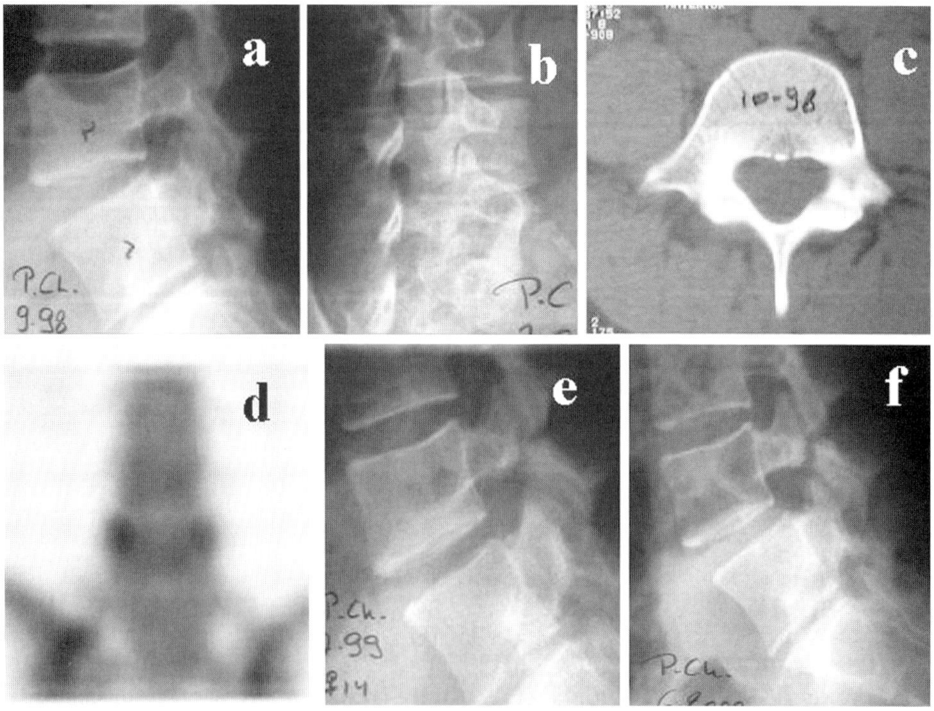

Fig. 6

A 14-year-old girl complained of backache; her involvement in sports suggested a possible spondylolysis which is not seen on initial radiographs (a) and (b). CT shows alterations in the isthmic regions (c) and bone scanning demonstrates hyperactivity (d). A few months later, bilateral spondylolysis became obvious (e and f).

spondylolisthesis in patients receiving a disability pension for musculoskeletal disorders. The incidence was similar to that in the general population, indicating that the disease is probably not connected to an increased risk of permanent disability in the lower back. A greater proportion of L4 defects suggests, however, that spondylolysis with or without spondylolisthesis above L5 could be at greater risk.

From personal experience, spondylolysis with or without spondylolisthesis ultimately requiring surgical management is a problem of the young adult. In a series of 176 patients, the mean age was 37 years (13 to 70).

GENERAL PRINCIPLES FOR TREATMENT

It is well accepted that asymptomatic patients presenting with spondylolysis and spondylolisthesis of grade 0 to grade 2 should not be prevented from sports activities and strenuous work as long as such activities do not induce pain. In symptomatic patients without neurological compromise, adaptation of the lifestyle, which can mean change of work and refraining from sports, in association with conservative management, is the cornerstone of treatment. Since most spondylolysis or spondylolisthesis is well tolerated, other causes of back pain should be considered and excluded. Fusion procedures, which will be described later, should only be performed in unusual cases in which a considerable risk of increased spondylolisthesis is present, whether the patient is symptomatic or not, and in cases in which conservative treatment has failed. There is, however, a place for surgery in patients who are relieved by adaptation of their lifestyle but who want to regain normal work or sporting activities. If a reasonable surgical procedure can be proposed, operative treatment, although invasive, may be considered in selected patients capable of making a well-understood decision with the surgeon.

A detailed description of conservative treatment is beyond the scope of this review. Options for treatment include restriction of activities, anti-inflammatory drugs and analgesia, isometric abdominal and paraspinal muscle strengthening, reduction of lumbar lordosis, symptomatic physiotherapy and temporary bracing.[43]

SURGICAL TREATMENT OF SPONDYLOLYSIS

Surgical options depend on the age of the patient, the existence or not of associated degenerative disc disease and the presence of true local instability. Usually some type of stabilisation procedure is performed. Possibilities include repair of the pars without fusion of a motion segment, different methods of posterior fusion and interbody fusion by a posterior or anterior approach. The number of motion segments to be fused should be estimated. The need for decompression of the nerve roots should be assessed. The differential diagnosis between referred pain and true radicular symptoms is sometimes difficult. Whether or not to reduce an associated spondylolisthesis and the role of internal fixation remain a matter of debate and must be discussed with each individual patient. Workers' compensation and litigation, as with other spinal procedures, are associated with a higher incidence of unsatisfactory results, especially if the symptoms are not neurological.[44]

Decompression procedures

The removal of the posterior arch to obtain adequate decompression of the nerve roots, if necessary, is a more aggressive procedure than the usual laminectomy for spinal degenerative stenosis. The entire posterior arch is removed together with all bulky fibrocartilaginous tissue present at the level of the pars defect. It is this fibrous tissue, in association with the slip, if present, which compresses the nerve roots. The operation is known as the Gill procedure.[45] Louis has described the most offending structure, which is the remnant of the proximal pars, as the *crochet isthmique* or isthmus hook. This particular structure may be responsible for stretching the nerve root. His views are confirmed by the findings of Edelson and Nathan[46] on skeletons and by MRI.[27] The Gill procedure must include a thorough removal of this structure and all offending tissue in order to be adjacent to the inferior and internal border of the pedicle. An isolated Gill procedure, without stabilisation, can increase the risk of progression[47] and should be avoided, except in some elderly patients in whom remodelling of the degenerative disc space induces some local stability.[48]

If a herniated disc is present and responsible for root compromise, it should be removed; isolated discectomy in a patient presenting with an otherwise asymptomatic spondylolisthesis may be considered.

Fusion procedures

The usefulness and indication for surgical stabilisation in spondylolysis and spondylolisthesis have been questioned by many authors and indisputable data remain scarce. Some authors, however, have shown that surgical treatment can alleviate pain and allow a more active lifestyle.[16-18,31] A classification of the most commonly performed surgical stabilisation procedures is given in Table I.

Posterior midline fusion. An onlay bone graft is applied to the laminae and spinous processes of the olisthetic and adjacent vertebrae. Successful results have been described in young patients even with severe slips,[3] but this technique has been associated with a high risk of nonunion and spinal stenosis; it did not prevent further slip in the series of Seitsalo et al.[49,50] For anatomical reasons, the fusion should at least be one level longer than posterolateral or interbody fusions and the procedure requires prolonged rest. It should be considered nowadays as a historical aspect of the surgical treatment of spondylolisthesis.

Posterolateral fusion with and without instrumentation. This remains probably the most common procedure performed in the lumbosacral area. Bone graft is applied between the transverse processes and the ala of the sacrum. This consists of iliac corticocancellous bone chips or chips trimmed from the posterior arch if a Gill procedure is

Table I. Classification of the most commonly performed surgical stabilisation procedures

Fusion without reduction	Posterior midline fusion Posterolateral intertransverse fusion Posterior interbody fusion Anterior interbody fusion Staged or combined anterior and posterior fusions (all of these procedures may include resection of the posterior arch and internal fixation)
Fusion with reduction	Posterior or posterolateral fusion with posterior reduction Posterior interbody fusion with posterior reduction Staged posterior and anterior approach with reduction and anterior interbody fusion (all of these procedures usually include the removal of the posterior arch and some type of internal fixation) Reduction can be achieved preoperatively or postoperatively by the use of progressive traction and repositioning using some type of traction table or Cotrel reduction frame
Fusion with resection of the olisthetic vertebra	
Pars defect reconstruction procedures	

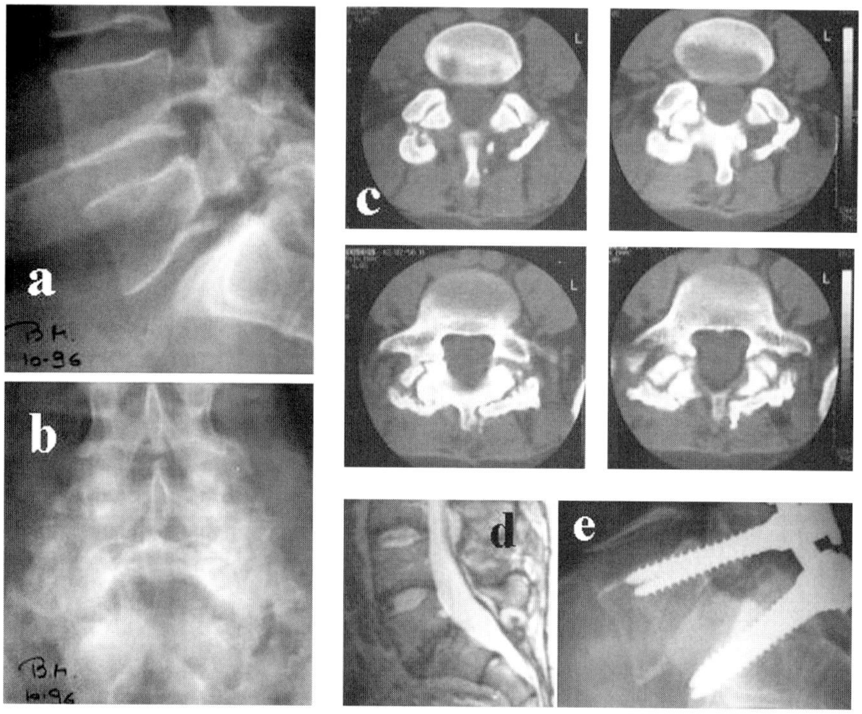

Fig. 7

A 40-year-old bricklayer complained of incapacitating back pain. He had undergone posterolateral arthrodesis ten years earlier with a satisfactory radiological appearance of the bone graft (a and b). CT shows that the graft has not fused to the transverse processes and sacral ala (c). MRI shows that the L5/S1 segment only is degenerative (d). The patient underwent posterior lumbar interbody fusion and Compact Cotrel Dubousset instrumentation. The bone graft was harvested from the abundant posterolateral graft (e). He returned to his former profession six months after surgery after disability for more than ten years.

performed. Bank bone and bone substitutes are sometimes used as an adjunct to or a substitute for autogenous bone graft. The length of the fusion depends on the degree of slip. In severe L5/S1 slips, an extension of the graft up to L4 has been traditionally recommended, but this is probably an inheritance from the time when non-instrumented fusion was performed. With modern techniques of instrumentation, it is more often possible to keep the fusion short. For L4 spondylolysis with olisthesis, L4/S1 fusions have been the rule but with adequate internal fixation, L4/L5 floating fusions may be successfully performed. Isolated interarticular fusion is unsatisfactory in spondylolysis since it will only provide immobilisation of the loose posterior arch, leaving the vertebral body mobile. Interarticular fusion may only be used in association with posterolateral fusion to augment the graft material and immobilise the arch, if the latter is not to be removed as part of a decompression procedure. Internal fixation is often used to allow early mobilisation and a short hospital stay and to avoid postoperative bracing. Pedicle fixation has become the rule. Screw placement can be safely performed with a meticulous technique. The pitfalls must be borne in mind.[51,52] Screws are used in combination with different types of plate or rod.[53-58] Posterior distraction devices such as Harrington rods or Knod rods do not offer enough stability to avoid postoperative immobilisation, require

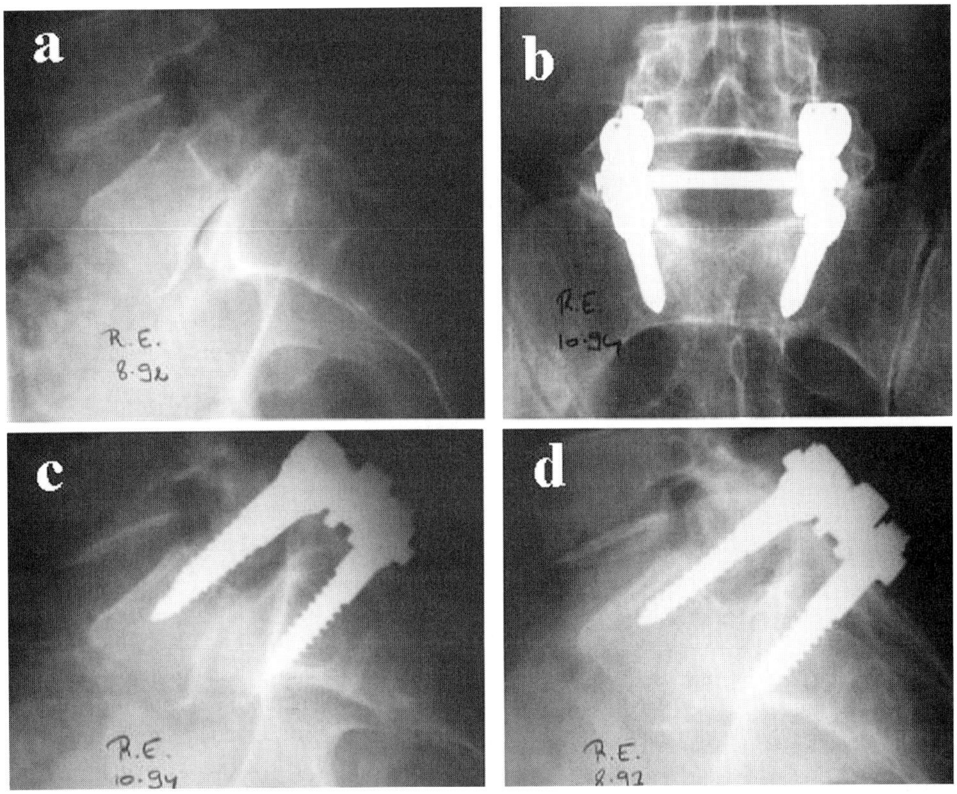

Fig. 8

An example of posterolateral fusion in situ with a Gill procedure in a 45-year-old disabled factory worker with grade-II spondylolisthesis (a). There was solid arthrodesis on AP views (b) and spontaneous interbody fusion after two years because of initial extreme narrowing of the disc space (compare c with d). He returned to work six months after surgery.

longer instrumentation and lead to local kyphosis. Better immobilisation by internal fixation should improve the rate of fusion and possibly the time to fusion especially in adult patients, but studies which could confirm this are scarce and the clinical relevance is unclear. Some studies specifically show that the use of internal fixation has not improved the clinical results.[6-18,57] Rigid internal fixation improves postoperative comfort as complementary bracing is not required,[58] but it is unclear if the benefits outweigh the potential risks, especially if reduction of the slip is not required.

A radiograph can give the impression that there is a solid posterolateral fusion, but bone may be present which does not fuse with the transverse processes and is not effective (Fig. 7). The diagnosis of nonunion is difficult. CT may help but requires perfect imaging with multiple thin slices; the presence of metal can reduce the quality of the images.

Posterolateral fusion in situ. Posterolateral fusion has been described as a successful form of treatment especially in young patients even in high-grade spondylolisthesis when performed in situ, i.e., without any attempt to improve the sagittal alignment of the lumbosacral junction.[35,49,59,60] Using gait analysis, Shelokov, Haideri and Roach[61] found no significant abnormalities of gait in a group of adult patients fused in situ for high-grade slip during adolescence; they did not complain about the cosmetic result and none reported missing work because of back pain. The authors concluded that fusion in situ should not be abandoned. It seems, however, that even if the clinical results are satisfactory, posterolateral fusion in situ does not prevent further progressive asymptomatic slip.[36] Even in the presence of mild nerve-root irritation, immobilisation of the pathological vertebra may suffice to alleviate the symptoms.[35] Severe neurological impairment would probably justify more aggressive procedures including adequate decompression of the nerve roots by removing all potentially offending structures, but this can further increase the local instability. Even partial reduction of the deformity can contribute to root decompression. Abdu, Wilber and Emery[62] reported lumbosacral fixation in situ by means of screws passing from S1 to L5 through the disc, associated with L4/S1 plating and posterolateral fusion. Posterolateral fusion in situ can be performed in adults with a favourable clinical and radiological outcome (Figures 8 to 10).

Posterolateral fusion with reduction of the spondylolisthesis. Reduction of the spondylolisthesis may be obtained preoperatively using traction tables as described

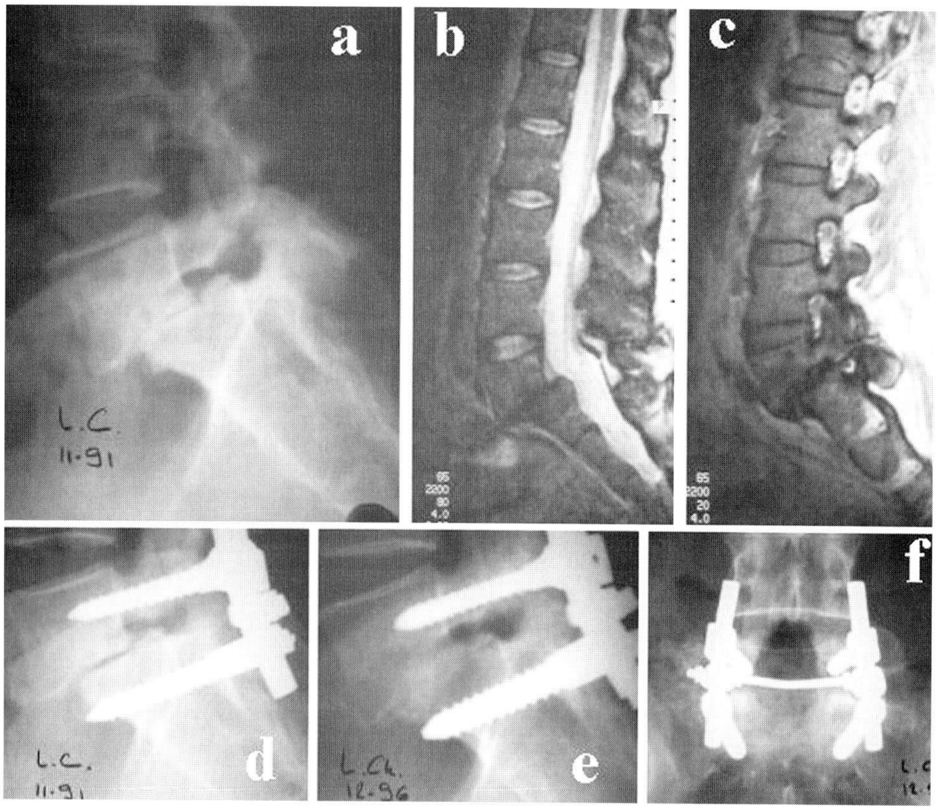

Fig. 9

The same situation as in Figure 8 in a 40-year-old woman (a). MRI shows an isolated L5/S1 degenerative disc (b) although foraminal encroachment was present (c). A Gill procedure only was carried out to free the L5 nerve roots, without any attempt to reduce the slip as the mechanical situation seemed stable. Posterolateral fusion in situ with CD instrumentation led to disappearance of back and leg pain with spontaneous interbody fusion (d, e and f).

by Scaglietti, Frontino and Bartolozzi[63] or postoperatively by using halo-pelvic or halo-femoral traction.[64] Aggressive perioperative and postoperative reduction by external fixation and traction has been described.[65] These procedures would probably no longer be considered since they are not accepted by patients. Correction of the deformity can be obtained intraoperatively by instrumentation. Reduction of the translational slip and of the slip angle or lumbosacral kyphosis has two aims. It seems logical that anatomical restoration of the lumbosacral sagittal balance should lead to better long-term results with regard to back and thigh pain. Restoration of normal or nearly normal anatomical relationships also favours radicular decompression, but in severe slips there can be a shortening of the L5 roots and they may be stretched during the reduction procedure, either closed or open, leading to neurological deficit. A compromise reduction of the deformity is often the best procedure. Correction of the kyphosis, when present, is more important than reducing the translational slip. It requires an angular correction, by trying to roll the sacrum anteriorly under the L5 vertebra more than by pulling the L5 vertebra backwards. Internal fixation has two aims: obtaining the desired reduction and providing immobilisation. In gross instability supplementary postoperative bracing must be considered. Harrington rods have been used to obtain reduction but require long fixation.[66-68] Knodt rods have also been used.[69,70] All techniques using distraction encourage loss of lumbosacral lordosis and should be abandoned. Pedicle screw fixation with plates or rods has been used to obtain and maintain correction keeping the length of fusion to a minimum.[52,54-59,71,72]

Instrumented reduction of severe spondylolisthesis in young patients remains controversial. Theoretical advantages include a reduction in postoperative pain due to immediate immobilisation, a lower risk of further slip, an improved rate of union and better sagittal clinical appearance. Disadvantages are a higher risk of neurological complications than with fusion in situ. Restoring normal sagittal alignment in this group has not proved necessary[73] and is even more debatable in adult patients.

It must be kept in mind that any attempt to obtain reduction of a spondylolisthesis may create further instability. The instrumentation is submitted to tremendous stress before bone fusion occurs with a risk of recurrence of the slip depending on the type of bone graft, the strength of the fixation and the postoperative behaviour of the patient. Reduction by plates and posterolateral fusion only is at risk of secondary loss of correction because of the lack of an

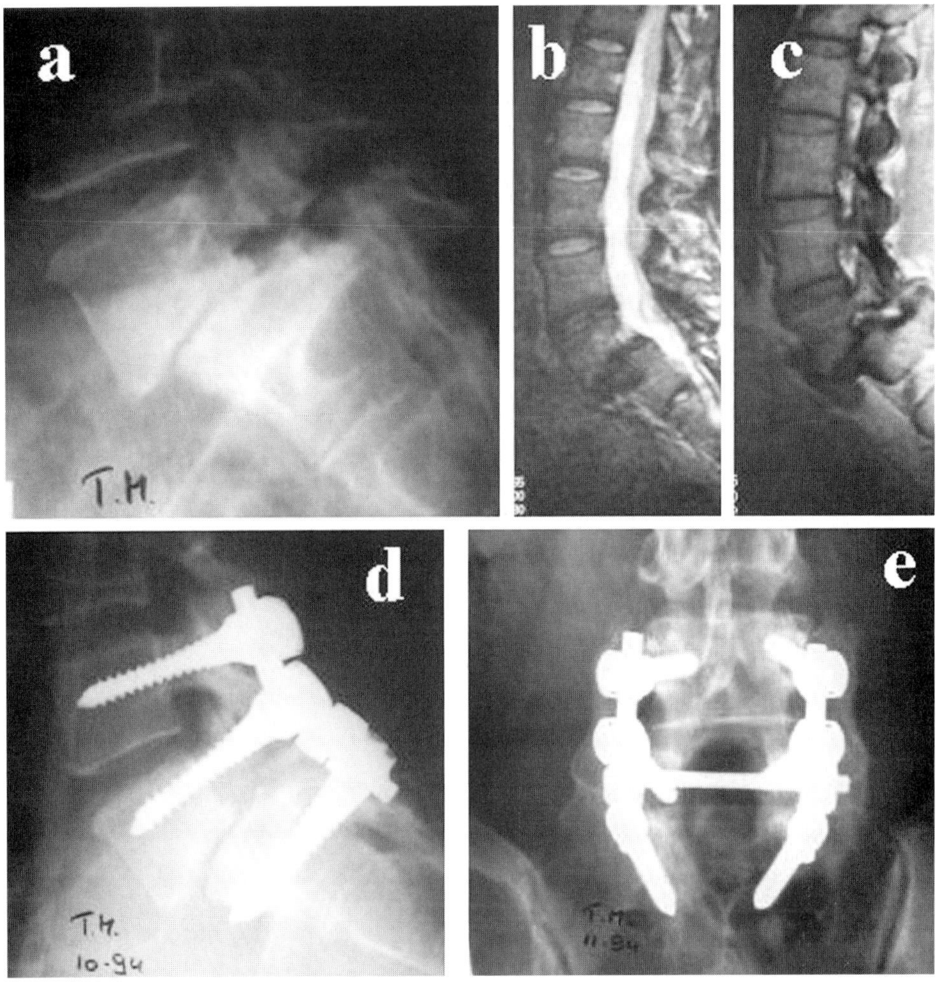

Fig. 10

Grade-I spondylolisthesis (a) in a 43-year-old woman with L4/L5 disc degeneration (b) and moderate foraminal root entrapment (c). A Gill procedure and L4/L5/S1 posterolateral fusion with Compact Cotrel Dubousset (CCD) instrumentation allowed her to return to a normal lifestyle with disappearance of back and leg pain. Radiographs show the fusion mass at 12 months (d,e).

anterior weight-bearing bone graft.[19] Rod constructs such as CD instrumentation give greater rigidity and lessen, but do not eliminate, the incidence of secondary loss of correction (Fig. 11).[54,55,58,74-78]

An extended Gill procedure should be performed whenever reduction is attempted in order to decompress and visualise the nerve roots throughout the procedure. Periradicular scarring is always a risk in such cases.

Interbody fusion. Posterolateral fusions can be criticised because they are submitted to tension and bending stresses. From the point of view of biomechanics, an interbody fusion is more logical since it is submitted to compression stress and only to shear stress if the lumbosacral junction is very oblique.[79] In the L5/S1 area, instability of L5 is relative, except in severe slips usually associated with some type of local dysplasia. The iliolumbar ligaments may contribute to this increased stability, although their role is questioned.[80] Intertransverse bone grafting has been shown to be a reliable technique at that level and remains the treatment of choice. In the case of L3 or L4 spondylolysis, the local instability is greater, especially if there is some spondylolisthesis with a normal height of the disc space. In such cases, posterolateral fusion techniques may not lead to complete immobilisation of the L3/L4 or L4/L5 segment, and nonunion or delayed bending and local kyphosis with subsequent narrowing of the disc space may occur, especially when using non-rigid instrumentation.[58]

Posterior lumbar interbody fusion (PLIF). This technique offers the opportunity to perform the whole surgical procedure through one approach. Removal of the posterior arch allows inspection of nerve roots and their decompression by removing the fibrous tissue which can obstruct the lateral recesses. It gives access to the disc which may be removed. The use of specific intradiscal instruments and pedicle screws with rods or plates allows the surgeon to reduce the slip if desired. Solid bone blocks or cages with cancellous bone graft can be introduced into the disc space, and instrumentation can be performed (Fig. 12). However,

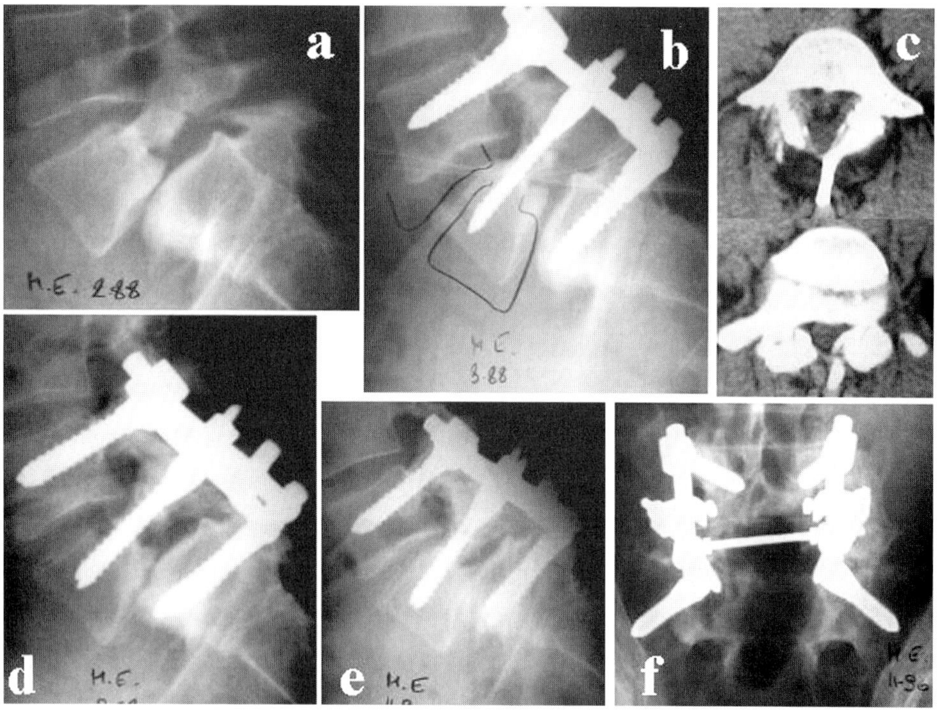

Fig. 11

Grade-II to grade-III spondylolisthesis in a 33-year-old blacksmith (a). Posterior reduction was attempted and partially obtained (b) but lost after three months (c, d) because of the lack of anterior bony support. Solid fusion was obtained (e and f), however, and the patient returned to full work and playing tennis.

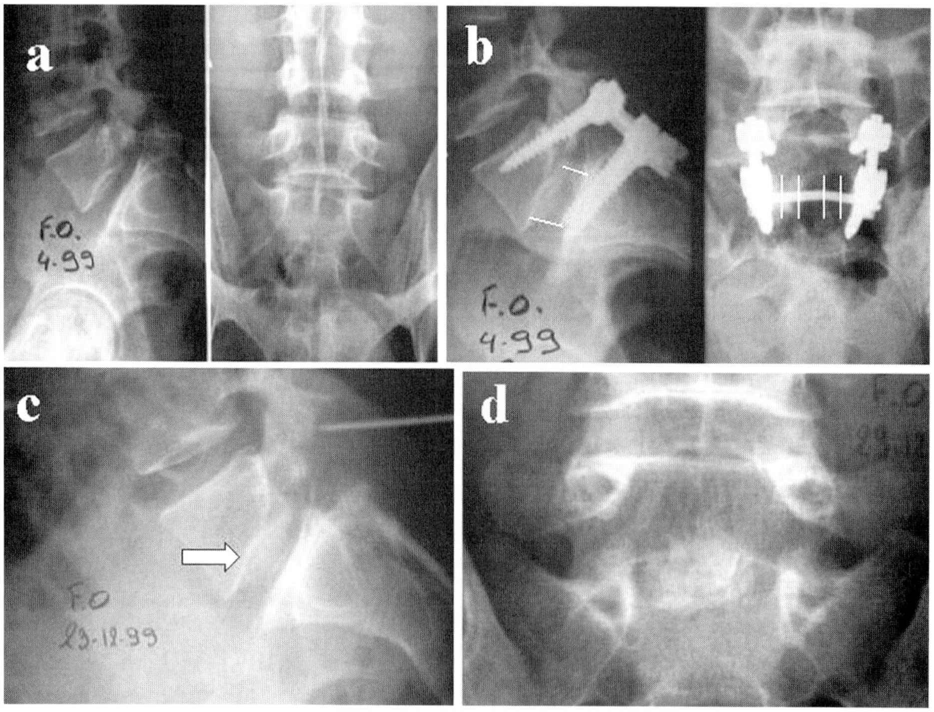

Fig. 12

Posterior lumbar interbody fusion performed in a 20-year-old factory worker with moderate grade-I slip. PLIF was chosen because of a normal disc height, although it appeared degenerated on MRI (a). Postoperative radiographs showed interbody grafts trimmed from the posterior arch (white lines) (b). Radiographs at one year after removal of the CD Horizon instrumentation because of sacral pain in a very slender patient showed the fused interbody graft (c and d). He returned to full work.

these techniques have drawbacks. Manipulation of the dural sac and nerve roots can lead to neurological injury, adhesions and dural leaks. Haemostasis of epidural veins may be difficult, as is adequate decortication of sclerotic endplates. The anterior longitudinal ligament and anterior border of the disc should be carefully respected in order to avoid injury to the great vessels.[81] Cloward[82] reported on uninstrumented PLIF, and more recently other authors have combined specific pedicle fixation with rods or plates with interbody fusion.[83-85] The use of Harrington rods with interbody fusion has been described but should be avoided since it carries the risk of lumbosacral kyphosis and requires longer instrumentation.[68] The use of internal fixation combined with interbody fusion to improve the rate of fusion and clinical results remains a matter of debate because few comparative studies have been reported, but some authors have shown better results with instrumentation.[83]

Anterior lumbar interbody fusion (ALIF). Anterior interbody bone grafting would rarely be performed as an isolated procedure according to current protocols since it requires aggressive postoperative bracing and bed rest. Instrumentation using some type of plate cannot safely be performed at the L5/S1 level from the front because of the proximity of the vascular structures. A fibular peg or an oblique screw from the anterosuperior border of L5 to the vertebral body of S1 through the disc space has been used by Louis.[86] Isolated anterior bone-grafting procedures have been described for the L5/S1 level, with or without reduction of the spondylolisthesis. Ghosez et al[87] reported superior functional results with anterior interbody fusion when compared with posterolateral fusion. Kim and Lee[88] described a similar outcome when using anterior interbody fusion and instrumented posterolateral fusion. Debeyre, Goutallier and Scheffer[89] described an anterior graft fixed in front of the sacrum. An isolated anterior approach to the lumbosacral spine avoids trauma to spinal muscles which could be advantageous. Newer, less invasive techniques and the use of some kind of cage offer new possibilities for an isolated anterior approach but their role remains to be defined. L3/L4 or L4/L5 floating fusions, if indicated, can be performed by an anterolateral retroperitoneal approach, allowing both bone grafting and instrumentation. With anterior interbody fusion, true decompression is not possible, and these techniques should be reserved for cases in which fusion without decompression is indicated. However, it should be borne in mind that the restoration of normal dimensions of the foramina by restoring disc height may sufficiently decompress offended nerve roots. The possible complications of the anterior approach to the lumbosacral spine have been described, and include vascular, bowel and urogenital injury.[90-92] Anterior approaches should only be performed after appropriate training and with the help of an abdominal or vascular surgeon. The true frequency of urogenital complications, such as retrograde ejaculation, sterility and erectile dysfunction, related to the anterior approach to the lumbosacral junction, is difficult to evaluate. Meticulous surgical technique should keep this risk to a minimum and use of the monopolar electrocautery should be avoided.[86,93]

Combined anterior and posterior fusion. Several authors[67,72,83,86,87,94,95] have described combined or staged anterior and posterior approaches for spondylolysis with spondylolisthesis, usually with severe slips. The aim of this two- or three-stage surgery is generally to obtain correction of the slip while improving the incidence of fusion. The anterior approach is used to perform interbody fusion and specific reduction instruments have been designed (Louis). The posterior approach allows a Gill procedure, supplementary posterolateral fusion and pedicle screw instrumentation (Fig. 13). All these combined procedures can be performed together or, more often, as staged operations, depending on the severity of the case, the surgical team and general health of the patient. Muschik et al[94] reported a better rate of fusion when using anterior fusion with posterior instrumentation compared with fusion without fixation, but the clinical results were identical in both groups.

Lehmer, Steffee and Gaines[96] have advocated a combined approach in spondyloptosis with removal of the vertebral body of L5 and the posterior arch and L4/S1 fusion.

Reconstruction of the pars defect

If degenerative disc disease is not present in association with the pars defect, the hypermobility of the loose posterior arch stimulates the formation of defect tissue which seems rich in nociceptive nerve endings, and relative instability with excessive stress on the underlying disc can account for the symptoms.[97,98] Removal of the soft tissue and bone grafting of the defect to restore the stabilising role of the posterior arch seem to be a logical form of treatment in this small group of patients, and avoid sacrifice of a motion segment.

'Isthmic reconstruction' or 'direct repair of the pars interarticularis' has been proposed by different surgeons since 1968. Kimura[99] used an isolated bone graft followed by postoperative bed rest and a cast. Most procedures include some sort of internal fixation in order to improve the rate of fusion and favour more rapid return to active life without external support. Buck[100] used a screw across the pars. Nicol and Scott[101] described a technique using the passage of wires under the laminae and transverse processes, and Salib and Pettine[102] and Songer and Rovin[103] similarly proposed wiring the posterior arch with fixation using a cable and pedicle screws. Morscher, Gerber and Fasel[104] designed a special screw-hook construct and Louis[86] proposed bone grafting of the pars combined with temporary fixation of the lumbosacral junction with his butterfly plate. We have described an original technique using a V-shaped rod and pedicle screws, combined with direct bone grafting of the pars defect using a universal rod-screw instrumentation such as the Compact Cotrel Dubousset (CCD) or CD Horizon instrumentation (Medtronic-Sofamor-Danek) (Figs 14 to 16).[105]

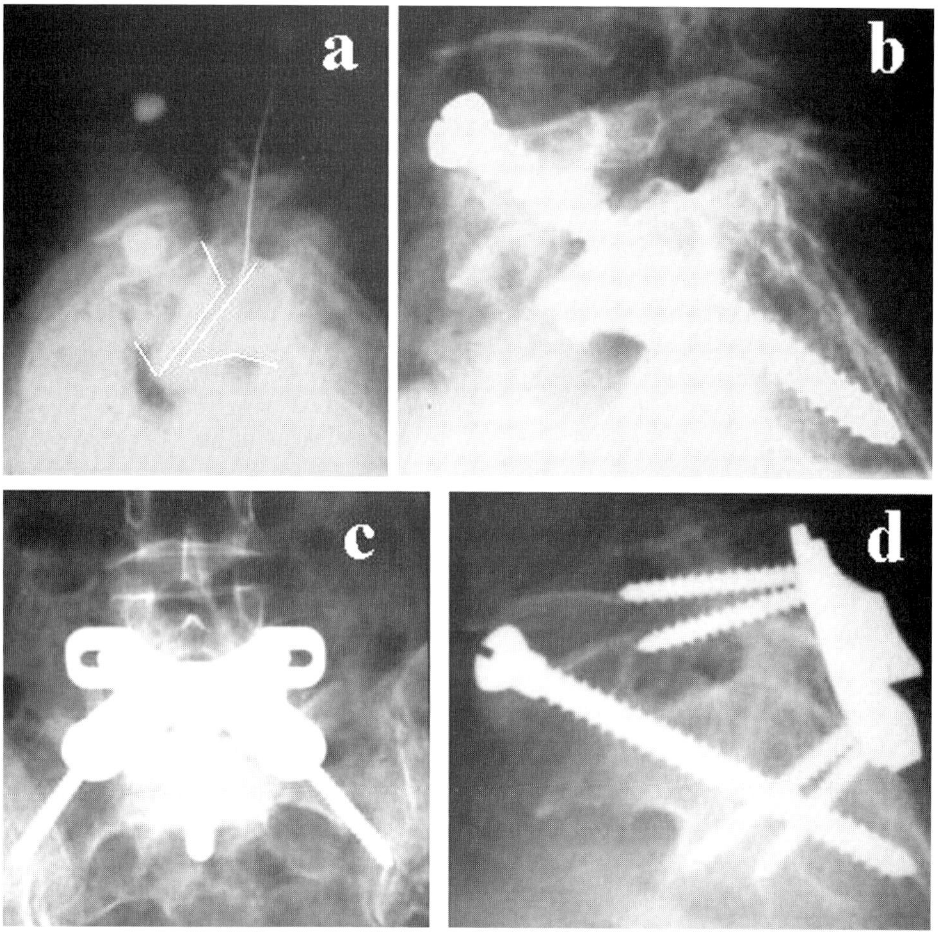

Fig. 13

Radiographs of a 50-year-old woman with grade-II slip (a) treated by a combined approach following the technique described by Louis, initial anterior interbody fusion and oblique lumbosacral fixation (b) followed by posterolateral fusion and plating (c and d). This patient was treated some years ago. Such a problem would now be treated in our hands by PLIF.

Unfortunately, although isthmic reconstruction is theoretically advantageous, Schlenzka et al[106,107] were unable to show better functional results or less degenerative disc disease on MRI at follow-up at five years compared with a group of patients treated by segmental fusion. The two groups, however, were not identical and the degree of slip was somewhat greater in the fused than in the repaired group. Further studies with longer follow-up are necessary to identify the possible protective role of isthmic repair for both the disc involved by the spondylolysis and the disc at the level above.

The author's usual procedures in adult and adolescent patients

The author has no significant experience in the management of severe spondylolisthesis in children and young adolescents. The following guidelines deal with the treatment of patients from 14 years of age to adulthood, presenting with symptomatic spondylolysis associated with spondylolisthesis of grade 0 to grade 3.

General rules. The presence of degenerative disc disease at the level of the motion segment involved by the spondylolysis or spondylolisthesis is first assessed by plain radiography. If obvious degenerative disc disease is present with loss of disc height, osteophytes and significant slip, fusion is chosen. If the disc seems normal, it is checked by MRI to decide whether a reconstruction procedure or a fusion should be performed.

If a fusion is required, its length must be defined. The author considers it unwise to stop a fusion at the level of a motion segment which is not strictly normal. Since the availability of MRI (T2-weighted images), an accurate estimation of the different lumbar motion segments can be made with one single non-invasive procedure. Thus, nowadays, in the author's practice, every patient considered for operative treatment for spondylolysis with or without spondylolisthesis has routine plain radiography and MRI of the lumbar spine. If the latter gives inadequate detail, a discogram is performed, under sterile conditions in an operating theatre and by the treating surgeon. Before the availability of MRI, a discogram was not routinely per-

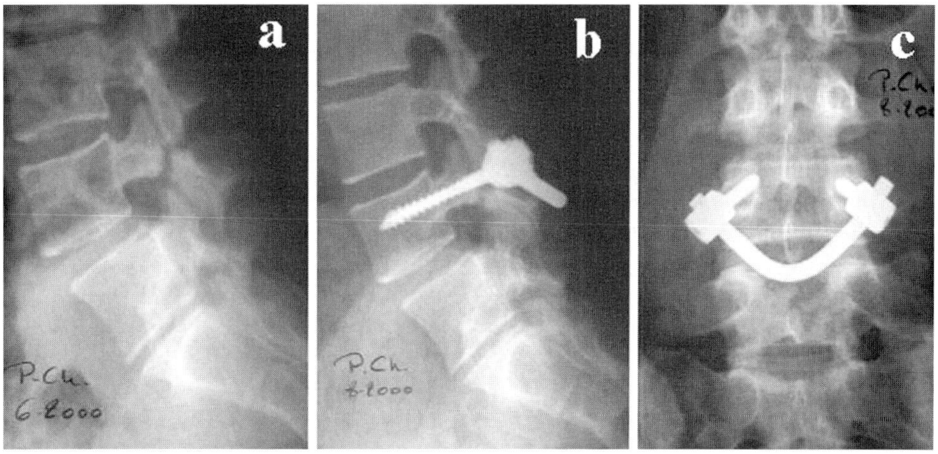

Fig. 14

Radiographs showing isthmic reconstruction using our technique with a V-shaped rod and pedicle screws in the patient described in Figure 6 (a). There is custom-made bending of the rod on the AP and lateral views (b and c). No brace was required.

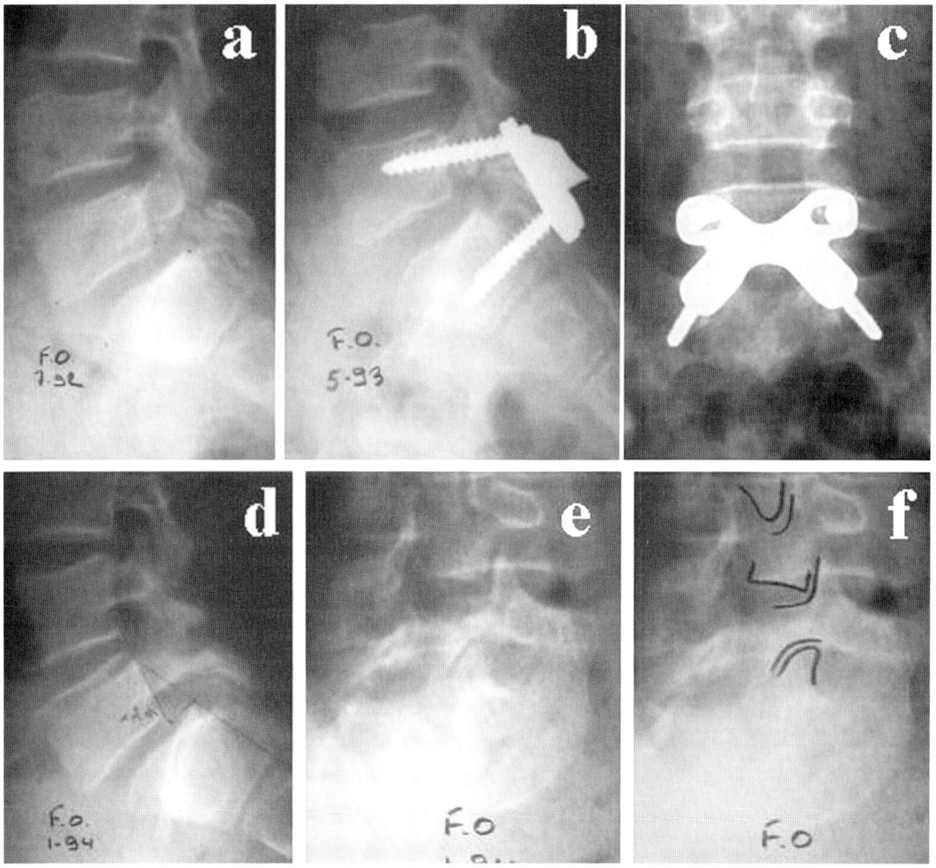

Fig. 15

Radiographs showing isthmic reconstruction of L5 spondylolysis (a) using the technique of Louis with a temporary butterfly plate (b and c) in a 14-year-old boy who was eager to return to sports. Fusion was obtained and instrumentation was removed after six months (d). The oblique views show the solid fusion and the removal of the tip of the inferior articular process of L4 to avoid recurrence of spondylolysis (e and f). Bracing was recommended for four months.

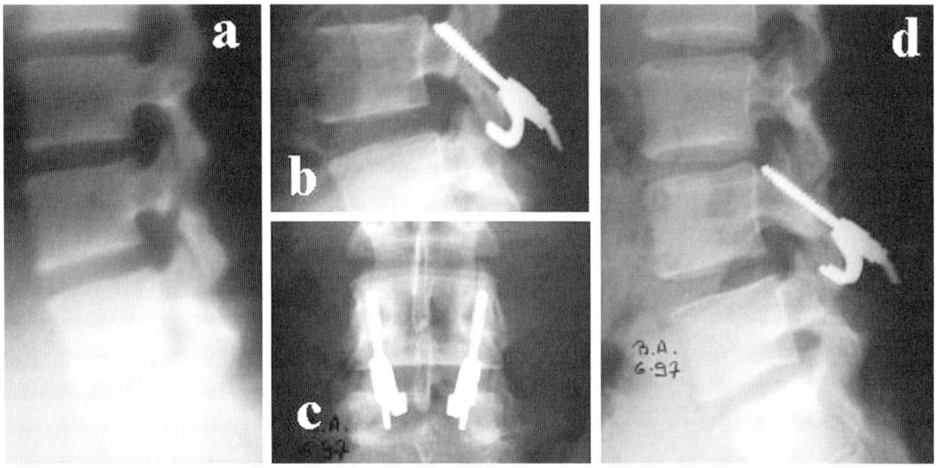

Fig. 16

Radiographs showing isthmic reconstruction in an 18-year-old handball player using Morscher hooks (a, b and c). There was solid fusion of the pars after six months (d) with return to competition level. A brace was worn for four months.

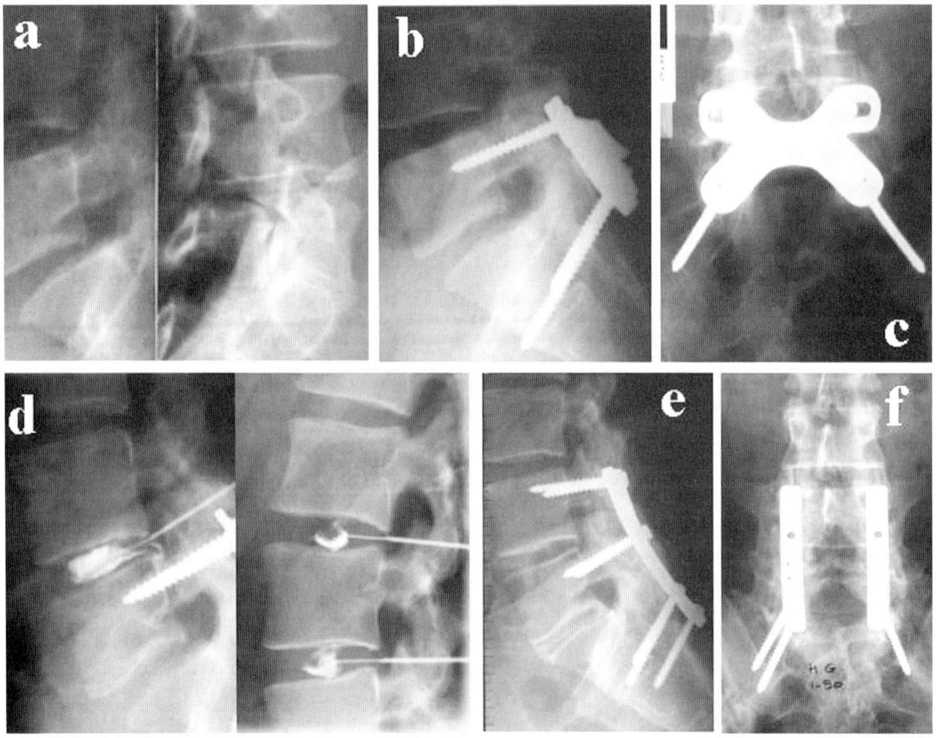

Fig. 17

Radiographs of a 31-year-old man who underwent a posterolateral fusion with a Louis butterfly plate for L5 spondylolysis. No discogram was performed and MRI was not available at the time. L5/S1 fusion seemed sufficient due to the young age of the patient and the small chance of the development of degenerative changes in the adjacent motion segment (a, b, c). He developed further symptoms after weaning off the brace. Discography showed L4/L5 degeneration and intact upper levels (d). Relief was obtained after L4/L5 complementary fusion (e and f) and has been maintained at follow-up for 13 years.

formed because it is an invasive procedure. Degenerative changes in adjacent discs, however, have occasionally been overlooked, even in young patients and an inaccurate length of fusion selected, with the need for subsequent secondary lengthening of the fusion (Fig. 17). Since the expectancy of patients who undergo surgery for spondylolysis is usually to return to normal or near normal lifestyle, precise evaluation seems mandatory.

In the case of a fusion, its length is important with regard to the activities which the patient expects to undertake after the operation. It is reasonable to assume that the longer the fusion, the more the residual free motion segments are at risk of overuse and progressive degenerative disease with possible recurrence of back pain. The requirements of the patient for work and sport must be considered when deciding on the length of the fusion. If it involves only one motion segment (lumbosacral or floating lumbar segment), all types of work or sports will be allowed, as with a reconstruction procedure. A fusion length that does not exceed two levels is considered to be acceptable in most cases, but strenuous work or sport would be discouraged and professional retraining would be suggested. If more than two motion segments are involved with degenerative changes, the decision becomes very difficult. Surgical treatment would not be advised except in the presence of significant pain which can definitely be related to the abnormalities. In order to evaluate the respective role of spondylolysis, spondylolisthesis and degenerative disc disease, discograms of the various motion segments involved may help, not so much because of the radiological image but for the provocative pain test which they allow. These must again be performed by the treating surgeon. In carefully selected cases, and with a good understanding by the patient of a potentially less than optimal result, 'compromise' reconstruction procedures or fusions may be considered, and may represent a more satisfactory surgical option than a fusion involving many motion segments.

Spondylolysis without associated disc disease or spondylolisthesis. In such cases, a reconstruction procedure preserving all motion segments is selected. In most cases, the technique used is as reported in a recent publication.[105] By a posterior midline approach, the lumbosacral junction is exposed from the spinous processes of L4 to S1 and laterally to the tips of the L5 transverse processes. To avoid stress on the isthmus of L5 by the overlying inferior L4 facets which could lead to a recurrence of the spondylolysis, described by Louis,[108] two or three millimetres of the distal aspect of these facets are removed with an osteotome. The soft tissue situated in the pars defect is removed with rongeurs. If the preoperative MRI has shown no root impingement, as is usually the case, a very thin layer of soft tissue is preserved at the bottom of the defect to avoid migration of bone graft into the foramen. The sides of the defect, the upper half of the laminae and the lateral, extra-articular aspect of the upper zygapophyseal joint are exposed down to bleeding bone and 35 mm length, 5 mm diameter CCD or Horizon lumbar screws are inserted in the L5 pedicles, avoiding encroachment upon the L4/L5 joint. Iliac bone graft is harvested and placed in the defect, and on the posterior aspect of the laminae and lateral aspect of the zygapophyseal processes. A 6 mm rod, usually 8 to 10 cm in length, is bent in a V shape and placed beneath the L5 spinous process, after the L5/S1 interspinous ligament has been removed. The rod is firmly fixed against the spinous process and the laminae, offering the possibility of compressing the graft in the defect and stabilising the posterior arch. Slight bending is performed in the sagittal plane if required to allow the rod to lie against the posterior arch of the vertebra and the grooves of the open pedicle screws. The pedicle screws have been placed with their grooves orientated 30° to 45° to the longitudinal axis of the patient. Finally, the blocking elements are firmly tightened against the rod to fix it to the pedicle screws. Care is taken to avoid any impingement between the rod and the superior aspect of the S1 spinous process during extension of the spine. Patients are allowed to sit and walk one or two days after operation and are usually discharged on the fourth day. No brace is required. The results of this technique were encouraging in preliminary studies and remain satisfactory with a longer follow-up and a greater number of cases. The same technique has been used for some patients with L4 spondylolysis. If, for anatomical reasons, the V-shaped rod and screw instrumentation cannot be used, Morscher hooks or the Louis technique with temporary plating may be employed. In these cases, protection with a brace is recommended for three or four months.

The optimal indication for reconstruction of the pars defect is isolated spondylolysis. We have not used the procedure if underlying disc degenerative disease was present, e.g. L5 spondylolysis with L5/S1 disc disease. In a few young adult patients, however, in whom L5 spondylolysis was present with an intact L5/S1 disc, but with disc degenerative changes at L4/L5, isthmic reconstruction of L5 has been attempted to avoid L4/S1 fusion, hoping that in such cases, the L5 spondylolysis was the main cause of back pain. The results were satisfactory but inferior to those in patients with isolated spondylolysis. Such a therapeutic option should be considered with caution and only in carefully selected cases (Fig. 18).

Spondylolysis with associated disc disease and grade-0 or grade-1 spondylolisthesis. In this situation the mechanical stress imposed on a posterolateral bone graft is not significant and this seems to be an appropriate method of fusion. It has been used with success in association with Louis plates and CD-type instrumentation. The bone graft is always harvested from the iliac crest. Decortication is thoroughly performed down to bleeding bone on the transverse processes, lateral extra-articular aspects of the articular processes of the upper vertebra and the ala of the sacrum. To obtain adequate decortication, it is advisable to perform it before putting the instrumentation in place as the latter may hinder access to the anatomical structures receiving bone grafts, and this can be a cause of nonunion.

If no thigh or leg pain is present, the posterior arch is not removed. Interarticular fusion of the loose arch is performed to avoid pain arising from persistent movement of the posterior arch. Isolated interarticular fusion of the posterior arch is, of course, an inappropriate procedure since it does not stabilise the intervertebral motion segment. This seems obvious but such procedures have been occasionally observed by the author.

If thigh or leg pain is present, a Gill procedure is

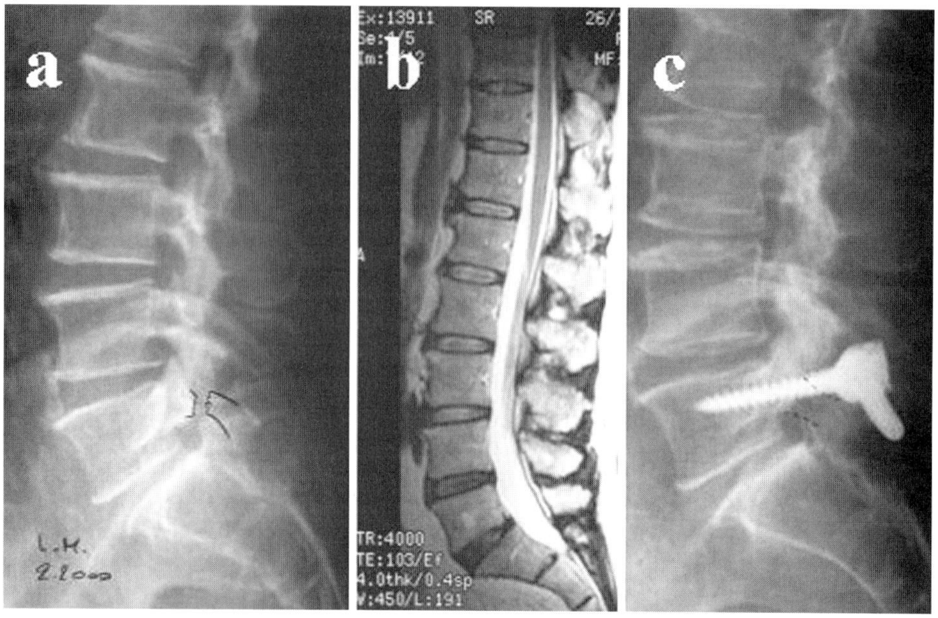

Fig. 18

Radiograph of a 51-year-old man scheduled for L4/L5/S1 posterolateral fusion because of L5 spondylolysis (a). There are degenerative changes at the two lower motion segments on MRI (b). Since standard radiographs showed multilevel alteration of the lumbar motion segments, rapid deterioration of the junctional disc after fusion was feared and a compromise L5 reconstruction was proposed (c), which appeared to be successful at follow-up at six months.

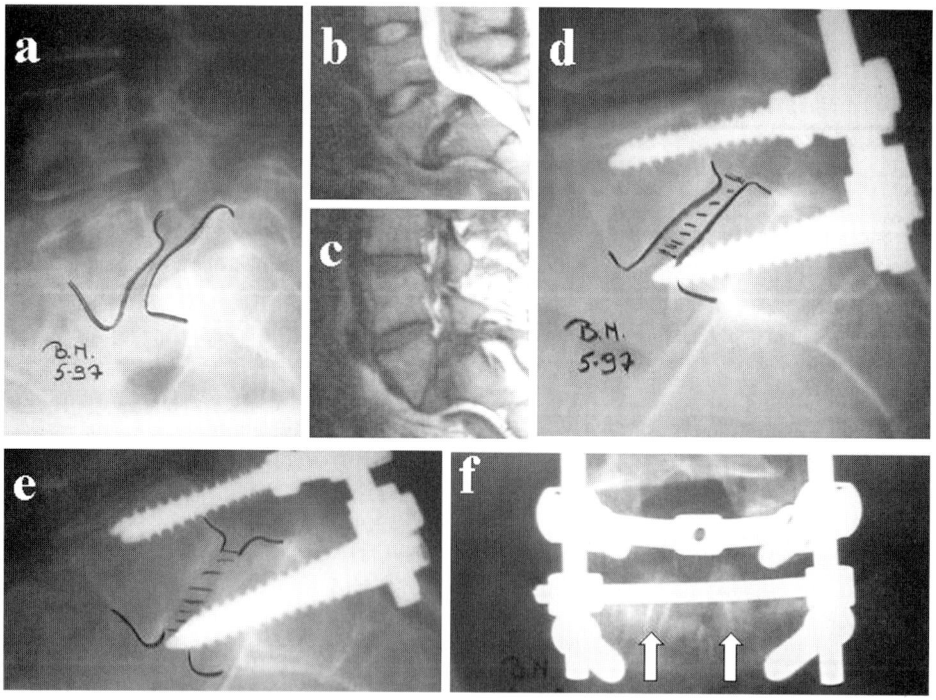

Fig. 19

Radiographs showing the reduction of a grade-II to grade-III spondylolisthesis in a 25-year-old housewife (a, b, c). Instrumental reduction was obtained and PLIF with CCD instrumentation performed (d). The clinical result was fair although the fusion seemed to be solid (e and f).

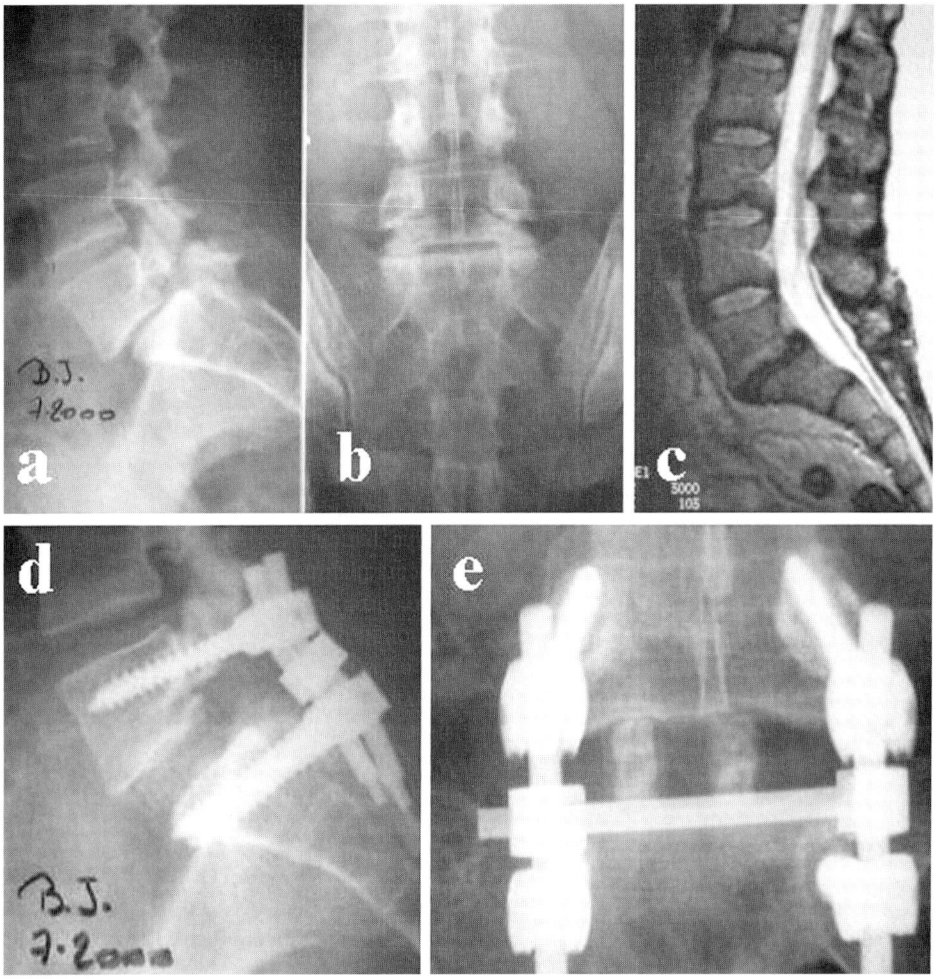

Fig. 20

Radiographs showing PLIF with radiolucent carbon cages filled with chips from the removed posterior arch (d and e) in grade-I spondylolisthesis (a, b, c). There is preservation of lumbosacral lordosis following the use of rods which can be bent appropriately.

routinely performed, but it should be emphasised that in many cases, no impingement of the nerve roots has been observed during surgery. Radicular pain can be the result of inflammation due to local hypermobility and true decompression is probably only required when obvious compression of the nerve roots, either by disc prolapse or by fibrous tissue present in the lysis, is recognised on MRI.

If severe bony and disc encroachment of the foramen is present, restoring normal disc height may help to decompress the nerve roots and a posterior lumbar interbody fusion should be considered. Reduction of the slip is not sought.

Posterior lumbar interbody fusion can also be undertaken when the patient has a degenerative but normal disc height and performs strenuous work, because it is thought that there is a greater risk of residual pain caused by compressive stresses imposed on the degenerated disc (Fig. 12).

The use of regular screw plates, such as those designed by Louis, or Cotrel-Dubousset type instrumentation has not changed the clinical or radiological results in L5/S1 or L4/L5/S1 fusions. However, when using routine plates, the patients wore a brace for three months and their activities were more restricted than with more rigid internal fixation.

Spondylolysis with associated disc disease and grade-2 or grade-3 spondylolisthesis. In the case of more significant spondylolisthesis, it is thought that mechanical stresses on a posterolateral fusion are greater and that this could compromise fusion. Such a theory encourages some surgeons to promote interbody fusion procedures. This depends upon whether the slip is corrected or not.

If no foraminal encroachment causing root impingement is present and if lumbosacral lordosis is satisfactory, in situ posterolateral fusion using iliac bone and pedicular type internal fixation has given the author satisfactory results.

If partial or complete correction of the spondylolisthesis is performed to correct lumbosacral sagittal alignment or obtain root decompression, an iatrogenic unstable condition is created. It has been the experience of the author that the correction of a slip in an adult patient creates a true void at the level of the disc space, and this view is shared by Argenson (personal communication). It is necessary to place a load-sharing interbody bone graft into the disc space in order to avoid secondary loss of correction and nonunion in these cases (Fig. 19). The risk is greatest when disc height is regained, and less if the slip is reduced while maintaining a narrow disc space. Nonunion after posterolateral fusion with reduction has been reported in a few cases using either Louis plates or Cotrel-Dubousset instrumentation, which illustrates that a stronger instrumentation device does not replace a mechanically sound bone-grafting procedure. When some correction of slip is desired, posterior lumbar interbody fusion is routinely performed. The correction is obtained with the help of intradiscal broaches which partially correct the slip while regaining disc height, and ancillary instruments with which it is possible to push forward the rods fixed to the sacral pedicle screws and pull back the lumbar pedicle screws. The bone graft used for PLIF is generally prepared from the loose posterior arch which has been removed *en bloc*. It is possible to obtain two or three solid corticocancellous bone grafts of about 2 cm in length, 1 cm in height and 6 to 10 mm in thickness from the laminae and spinous process, depending on the size of the posterior arch. If necessary, corticocancellous bone blocks are harvested from the iliac crest. Another option is the use of cages filled with bone chips trimmed from the posterior arch or iliac crest (Fig. 20).

It is advised to supplement PLIF by posterolateral fusion, but in most cases, when PLIF could be undertaken incorporating the posterior arch, the author did not use the iliac crest in order to avoid a further possible cause of pain. This did not seem to cause nonunion. An option is the use of some type of bone substitute to perform the supplementary posterolateral fusion.

Lysis at the level of the pedicle. If unilateral pedicle lysis associated with contralateral spondylolysis or bilateral pedicle lysis is present, the only option is interbody fusion since a posterolateral bone graft will not stabilise the vertebral body and the motion segment.

CONCLUSIONS

The surgical treatment of spondylolysis with or without spondylolisthesis remains a matter of debate, both with regard to indications and techniques. The literature lacks indisputable comparative studies proving the advantage of one method over another. Spondylolysis and spondylolisthesis rarely require invasive treatment and when the latter is needed, techniques which could seem old-fashioned still have their place in our armamentarium as well as procedures that are more in vogue. It is the responsibility of surgeons not to adopt the latest technique but to choose one that is sufficiently documented. The quality of the bone graft is more important than any instrumentation. We must avoid the most aggressive procedures which carry the greatest risks to the patient, particularly if they are not required to obtain a better functional result. Good postoperative radiographs with adequate correction of the deformity often offer a greater reward to our pride than benefit to our patients.

REFERENCES

1. **Wiltse LL, Newman PH, Macnab I.** Classification of spondylolysis and spondylolisthesis. *Clin Orthop* 1976;117:23-9.
2. **Wiltse L, Jackson D.** Treatment of spondylolisthesis and spondylolysis in children. *Clin Orthop* 1976;117:92-100.
3. **Borkow S, Kleiger B.** Spondylolisthesis in the newborn: a case report. *Clin Orthop* 1971;81:73-6.
4. **Fredrickson BE, Baker D, McHolick WJ, Yuan HA, Lubicky JP.** The natural history of spondylolysis and spondylolisthesis. *J Bone Joint Surg [Am]* 1984;66-A:699-707.
5. **Tower SS, Pratt WB.** Spondylolysis and associated spondylolisthesis in Eskimo and Athabascan populations. *Clin Orthop* 1990;250:171-5.
6. **Lonstein JE.** Spondylolisthesis in children: cause, natural history and management. *Spine* 1999;24:2640-8.
7. **Farfan H, Osteria M, Lamy C.** The mechanical etiology of spondylolysis and spondylolisthesis. *Clin Orthop* 1976;117:40-55.
8. **Hadley L.** Fatigue fracture of the fifth lumbar neural arch: is spondylolysis a stress fracture? *Clin Orthop* 1955;6:110-3.
9. **Taillard W.** Les spondylolyses acquises. *Rev Chir Orthop* 1960; 46:617.
10. **Taillard W.** Trauma and spondylolisthesis. *Acta Orthop Belg* 1969;35:703-16.
11. **Taillard WF.** Etiology of spondylolisthesis. *Clin Orthop* 1976; 117:30-9.
12. **Wiltse LL, Widell EH Jr, Jackson DW.** Fatigue fracture: the basic lesion in isthmic spondylolisthesis. *J Bone Joint Surg [Am]* 1975;57-A:17-22.
13. **Jackson DW, Wiltse LL, Cirincione RJ.** Spondylolysis in the female gymnast. *Clin Orthop* 1976;117:68-73.
14. **Congeni J, McCulloch J, Swanson K.** Lumbar spondylolysis: a study of natural progression in athletes. *Am J Sports Med* 1997;25:248-53.
15. **Micheli LJ, Wood R.** Back pain in young athletes: significant differences from adults in causes and patterns. *Arch Pediatr Adolesc Med* 1995;149:15-8.
16. **Möller H, Sundin A, Hedlund R.** Symptoms, signs and functional disability in adult spondylolisthesis. *Spine* 2000;25:683-9.
17. **Möller H, Hedlund R.** Instrumented and noninstrumented posterolateral fusion in adult spondylolisthesis: a prospective, randomized study, part 2. *Spine* 2000;25:1716-21.
18. **Möller H, Hedlund R.** Surgery versus conservative management in adult isthmic spondylolisthesis: a prospective, randomized study, part 1. *Spine* 2000;25:1711-5.
19. **Nazarian S.** Spondylolysis and spondylolytic spondylolisthesis: a review of current concepts on pathogenesis, natural history, clinical symptoms, imaging and therapeutic management. *Eur Spine J* 1992;1:62-83.
20. **Wood KB, Popp CA, Transfeldt EE, Geissele AE.** Radiographic evaluation of instability in spondylolisthesis. *Spine* 1994;19: 1697-703.
21. **Van den Oever M, Merrick M, Scott J.** Bone scintigraphy in symptomatic spondylolysis. *J Bone Joint Surg [Br]* 1987;69-B: 453-6.
22. **Maldague B, Malghem J.** Dynamic radiologic aspects of lumbar spondylolysis. *Acta Orthop Belg* 1981;47:441-57.
23. **Maldague B, Malghem J.** Developmental spondylolysis. *J Radiol* 1985;66:263-74.
24. **McAfee PC, Yuan HA.** Computed tomography in spondylolisthesis. *Clin Orthop* 1982:166:62-71.
25. **Linson MA, Crowe CH.** Comparison of magnetic resonance imaging and lumbar discography in the diagnosis of disc degeneration. *Clin Orthop* 1990;250:160-3.
26. **Deutman R, Diercks R, de Jong E, van Woerden HH.** Isthmic lumbar spondylolisthesis with sciatica: the role of the disc. *Eur Spine J* 1995;4:136-8.

27. **Jinkins JR, Matthes JC, Sener RN, Venkatappan S, Rauch R.** Spondylolysis, spondylolisthesis and associated nerve root entrapment in the lumbosacral spine: MR evaluation. *AJR Am J Roentgenol* 1992;159:799-803.

28. **Danielsson BI, Frennered AK, Irstam IK.** Radiologic progression of isthmic lumbar spondylolisthesis in young patients. *Spine* 1991;16:422-5.

29. **Freeman BL 3rd, Donati NL.** Spinal arthrodesis for severe spondylolisthesis in children and adolescents: a long-term follow-up study. *J Bone Joint Surg [Am]* 1989;71-A:594-8.

30. **Frennered AK, Danielson BI, Nachemson AL, Nordwall AB.** Midterm follow-up of young patients fused in situ for spondylolisthesis. *Spine* 1991;16:409-16.

31. **Harris IE, Weinstein SL.** Long-term follow-up of patients with grade III and IV spondylolisthesis: treatment with and without fusion. *J Bone Joint Surg [Am]* 1987;69-A:960-9.

32. **Österman K, Schlenzka D, Poussa M, Seitsalo S, Virta L.** Isthmic spondylolisthesis in symptomatic and asymptomatic subjects, epidemiology and natural history with special reference to disk abnormality and mode of treatment. *Clin Orthop* 1993;297:65-70.

33. **Saraste H.** Long-term clinical and radiological follow-up of spondylolysis and spondylolisthesis. *J Pediatr Orthop* 1987;7:631-8.

34. **Seitsalo S, Osterman K, Poussa M.** Scoliosis associated with lumbar spondylolisthesis: a clinical survey of 190 young patients. *Spine* 1988;13:899-904.

35. **Seitsalo S.** Operative and conservative treatment of moderate spondylolisthesis in young patients. *J Bone Joint Surg [Br]* 1990;72-B:908-13.

36. **Seitsalo S, Osterman K, Hyvarinen H, et al.** Progression of spondylolisthesis in children and adolescents: a long-term follow-up of 272 patients. *Spine* 1991;16:417-21.

37. **Seitsalo S, Schlenzka D, Poussa M, Osterman K.** Disc degeneration in young patients with isthmic spondyolisthesis treated operatively or conservatively: a long-term follow-up. *Eur Spine J* 1997;6:393-7.

38. **Lindholm TS, Ragni P, Ylikoski M, Poussa M.** Lumbar isthmic spondylolisthesis in children and adolescents: radiologic evaluation and results of operative treatment. *Spine* 1990;15:1350-5.

39. **Dubousset J.** Treatment of spondylolysis and spondylolisthesis in children and adolescents. *Clin Orthop* 1997;337:77-85.

40. **Apel D, Lorenz MA, Zindrick MR.** Symptomatic spondylolisthesis in adults: four decades later. *Spine* 1989;14:345-8.

41. **Floman Y.** Progression of lumbosacral isthmic spondylolisthesis in adults. *Spine* 2000;25:342-7.

42. **Frennered K.** Isthmic spondylolisthesis among patients receiving disability pension under the diagnosis of chronic low back pain syndrome. *Spine* 1994;19:2766-9.

43. **O'Sullivan PB, Phyty GD, Twomey LT, Allison GT.** Evaluation of specific stabilizing exercise in the treatment of chronic low back pain with radiologic diagnosis of spondylolysis or spondylolisthesis. *Spine* 1997;22:2959-67.

44. **Vaccaro A, Ring D, Scuderi G, Cohen D, Garfin S.** Predictors of outcome in patients with chronic back pain and low-grade spondylolisthesis. *Spine* 1997;22:2030-4.

45. **Gill GG, Manning JG, White HL.** Surgical treatment of spondylolisthesis without spine fusion: excision of the loose lamina with decompression of the nerve roots. *J Bone Joint Surg [Am]* 1955;37-A:493-520.

46. **Edelson JG, Nathan H.** Nerve root compression in spondylolysis and spondylolisthesis. *J Bone Joint Surg [Br]* 1986;68-B:596-9.

47. **Amuso SJ, Neff RS, Coulson DB, Laing PG.** The surgical treatment of spondylolisthesis by posterior element resection: a long-term follow-up study. *J Bone Joint Surg [Am]* 1970;52-A:529-36.

48. **Österman K, Lindholm TS, Laurent LE.** Late results of removal of the loose posterior element (Gill's operation) in the treatment of lytic lumbar spondylolisthesis. *Clin Orthop* 1976;117:121-8.

49. **Seitsalo S, Schlenzka D, Poussa M, Hyvarinen H, Osterman K.** Solid fusion vs nonunion in long-term follow-up of in situ fusion without internal fixation in symptomatic spondylolisthesis in young patients. *Eur Spine J* 1992;1:163-6.

50. **Seitsalo S, Osterman K, Hyvarinen H, Schlenzka D, Poussa M.** Severe spondylolisthesis in children and adolescents: a long-term review of fusion in situ. *J Bone Joint Surg [Br]* 1990;72-B:259-65.

51. **Boos N, Webb JK.** Pedicle screw fixation in spinal disorders: a European view. *Eur Spine J* 1997;6:2-18.

52. **Weinstein JN, Rydevik BL, Rauschning W.** Anatomic and technical considerations of pedicle screw fixation. *Clin Orthop* 1992;284:34-46.

53. **Louis R, Maresca C.** Stabilisation chirurgicale avec réduction des spondylolyses et des spondylolisthésis. *Int Orthop* 1977;1:215-25.

54. **Roy-Camille R, Saillant G, Boucher T, Saldago V, Suarez H.** Spondylolisthesis. *Cahiers d'enseignement de la SOFCOT. Expansion Scientifique Française.* 1986;26:89-101.

55. **Boos N, Marchesi D, Aebi M.** Treatment of spondylolysis and spondylolisthesis with Cotrel-Dubousset instrumentation: a preliminary report. *J Spinal Disord* 1991;4:472-9.

56. **Boos D, Marchesi D, Zuber K, Aebi M.** Treatment of severe spondylolisthesis by reduction and pedicular fixation. *Spine* 1993;18:1655-61.

57. **McGuire RA, Amundson GM.** The use of primary internal fixation in spondylolisthesis. *Spine* 1993;18:1662-72.

58. **Gillet P, Bayaux M.** Retrospective review of lumbar fusion in spondylolysis comparing instrumentation with standard plates and Cotrel-Dubousset or Compact C-D rods with pedicular rods. *J Bone Joint Surg [Br]* 1995;77-B Suppl II:158.

59. **Poussa M, Schlenzka D, Seitsalo S, et al.** Surgical treatment of severe isthmic spondylolisthesis in adolescents: reduction or fusion in situ. *Spine* 1993;18:894-901.

60. **Grzegorzewski A, Kumar SJ.** In situ posterolateral spine arthrodesis for grades III, IV and V spondylolisthesis in children and adolescents. *J Pediatr Orthop* 2000;20:506-11.

61. **Shelokov A, Haideri N, Roach J.** Residual gait abnormalities in surgically treated spondylolisthesis. *Spine* 1993;18:2201-5.

62. **Abdu WA, Wilber RG, Emery SE.** Pedicular transvertebral screw fixation of the lumbosacral spine in spondylolisthesis: a new technique for stabilization. *Spine* 1994;19:710-5.

63. **Scaglietti O, Frontino G, Bartolozzi P.** Technique of anatomical reduction of lumbar spondylolisthesis and its surgical stabilization. *Clin Orthop* 1976;117:164-75.

64. **Bradford D, Boachie-Adjei O.** Treatment of severe spondylolisthesis by anterior and posterior reduction and stabilization: a long-term follow-up study. *J Bone Joint Surg [Am]* 1990;72-A:1060-6.

65. **Snijder JGN, Seroo JM, Snijder CJ, Schijvens AWM.** Therapy of spondylolisthesis by repositioning and fixation of the olisthetic vertebra. *Clin Orthop* 1976;117:149-56.

66. **Harrington PR, Dickson JH.** Spinal instrumentation in the treatment of severe progressive spondylolisthesis. *Clin Orthop* 1976;117:157-63.

67. **Vidal J, Allieu Y, Fasio B, Adrey J, Goalard C.** Spondylolisthesis: reduction with Harrington's rod. *Rev Chir Orthop Reparatrice Appar Mot* 1973;59:21-41.

68. **Vidal J, Fassio B, Buscayret Ch, Melka J.** Surgical treatment of spondylolisthesis L5-S1: 12 years' experience in instrument reduction using the Harrington method. *Acta Orthop Belg* 1981;47:487-501.

69. **Selby D.** Internal fixation with Knodt's rods. *Clin Orthop* 1986;203:179-84.

70. **Johnson LP, Nasca RJ, Dunham WK.** Surgical management of isthmic spondylolisthesis. *Spine* 1988;13:93-7.

71. **Schöllner D.** Ein neues Verfahren zur Reposition und Fixation bei Spondylolisthesis. *Orthop Praxis* 1975;11:270-4.

72. **Matthiass HH, Heine J.** The surgical reduction of spondylolisthesis. *Clin Orthop* 1986;203:34-44.

73. **Edwards CC, Bradford DS.** Instrumented reduction of spondylolisthesis. *Spine* 1994;19:1535-7.

74. **Passuti N, Cistac C, Allioux J, et al.** CD instrumentation and spondylolisthesis: results about 40 cases. *Procs of the 6th International GICD* Sauramps Médical, 1989:169-73.

75. **Passuti N, Delécrin J, Takahashi S.** CCD: concepts and strategy. *Instrumented fusion of the degenerative lumbar spine: state of the art, questions and controversies.* Philadelphia: Lippincot-Raven, 1996:201-9.

76. **Steib J, Lang G, Kehr P, Leculee F.** Spondylolisthesis, scoliosis and CD. *Procs of the 7th International GICD* Sauramps Médical, 1990:113-6.

77. **Steib J.** Traitement chirurgical du spondylolisthésis L5-S1. *Imagerie des spondylolisthésis.* Paris: Masson, 1995:116-25.

78. **Gillet P.** Utilization of the Compact Cotrel-Dubousset system. *Current techniques in spinal stabilization.* New York:McGraw Hill, 1996:297-308.

79. **Schlegel KF, Pon A.** The biomechanics of posterior lumbar interbody fusion (PLIF) in spondylolisthesis. *Clin Orthop* 1985;193:115-9.

80. **Grobler IJ, Novotny JE, Wilder DG, Frymoyer JW, Pope MH.** L4-5 isthmic spondylolisthesis: a biomechanical analysis comparing stability in L4-5 and L5-S1 isthmic spondylolisthesis. *Spine* 1994;19:222-7.

81. **Lin P.** Posterior lumbar interbody fusion technique: complications and pitfalls. *Clin Orthop* 1985;193:90-102.

82. **Cloward RB.** Spondylolisthesis: treatment by laminectomy and posterior interbody fusion. Review of 100 cases. *Clin Orthop* 1981;154:74-82.

83. **Suk SI, Lee CK, Kim WJ, et al.** Adding posterior lumbar interbody fusion to pedicle screw fixation and posterolateral fusion after decompression in spondylolytic spondylolisthesis. *Spine* 1997; 22:210-20.

84. **Enker P, Steffee AD.** Interbody fusion and instrumentation. *Clin Orthop* 1994;300:90-101.

85. **Roca J, Ubierna MT, Caceres E, Iborra M.** One-stage decompression and posterolateral and interbody fusion for severe spondylolisthesis: an analysis of 14 patients. *Spine* 1999;24:709-14.

86. **Louis R.** Fusion of the lumbar and sacral spine by internal fixation with screw plates. *Clin Orthop* 1986;203:18-33.

87. **Ghosez JP, Himmer O, Devyer B, et al.** Surgical treatment of isthmic spondylolisthesis: a comparative study of 3 types of arthrodesis. *Rev Chir Orthop Reparatrice Appar Mot* 1992;78:515-28.

88. **Kim NH, Lee JN.** Anterior interbody fusion versus posterolateral fusion with transpedicular fixation for isthmic spondylolisthesis in adults: a comparison of clinical results. *Spine* 1999;24:812-6.

89. **Debeyre J, Goutallier D, Scheffer JC.** L'arthrodèse console dans le traitement des spondylolisthésis. *Rev Chir Orthop Reparatrice Appar Mot* 1976;62:793-803.

90. **Berchuck M, Garfin SR, Bauman T, Abitbol JJ.** Complications of anterior intervertebral grafting. *Clin Orthop* 1992;284:54-62.

91. **Rajaraman V, Vingan R, Roth P, et al.** Visceral and vascular complications resulting from anterior lumbar interbody fusion. *J Neurosurg Spine* 1999;91:60-4.

92. **Watkins R.** Anterior lumbar interbody fusion surgical complications. *Clin Orthop* 1992;284:47-53.

93. **Johnson R, McGuire E.** Urogenital complications of anterior approaches to the lumbar spine. *Clin Orthop* 1981;154:114-8.

94. **Muschik M, Zippel H, Perka C.** Surgical management of severe spondylolisthesis in children and adolescents: anterior fusion in situ versus anterior spondylodesis with posterior transpedicular instrumentation and reduction. *Spine* 1997;22:2036-42.

95. **O'Brien J, Mehdian H, Jaffray D.** Reduction of severe lumbosacral spondylolisthesis: a report of 22 cases with a ten-year follow-up period. *Clin Orthop* 1994;300:64-9.

96. **Lehmer SM, Steffee AD, Gaines RW Jr.** Treatment of L5-S1 spondyloptosis by staged L5 resection with reduction and fusion of L4 onto S1 (Gaines procedure). *Spine* 1994;19:1916-25.

97. **Eisenstein SM, Ashton IK, Roberts S, et al.** Innervation of the spondylolysis 'ligament'. *Spine* 1994;19:912-6.

98. **Nordström D, Santavirta S, Seitsalo S, et al.** Symptomatic lumbar spondylolysis: neuroimmunologic studies. *Spine* 1994;19:2752-8.

99. **Kimura M.** My method of filling the lesion with spongy bone in spondylolysis and spondylolisthesis. *Seikei Geka* 1968;19:285-96.

100. **Buck JE.** Direct repair of the defect in spondylolisthesis: preliminary report. *J Bone Joint Surg [Br]* 1970;52-B:432-7.

101. **Nicol RO, Scott JH.** Lytic spondylolysis: repair by wiring. *Spine* 1986;11:1027-30.

102. **Salib RM, Pettine KA.** Modified repair of a defect in spondylolysis or minimal spondylolisthesis by pedicle screw, segmental wire fixation, and bone grafting. *Spine* 1993;18:440-3.

103. **Songer MN, Rovin R.** Repair of the pars interarticularis defect with a cable-screw construct: a preliminary report. *Spine* 1998;23:263-9.

104. **Morscher E, Gerber B, Fasel J.** Surgical treatment of spondylolisthesis by bone grafting and direct stabilization of spondylolysis by means of a hook screw. *Arch Orthop Trauma Surg* 1984;103:175-8.

105. **Gillet P, Petit M.** Direct repair of spondylolysis without spondylolisthesis using a rod-screw construct and bone grafting of the pars defect. *Spine* 1999;24:1252-6.

106. **Schlenzka D, Poussa M, Seitsalo S, Österman K.** Intervertebral disc changes in adolescents with isthmic spondylolisthesis. *J Spinal Disord* 1991;4:344-52.

107. **Schlenzka D, Seitsalo S, Poussa M, Österman K.** Operative treatment of symptomatic lumbar spondylolysis and mild isthmic spondylolisthesis in young patients: direct repair of the defect or segmental spinal fusion? *Eur Spine J* 1993;2:104-12.

108. **Louis R.** Pars interarticularis reconstruction for spondylolysis by plates and screws with grafting without arthrodesis. *Rev Chir Orthop Reparatrice Appar Mot* 1988;74:549-57.

INSTABILITY OF THE SHOULDER

PANAYOTIS P. SYMEONIDES

From the Aristotle University of Thessaloniki, Greece

The shoulder, or more precisely the glenohumeral joint, is inherently unstable. In contrast to the hip it does not have bony support. The glenoid cavity is shallow and normally contains one-third of the articular surface of the humerus in the various positions which occur during the movement of the joint. The glenoid labrum increases the depth of the glenoid cavity slightly but is not responsible for stability which is dependent mainly on the ligaments, capsule, the muscles and tendons which surround the joint, on the negative intra-articular atmospheric pressure[1] and on proprioception.[2]

The ligaments and capsule are the passive and the muscles the dynamic stabilising structures.

Concerning the role of the ligaments in the stability of the joint it has been pointed out[3,4] that the superior glenohumeral ligament (SGHL) and the coracohumeral ligament run a parallel course and resist inferior translation of the humeral head in forward flexion, adduction and internal rotation.[5]

The middle glenohumeral ligament (MGHL), although absent in nearly 40% of shoulders, seems to limit anterior translation of the humeral head between 60° and 90° of abduction. In this range it appears that the cuff muscles are stabilising the glenohumeral joint. The inferior glenohumeral ligament (IGHL) seems to prevent anterior translation of the humeral head in external rotation and posterior translation in internal rotation between 60 and 90° of abduction.[3,5] Plain radiography shows that the surface of the glenoid appears to be flatter than the articular surface of the humeral head. MRI demonstrates that the concavity of the glenoid closely matches the convexity of the humeral head.

CLASSIFICATION OF GLENOHUMERAL INSTABILITY

There is no general agreement concerning a classification scheme for instability of the shoulder. There are two main categories of instability, namely traumatic and atraumatic. According to Neer[6] they were described by Hippocrates, who also recognised that voluntary dislocation of the shoulder could occur at will. Neer[6] added a third category, which he called 'acquired instability'. This group is large and comprises patients who have had neither a significant injury nor generalised joint laxity. Their instability is the result of repetitive microtrauma which leads to an enlarged joint capsule.

Traumatic instability is always caused by significant injury. It is usually unidirectional and it may be anterior (95%) or posterior (5%). More precisely, the dislocation is anteroinferior. Pure anterior or posterior dislocation is very rare (Fig. 1). By contrast, atraumatic instability may be multidirectional (MDI), that is anterior, posterior or inferior. In addition, it may be involuntary or voluntary (Table I).

PATHOGENESIS OF SHOULDER INSTABILITY

Traumatic instability. If anterior or posterior glenohumeral dislocation recurs within one to two years the joint becomes unstable. There are several factors responsible for

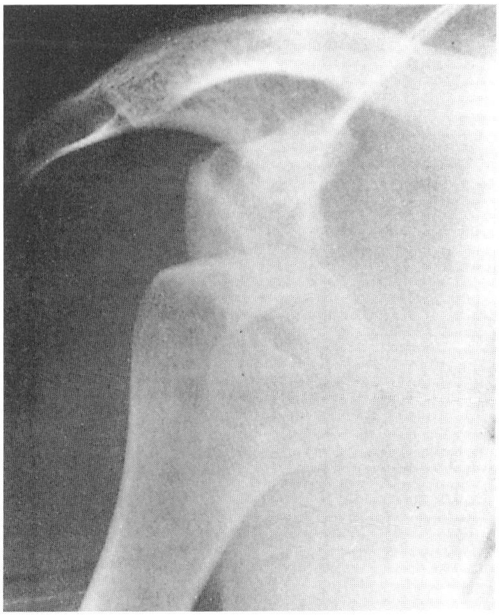

Fig. 1

Radiograph of a typical anterior dislocation of the shoulder which is clearly anteroinferior.

Table I. Classification of glenohumeral instability

Traumatic	Unidirectional Anterior (frequent) (anteroinferior) Posterior (rare) (posteroinferior)
Atraumatic	Multidirectional (anteroposterior inferior) Involuntary Voluntary
Acquired	Unidirectional Anterior (anteroposterior) Posterior (posteroinferior)

the instability and they may be classified as follows: 1) predisposing factors; 2) those related to the acute dislocation *per se*; and 3) those arising after an acute dislocation.

Predisposing factors. These include: 1) reduced retroversion of the humeral head; 2) reduced retroversion of the glenoid cavity or even anteversion; and 3) a gap between subscapularis and supraspinatus (the rotator-cuff interval).

Factors related to the acute dislocation. These are: 1) age – the younger the patient the greater is the likelihood of the joint becoming unstable; 2) the severity of the first dislocation – the more severe the initial injury the less is the probability of resultant instability; and 3) limited or no immobilisation of the joint after the first dislocation.

Factors arising after an acute dislocation. These may be: 1) fracture of the greater tuberosity of the humerus in combination with the first dislocation which reduces the risk of recurrence; 2) fracture of the anterior glenoid rim which increases instability; 3) detachment of the anterior glenoid labrum (Bankart lesion) which increases the rate of recurrence; 4) a defect on the posterolateral surface of the humeral head (Hill-Sachs lesion) which increases the instability; and 5) post-traumatic laxity of the subscapularis from non-immobilisation of the shoulder after the first dislocation which increases the risk of recurrence.

Atraumatic instability. The predisposing factors are: 1) generalised joint laxity; 2) a shallow or hypoplastic glenoid cavity; 3) hypoplasia of the ligaments; and 4) psychological disorders.

CLINICAL EXAMINATION AND DIAGNOSIS

When a patient with instability of the shoulder is examined it is most important to establish whether the instability is atraumatic or traumatic. Table II gives the characteristics for differentiation.

If the instability is atraumatic the next step is to determine whether it is involuntary or voluntary and whether it is multidirectional (MDI) (Fig. 2). In patients with involuntary instability their shoulders can be dislocated against their will, most often as a posterior dislocation in flexion, adduction and internal rotation[7] (Fig. 3). Most patients, but not all, with voluntary instability, have psychological problems. They dislocate their shoulders at will by asymmetrical muscle contractions usually with the arm in contact with the thoracic wall (Fig. 4).

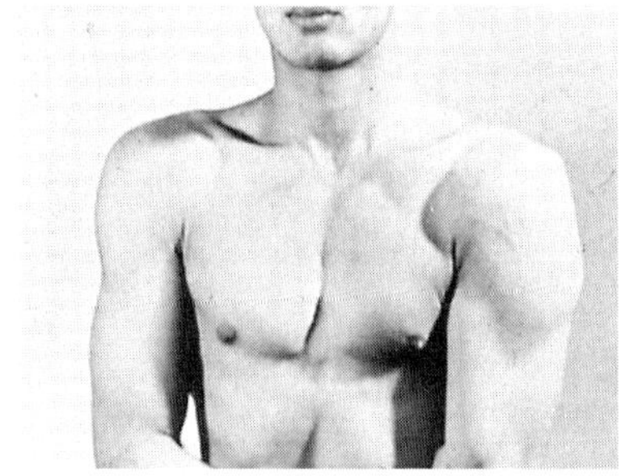

Fig. 2a

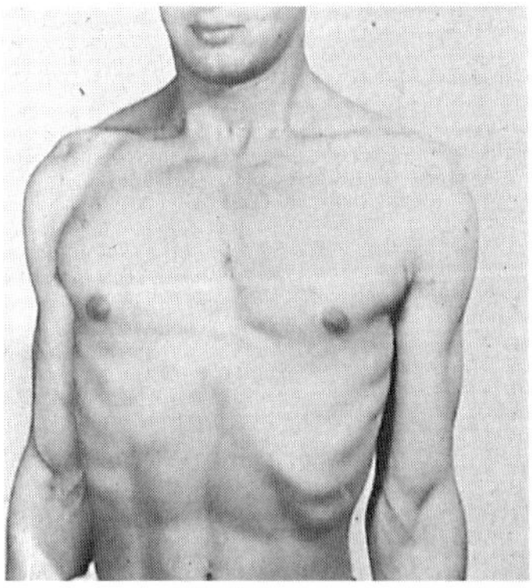

Fig. 2b

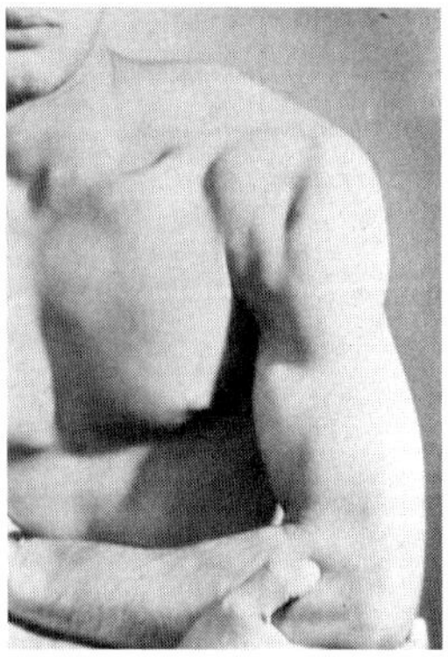

Fig. 2c

Photographs showing a) anterior, b) inferior and c) posterior voluntary MDI of the left glenohumeral joint.

Table II. Characteristics of traumatic and atraumatic instability

Atraumatic	Traumatic
First dislocations without injury	First dislocation after injury
Dislocation multidirectional	Dislocation unidirectional
Frequent bilateral dislocation	Bilateral dislocation very rare
Frequent voluntary dislocation	Voluntary dislocation very rare
Dislocation usually painless and may be reduced without aid	Dislocation usually painful and requires reduction by a physician
Usually generalised joint laxity	Generalised joint laxity rare
Age of onset below 16 years	Age of onset above 16 years
Frequent associated psychiatric problems	Associated psychiatric problems rare

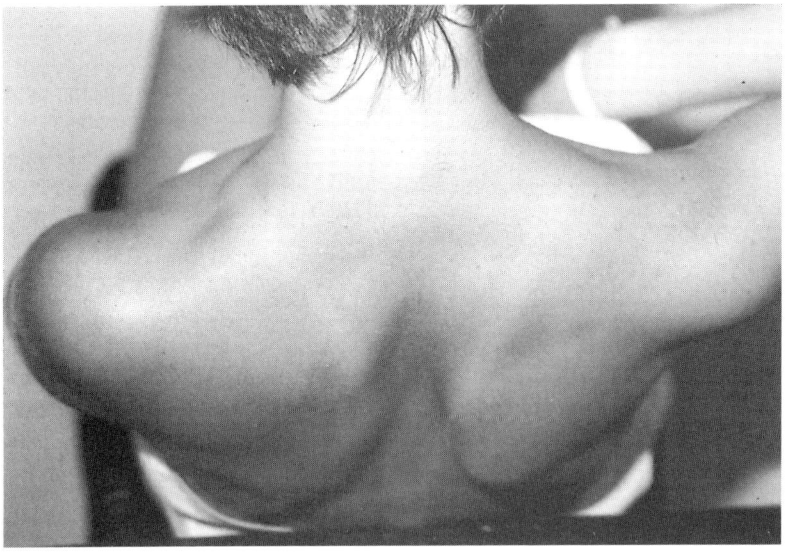

Fig. 3

Photograph of an 18-year-old patient with involuntary posterior dislocation of the right shoulder which she could produce only by placing her arm in flexion, slight abduction and internal rotation.

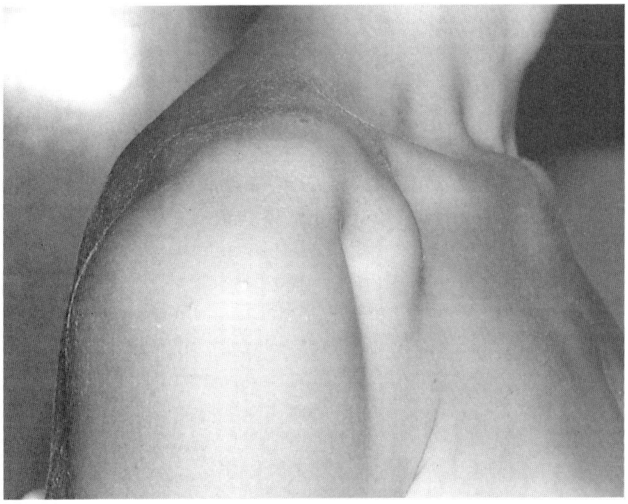

Fig. 4

Photograph of a 28-year-old woman who could produce posterior dislocation of the right shoulder at will by muscle contraction keeping her arm in contact with the chest wall.

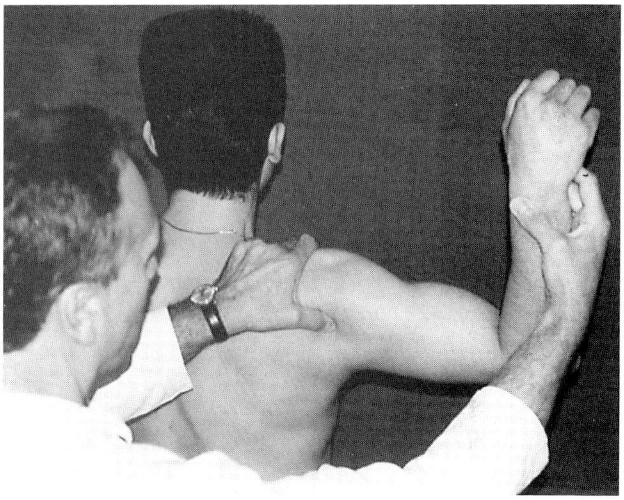

Fig. 5

The apprehension test (anterior).

Many patients in the atraumatic group present with generalised joint laxity. Gerber[8] stressed that MDI must be distinguished from multidirectional laxity. The latter "is a character trait of an individual. It is not a pathologic entity." Multidirectional laxity is a risk factor for the development of MDI.

Evaluation of traumatic instability. Clinically, a thorough examination of the range of movement of both shoulders, the neurovascular condition of the unstable shoulder, the cuff and deltoid muscles and the presence or absence of joint laxity are of paramount importance.

The physician will rely on the following:

1) The description by the patient of the mechanism of the first and subsequent dislocations.

2) Radiographs to determine the presence of a Hill-Sachs lesion,[9] a defect at the posterolateral or anterolateral aspect of the head of the humerus.

3) The apprehension test (anterior) (Fig. 5).

4) Apprehension test (posterior).[10,11] The arm is placed in adduction, internal rotation and 90° of flexion. A posterior force is applied along the axis of the arm. The patient with posterior instability experiences subluxation or pain.

5) The sulcus test[12] (Fig. 6). This is performed with the patient standing or sitting, either by pulling down on the adducted arm at the side of the body or by pressing down on the abducted humerus.

6) The relocation test.

7) Arthroscopy.

8) Examination under general anaesthesia.

Radiological evaluation. This always includes plain radio-

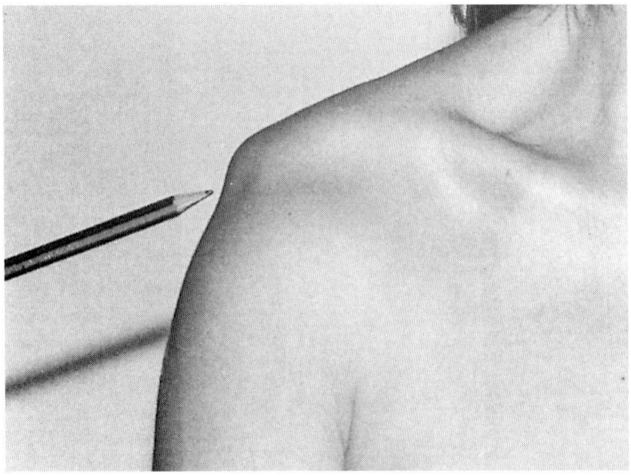

Fig. 6

The sulcus test.

graphy and often CT and MRI. As regards the former AP, axillary and lateral scapular views are of the utmost importance. The axillary view is essential in order to exclude, especially in acute cases, posterior dislocation, which is often missed. An AP view with the arm in internal rotation is useful to demonstrate a Hill-Sachs lesion. A west-point view may occasionally be used for the diagnosis of antero-inferior glenoid fractures.

CT is useful in clarifying the existence and size of fractures of the glenoid rim and compression fractures (Hill-Sachs lesion). CT arthrography may show an excessive capsular volume as well as glenoid hypoplasia and retroversion.

MRI occasionally may be used in evaluating shoulder instability by demonstrating associated soft-tissue injuries. It is particularly useful in patients over 40 years of age in order to show a concomitant rupture of the rotator cuff.[13] MRI arthrography is more than 90% sensitive in demonstrating capsular laxity as well as labral lesions.

TREATMENT OF SHOULDER INSTABILITY

Traumatic. The shoulder is considered to be unstable if at least a second dislocation occurs within one to two years. Recurrence which takes place after a long time after further significant injury, may be considered as a new dislocation of a normal joint which had healed after the first dislocation.

The treatment of primary acute shoulder dislocation consists of closed reduction, immobilisation for three to six weeks, followed by a rehabilitation programme, consisting of exercises to strengthen the rotator cuff and scapular stabilisers. There is a continuing debate concerning the value of post-reduction immobilisation after an acute primary dislocation. Many authors believe that immobilisation for three to six weeks after reduction of an acute dislocation does not reduce the rate of recurrence[14,15] whereas others believe that it does. The length of the period of immobilisation may be gradually reduced to one week for individuals aged over 40 years. Age is the most important factor in the rate of recurrence.

Those who believe that in young athletic individuals the rate of recurrence is 90%, regardless of post-reduction immobilisation of the shoulder, recommend immediate arthroscopic stabilisation.

In a recent prospective study[16] military cadets below the age of 24 years with primary anterior dislocation of the shoulder were treated according to their wish by immobilisation in a sling for four weeks followed by rehabilitation as against immediate arthroscopic suture repair. After four months the conservatively-treated group had a rate of recurrence of 80% compared with 14% in those managed arthroscopically. Despite these satisfactory results with arthroscopic repair it is not usually recommended for the following reasons. The rate of recurrence in the young athletic group treated by immobilisation is about 70% to 80%. This means that one in four or five individuals in this group is having an unjustifiable procedure. The recurrences in the arthroscopically-treated group are not necessarily within the 80% of the conservatively-treated group with a recurrence, but are part of the whole group i.e., including the 20% of individuals who did not have a recurrence. Thus, three of the 20 individuals who were not going to have a recurrence with conservative treatment have become unstable after failed arthroscopic treatment. Infection after the arthroscopic procedure or other complications related to anaesthesia, although rare, may occur in individuals who did not need to have arthroscopic treatment.

Arthroscopic lavage. This is a new method described by Wintzell et al.[17,18] They performed arthroscopic lavage after acute anterior dislocation of the shoulder in 30 athletic individuals under the age of 25 years. Redislocations occurred only in 12% compared with 65% of a control group. Although the follow-up was only for one year, and the rate of recurrence is expected to increase in both groups, it appears that the Bankart lesions may have healed in several of the patients treated with lavage. More control studies with longer follow-up should be carried out before this method of treatment is accepted.

Operative. This can be open or closed (arthroscopic).

Open. More than a hundred operative procedures have been described for traumatic anterior instability of the shoulder. They can be classified into four groups[19] as follows:

1) Procedures which limit external rotation by tightening the anterior structures such as the Magnuson-Stack and the Putti-Platt techniques.

2) Bony blocks which prevent anterior translation of the humeral head such as the Bristow procedure.

3) Osteotomies either of the glenoid or the humerus to change their version.

4) Anatomical reconstruction of the disrupted antero-inferior capsulolabral complex, such as the Bankart procedure.[20]

All these techniques have stood the test of time and have a high rate of success in restoring stability of the shoulder. These operations, however, often do not meet the currently accepted criteria for evaluation of a shoulder procedure by not restoring movement and function, as well as providing stability. The Magnuson-Stack[21,22] and Putti-Platt procedures produce limitation of external rotation which may lead to secondary osteoarthritis of the glenohumeral joint. This incidence has been reduced after the introduction of the simplified Putti-Platt technique,[23,24] in which the lateral inelastic part of the divided subscapularis tendon is not sutured to the anterior glenoid rim resulting in limitation of external rotation. Instead, the two parts of the divided subscapularis tendon are simply overlapped and sutured, thus shortening the subscapularis muscle by 1 to 1.5 cm. The shortening restores the traumatically stretched and lax subscapularis and produces minimal limitation of external rotation. This simplified technique is easy to perform, short in duration (30 to 45 minutes) and has given very satisfactory results with a success rate of over 95% in terms of function and stability.[23,25] It may be used in non-athletic young individuals as well as in older patients.

The Bankart procedure remains the procedure of choice for young athletes, as it restores normal glenohumeral anatomy and function.[26]

The indications for the surgical treatment of glenohumeral instability are pain, recurrent dislocation and limitation of sporting activity. The time interval between injury and arthroscopic or open stabilisation is an important factor for achieving good results. This is more so after an acute anterior primary dislocation than after recurrences. It has been suggested[27] that fresh haemarthrosis and associated inflammatory mediators provide the optimal environment for wound healing after a Bankart repair.

The Bankart procedure and its modifications[26] have provided excellent results in terms of stabilisation and restoration of function. It is, however, a relatively difficult procedure with regard to the positioning of the sutures in the anterior glenoid rim and in stabilising the detached labrum. Rowe,[26] a surgeon with extensive experience of the Bankart procedure, has stated that the mean duration of this operation in his hands is 2.5 hours.

With the introduction of bioabsorbable implants and suture anchors for the fixation of the glenoid labrum the operation has become easier and safer.

We have used suture anchors (MITEK) for the last five years in a mixed population of 32 individuals aged between 18 and 36 years of age with traumatic anterior instability of the shoulder. After a follow-up of one to four years we have had one recurrence in a football player after a further significant injury.

Closed (arthroscopic). Since the first account of arthroscopic stabilisation in 1982 by Johnson[28] there have been many further reports.[29,30] These have used a variety of stabilisation techniques and devices, such as staples, transglenoid sutures, bioabsorbable materials and anchor sutures.

The rate of recurrence is high at between 10% and 20%[29,31] compared with that for open surgical procedures which is below 5%.[26]

There are three possible reasons for this high rate of failure. First, arthroscopy cannot correct the deformity of the glenohumeral ligament-labrum complex.[13] Thus an arthroscopic Bankart repair should be performed only in young athletic patients with unidirectional anterior instability, a clear-cut Bankart lesion with capsular laxity, and a well-developed IGHL. Secondly, a Bankart lesion is part of a wide spectrum of pathology including lesions of muscle, ligament, capsule and bone.[32] Thirdly, the quality and strength of the capsule are not the same in all shoulders after traumatic anterior dislocation.

Therefore our philosophy is in accord with that of Cole and Warner[13] that shoulder surgeons should not hesitate to convert to an open stabilisation if the arthroscopic technique does not address all the pathology identified at the time of the procedure.

Regardless of the above-mentioned possible disadvantages, arthroscopists should continue their endeavours to improve the results in view of the advantages of the procedure which include a lower surgical morbidity, better postoperative movement, earlier return to previous activities and a smaller scar.

Traumatic posterior instability of the shoulder. This is seen infrequently and represents less than 5% of patients with traumatic shoulder instability. Acute posterior dislocation evades diagnosis in many cases.

A prominent coracoid process anteriorly with the arm internally rotated and complete elimination of external rotation are the main clinical signs of this condition. An axillary view radiograph is of the utmost importance in establishing the diagnosis.

The initial treatment is non-operative. Exercises to strengthen external rotation as well as other shoulder and scapular stabilisers may be adequate. If this treatment fails surgical repair is indicated.

A variety of surgical techniques has been used, i.e., posterior bone block, osteotomy of the glenoid or of the neck of the humerus, posterior capsular plication and posterior capsulorrhaphy. Since the condition is rare the number of published papers is limited and evaluation of the best procedure to use is difficult. It appears that posteroinferior capsulorrhaphy with reduction of the capsular volume is the preferred procedure.[6,33]

Atraumatic multidirectional instability (MDI). This is a complex problem concerning both diagnosis and treatment. The surgeon should establish the exact diagnosis taking into consideration the history of the instability, physical examination and the radiological findings. More details may be obtained from CT, MRI and arthro-MRI, examination under general anaesthesia and arthroscopy. With this information the surgeon should establish to which of the following categories the instability belongs: 1) involuntary; 2) voluntary with an involuntary component;[34] 3) voluntary without psychological disorder; and 4) voluntary with psychological disorder. Treatment of MDI may be conservative or operative, but there is a consensus of opinion that initially it should be non-operative regardless of whether the type of instability is involuntary or voluntary.[6,7,35-37] Conservative treatment consists of a prolonged rehabilitation programme to strengthen the deltoid and rotator-cuff muscles and the scapular stabilisers. The duration of this programme may range from six months[12,37] to one year. During this time the surgeon evaluates the patient's motivation and ability to co-operate with treatment. A variety of rehabilitation programmes has been described of which that of Rockwood and Burkhead[38] is the most generally accepted (Fig. 7). They treated 115 patients with 140 unstable shoulders using their specific programme of exercises. Of these, 80% of the atraumatic group responded favourably to this programme compared with 16% in the traumatic group.[39]

Operative treatment is indicated for patients with atraumatic involuntary instability who fail to respond to conservative management. Patients with voluntary dislocation and psychiatric disorders should be excluded from operative treatment regardless of the failure of any prolonged exercise programme. Not all patients with voluntary dislocation, however, have psychiatric problems.[40]

Inferior capsular shift. This was described by Neer and Foster[12] in 1980 and continues to be the operation of choice in the treatment of MDI. It aims at the global reduction of the volume of the redundant capsule.

Before operation it is of the utmost importance to determine the direction of greatest instability. By approaching the unstable shoulder from this side, which is usually anterior, the surgeon may tighten all sides of the capsule including the posterior and obliterate the inferior capsular pouch. The results of inferior capsular shift have been satisfactory in over 80% of cases.[41-43]

Modifications to inferior capsular shift. Since the original description a variety of modifications has been described. They differ from the original mainly in the position of the vertical limb of the T-shaped incision of the capsule in three ways.

First, the approach and division of the subscapularis tendon 1 cm medial to its insertion into the lesser tuberosity of the humerus are the same as in the original procedure. Similarly, a thin layer of the deep surface of the tendon is retained with the capsule for subsequent reinforcement. The vertical limb of the T-shaped opening of the capsule is located 0.15 to 1 cm medial to the level of the divided subscapularis tendon and the insertion of the capsule into the neck of the humerus. This narrow part of the capsule allows safer suturing of the inferior capsular flap.[7]

Secondly, the vertical limb of the T-shaped opening of the capsule is positioned midway between its attachment to the humerus and that to the glenoid rim, as described by Rockwood.[37] The medial flap is brought superiorly and laterally under the lateral capsular flap.

Thirdly, the capsule is approached by dividing subscapularis horizontally along its fibres at the junction of its upper two-thirds and lower one-third. The horizontal limb of the T-shaped incision into the capsule follows the direction of the split in subscapularis. The vertical limb is made parallel to the edge of the glenoid process just medial to the labrum. The inferior capsular flap is shifted superiorly and sutured to the glenoid, and the superior flap is overlapped onto the inferior flap and is also sutured onto the glenoid.[44]

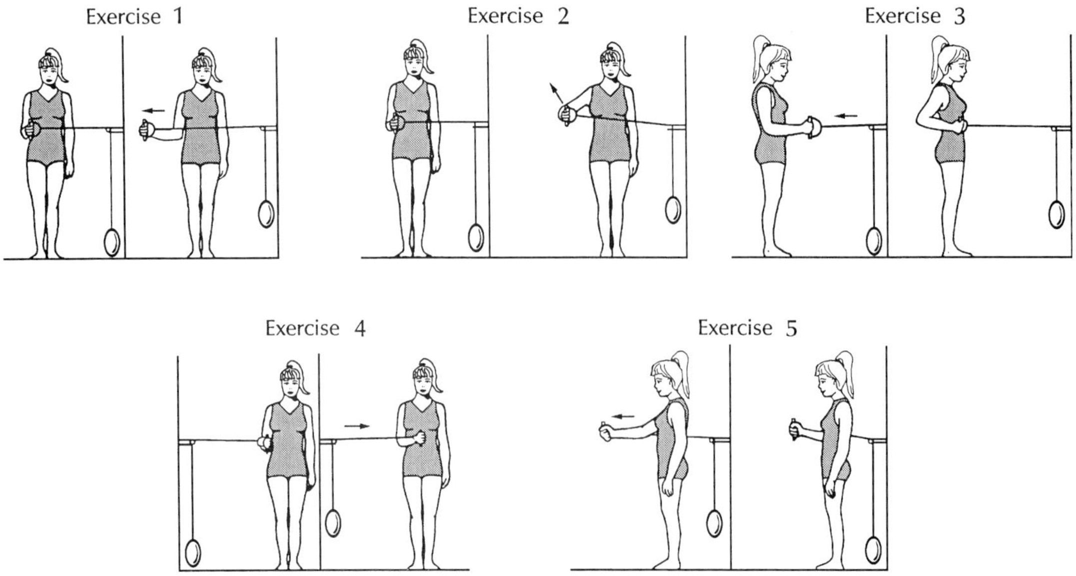

Fig. 7

The exercise system of Rockwood and Burkhead[38] in patients with atraumatic multidirectional instability.

Glenoid osteotomy. This is a completely different procedure from the inferior capsular shift. It has been described by Nobuhara and Ikeda[45] for the treatment of MDI and aims to change the inclination of the glenoid cavity so that it faces more superiorly. This change in the orientation of the glenoid cavity controls the tendency of the humeral head to displace inferiorly and establishes a new fulcrum for the shoulder muscles. They have reviewed 100 of the 111 patients who have undergone this procedure over a period of 14 years, with a follow-up of more than one year. Symptomatic instability decreased in all except three. More studies with larger series and longer follow-up are needed to evaluate the efficacy of this rather difficult operation.

Arthroscopic treatment. This has significantly advanced in the past few years. Duncan and Savoie[46] reported the results after arthroscopic inferior capsular shift for MDI. They performed a superomedial shift of the capsule on ten patients with satisfactory results at a follow-up of one to three years.

McIntyre, Gaspari and Savoie[47] treated 19 patients with MDI using an arthroscopic capsular shift in an outpatient setting. All except one returned to their previous level of athletic performance after a follow-up of at least 24 months (mean 34).

Treacy, Savoie and Field[48] reported the results of arthroscopic capsular shift in 25 patients with involuntary MDI of the shoulder; 21 (88%) had a satisfactory result according to the grading system of Neer and Foster[12] after a mean follow-up of 60 months. Thus, it appears that the arthroscopic inferior capsular shift procedure gives results in patients with involuntary MDI which are comparable to those treated by an open operation.

Thermal capsular shrinkage. The arthroscopic application of thermal energy in the form of laser or radiofrequency to shrink the redundant capsule is a new form of treatment of MDI of the shoulder. Most of the relevant studies, however, have been performed on animals.[49] The procedure is relatively safe; over 30 000 have been performed in North America[50] and many in Europe.[51] The early results are encouraging. There is, however, a potential risk to the axillary nerve during this procedure. In a recent round-table discussion at the American Academy of Orthopaedic Surgeons Meeting (Orlando 2000), a show of hands of the surgeons present revealed that about 20 had seen damage to the axillary nerve related to thermal therapy.[52] More controlled clinical studies with a long follow-up are needed to evaluate the natural history of the shrunken capsule in the long term.

REFERENCES

1. **Kumar VP, Balasubramaniam P.** The role of atmospheric pressure in stabilising the shoulder: an experimental study. *J Bone Joint Surg [Br]* 1985;67-B:719-21.
2. **Warner JJ, Lephart S, Fu FH.** Role of proprioception in pathoetiology of shoulder instability. *Clin Orthop* 1996;330:35-9.
3. **Bigliani LU, Pollock RG, Soslowsky LJ, et al.** Tensile properties of the inferior glenohumeral ligament. *J Orthop Res* 1992;10:187-97.
4. **Boardman ND, Debski RE, Warner JJ, et al.** Tensile properties of the superior glenohumeral and coracohumeral ligaments. *J Shoulder Elbow Surg* 1996;5:249-54.
5. **O'Brien SL, Schwarz RS, Warren RF, Torzilli PA.** Capsular restraints to anterior posterior motion of the abducted shoulder: a biomechanical study. *J Shoulder Elbow Surg* 1995;4:298-308.
6. **Neer SC II.** *Shoulder reconstruction.* Philadelphia, etc: WB Saunders, 1990:273-41.
7. **Flatow EL.** Glenohumeral instability. In: Post M, Bigniali L, Flatow E, Pollock R, eds. *The shoulder: operative technique.* Baltimore: Williams and Wilkins, 1998:167-200.
8. **Gerber C.** Observations on the classification of instability. In: Warner JJP, Iannotti JP, Gerber C, eds. *Complex and revision problems in shoulder surgery.* Philadelphia: Lippincott Raven, 1997:9-18.
9. **Hill HA, Sachs MD.** The grooved, defect of the humeral head: a frequently unrecognized complication of dislocations of shoulder joint. *Radiology* 1940;35:690-700.
10. **Hawkins RJ, Koppert G, Johnston G.** Recurrent posterior instability (sublucation) of the shoulder. *J Bone Joint Surg [Am]* 1984;66-A:169-74.
11. **Pollock RG, Bigliani LU.** Recurrent posterior shoulder instability: diagnosis and treatment. *Clin Orthop* 1993;291:85-96.
12. **Neer CS II, Foster CR.** Inferior capsular shift for involuntary inferior and multidirectional instability of the shoulder. *J Bone Joint Surg [Am]* 1980;62-A:897-908.
13. **Cole BJ, Warner JJP.** Arthroscopic versus open Bankart repair for traumatic anterior shoulder instability. *Clin Sports Med* 2000;19:19-48.
14. **Hovelius L, Augustini BG, Fredin H, et al.** Primary anterior dislocation of the shoulder in young patients: a ten-year prospective study. *J Bone Joint Surg [Am]* 1996;78-A:1677-84.
15. **Rowe C, Sakellaridis H.** Factors related to recurrences of anterior dislocations of the shoulder. *Clin Orthop* 1961;20:40-8.
16. **Archiero RA, Wheeler JH, Ryan JB, et al.** Arthroscopic Bankart repair versus nonoperative treatment for acute, initial anterior shoulder dislocation. *Am J Sports Med* 1994;22:589-94.
17. **Wintzell G, Haglund-Akerlind Y, Tidermark J, Wredmark T, Erisksson E.** A prospective controlled randomized study of arthroscopic lavage in acute primary anterior dislocation of the shoulder: one-year follow-up. *Knee Surg Sports Traumatol Arthrosc* 1996;4:43-7.
18. **Wintzell G, Hovelius L, Wikblad L, Saebo M, Larson S.** Arthroscopic lavage speeds reduction in effusion in the glenohumeral joint after primary anterior shoulder dislocation: a controlled randomized ultrasound study. *Knee Surg Sports Traumatol Arthrosc* 2000;8:56-60.
19. **Payne LZ, Altchek DW.** The surgical treatment of anterior shoulder instability. *Clin Sports Med* 1995;14:863-83.
20. **Bankart ASB.** The pathology and treatment of recurrent dislocation of the shoulder joint. *Br J Surg* 1938;26:23-9.
21. **Karadimas J, Rentis G, Varouchas G.** Repair of recurrent anterior dislocation of the shoulder using transfer of the subscapularis tendon. *J Bone Joint Surg [Am]* 1988;62-A:1147-9.
22. **Magnuson PB, Stack JK.** Recurrent dislocation of the shoulder. *JAMA* 1943;23:889-92.
23. **Symeonides PP.** Reconsideration of the Putti-Platt procedure and its mode of action in recurrent traumatic anterior dislocation of the shoulder. *Clin Orthop* 1989;246:8-15.
24. **Symeonides PP.** Surgical management of the unstable shoulder. In: Watson MS, ed. *Practical shoulder surgery.* London: Grune and Straton, 1984:67-127.
25 **Caira SF.** The Symeonides procedure for the recurrent anterior inferior dislocation of the shoulder. In: Willems J, et al eds. *Abstract book 13th Congress of ESSE (SECEC).* The Hague, 1999:186.
26. **Rowe C, Patel D, Southmayd W.** The Bankart procedure: a long-term end-result study. *J Bone Joint Surg [Am]* 1978;60-A:1-16.
27. **Wen DY.** Current concepts in the treatment of anterior shoulder dislocations. *Am J Emerg Med* 1999;17:401-7.
28. **Johnson LL.** *Diagnostic and surgical arthroscopy of the shoulder.* St Louis: Mosby, 1993;276-52.
29. **Resch H, Povacz P, Wambacher M, Sperner G, Golser K.** Arthroscopic extra-articular Bankart repair for the treatment of recurrent anterior shoulder dislocation. *Arthroscopy* 1997;13:188-200.

30. **Walch G, Boileau P, Levigne C, et al.** Arthroscopic stabilization for recurrent anterior shoulder dislocation: results of 59 cases. *Arthroscopy* 1995;11:173-9.

31. **Hawkins RB.** Arthroscopic stapling repair for shoulder instability: retrospective study of 50 cases. *Arthroscopy* 1989;5:122-8.

32. **Symeonides PP.** The significance of the subscapularis muscle in the pathogenesis of recurrent anterior dislocation of the shoulder. *J Bone Joint Surg [Br]* 1972;54-B:476-83.

33. **Bigliani LU, Pollock RG, McIlveen SJ, et al.** Shift of the posteroinferior aspect of the capsule for recurrent posterior glenohumeral instability. *J Bone Joint Surg [Am]* 1995;77-A:1011-20.

34. **Cofield RH, Irving JF.** Evaluation and classification of shoulder instability with special reference to examination under anaesthesia. *Clin Orthop* 1987;223:32-43.

35. **Mallon WJ, Speer KP.** Multidirectional instability: current concepts. *J Shoulder Elbow Surg* 1995;4:54-64.

36. **Matsen FA, Thomas SC, Rockwood CA.** Anterior glenohumeral instability. In: Rockwood CA, Matsen FA, eds. *The shoulder.* Philadelphia: W B Saunders, 1990.

37. **Rockwood CA.** Approach to treatment of atraumatic and multidirectional glenohumeral instability. In: Rockwood CA, Matsen FA III, eds. *The shoulder.* Philadelphia: WB Saunders, 1990;1:608-12.

38. **Rockwood CA, Burkhead WZ.** Subluxation of the glenohumeral joint: response to rehabilitative exercise: traumatic versus atraumatic instability. Procs 3rd International Conference on Surgery of the Shoulder, 1986:293-8.

39. **Burkhead WZ Jr, Rockwood CA Jr.** Treatment of instability of the shoulder with an exercise program. *J Bone Joint Surg [Am]* 1992;74-A:890-6.

40. **Rowe C, Pierce DS, Clark JG.** Voluntary dislocation of the shoulder: a preliminary report on a clinical electromyographic and psychiatric study of twenty-six patients. *J Bone Joint Surg [Am]* 1973;55-A:445-60.

41. **Bigliani LU, Pollock RG, Owens JM, et al.** The inferior capsular shift procedure for MDI of the shoulder. *Orthop Trans* 1993;17:576.

42. **Cooper RA, Brems AA.** The inferior capsular shift procedure for multidirectional instability of the shoulder. *J Bone Joint Surg [Am]* 1992;74-A:1516-21.

43. **Hamada K, Fukuda H, Nakajima T, Yamada N.** The inferior capsular shift operation for instability of the shoulder: long-term results in 34 shoulders. *J Bone Joint Surg [Br]* 1999;81-B:218-25.

44. **Rubenstein DL, Jobe FW, Glousman RE, et al.** Anterior capsulolabral reconstruction of the shoulder in athletes. *J Shoulder Elbow Surg* 1992;1:229-73.

45. **Nobuhara K, Ikeda H.** *Glenoid osteotomy for loose shoulder. In: Watson MS, ed. Surgical disorders of the shoulder.* Edinburgh: Churchill Livingstone, 1991:44-50.

46. **Duncan R, Savoie FH III.** Arthroscopic inferior capsular shift for multidirectional instability of the shoulder: a preliminary report. *Arthroscopy* 1993;9:24-7.

47. **McIntyre LF,Gaspari RB, Savoie FH III.** The arthroscopic treatment of multidirectoral shoulder instability: two-year results of a multiple suture technique. *Arthroscopy* 1997;13:418-25.

48. **Treacy SH, Savoie FH III, Field LD.** Arthroscopic treatment of multidirectional instability. *J Shoulder Elbow Surg* 1999;8:345-50.

49. **Levy O, Copeland S.** Thermal capsular shrinkage. In: Williams J, et al, ed. *Abstract Book 13th Congress of ESSE (SECEC).* The Hague, 1999:120-36.

50. **Wallace AI.** Effects of thermal shrinkage on cellular responses and mechanical behaviour of ligament tissue. In: Williams J, et al, eds. *Abstract Book 13th Congress of ESSE (SECEC).* The Hague, 1999:112-5.

51. **Frostick SP, Sinopidis CT, Maskari SA, Richmont JC.** Arthroscopic capsular shrinkage of the shoulder: 2 years follow-up. Procs American Academy Orthopaedic Surgeons, 67th Annual Meeting, Orlando, 2000:427.

52. **Gryler EC, et al.** Temperatures along the axillary nerve during radiofrequency induced thermal capsular shrinkage of the shoulder. Procs American Academy of Orthopaedic Surgeons, 67th Annual Meeting, Orlando, 2000.

REPAIR OF RUPTURES OF THE ROTATOR CUFF

INFLUENCE OF THE STATUS OF MUSCLE AND TENDON ON THE RESULTS

D. GOUTALLIER, J. M. POSTEL, P. LEGUILLOUX

From the Henri Mondor Hospital, Créteil, France

The rotator cuff is essential for normal function and strength of the shoulder. Ruptures of the rotator cuff reduce the strength of the joint and lead to arthritis. It is therefore logical to attempt to repair them. Further ruptures often occur, however, and the larger the preoperative defect, the more frequent are recurrent tears.[1-4] The fact that further ruptures are less extensive than previously treated tears and that the functional results in the short and medium term are satisfactory[5] does not justify performing reconstructive surgery. This surgery may be criticised as palliative surgery, involving arthrolysis and decompression, and may give good functional results despite being illogical. Furthermore, rehabilitation after palliative surgery, easily performed arthroscopically, is much more simple than after reconstructive procedures. Degenerative changes in the short or medium term, however, are accorded different significance by various authors; the reduction of the subacromial space is deemed important by Kempf et al,[6] but much less so by Thomazeau et al.[7]

To be objective about whether repair should be performed it is necessary to establish which ruptures require repair, and which technique is appropriate in order to restore function.

ANATOMY AND PHYSIOLOGY

The rotator cuff consists of three main musculotendinous elements: supraspinatus, infraspinatus and subscapularis. To these should be added teres minor and the long head of biceps.

The rotator cuff ensures that the head of the humerus is centred in relation to the glenoid. It should be emphasised that infraspinatus is almost the only muscle responsible for external rotation of the shoulder. It may be helped in this activity by teres minor.[8] The supraspinatus ensures, passively and actively, that the humeral head is centred in the frontal plane, but subscapularis and infraspinatus[9] are also actively involved. They prevent upward displacement of the head towards the coracoacromial arch during active elevation of the arm. The importance of the function of both infraspinatus and subscapularis is confirmed by daily experience: an isolated rupture of supraspinatus leaves a shoulder adequately centred[10] with normal or almost normal function and satisfactory strength, provided that the pain caused by impingement of the ruptured tendon within the subacromial space can be overcome. There is minimal development of degenerative changes under these circumstances. On the other hand, a rupture of the cuff which spreads beyond the supraspinatus is much more detrimental to the shoulder. Rupture of infraspinatus weakens active external rotation and is associated with considerable loss of strength and function of the shoulder. The disappearance of the posterior stabiliser of the glenohumeral joint and of external rotation allows increased internal rotation and progressive posterior subluxation which becomes irreducible and associated with posterior glenohumeral degenerative changes.

A serious rupture of subscapularis, which is painful because of impingement of the stump of the muscle against the coracoid process, is associated with progressive anterior subluxation of the head of the humerus. This anterior subluxation also may become irreducible and is associated with anterior glenohumeral degenerative changes. The superior facet of the greater tuberosity migrates from the supraspinous fossa[11] which increases the risk of secondary rupture by stretching the repaired supraspinatus.

Thus ruptures spreading beyond the supraspinatus should be repaired, at least in active patients, for both anatomical and physiological reasons. Repair of an isolated rupture of the supraspinatus, however, is not justified on these grounds except to prevent progressive enlargement of the tear with involvement of adjacent tendons. There is not sufficient evidence to show that progressive enlargement occurs and the repair of a torn supraspinatus is not always successful.

MUSCULAR LESIONS OF TENDINOUS RUPTURES OF THE CUFF

The tendons of the cuff muscles which rupture undergo progressive fatty infiltration termed 'fatty muscular degeneration'.[12] Fat replaces atrophied muscle fibres. This degeneration is seen on CT horizontal slices with soft-tissue windows and fatty degeneration has been quantified

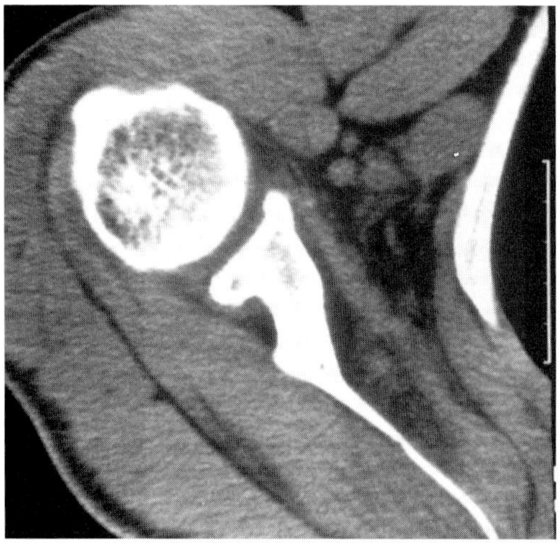

Fig. 1

CT (soft-tissue windows) showing fatty degeneration according to the scale of Goutallier et al[12]: infraspinatus, stage 1; and subscapularis, stage 2.

according to the percentage of the muscle which it occupies. The normal layer of fat between the muscles and the scapula is accounted for in this estimate. Quantification can be made in five stages according to the scale of Goutallier et al[12] (Fig. 1). Fatty degeneration may also be evaluated by MRI and when it occurs[13] in supraspinatus is accompanied by atrophy of the muscle. This atrophy was first quantified on sagittal MRI sections by Thomazeau et al,[14] and can now also be demonstrated by means of CT reconstruction.

Fatty degeneration around shoulders without degenerative or neurological pathology is not due to old age; it appears only in cases of rupture of the rotator cuff.[12] It affects the muscles with tendons which have been ruptured, and sometimes increases rapidly as the ruptured tendinous stump migrates proximally.[3] It is associated with a reduction of muscle function, as assessed by determination of the amplitude of active external rotation in the case of anterosuperior ruptures of the cuff which involve both supraspinatus and subscapularis but leave an intact infraspinatus, the only case when a muscle with a non-ruptured tendon can receive fat. It is significant that the fatty degeneration of the muscle with a repaired tendon seems to decrease only after four to five years. Fatty degeneration of supraspinatus becomes important above stage 2, only if rupture of the supraspinatus tendon is associated with that of one or several adjacent tendons. It is therefore necessary to quantify not only the fatty degeneration of each of the muscles of the shoulder individually, but also the overall fatty degeneration of the shoulder by means of the global degeneration index (GDI)[15] which is a measurement of the mean of the fatty degeneration of each muscle (supraspinatus, infraspinatus and subscapularis).

Thus an infraspinatus muscle with a ruptured tendon and heavy fatty infiltration would not recover its functional potential after tendinous repair for several years. During that period, it cannot efficiently lower the humeral head. There is mechanical conflict between a repaired supraspinatus and the coracoacromial arch, and further rupture of the repaired supraspinatus seems almost certain. Similarly, repair of subscapularis with significant fatty degeneration would not be able to reduce or prevent anterior subluxation of the head and progressive stretching followed by rupture of a repaired supraspinatus tendon. A multicentre study conducted by the French Society of Orthopaedics and Traumatology (SOFCOT), directed by Augereau and Gazielly,[16] on repair of ruptures of the cuff confirmed that the incidence of ruptured tendinous cuff repairs depended on the fatty degeneration of the muscles and particularly on the preoperative GDI.[15] In this study 231 ruptures of the cuff repaired by tendon-bone suture without tendino-muscular plastic surgery were studied at a mean follow-up of three years after operation, half by MRI and half by arthroCT. Of these, 79 (34%) had further ruptures and 152 (66%) remained intact. The postoperative security of the repair of the tendinous cuff depended statistically on the preoperative GDI whatever the type of rupture, that is, isolated rupture of supraspinatus, associated ruptures of supraspinatus and infraspinatus, associated ruptures of supraspinatus and subscapularis or ruptures of all tendons. The more the muscles were infiltrated with fat preoperatively, the more common were further ruptures. Further ruptures (Fig. 2) occurred in 100% of shoulders with a

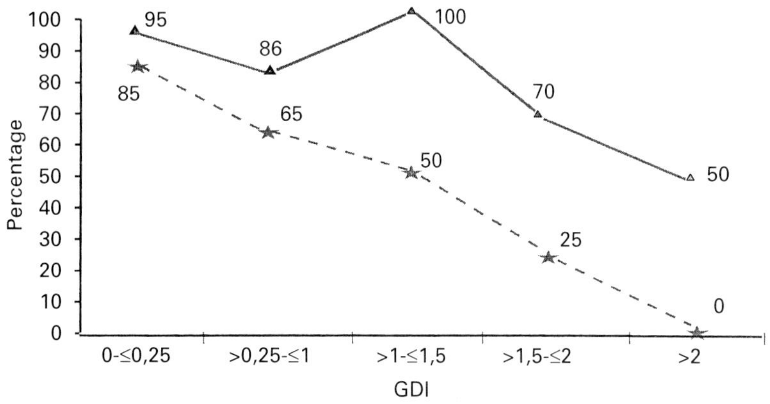

Fig. 2

Percentage of postoperative secure cuffs according to the preoperative global degenerative index (GDI) in the series of Augereau and Gazielly[16] (—★— simple repairs; —▲— repairs with plastic surgery (without tension)).

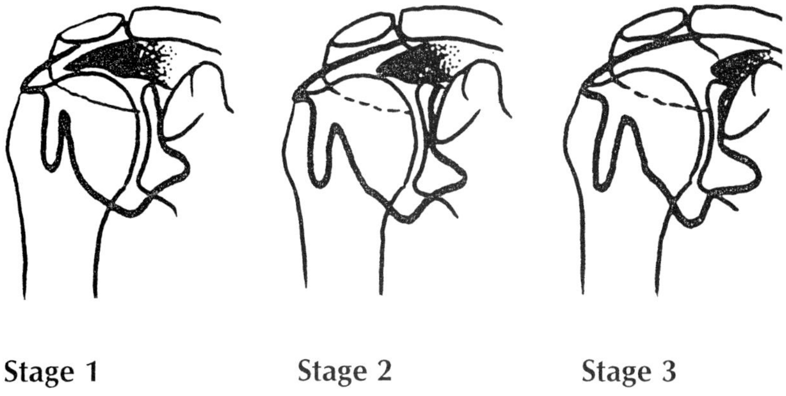

Fig. 3

Diagram of the scale of Bernageau[18] for quantifying the position of a torn supraspinatus tendon.

preoperative GDI>2, in 50% of those with a more moderate preoperative GDI (>1 to ≤1.5), and in only 15% of shoulders with very weak preoperative GDI (0 to ≤ 0.25). In addition, our study confirmed that shoulders with repaired secure cuffs had statistically better functional results than those with further ruptures. Constant's score decreased, however, as the preoperative GDI increased.

Of the different cuff muscles, it seems that the fatty state of infraspinatus is most indicative of the evolution of the repaired cuff. A study at the Henri Mondor Hospital[3] of 74 ruptures of the cuff, all of which were reviewed by arthroCT at a mean of one year after repair, showed no further rupture when the value for fatty preoperative degeneration of infraspinatus was less than 2.

Ruptures spreading beyond the supraspinatus therefore must be repaired rapidly before fatty infiltration of infraspinatus and subscapularis develops. On the other hand, as regards the muscle, there is no reason to repair an isolated rupture of the supraspinatus quickly. If it is repaired there is no threat of further rupture because of muscular problems, since the main 'depressors' and the main anteroposterior 'centerers' of the humeral head retain their ability to function.

Nevertheless, slight preoperative fatty degeneration does not preclude a secure cuff postoperatively. In the SOFCOT series,[15] the incidence of further rupture in tears repaired without significant fatty muscular degeneration (GDI 0 to ≤0.25) was 15%. Moreover, Kempf, Marcillou and Schlemmer[17] noted further ruptures in 28% of repairs of isolated ruptures of supraspinatus with a slightly retracted tendinous stump, stage 1 of Bernageau[18] (Fig. 3), and without significant fatty degeneration (<2). Another factor other than muscular degeneration must be responsible for further ruptures.

HISTOLOGY OF RUPTURED TENDONS

Are reinserted ruptured tendons normal enough to heal well to bone and to have the mechanical qualities necessary for normal function?

We usually resect the tendinous stumps which seem to be too thin or macroscopically disorganised (cleaved or fissured) before reinsertion to bone. By resecting the stump, we seek to reach a macroscopically healthy tendon, slightly bleeding and thick enough to hold sutures. Thus between 1998 and 1999 we resected 32 supraspinatus tendons over a length of more than 1 cm. The mean age of the patients at operation was 59.5 years (49 to 72). In four cases the ruptures involved only one tendon, in 13 two tendons and in 15 three tendons. In 17 cases the stump of supraspinatus before resection was located near the greater tuberosity of the humerus (stage 1 of Bernageau) (Fig. 3), in ten above the humeral head (stage 2) and in only five within the humeral head (stage 3). The resected tendons were sent for histological examination. The mean length was 2.2 cm (1.2 to 3.5) and that of the histologically abnormal tendon 1.8 cm (0.8 to 3). All the resected tendons were found to be histologically abnormal and in 17 cases this involved the whole length of the tendon. The connective tissue was abnormal with disorganisation, necrosis and fatty infiltration (Fig. 4). Tendinous necrosis was rarely seen (six cases) and was mainly found (five cases) in ruptures with tendinous stumps remaining near the greater tuberosity. Fatty infiltration was found in seven elderly patients with a mean age of 63 years (58 to 72) in five of whom the infiltration of the supraspinatus muscle was ≥2.

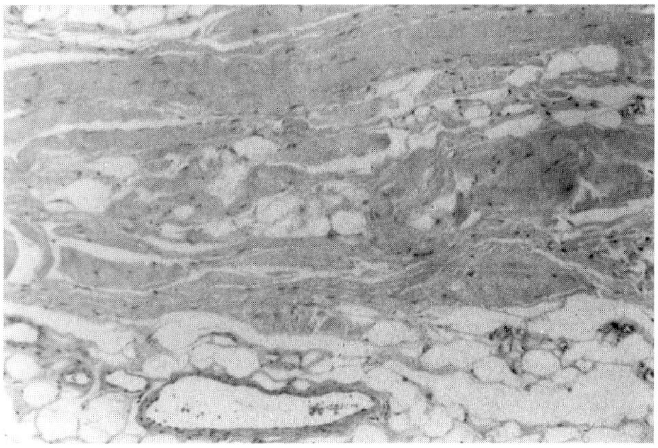

Fig. 4

Photomicrograph showing fatty infiltration of a torn supraspinatus tendon.

Extension of tendinous resection to macroscopically healthy tissue is essential for secure holding of the sutures in the tendon stumps and for a mechanically satisfactory tendinous cuff.[19]

HOW TO REPAIR THE ROTATOR CUFF

As in any tendinous repair, suture of ruptures of the cuff must be performed without tension. It is essential that the sutures have a good hold on the humeral cortex as well as on the stump of the tendon. Reinsertion of the tendinous stump into an osseous trough with haemorrhagic cancellous bone is satisfactory. It is not certain that the tendinous stump after resection is histologically sound since 50% of the resected tendons in our series were histologically abnormal. From an experimental study on goats Pierre et al[20] concluded that tendon-bone healing after repair of the cuff is as good when either the tendon is fixed close to cortical bone or fixed in a cancellous trough.

Cuff repair by simple suture is therefore satisfactory only if the shoulder muscles and particularly infraspinatus have no fatty degeneration, and if operative tendinous resection, which eliminates the macroscopically abnormal part of the stump to be repaired, is minor enough to enable the stump to be brought to the humerus without tension. This is relatively rare. It is to be found only in ruptures of the cuff after injury when the tendons are healthy and the trauma recent enough for there to be little retraction of the tendons and for the muscles still to be normal. The more the tears are of degenerative origin in elderly patients, with no clear injury, the smaller is the possibility of a satisfactory simple repair. Two factors are likely to make a simple repair without tension either impossible or precarious; first, the necessity of tendinous resection to obtain a healthy tendon capable of holding sutures and having good mechanical qualities, and secondly the usual delay in making a surgical decision and the development of fatty degeneration within the muscles.

In order to improve the outcome after repairs on the tendon it is necessary for the surgeon to be familiar with all the techniques available.[21] The correct resection of tendinous stumps requires plastic surgical techniques. If muscles, and particularly the infraspinatus, are too degenerate, they must either be reinforced by a rhomboid flap[22] or replaced by healthy muscles as with a latissimus dorsi flap,[23] a deltoid flap,[24] a trapezius flap,[25] or a pectoralis major flap.[26] We perform plastic surgical techniques for supraspinatus and infraspinatus by musculotendinous advancement. This does not cause lesions of the suprascapular nerve on the clinical level,[27] contrary to the findings of Warner et al[28] in experimental studies on cadavers with normal cuffs. The infraspinatus muscle with fatty degeneration is reinforced by rhomboid major, which is detached from the border of the spine of the scapula and kept tied to the superficial aponeurosis of the advanced infraspinatus. A subscapularis muscle in which the tendon is much retracted and the muscle of which has fatty degeneration is replaced by an osteotendinomuscular flap from the superior part of trapezius.

A study of two series confirmed the anatomical soundness of these procedures. The first consisted of 45 shoulders reported by Goutallier et al.[15] Recurrent ruptures of the cuff (Fig. 2) were rare (5%) if the GDI was very low (≤ 0.25) as compared with 15% in tears with simple sutures. Thus, the tendinous aspect of these ruptures had been eliminated by macroscopically appropriate tendinous resection. When the GDI is >1 and ≤ 1.5, the percentage of further ruptures is 0%, significantly less than the 50% with simple repairs. With a GDI >2, the incidence of further ruptures was 50% which is significantly less than the 100% found with simple repair. This shows that even utilising these technical advances, a GDI of more than 2 is a contraindication to repair. The second series was a study of the histological lesions of tendons in 19 repaired cuffs after total resection of the abnormal tendon assessed by arthroCT one year after operation. Only one tear affected supraspinatus. Six ruptures affected two tendons, and 11 three tendons. The mean GDI was more than 2 in one case. Fatty degeneration of the infraspinatus was ≥ 2 in two cases. Fifteen advancements of only supraspinatus, four advancements of both supraspinatus and infraspinatus and two trapezius flaps were performed. We noted only three cases (16%) of further ruptures. We assume that the functional results improve with time, often until the first or the second postoperative year when the cuff has remained secure.

INDICATIONS FOR CUFF RUPTURE REPAIR

Isolated ruptures of supraspinatus do not necessarily need to be repaired. Nevertheless, it seems wise to do so in young patients. If plastic surgery is necessary for a sound repair, it should be performed. In older patients, repair of isolated ruptures of the supraspinatus should be done only if the shoulders remain symptomatic after conservative treatment. In such cases, however, palliative surgery can also be recommended.

Symptomatic rupture which spreads beyond supraspinatus should be repaired, particularly if the patients are active and well motivated. In these cases, the repair should be performed without loss of time. A long period of preoperative physiotherapy in these often stiffened shoulders serves no purpose. It rarely allows the recovery of more movement and wastes time. Postoperative physiotherapy, however, almost always allows the recovery of good movement and function. Reconstructive surgery must use techniques which include the reinsertion of healthy tendon without tension with healthy or reinforced muscle. The patient must be warned of the difficulty of postoperative physiotherapy and of slow recovery. It is better, however, to perform major surgery which has been explained carefully and is well accepted by the patients than to propose a lesser procedure which is more likely to fail. Palliative surgery should be offered to patients who are not motivated or are too elderly to benefit from long postoperative rehabilitation.

REFERENCES

1. **Bellumore Y, Mansat M, Assoun J.** Résultats de la chirurgie réparatrice de la coiffe des rotateurs: corrélation radio-clinique. *Rev Chir Orthop* 1994;80:582-94.
2. **Gazielly DF, Gleyze P, Montagnon C, Bruyère G, Prallet B.** Résultats fonctionnels et anatomiques après traitement chirurgical des ruptures de la coiffe des rotateurs. *Rev Chir Orthop* 1995;81:8-16.
3. **Goutallier D, Postel JM, Lavau L, Bernageau J.** Influence de la dégénérescence graisseuse des muscles supra-épineux et infra-épineux sur le pronostic des réparations chirurgicales de la coiffe des rotateurs. *Rev Chir Orthop* 1999;85:668-76.
4. **Harryman DT II, Mack LA, Wang KY, et al.** Repairs of the rotator cuff: correlation of functional results with integrity of the cuff. *J Bone Joint Surg [Am]* 1991;73-A:982-9.
5. **Jost B, Pfirrmann CH, Gerber CH.** Clinical outcome after structural failure of rotator cuff repairs. *J Bone Joint Surg [Am]* 2000;82-A:304-14.
6. **Kempf JF, Gleyze P, Bonnomet F, et al.** A multicentric study of 210 rotator cuff tears treated by arthroscopic acromioplasty. *Arthroscopy* 1999;15:56-66.
7. **Thomazeau H, Gleyze P, Frank A, et al.** Le débridement endoscopique des ruptures transfixiantes de la coiffe des rotateurs: étude rétrospective multicentrique de 283 cas á plus de 3 ans de recul. *Rev Chir Orthop* 2000;86:136-42.
8. **Walch G, Boulahia A, Calderone S, Robinson A.** The 'dropping' and 'hornblower's signs' in evaluation of rotator cuff tears. *J Bone Joint Surg [Br]* 1998;80-B:624-8.
9. **Blaimont P, Tacheri A.** Contribution à la biomécanique de l'articulation gléno-humérale. *Rev Chir Orthop* 1992;78:Suppl I:174-5.
10. **Loehr JF, Helmig P, Sojbjerg J-O, Jung A.** Shoulder instability caused by rotator cuff lesions: an in vitro study. *Clin Orthop* 1994;304:84-90.
11. **Hernigou Ph, Duparc F.** Rupture du sus épineux et retroversion de l'humérus. *Rev Rhum* 1997;64:859-60.
12. **Goutallier D, Postel JM, Bernageau J, Lavau L, Voisin MC.** Fatty muscle degeneration in cuff ruptures: pre and postoperative evaluation by CT scan. *Clin Orthop* 1994;304:78-83.
13. **Fuchs B, Weishaupt D, Zanetti M, Holder J, Gerber CH.** Fatty degeneration of the muscles of the rotator cuff: assessment by computed tomography versus magnetic resonance imaging. *J Shoulder Elbow Surg* 1999;8:599-605.
14. **Thomazeau H, Boukobza E, Morcet N, Chaperon J, Langlais F.** Prédiction of rotator cuff repair results by magnetic resonance imaging. *Clin Orthop* 1997;344:275-83.
15. **Goutallier D, Leguilloux P, Postel JM, Gleyze P.** La dégénérescence musculaire graisseuse. *Rev Chir Orthop* 1999;85:Suppl II:132-6.
16. **Augereau B, Gazielly DF.** Les ruptures transfixiantes de la coiffe des rotateurs, subscapularis inclus: symposium. *Rev Chir Orthop* 1999;85:Suppl II:87-139.
17. **Kempf JF, Marcillou Ph, Schlemmer B.** Résultats du traitement chirurgical des ruptures isolées du supraspinatus distales, intermédiaires, à la glène. *Rev Chir Orthop* 1999;85;Suppl II:105-9.
18. **Bernageau J.** Étude radiologique de la coiffe des rotateurs. *Rev Chir Orthop* 1984;74:282-7.
19. **Sano H, Uhthoff HK, Backman DS, et al.** Structural disorders at the insertion of the supraspinatus tendon: relation to tensile strength. *J Bone Joint Surg [Br]* 1998;80-B:720-5.
20. **Pierre St P, Olson EJ, Elliott JJ, et al.** Tendon healing to cortical bone compared with healing to a cancellous trough: a biomechanical and histological evaluation in goats. *J Bone Joint Surg [Br]* 1995;77-A:1858-66.
21. **Goutallier D, Postel JM, Leguilloux P.** *Fermeture chirurgicale des coiffes non réparables par suture simple.* Paris: Elsevier SAS 2000. Techniques chirurgicales - Orthopédie -Traumatologie, 44:285, 14p.
22. **Goutallier D, Postel JM.** Infraspinatus reinforcement by a rhomboid flap in the management of massive tears of the rotator cuff. *J Bone Joint Surg [Br]* 1992;74-B:Suppl I:18.
23. **Gerber CH.** Latissimus dorsi transfer for treatment of irreparable tears of the rotator cuff. *Clin Orthop* 1992;275:152-60.
24. **Apoil A, Augereau B.** Réparation par lambeau de deltoide des grandes pertes de substances de la coiffe des rotateurs de l'épaule. *Chirurgie* 1985;111:287-90.
25. **Goutallier D, Lavau L, Postel JM.** The trapezius flap in non-reinsertable tears of the subscapularis. In: Vastamaki M, Jalovaara P, eds. *Surgery of the shoulder.* Amsterdam: Elsevier Science, 1995:79-83.
26. **Wirth MA, Rockwood CA.** Operative treatment of irreparable rupture of the subscapularis. *J Bone Joint Surg [Am]* 1997;79-A:722-31.
27. **Goutallier D, Postel JM, Boudon R, Lavau L, Bernageau J.** Étude du risque neurologique à l'avancement tendinomusculaire des supra-épineux et infra-épineux dans les réparations des larges ruptures de coiffe. *Rev Chir Orthop* 1996;82:299-305.
28. **Warner JP, Krushell RJ, Masquelet A, Gerber Ch.** Anatomy and relationships of the suprascapular nerve: anatomical constraints to mobilization of the supraspinatus and infraspinatus muscles in the management of massive rotator cuff tears. *J Bone Joint Surg [Am]* 1992;74-A:36-45.

THE PAINFUL HIP IN A WELL-FIXED TOTAL HIP REPLACEMENT

K. KNAHR, W. SCHNEIDER, J. KRUGLUGER, M. KASPAREK

From the Orthopaedic Hospital, Vienna, Austria

A painful hip after total hip arthroplasty (THA) is an unsatisfactory outcome. We have therefore reviewed the numerous situations in which hip or thigh pain may occur, despite a well-fixed implant, classifying them according to the site of origin of the pain (Table I).

INTRA-ARTICULAR ORIGIN

The major intra-articular causes of hip pain are wear and infection, but impingement of components has recently gained importance because of the increased recognition of the role of the range of motion and the use of the so-called 'hard bearing' articulations such as metal-on-metal or ceramic-on-ceramic.

Wear. Adverse biological reaction to wear particles from the articulating surfaces of THAs are now recognised as the major cause of long-term failure of cementless artificial joints.[1] Thus far, the standard implant has been polyethylene on the acetabular side and a metal or ceramic head on the femoral side with a life span of approximately 10 to 15 years (Fig. 1). Minakawa et al[2] demonstrated that the ceramic femoral head retains its surface finish better than the metal head, and that it produces lower long-term rates of polyethylene wear. Currently, there is competition between ceramic-on-ceramic and metal-on-metal implants as to which are best.[3,4] Recently, new zirconia-on-zirconia and cross-linked implants have been introduced.[5,6]

Despite the effectiveness of these materials, all produce wear particles which have biological reactions in the body. Some of these are well known, especially those from polyethylene particles, but the biological response to metal or ceramic debris is still being evaluated. Therefore, if patients present with pain in their joint without signs of osteolysis, loosening or infection, irritation due to wear particles must be included in the differential diagnosis (Fig. 2).

Table I. Classification of the painful hip in a well-fixed total hip arthroplasty according to the site of origin of the pain

Intra-articular	Wear
	Infection
	Impingement of components
Periarticular	Bony structures
	Fatigue (stress) fractures
	Wear fractures
	Heterotopic ossification
	Trochanteric osteotomy
	Soft tissues
	Irritation of bursae
	Irritation of tendons and muscles
	Tumours
	Nerve-entrapment syndromes
	Muscular inbalance - leg length, offset
	Impingement of soft tissue or bone
Thigh pain	Shape/size component
	Fixation
	Muscle hernia
	Stress fractures
Lumbar spine	Radicular symptoms
	Spinal stenosis
	Spinal lesions with pseudoradicular pain syndromes
	Referred pain in the groin
Intra-abdominal	Urological
	Gynaecological
	Gastrointestinal

Infection. It is often difficult to differentiate the pain caused by aseptic loosening from that resulting from deep infection. Since many of these patients will need revision surgery, a preoperative diagnostic technique would be useful to differentiate infection from loosening.

In their prospective multicentre study Levitsky et al[7] evaluated plain radiography, three-phase bone scintigraphy, the ESR, aspiration of the joint for culture, and multiple intraoperative cultures at the time of revision. Intraoperative cultures and the operative appearance were used to form a diagnosis of definite infection (unequivocal microbiology and gross sepsis), possible infection (positive microbiology or gross sepsis) or no infection (neither positive microbiology nor gross sepsis). For the preoperative diagnosis of infection, as opposed to aseptic loosening, three-phase bone scintigraphy alone had a sensitivity of 33% and a specificity of 86%. In conjunction with plain radiography, a minimal improvement in accuracy was seen. A preoperative ESR greater than 30 mm/hr had a low sensitivity (60%) and a specificity of 65%, but the ESR was statistically significantly higher in hips with definite infection compared with those without. Preoperative joint aspiration had a sensitivity of 67% and a specificity of 96%

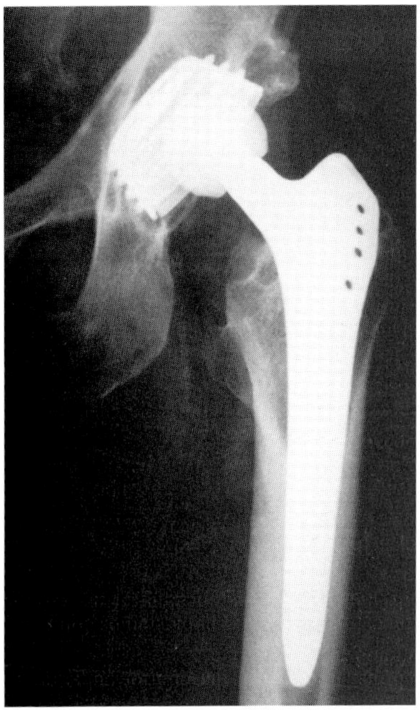

Fig. 1a

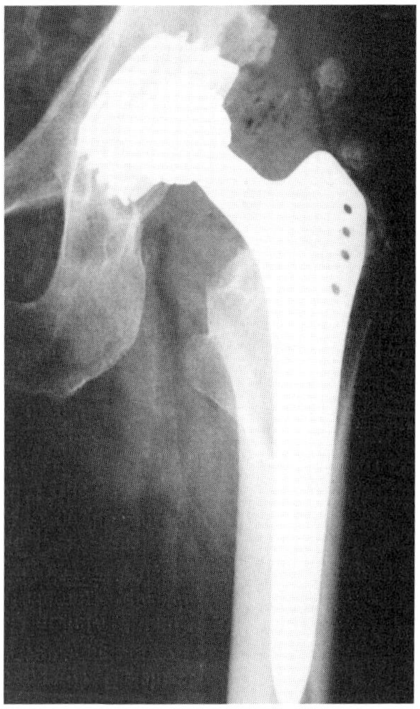

Fig. 1b

Figure 1a – Radiograph showing cementless implantation of a threaded cup with a polyethylene inlay articulating with a 32 mm ceramic head. There is severe wear of the polyethylene after ten years with osteolysis around the acetabular and femoral components. Both implants are stable without signs of loosening but with increasing pain in the groin. Figure 1b – Radiograph showing revision of the polyethylene inlay and the ceramic head with reimplantation of a metal-on-metal articulation. After revision there was complete relief of pain.

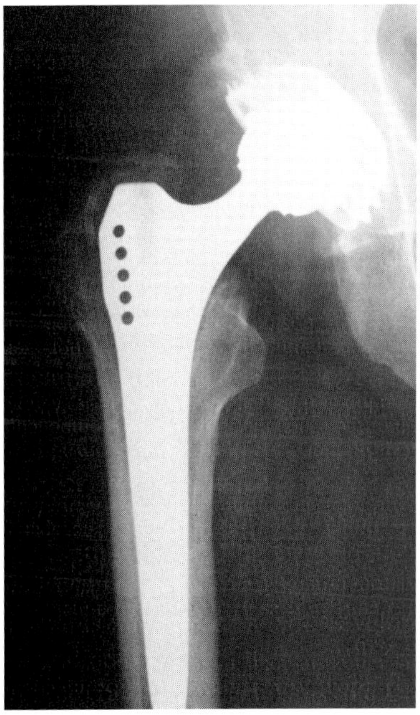

Fig. 2a

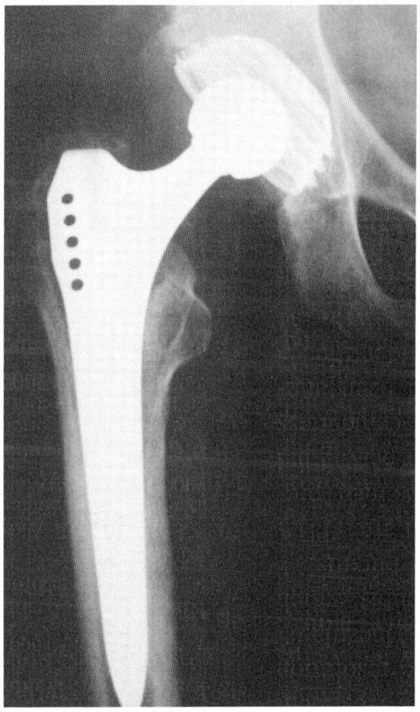

Fig. 2b

Figure 2a – Radiograph showing a threaded Bicon-cup with metal inlay, and a Zweymüller stem with a metal head 28 mm in diameter. Seven months after operation the patient had increasing pain in the groin. Because of a urinary infection, she was treated with antibiotics, but the pain persisted and an infection of the THA was suspected. Figure 2b – Radiograph three months after exchange of the metal inlay and the femoral stem. Histological evaluation showed no signs of bacterial infection but there was a massive lymphocyte reaction to macrophages, including wear particles which suggested an allergic reaction to metal wear.

and therefore appeared to be the most useful single test in the assessment of a painful THA.

A prerequisite of every evaluation is a careful history, particularly in regard to possible areas of infection within the body. Recently LaPorte et al[8] pointed out the importance of dental infection as a cause of concomitant infection of THA. Their findings showed that infection of THA may be more common than has been previously suspected and they recommended that patients with systemic diseases or those undergoing extensive dental procedures should be considered for prophylactic treatment with antibiotics before having dental treatment.

Impingement of components. Impingement between the acetabular and femoral components produces wear debris and results in osteolysis around the implant.[9] In their evaluation of 111 retrieved acetabular components from a single manufacturer, Yamaguchi et al[10] identified evidence of impingement in 39%. In all cases the posterior portion of the acetabulum was involved. They concluded that excessive anteversion of the cup combined with a relatively

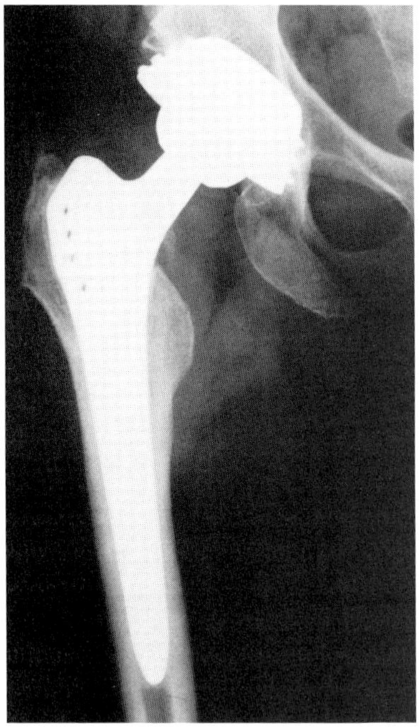

Fig. 3a

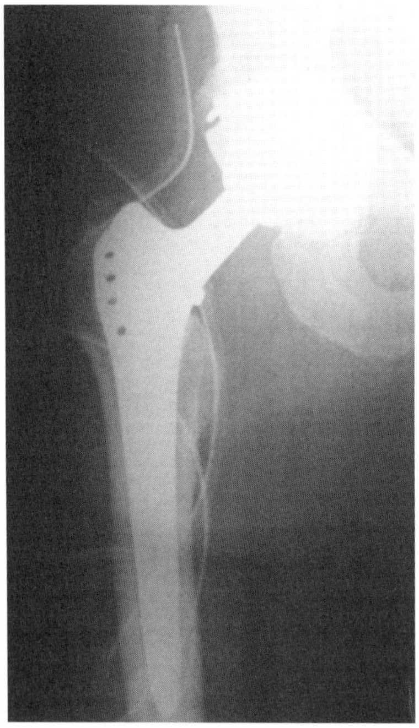

Fig. 3b

Figure 3a – Radiograph of a cementless threaded cup (Hofer-Imhof) metal inlay articulating with a 32 mm metal head of a cementless Alloclassic femoral prosthesis. Groin pain occurred in flexion of more than 100° and revision was indicated. Figure 3b – Intraoperative exposure of the joint showed impingement of the neck at 100° flexion because of neutral anteversion of the cup. The acetabular cup was changed to an Alloclassic cup, again using a metal inlay, but this time the cup was implanted in 20° of anteversion. The foreign body seen at the femoral neck is a broken part of the extraction instrument for the metal inlay.

small ratio of the head-to-neck diameter of the femoral components were the main factors involved. Similar results were presented by D'Lima et al[11] concerning the effect of the orientation of acetabular and femoral components on the range of motion of the hip. Bader and Willmann[12] evaluated failure of THA caused by a limited range of motion according to the design, positioning and wear of the implants. Iida et al[13] reported a case of metallosis resulting from impingement between the socket and the femoral neck in a metal-on-metal-bearing THA. They concluded that although every effort can be made to prevent impingement by positioning the components properly during the operation, it is impossible to avoid this complication in every patient, especially in those with a good preoperative range of motion. Therefore, in any case of unexplained pain in the hip, impingement of components should be considered as being responsible (Fig. 3).

PERIARTICULAR ORIGIN

The periarticular anatomical structures offer a variety of diagnostic possibilities and pitfalls in the diagnosis of a painful hip because of their complexity, especially in the inguinal region.[14] Pain after THA may be caused by affections of bone or soft tissues, tumours, nerve-entrapment syndromes, muscle imbalance due to different leg lengths or offset and impingement of soft tissue or bone.

Bony structures

Fatigue (stress) fractures. Those occurring in the pubic ramus after THA are rare complications.[15-19] McElfresh and Coventry[20] found two cases in their series of 5400 THAs. These stress fractures are often not apparent on the initial radiographs, but bone scanning can detect increased turnover in the fractured pubis. They are mostly of the compression type and heal quickly with non-weight-bearing. Adverse results were reported by Miller.[17] In his series of nine stress fractures of the ischiopubic region, none united. Rare cases of distraction-type fractures show delayed healing without sufficient formation of callus.[19]

Wear fractures. Periprosthetic wear-induced fractures of the acetabulum were reported by Sanchez-Sotelo, McGrory and Berry[21] around uncemented porous-coated acetabular components associated with osteolytic lesions. Because of the absence of injury or evidence of loosening, they can also be described as fatigue fractures, promoted by pelvic osteolysis. The osteolytic lesion is the first and only initial radiographic clue, and the classic signs of fracture may be missing. Chatoo, Parfitt and Pearse[22] described a case of a non-traumatic periprosthetic acetabular fracture associated with considerable osteolysis, which was managed successfully by addressing the osteolysis independently.

Osteolysis as a cause of periprosthetic fracture of the femur was described by Heekin, Engh and Herzwurm[23] in four patients who had sudden onset of hip pain 7 to 11 years after successful porous-coated cementless THA. Callaghan[24] reported an increase in the number of fractures because of long-term problems associated with osteolysis. Wirganowicz and Thomas[25] described a 66-year-old woman who sustained a pathological fracture of the femur secondary to extensive osteolysis distal to a press-fit femoral stem with a ceramic-on-ceramic bearing surface.

Heterotopic ossification. Periarticular ossification is a well-known cause of pain and impaired function after THA. Routine prophylaxis, including the use of non-steroidal

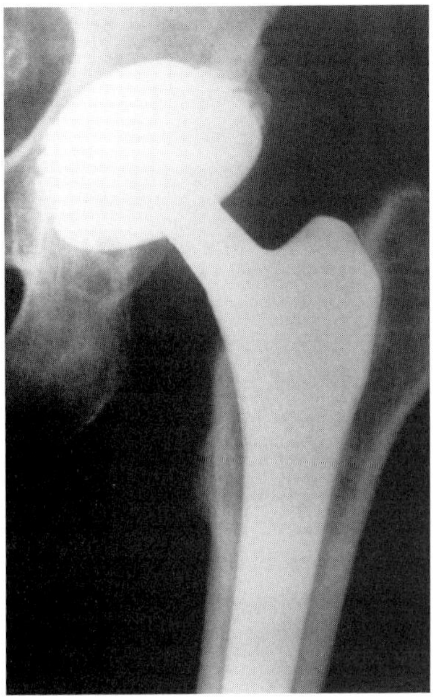

Fig. 4a

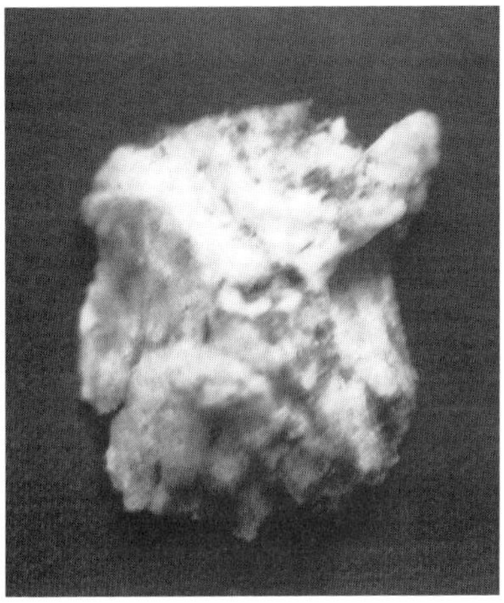

Fig. 4b

Figure 4a – Radiograph of a cementless THA of the left hip. Because of persistent pain at the greater trochanter despite numerous infiltrations of cortisone revision surgery was indicated. Osteolysis was demonstrated radiologically at the lateral trochanteric area. Figure 4b – Specimen of the resected part of the greater trochanter shows irregularity of the bony surface with sharp bony exostoses responsible for pain during movement. After surgery there was complete relief of pain.

antirheumatic drugs or radiation therapy, has reduced the incidence of these complications.[26-28] The ossification is easy to detect and classify on plain radiographs.[29]

Heterotopic ossification does not usually cause pain after maturation is complete and therefore there should be no indication for surgery within the first year after THA. There is evidence that pain and function improve after surgical revision with removal of the heterotopic bone. Wick et al[30] reported that over 90% of their patients had excellent relief from pain after excision of heterotopic bone followed by treatment with oral indomethacin, and Warren and Brooker[31] described 12 patients all of whom were free from pain after excision and low-dose radiation. By contrast, Cobb et al[32] reported unpredictable alleviation of pain in their series of 53 cases of symptomatic heterotopic ossification. Nevertheless, all of these studies described an improvement of function and range of motion.

Trochanteric osteotomy. The main risks of trochanteric osteotomy after the classical Charnley technique are proximal migration of the bone fragment, fibrous union and a painful limp. Although nonunion may be a cause of pain requiring revision, Hawkins, Midwinter and Macdonald[33] found no difference between patients with or without nonunion in terms of pain, function and general satisfaction. By contrast, other authors[34,35] view trochanteric osteotomy as a cause of persisting pain, partly from the nonunion itself and partly from trochanteric exostoses after the osteotomy.[36] To what extent painful trochanteric bursitis may be directly related to the presence of prominent fixation devices is still under discussion.[37] Trochanteric osteotomy should be reserved only for difficult cases and revision surgery.[36]

Soft tissues

Irritation of bursae. The most frequent location of painfully irritated bursae after THA is the greater trochanteric region, followed by the supra-acetabular area and the iliopsoas.[38] These bursae can be visualised by arthrography or injection of contrast media directly into the bursa. In most cases, MRI can detect irritated and therefore fluid-filled bursae. Diagnostic injection of local anaesthetic or corticosteroids gives additional information about the involvement of bursal structures in painful THA.

Bony spurs on the greater trochanter may also give rise to painful irritations of the bursa (Fig. 4). The reasons could be excessive scar formation after a lateral approach or increase of the offset after THA which produces higher pressure between the greater trochanter and tensor fasciae lata.

Bursitis of the iliopsoas is a clinical entity which is rarely encountered. It is most commonly observed in conjunction with rheumatoid arthritis or osteoarthritis of the hip.[39] Although there are no reports of this condition in conjunction with THA, it should be borne in mind for patients with hip pain of unknown origin.

Irritation of tendons and muscles. Impingement between the iliopsoas tendon or muscle and the anteromedial part of the acetabular component was reported by Lequesne et al[40] in six patients and Trousdale, Cabanela and Berry[41] in two. In both series the cause was a malpositioned cementless acetabular component. The symptoms can be provoked by active elevation of the lower limb, while passive mobility is normal and painless.

Kingzett Taylor et al[42] reported the results of an MRI study of patients presenting with pain in the buttock, lateral hip or groin. In most they found either tendinosis or partial or complete tears of the gluteus medius or minimus as the primary findings. Although this study was made in patients without THA, its importance is obvious especially for patients who have had THA in whom surgical exposure has taken place in this muscular region.

Tumours. Several reports deal with malignant tumours around a THA. These have included primary soft-tissue tumours such as malignant fibrous histiocytoma[43-45] malignant lymphoma[46,47] and soft-tissue sarcoma[48] as well as locally aggressive benign soft-tissue tumours, for example desmoid tumours.[49] Metastases at the site of a previous THA have been found to be responsible for thigh pain[50] and painful loosening of a cemented endoprosthesis.[51] When plain radiographs fail to detect osteolysis caused by malignant tissue, radionucleide bone scans or MRI may help to diagnose the malignant disease.[52] Aspiration of bone marrow or soft-tissue biopsy provides a definite diagnosis.

Nerve-entrapment syndromes. Delayed onset of palsy of the sciatic nerve after THA is rare, but there are case reports of various causes for nerve entrapment which range from fragments of methylmethacrylate, migrating trochanteric wires or entrapment after reconstruction with a pelvic plate.[53] Furthermore, cases have been reported of palsy of the obturator nerve in association with fixation of an acetabular reinforcement ring with transacetabular screws,[54] compression of the femoral nerve caused by extruded bone cement and meralgia paraesthetica (entrapment of the lateral cutaneous nerve) secondary to limb-length discrepancy.[55]

A painful bilateral piriformis syndrome was reported by Uchio et al[56] after THA. This syndrome is commonly attributed to entrapment of the sciatic nerve by a tense piriformis muscle with pain in the hip and especially the buttock. McCrory and Bell[57] suggested renaming the syndrome the 'deep gluteal syndrome' to take account of all the observed phenomena since they found that all the local symptoms were more likely to be due to compression of structures other than the sciatic nerve.

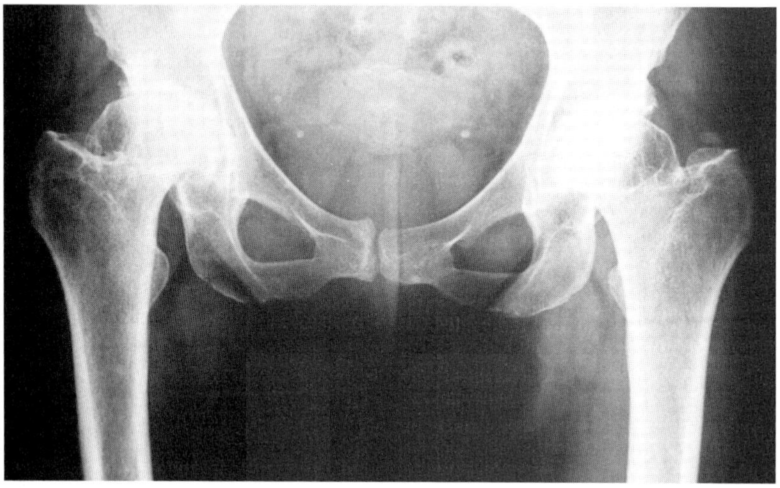

Fig. 5a

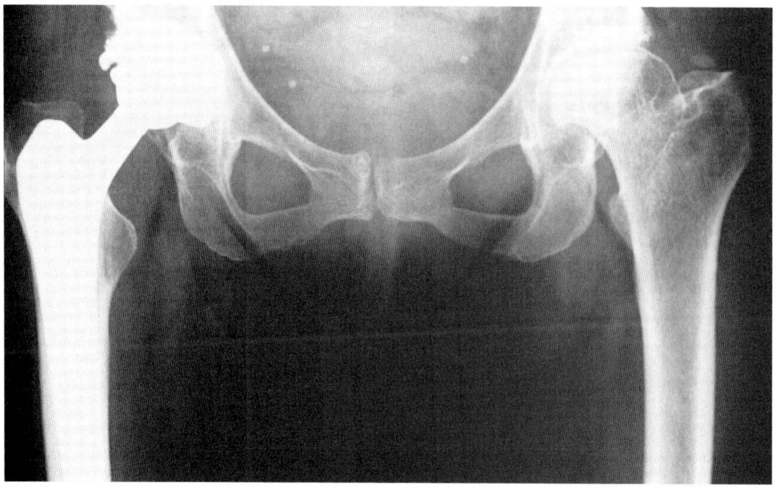

Fig. 5b

Figure 5a – Radiograph showing osteoarthritis of the right hip with narrowing of the joint space. Figure 5b – There was persistent pain in the hip after THA because of increased offset.

Muscular imbalance – leg length, offset. Marked increase in the femoral offset after THA may lead to pain probably caused by high pressure between the greater trochanter and the tensor fasciae lata as well as a higher tension within gluteus medius (Fig. 5).

Turula et al[58] reported that postoperative leg-length inequality was not only a cause of aseptic loosening, but also of otherwise unexplained pain.

Impingement of soft tissue or bone. Pain which persists in a hip after an otherwise successful THA may be due to impingement of soft tissues between bony prominences. Johnson[59] described two patients who had painful impingement between the lesser trochanter and the ischial ramus and who were relieved of their pain by excision of the lesser trochanter. We have recently found a similar case when pain was caused by impingement of the lesser trochanter after THA in a high dysplastic hip (Fig. 6).

A unique case concerning capsular impingement as a source of pain was seen by Schaffer, Wilson and Scott[60] in a bipolar THA. There are concerns regarding the extent and predictability of the relief of pain by this method. Although the source of postoperative pain is difficult to determine, in this case the authors achieved relief from the groin pain after capsulectomy since it was found intraoperatively that restricted movement was caused by prominent local fibrous tissue.

THIGH PAIN

Thigh pain is predominantly a problem after cementless THA. Its incidence with uncemented femoral components has been reported to be as high as 40%, mainly occurring in the first and second year after surgery with a steady decrease in symptoms with the passage of time.[61] The aetiology is unknown. Theories include inadequate fit or fixation of the femoral component within the femoral canal allowing micromovement, or excessive stress because of the rigidity of the implant.

Shape/size component. Using a wedge-shaped uncemented femoral component, Vresilovic, Hozack and Rothman[62] found that the incidence of thigh pain was significantly influenced by the size of the prosthesis and that in general thigh pain increased with stem size. They concluded that thigh pain has a high degree of correlation with the bending stiffness of the component. Increased stiffness of the prosthesis has the potential to create a more abrupt transmission of femoral bending at the top of the component. The importance of the shape of the implant was stressed by Burkart et al.[63] The results of their short-term clinical comparison suggested that a long, straight tapered design offered better initial stability than its anatomical counterparts, as reflected by the much lower incidence of thigh pain.

Fixation. Adequate fixation is one of the keys of successful cementless femoral stems. In the series reported by Engh and Massin[64] the incidence of thigh pain associated with a prosthesis which was stabilised by bone ingrowth was approximately 8%, whereas when stabilised by fibrous tissue it was 35%. To achieve stable fixation, many types of cementless endoprosthesis have been tried such as anatomical and straight stems either fully or proximally coated with hydroxyapatite, titanium or cobalt-chrome alloys, spherical beads, mesh, plasma-sprayed surfaces, fibre, metal and various textured surfaces.[65]

The importance of the shape, material and surface can be demonstrated by our own experience. For cementless stems we used first-generation tapered Zweymüller stems which had an incidence of thigh pain of approximately 15%. After modification of the design (SL-stem) this decreased to 1% to 2%.

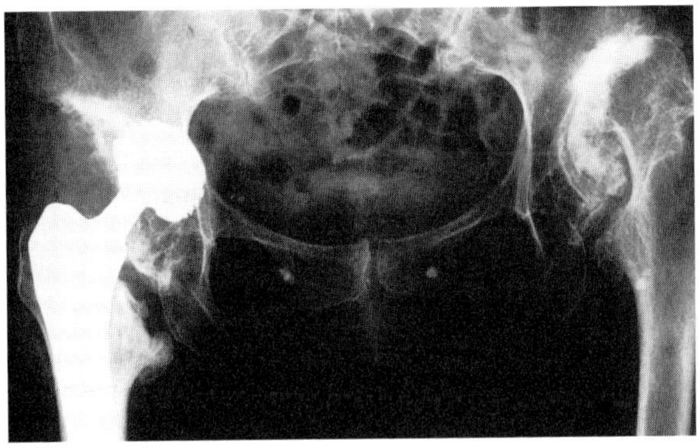

Fig. 6a

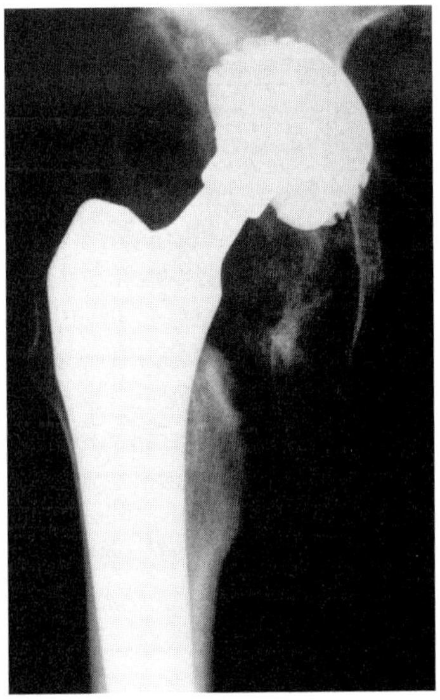

Fig. 6b

Figure 6a – Radiograph showing a THA in severe dysplastic osteoarthritis. There was a "feeling of impingement" in adduction and external rotation. Figure 6b – Radiograph showing revision to resect parts of the lesser trochanter and osteophytes of the lower part of the acetabulum. After the procedure the patient was free from pain in every position of movement.

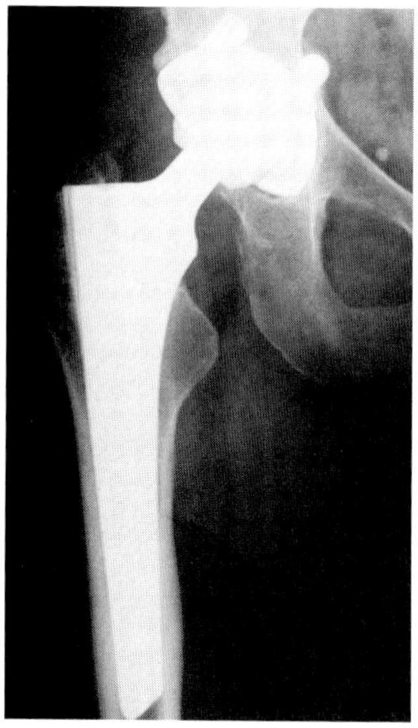

Fig. 7a

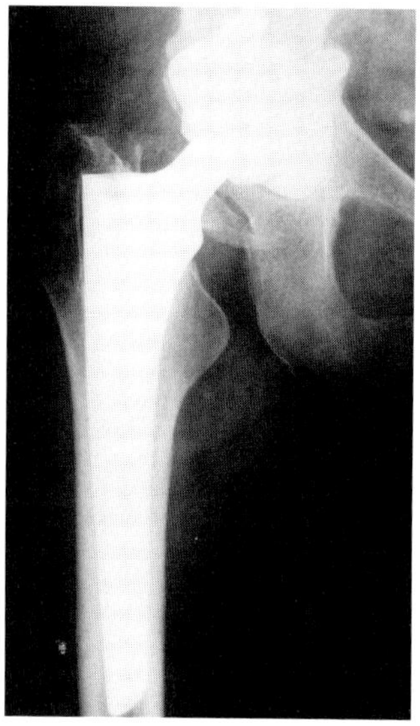

Fig. 7b

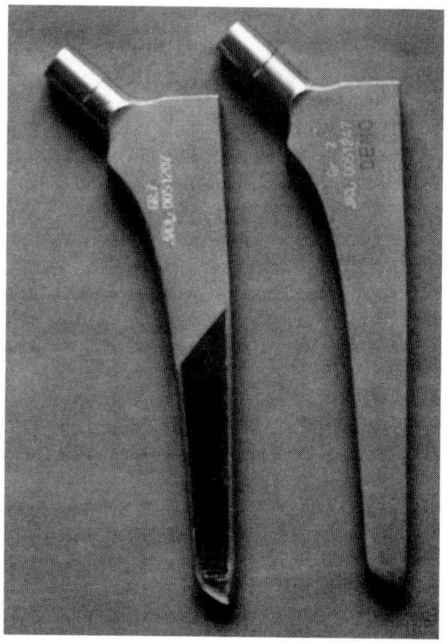

Fig. 7c

Figure 7a – Radiograph showing implantation of a cementless tapered titanium femoral stem, the proximal half rough-blasted, the distal half-polished. Because of resistant thigh pain without radiological signs of loosening revision was performed after two years. Figure 7b – At surgery the femoral stem was stable but easy to remove. After implantation of the same type and size of stem but fully rough-blasted, the patient reported complete relief from thigh pain. Figure 7c – Photograph of both stems.

We have also demonstrated the importance of adequate fixation in preventing thigh pain. We have used a proximally rough titanium stem which was polished distally. This gave an incidence of thigh pain of 20%. When revising some of these cases we found an implant which could be easily removed compared with totally rough-blasted stems. These implants were revised to a stem which was completely roughened. This was the only modification required to eliminate the thigh pain (Fig. 7).

Muscle hernia. This is a cause of disabling thigh pain that is relatively easy to diagnose and to prevent. Higgs et al[66] reported six patients who had thigh pain after THA which was due to a defect of the fascia lata and subsequent hernia of vastus lateralis. The patients complained of localised pain with activity including standing. They are able to localise the pain exactly and physical examination revealed a palpable defect in the fascia lata. Surgical repair gave immediate relief of symptoms in all patients.

Stress fractures. Eschenroeder and Krackow[67] described a case of late-onset stress fracture after THA caused by a cortical defect occupied by extruded polymethylmethacrylate. Pain started about 18 months after surgery. The patient was treated by removal of the extramedullary mass of cement and the bony defect was grafted with autogenous iliac bone.

Rare cases of stress fracture of the femur have been noted by Gill et al[68] and Lotke, Wong and Ecker.[69] In one, insufficiency fractures on the lateral femur occurred as a result of osteopenia and varus malposition of the femoral component with unexplained thigh and groin pain, and in the other a stress fracture occurred about a cortical window after revision of a THA.[69] Because of insufficient diagnostic information on plain radiography, tomography and radionucleide bone scanning were necessary to reveal the fracture.

LUMBAR SPINE

Concurrent disease of the hip and spine is common in the older population. For this reason the spine is one of the first areas to be examined if pain in the groin does not subside after THA. The term 'hip-spine syndrome' was created to describe this situation.[70] Symptoms from both sites give a confusing clinical picture and may require ancillary investigations to diagnose the major source of disability. Failure to recognise concurrent disease at both the hip and the spine may lead to misdiagnosis and possibly erroneous treatment. Obvious reasons may be nerve injury during THA or leg-length differences resulting in pelvic obliquity and consequent painful scoliosis. Less striking reasons which are not direct sequelae of surgery include radicular symptoms originating at L1 and L2,[71] spinal stenosis causing continued pain and disability,[72] spinal lesions with a pseudoradicular pain syndrome,[73] and referred pain in the groin.[74]

Radicular symptoms. The neurological evaluation of the hip must include the D12 level since sensory disturbances of the groin may be attributed to this source. Motor weakness of the iliopsoas muscle is seen in severe radicular lesions of D12 to L2. Any segmental pathology at these levels, such as disc prolapse, infection or tumour, simulates hip disease.[71] Sciatica is common after THA.[72] Evaluation

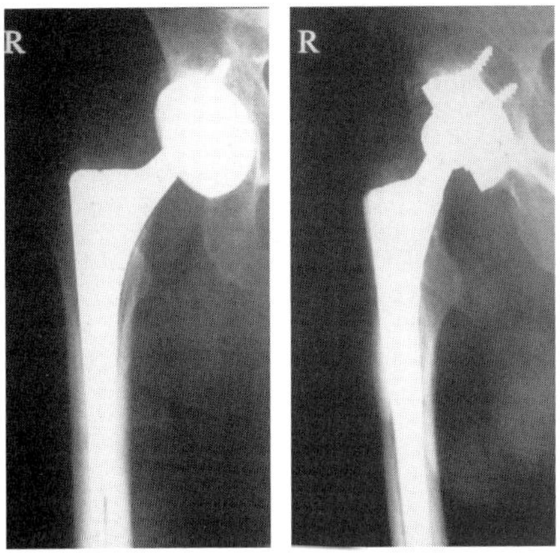

Fig. 8a

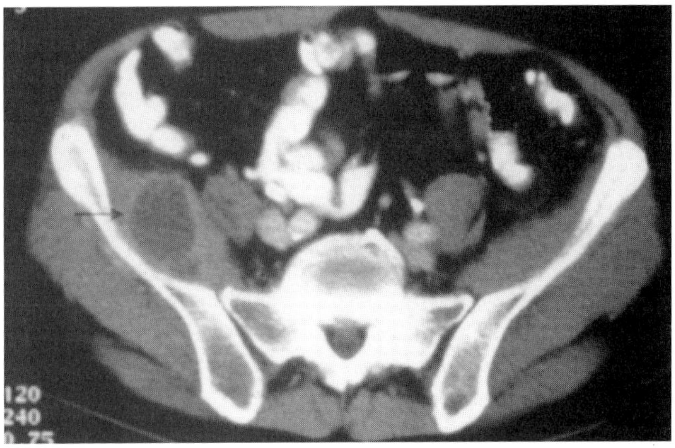

Fig. 8b

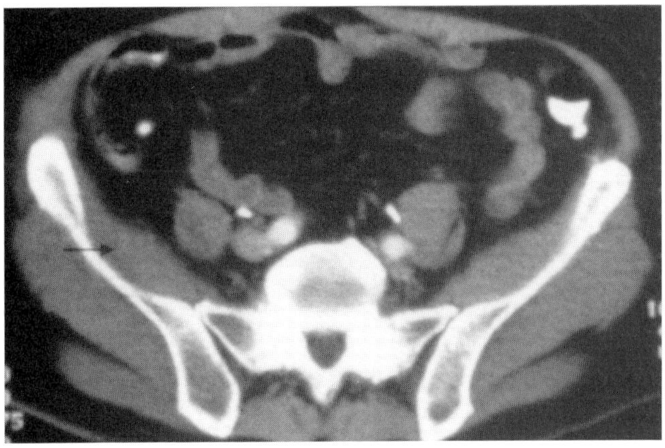

Fig. 8c

Figure 8a – Radiographs of a cementless THA two years after operation. There was hip pain with clinical signs of infection but joint aspiration was negative. Figure 8b – CT shows a cystic lesion within the iliacus muscle. Figure 8c – CT-guided drainage of the cyst (arrows) gave relief from pain.

should be supported by precise neurological examination including electrophysiological diagnosis to exclude particular nerve lesions or root pathology.

Spinal stenosis. Stenosis of the vertebral canal with clinical symptoms radiating to both legs and decreased walking distance is a well-known condition. If symptoms are not typical, or mainly unilateral, confusion with hip abnormality is possible,[72] and treatment of the hip is carried out first instead of the spine.[75] In lumbar spinal stenosis nerve injury after THA is more common.[76] It is suggested that a double-crush injury at the spine and hip will be symptomatic, even when each injury alone may not produce a sufficient reduction in axoplasmatic flow. Spinal decompressive surgery is an option for some patients with persistent pain after THA. Even nerve injuries may benefit from root decompression at stenotic levels.[76]

Spinal lesions with pseudoradicular pain syndromes. Pseudoradicular pain arises in soft tissue such as ligaments, muscles, joint capsules and other structures. It usually radiates to both legs if its origin is in the lumbar spine. There is no clear radicular distribution, but it often occurs along connected muscle and fascial layers.[73] The pain drawings done in patients with pseudoradicular pain are often very similar to those of radicular symptoms, but the patients lack definite neurological dysfunction. Radiation along the dorsal hip and lateral thigh to the knee is very common, thus simulating hip pathology. Only meticulous clinical investigation allows differentiation of these symptoms.

Referred pain in the groin. Stimulation of the ventral annulus fibrosus and the ventral longitudinal ligament has been shown to cause pain in the groin.[74] The exact mechanism of this referred pain is not known. There is evidence that it follows the embryological sclerotome, but there are many different schemata of these and none of the authors described methods of investigating them.[77-80] Pain at the hip is attributed to stimulation from the segmental units L3 to L5.[81] The capsule of the facet joint is another structure which causes pain radiating to the hip and greater trochanter.[82]

INTRA-ABDOMINAL

Intra-abdominal conditions can be the cause of referred patterns of pain in the hip. Therefore, if all other reasons for pain are excluded, careful examination and selective diagnostic assessment of this area should be performed.

Urological. Urological complications associated with THA have been reported mainly as single case reports. Tremps Velazquez et al[83] described a case of ureterohydronephrosis arising from extrinsic compression of the ureter by the cement used in THA in a patient with a solitary kidney. They concluded that the risk of acetabular perforation and subsequent migration of the cement into the pelvic cavity must be taken into account in patients undergoing THA. Waters et al[84] reported the delayed presentation of ureteric injury after thermal damage at THA, and Bamelis, De Graeve and Baert[85] presented a case of ureteric obstruction secondary to THA. Sheafor et al[86] discussed the possibility of scrotal pathology as a cause of hip pain and described three cases.

Gynaecological. Endometriosis is a disorder caused by actively growing and functioning endometrial tissue in aberrant sites outside the uterus, and endometriosis of the pelvis should be included into the differential diagnosis of hip pain. Silver and Jokl[87] presented a premenopausal woman in whom MRI showed evidence of bilateral intrapelvic endrometriosis adjacent to both acetabula. Treatment with cyclic hormonal suppressive therapy gave resolution of her symptoms. Pellegrini, Pasternak and Macaulay[88] reported two cases of endometrioma of the pubis which were erroneously misdiagnosed as iliopectineal bursitis.

A rare case of a gynaecological complication after THA was described by Howell.[89] A 77-year-old woman presented with right-sided pelvic pain and irregular pervaginal bleeding. Ten years earlier she had had a right cementless THA. The press-fit acetabular component had been augmented by screws. Radiological investigation identified a mass in the right iliac fossa. This communicated with the hip joint via a track formed by a fixation screw that had penetrated the medial wall of the acetabulum at the THA.

Gastrointestinal. The most common intra-abdominal lesion mimicking hip pain is an inguinal hernia. Chronic pain in the area of the hip is not only a preoperative symptom of a typical hernia, but may also be a problem after its surgical repair.[90]

An intra-abdominal septic cyst of the iliacus muscle with pain in the hip after THA was reported by Ascherl.[91] Needle biopsy and bone scanning provided no evidence of infection at the site of the implant and CT was performed. Surprisingly, the authors found a huge cystic lesion in the iliacus muscle. Needle biopsy and drainage gave immediate relief of pain. Culture confirmed infection with *Staphylococcus aureus* (Fig. 8).

CONCLUSIONS

Well-fixed components in THA do not guarantee a pain-free hip. Although radiological evaluation confirms a stable implant, there are many reasons why patients report pain and tenderness in the groin and thigh. Evaluation should include clinical examination, radiography, CT, MRI, scintigraphy, needle biopsy (joint, soft tissues) and bacteriological cultures which will determine the cause. Only rare cases of enigmatic pain will remain unsolved.

REFERENCES

1. **Fisher J, Ingham E, Stone MH, et al.** Wear particle morphologies in artificial hip joints: particle size is critical in the response of macrophages. In: Rieker C, Windler M, Wyss U, eds. *Metasul, a metal-on-metal bearing.* Bern: Hans Huber, 1999:121-4.
2. **Minakawa H, Stone MH, Wroblewski BM, Ingham E, Fisher J.** Quantification of third body damage and its effect on UHMWPE wear with different types of femoral heads. *Trans ORS* 1997.
3. **Rieker C, Windler M, Wyss U.** *Metasul, a metal-on-metal bearing.* Bern: Hans Huber, 1999.
4. **Maury Ph, Gagneux E, Gautier F, Didelot S.** Why selecting the ceramic on ceramic bearing couple? In: Willmann G, Zweymüller K, eds. *Bioceramics in hip joint replacement.* Procs 5th International Ceram Tec Symposium. 2000:16-8.
5. **Clarke IC, Good V, Schuldies J, Schroeder D, Gustafson A.** *Zirconia simulated wear performance up to 15 Mc in serum lubricant.* Zirconia Femoral Heads Symposium, Society for Biomaterials Hawaii, 2000.
6. **Harris WH.** Global overview of highly cross-linked PE. *World Tribology Forum,* Montreux-Switzerland, 2000.
7. **Levitsky KA, Hozack WJ, Balderston RA, et al.** Evaluation of the painful prosthetic joint: relative value of bone scan, sedimentation rate, and joint aspiration. *J Arthroplasty* 1991;6:237-44.
8. **LaPorte DM, Waldman BJ, Mont MA, Hungerford DS.** Infections associated with dental procedures in total hip arthroplasty. *J Bone Joint Surg [Br]* 1999;81-B:56-9.
9. **Klapperich C, Graham J, Pruitt L, Ries MD.** Failure of a metal-on-metal total hip arthroplasty from progressive osteolysis. *J Arthroplasty* 1999;14:877-81.
10. **Yamaguchi M, Akisue T, Bauer TW, Hashimoto Y.** The spatial location of impingement in total hip arthroplasty. *J Arthroplasty* 2000;15:305-13.
11. **D'Lima DD, Urquhart AG, Buehler KO, Walker RH, Colwell CW.** The effect of the orientation of the acetabular and femoral components on the range of motion of the hip at different head-neck ratios. *J Bone Joint Surg [Am]* 2000;82-A:315-21.
12. **Bader R, Willmann G.** Einschränkung der Range of Motion von Hüftendoprothesen durch Design, Position und Pfannenabrieb. In: Willmann G, Zweymüller K, eds. *Bioceramics in hip joint replacement.* Procs 5th International Ceram Tec Sympsoium, 2000:66-74.
13. **Iida H, Kaneda E, Takada H, et al.** Metallosis due to impingement between the socket and the femoral neck in a metal-on-metal bearing total hip prosthesis: a case report. *J Bone Joint Surg [Am]* 1999;81-A:400-3.
14. **Van den Berg JC, Rutten MJ, de Valois JC, Jansen JB, Rosenbusch G.** Masses and pain in the groin: a review of imaging findings. *Eur Radiol* 1998;8:911-21.
15. **Launder WJ, Hungerford DS.** Stress fracture of the pubis after total hip arthroplasty. *Clin Orthop* 1981;159:183-5.
16. **Oh I, Hardacre JA.** Fatigue fracture of the inferior pubis ramus following total hip replacement for congenital hip dislocation. *Clin Orthop* 1980;147:154-6.
17. **Miller AJ.** Late fracture of the acetabular after total hip replacement. *J Bone Joint Surg [Br]* 1972;54-B:600-6.
18. **Resnick D, Guerra J Jr.** Stress fractures of the inferior pubic ramus following hip surgery. *Radiology* 1980;137:355-8.
19. **Hallel T, Malkin C.** Fatigue fracture of the pubic ramus following total hip arthroplasty with unusual delayed healing. *Clin Orthop* 1982;166:162-4.
20. **McElfresh EC, Coventry MB.** Femoral and pelvic fractures after total hip arthroplasty. *J Bone Joint Surg [Am]* 1974;56-A:483-92.
21. **Sanchez-Sotelo J, McGrory BJ, Berry DJ.** Acute periprosthetic fracture of the acetabulum associated with osteolytic pelvic lesions: a report of 3 cases. *J Arthroplasty* 2000;15:126-30.
22. **Chatoo M, Parfitt J, Pearse MF.** Periprosthetic acetabular fracture associated with extensive osteolysis. *J Arthroplasty* 1998;13:843-5.
23. **Heekin RD, Engh CA, Herzwurm PJ.** Fractures through cystic lesions of the greater trochanter: a cause of late pain after cementless total hip arthroplasty. *J Arthroplasty* 1996;11:757-60.
24. **Callaghan JJ.** Periprosthetic fractures of the acetabulum during and following total hip arthroplasty. *J Bone Joint Surg [Am]* 1997;79-A:1416-21.
25. **Wirganowicz PZ, Thomas BJ.** Massive osteolysis after ceramic on ceramic total hip arthroplasty. *Clin Orthop* 1997;338:100-4.

26. **Knahr K, Salzer M, Eyb R, Frank P, Blauensteiner W.** Heterotopic ossification with total hip endoprostheses in various models of thrombosis prophylaxis. *J Arthroplasty* 1988;3:1-8.

27. **Kjaersgaard-Andersen P, Ritter MA.** Prevention of formation of heterotopic bone after total hip arthroplasty. *J Bone Joint Surg [Am]* 1991;73-A:942-7.

28. **Maloney WJ, Jasty M, Willett C, Mulroy RD Jr, Harris WH.** Prophylaxis for heterotopic bone formation after total hip arthroplasty using low-dose radiation in high-risk patients. *Clin Orthop* 1992;280:230-4.

29. **Brooker AF, Bowerman JW, Robinson RA, Riley LH Jr.** Ectopic ossification following total hip replacement: incidence and method of classification. *J Bone Joint Surg [Am]* 1973;55-A:1629-32.

30. **Wick M, Muller EJ, Hahn MP, Muhr G.** Surgical excision of heterotopic bone after hip surgery followed by oral indomethacin application: is there a clinical benefit for the patient? *Arch Orthop Trauma Surg* 1999;119:151-5.

31. **Warren SB, Brooker AF Jr.** Excision of heterotopic bone followed by irradiation after total hip arthroplasty. *J Bone Joint Surg [Am]* 1992;74-A:201-10.

32. **Cobb TK, Berry DJ, Wallrichs SL, Ilstrup DM, Morrey BF.** Functional outcome of excision of heterotopic ossification after total hip arthroplasty. *Clin Orthop* 1999;361:131-9.

33. **Hawkins A, Midwinter K, Macdonald DA.** Trochanteric nonunion in revision total hip arthroplasty: does it matter? *Ann R Coll Surg Engl* 2000;82:39-42.

34. **Simank HG, Chatzipanagiotis C, Kaps HP.** Complication rate following trochanteric osteotomy in total hip endoprosthesis: a retrospective study with failure analysis. *Z Orthop Ihre Grenzgeb* 1996;134:457-64.

35. **Volz RG, Brown FW.** The painful migrated ununited greater trochanter in total hip replacement. *J Bone Joint Surg [Am]* 1977;59-A: 1091-3.

36. **Needoff M, Milligan GF.** Trochanteric exostoses following total hip arthroplasty: a complication of trochanteric osteotomy. *J Arthroplasty* 1991;6 Suppl:83-4.

37. **Glassman AH.** Complications of trochanteric osteotomy. *Orthop Clin North Am* 1992;23:321-3.

38. **Berquist TH, Bender CE, Maus TP, Ward EM, Rand JA.** Pseudobursae: a useful finding in patients with painful hip arthroplasty. *AJR Am J Roentgenol* 1987;148:103-6.

39. **Fortin L, Belanger R.** Bursitis of the iliopsoas: four cases with pain as the only clinical indicator. *J Rheumatol* 1995;22:1971-3.

40. **Lequesne M, Dang M, Montagne P, Lemoine A, Witvoet J.** Conflict between psoas and total hip prosthesis. *Rev Rhum Mal Osteoartic* 1991;58:559-64.

41. **Trousdale RT, Cabanela ME, Berry DJ.** Anterior iliopsoas impingement after total hip arthroplasty. *J Arthroplasty* 1995;10:546-9.

42. **Kingzett Taylor A, Tirman PF, Feller J, et al.** Tendinosis and tears of gluteus medius and minimus muscles as a cause of hip pain: MR imaging findings. *AJR Am J Roentgenol* 1999;173:1123-6.

43. **Tait NP, Hacking PM, Malcolm AJ.** Case reports: malignant fibrous histiocytoma occurring at the site of a previous total hip replacement. *Br J Radiol* 1988;61:73-6.

44. **Swann M.** Malignant soft-tissue tumour at the site of a total hip replacement. *J Bone Joint Surg [Br]* 1984;66-B:629-31.

45. **Cole BJ, Schultz E, Smilari TF, Hajdu SI, Krauss ES.** Malignant fibrous histiocytoma at the site of a total hip replacement: review of the literature and case report. *Skeletal Radiol* 1997;26:559-63.

46. **Ito H, Shimizu A.** Malignant lymphoma at the site of a total hip replacement. *Orthopedics* 1999;22:82-4.

47. **Radhi JM, Ibrahiem K, al-Tweigeri T.** Soft tissue malignant lymphoma at sites of previous surgery. *J Clin Pathol* 1998;51:629-32.

48. **Langkamer VG, Case CP, Collins C, et al.** Tumors around implants. *J Arthroplasty* 1997;12:812-8.

49. **Gebhart M, Fourmarier M, Meymans O, et al.** Development of a desmoid tumor at the site of a total hip replacement. *Acta Orthop Belg* 1999;65:230-4.

50. **Jeffery JA, McCullough CJ.** Metastasis as a cause of pain after total hip arthroplasty: a case report. *Orthopaedics Int* 1995;4:341-2.

51. **Allain J, Le Mouel S, Voicin MC, Delepine G, Goutallier D.** The importance of systematic histological examination after loosening of an implant. *J Bone Joint Surg [Br]* 1998;80-B:591-4.

52. **Czerny C, Krestan C, Imhof H, Trattnig S.** Magnetic resonance imaging of the postoperative hip. *Top Magn Reson Imaging* 1999;10:214-20.

53. **Stiehl JB, Stewart WA.** Late sciatic nerve entrapment following pelvic plate reconstruction in total hip arthroplasty. *J Arthroplasty* 1998;13:586-8.

54. **Fricker RM, Troeger H, Pfeiffer KM.** Obturator nerve palsy due to fixation of an acetabular reinforcement ring with transacetabular screws: a case report. *J Bone Joint Surg [Am]* 1997;79-A:444-6.

55. **Goel A.** Meralgia paresthetica secondary to limb length discrepancy: case report. *Arch Phys Med Rehabil* 1999;80:348-9.

56. **Uchio Y, Nishikawa U, Ochi M, Shu N, Takata K.** Bilateral priformis syndrome after total hip arthroplasty. *Arch Orthop Trauma Surg* 1998;117:177-9.

57. **McCrory P, Bell S.** Nerve entrapment syndromes as a cause of pain in the hip, groin and buttock. *Sports Med* 1999;27:261-74.

58. **Turula KB, Friberg O, Lindholm TS, Tallroth K, Vankka E.** Leg length inequality after total hip arthroplasty. *Clin Orthop* 1986;202:163-8.

59. **Johnson KA.** Impingement of the lesser trochanter on the ischial ramus after total hip arthroplasty. *J Bone Joint Surg [Am]* 1977;59-A:268-9.

60. **Schaffer JL, Wilson MG, Scott RD.** Capsular impingement as a source of pain following bipolar hip arthroplasty. *J Arthroplasty* 1991;6:163-8.

61. **Hellman EJ, Capello WN, Feinberg JR.** Omnifit cementless total hip arthroplasty: a 10-year average follow-up. *Clin Orthop* 1999; 364:164-74.

62. **Vresilovic EJ, Hozack WJ, Rothman RH.** Incidence of thigh pain after uncemented total hip arthroplasty as a function of femoral stem size. *J Arthroplasty* 1996;11:304-11.

63. **Burkart BC, Bourne RB, Rorabeck CH, Kirk PG.** Thigh pain in cementless total hip arthroplasty: a comparison of two systems at 2 years' follow-up. *Orthop Clin North Am* 1993;24:645-53.

64. **Engh CA, Massin P.** Cementless total hip arthroplasty using the anatomic medullary locking stem: results using a survivorship analysis. *Clin Orthop* 1989;249:141-58.

65. **Mont MA, Hungerford DS.** Proximally coated ingrowth prostheses: a review. *Clin Orthop* 1997;344:139-49.

66. **Higgs JED, Chong A, Haertsch P, Sekel R, Leicester A.** An unusual cause of thigh pain after total hip arthroplasty. *J Arthroplasty* 1995;10:203-4.

67. **Eschenroeder HC, Krackow KA.** Late onset femoral stress fracture associated with extruded cement following hip arthroplasty: a case report. *Clin Orthop* 1988;236:210-3.

68. **Gill TJ, Sledge JB, Orler R, Ganz R.** Lateral insufficiency fractures of the femur caused by osteopenia and varus angulation: a complication of total hip arthroplasty. *J Arthroplasty* 1999;14:982-7.

69. **Lotke PA, Wong RY, Ecker ML.** Stress fractures as a cause of chronic pain following revision total hip arthroplasty: report of two cases. *Clin Orthop* 1986;206:147-50.

70. **Offierski CM, MacNab I.** Hip-spine syndrome. *Spine* 1983;8: 316-21.

71. **Austin RT.** Spinal lesions simulating hip joint disorders. *Clin Rheumatol* 1990;9:414-20.

72. **Bohl WR, Steffee AD.** Lumbar spinal stenosis: a cause of continued pain and disability in patients after total hip arthroplasty. *Spine* 1979;4:168-73.

73. **Breck LW.** Preliminary report on total hip joint replacement with Urist-Thompson unit without cement. *Clin Orthop* 1970;72:174-6.

74. **Takahashi Y, Sato A, Nakamura SI, Suseki K, Takahashi K.** Regional correspondence between the ventral portion of the intervertebral disc and the groin mediated by a spinal reflex: a possible basis of discogenic referred pain. *Spine* 1998;23:1853-8.

75. **De la Caffiniere JY, Rocolle J.** Arthrotic lumbar spinal canal stenosis and total hip prosthesis. *Rev Chir Orthop Rep Appar Mot* 1983;69:323-31.

76. **Pritchett JW.** Lumbar decompression to treat foot drop after hip arthroplasty. *Clin Orthop* 1994;303:173-7.

77. **Inman VT, Saunders JB de CM.** Referred pain from skeletal structures. *J Nerv Ment Dis* 1944;99:660-7.

78. **De Palma A, Rothman RH.** *The intervertebral disc.* In: Krämer J, ed. Bandscheiben-bedingte Erkrankungen. Stuttgart:Verlage Thieme, 1978.

79. **Maitland GD.** *Manipulation der Wirbelsäule 2.* Aufl. Berlin, Heidelberg, New York: Verlag Springer, 1994.

80. **König G, Wancura I.** *Praxis und Theorie der neuen chinesischen Akupunktur.* Bd. 1, 3.Aufl. Wien, München, Bern: Maudrich, 1995:57-60.

81. **Rhode J.** Zervikales und lumbales Radikulärsyndrom. *Manuelle Medizin* 1997;35:313-8.

82. **Mooney V, Robertson J.** The facet syndrome. *Clin Orthop* 1976;115:149-56.

83. **Tremps Velazquez E, Ramon Dalmau M, Garcia Rojo D, Cardona Carbonell S.** Ureteral stenosis secondary to methacrylate used in total hip arthroplasty. *Arch Esp Urol* 1995;48:741-3.

84. **Waters E, Bouchier Hayes DM, Hickey D.** Delayed presentation of ureteric injury after thermal insult at total hip replacement. *Br J Urol* 1998;82:594.

85. **Bamelis BF, De Graeve NR, Baert LV.** Ureteric obstruction secondary to total hip prosthesis. *Br J Urol* 1998;81:333.

86. **Sheafor DH, Holder LE, Thompson D, et al.** Scrotal pathology as the cause for hip pain: diagnostic findings on bone scintigraphy. *Clin Nucl Med* 1997;22:287-91.

87. **Silver MD, Jokl P.** Endometriosis of the pelvis presenting as hip pain: a case report. *Clin Orthop* 1999;368:207-11.

88. **Pellegrini VD, Pasternak HS, Macaulay WP.** Endometrioma of the pubis: a differential in the diagnosis of hip pain. *J Bone Joint Surg [Am]* 1981;63-A:1333-4.

89. **Howell GE.** Pelvic synovial cyst formation secondary to perforation of the quadrilateral plate: a case report. *J R Nav Med Serv* 1999;85:172-3.

90. **Callesen T, Bech K, Kehlet H.** Prospective study of chronic pain after groin hernia repair. *Br J Surg* 1999;86:1528-31.

91. **Ascherl R.** Der BEO-Schaft: 3-Jahresergebnisse: Möglichkeiten, Grenzen und Differentialindikationen. *Syposium: Evolution in der zementfreien Hüftendoprothetik.* München, 2000.

RECONSTRUCTION OF CONGENITALLY DISLOCATED HIPS IN ADULTS BY AN ARTHROPLASTY

THEODORE A. XENAKIS

From the University of Ioannina, Greece

The treatment of neglected congenital dislocation of the hip (CDH) by replacement arthroplasty is now well established, but the indications for this type of surgery, the technique to be followed and the subsequent rehabilitation are still open to debate.

There is considerable uncertainty regarding the term 'CDH'. Given that the dislocation comprises only one part of the pathology of the joint, the term 'congenital hip disease' with the consequent classification into dysplasia and higher and lower dislocation (Fig. 1) is preferred, as proposed by Hartofilakidis, Stamos and Ioannidis.[1] The surgical treatment is much more difficult in dislocation than in dysplasia.

The orthopaedic surgeon should bear in mind that he or she is not treating an anatomically normal hip but one which has many diverse abnormalities and even absence of the joint. These anatomical abnormalities affect the muscles as well as the skeleton. The spine and the knees may also present with abnormalities secondary to the condition of the hip. The surgeon may have to remodel the affected joint and also the skeleton of the lower limbs.

INDICATIONS FOR ARTHROPLASTY

Pain in the affected hip is not the only indication for surgery. The problems of abnormal gait and the effects of the limb-length discrepancy on the spine, the knees and the other hip, as well as on the patient's quality of life, should be seriously considered. The advantages and disadvantages of surgery as well as its complications should be discussed with the patient so that he or she is fully aware of the related problems.

The patient's age is an important factor in this decision. Increased wear in hip arthroplasty is well established in patients less than 50 years of age and it is reasonable to anticipate similar problems in patients who have had arthroplasty for CDH.[2-5] Because of the small numbers of such patients in reported series, it is not easy to draw conclusions about the survivorship of these operations and there is still intense speculation about the difficulties of their revision. However, young age remains a strong negative indication. Regular follow-up is of value and if the pain is treatable, the limp is not severe and there are no or only mild effects on other joints, it is best to delay the operation and to advise the patient to follow a conservative way of life, keep a low body-weight and undergo a programme of continuing physiotherapy, especially swimming.

PREOPERATIVE PLANNING

The clinical examination of the patient is most important. This should include evaluation and recording of the range

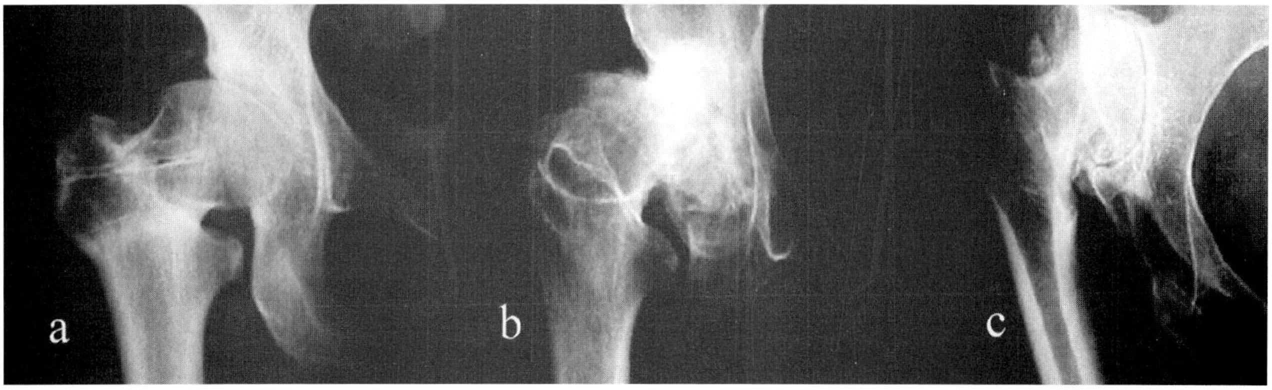

Fig. 1

Radiographs showing the classification of Hartofilakidis et al[1] into a) dysplasia, b) low dislocation and c) high dislocation.

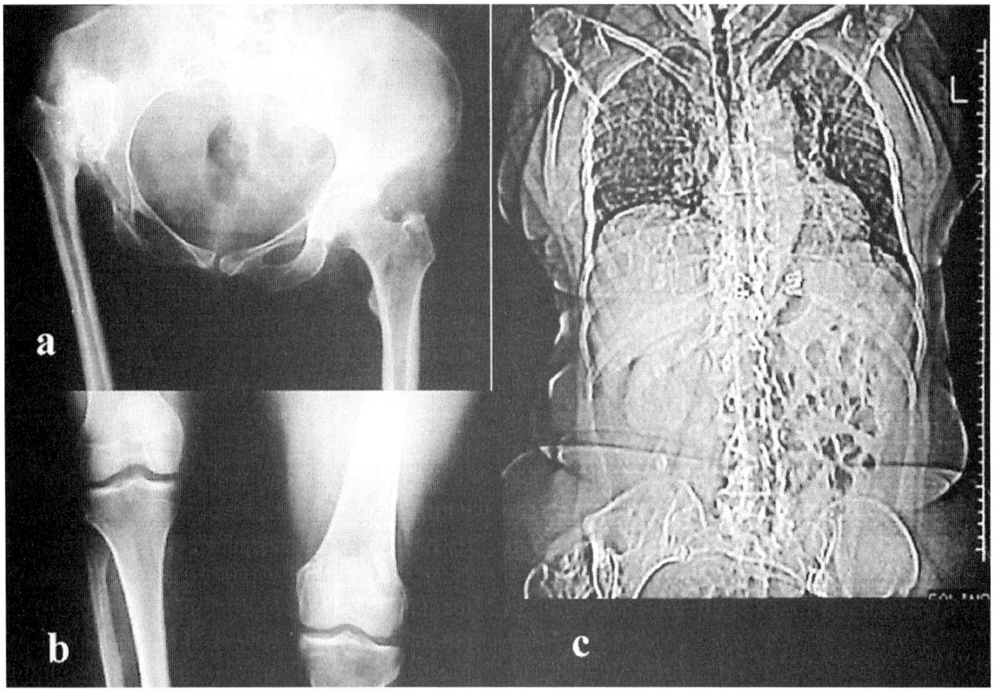

Fig. 2

Radiographs showing a) high dislocation of the right hip, b) the position of the knees and c) tilting of the pelvis and scoliosis of the spine.

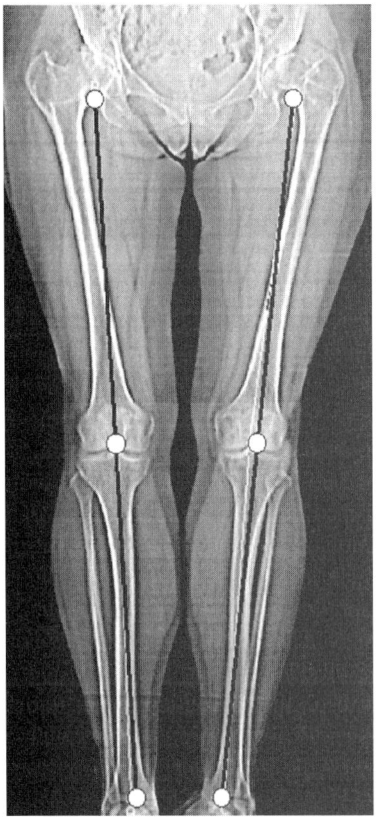

Fig. 3

Electronically reconstructed image of the skeleton of the lower limbs (topogram). This allows accurate measurement of bone length.

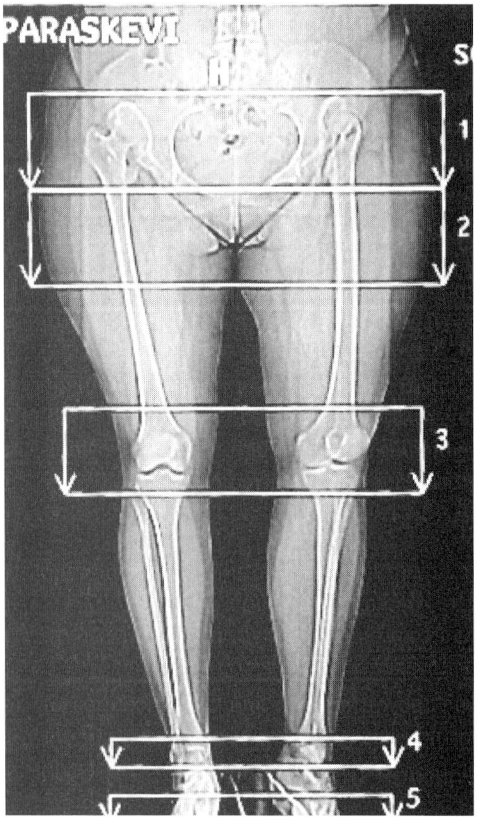

Fig. 4

The regions of transverse slices taken by CT. At region 1 the interval between slices is every 5 mm and in others every 10 mm.

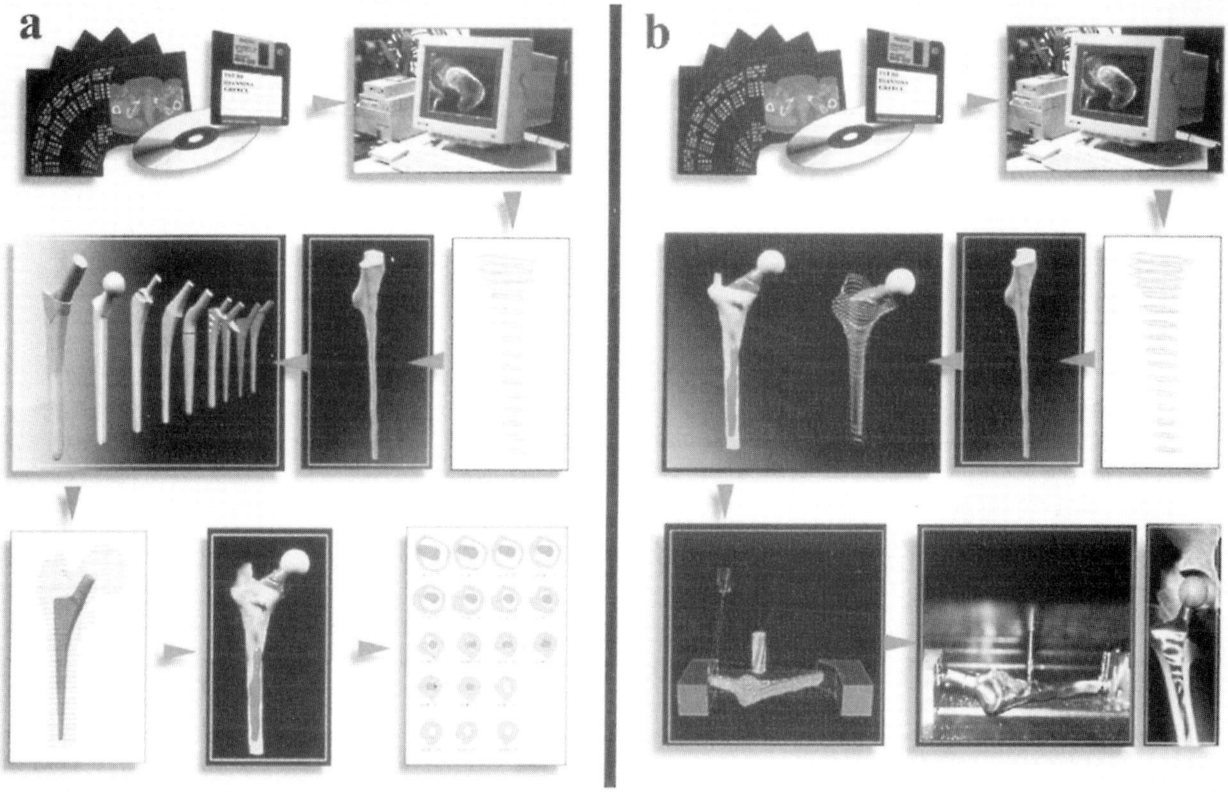

Fig. 5

Computerised procedure for a) selection of the femoral stem and simulated implantation and b) the manufacture of a customised stem (with permission of TST Ltd, Ioannina, Greece).

of movement of the joints, the muscle strength, the pain noted during examination, the position at rest of each joint and the difference in limb length. Careful examination of the spine is absolutely essential and the presence of scoliosis should be noted with possibilities for its correction in relation to the difference in leg length, the degree of lumbar lordosis and the position of the pelvis. Flexion deformity of the hip and the vascular and neurological status of the lower limbs should be noted.

Radiological examination (Fig. 2). This should include AP radiographs of the hips and pelvis, lateral radiographs of the hips, AP and lateral views of the lumbar spine and AP radiographs of the spine in flexion to the right and left as well as views in forward flexion and extension in order to examine the flexibility of the spine and the potential for correction of scoliosis. Finally, radiographs should be taken of the entire lower limb so that the axial deviations of the knees can be calculated and the length of each limb checked.

Examination by CT. Measurement of the lengths is better performed by CT (Fig. 3) and the use of this imaging is of much value in the detailed planning of the operation.[6-8] Patients are examined in the supine position. The slices to be taken, the patient's position on the tomograph table and the elements of the images taken follow a stringent protocol as there is a great potential for error. The patient must be correctly placed in a supine, comfortable and stable position on the table, using foam pillows and straps so that he or she should not move during the examination.

The pelvis and the skeleton of the lower limbs down to the feet are examined (Fig. 4). Serial transverse slices are taken at the area of the dislocated hip, the site of the true acetabulum and at a distance of 5 cm from the lesser trochanter in 5 mm intervals. This is followed by scanning at 10 mm intervals to the middle of the femur. Sections are taken at 10 mm intervals in the area of the femoral condyles, the ankle and the toes. This last series is required in order to assess accurately the rotational deformity of the limb. For reasons of clarity in the imaging and accuracy in the measurements, the scanning thickness of each slice is set at 1 mm.

Use of the CT scanning data. The initial data derived from CT are further used after appropriate processing at a three-dimensional level[9] to determine the mechanical parameters in order to plan the operation, to decide on the prosthesis or the design and to construct a customised arthroplasty (Fig. 5).[6,9]

Initially, the true length of the bones of both lower limbs is calculated. These measurements include the distance from the lesser trochanter to the centre of the knee and from there to the centre of the ankle.

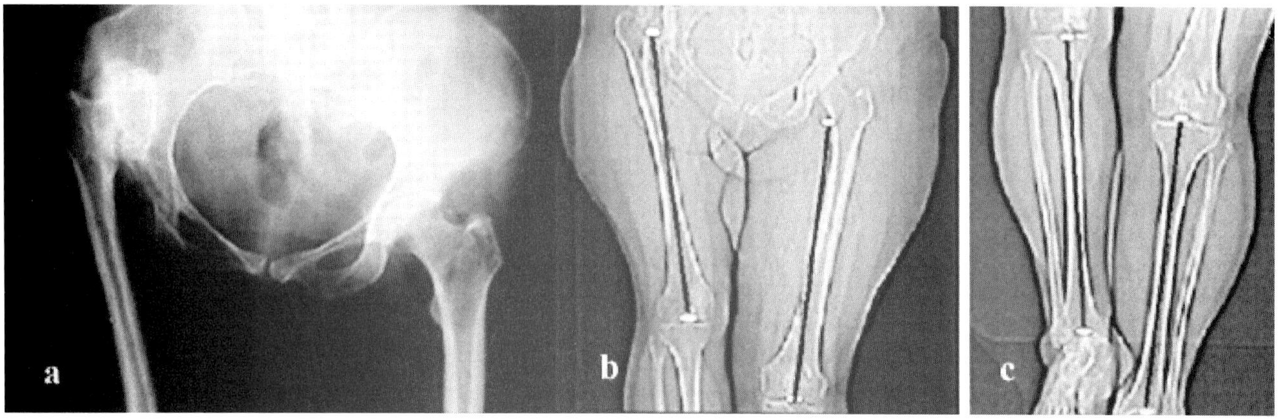

Fig. 6

Radiograph of a high dislocated right hip a) and the accurate electronic measurement of the bone length (b and c).

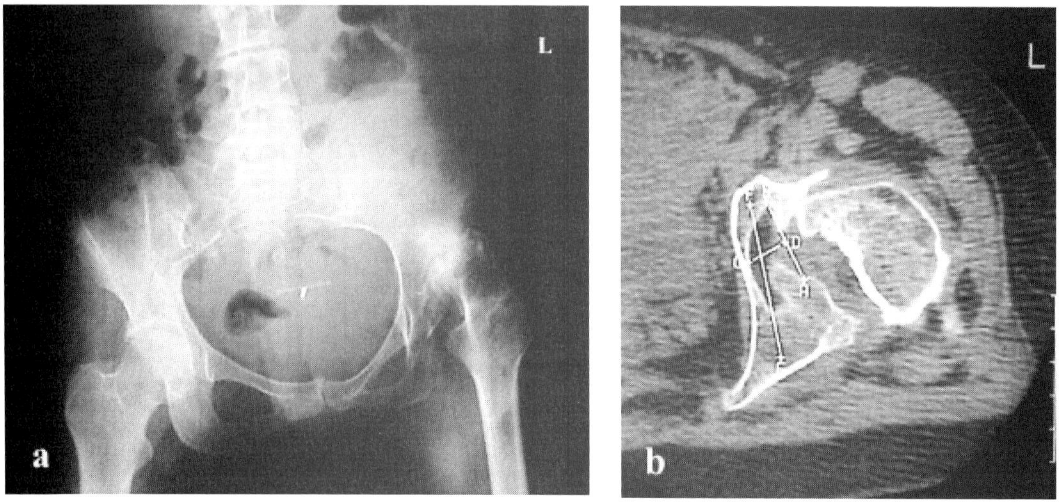

Fig. 7

Figure 7a – Radiograph of dislocation of the left hip. Figure 7b – The measurement of the dimensions of the true acetabulum by CT. The distance C-D indicates the shallow acetabulum.

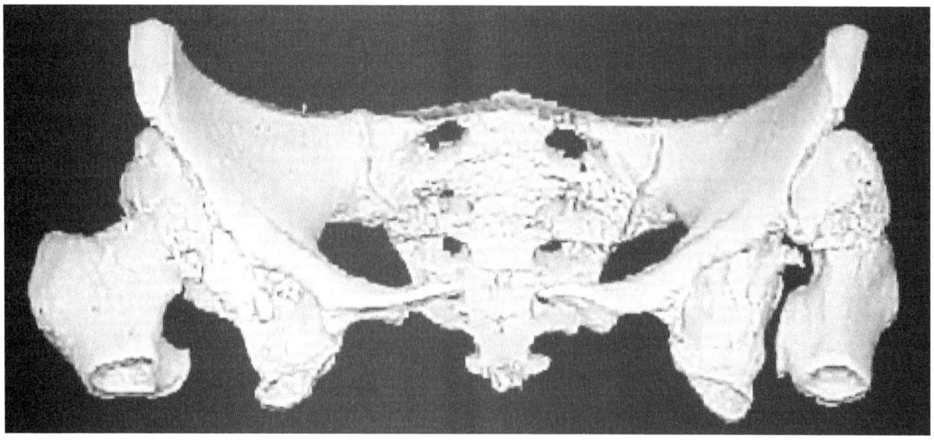

Fig. 8

3-D CT reconstruction of a pelvis with bilateral CDH. The position of the true acetabulum in relation to the luxation is clearly indicated.

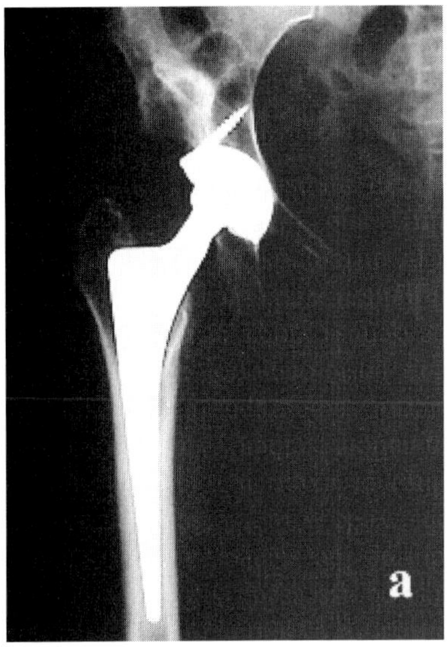

Fig. 9a

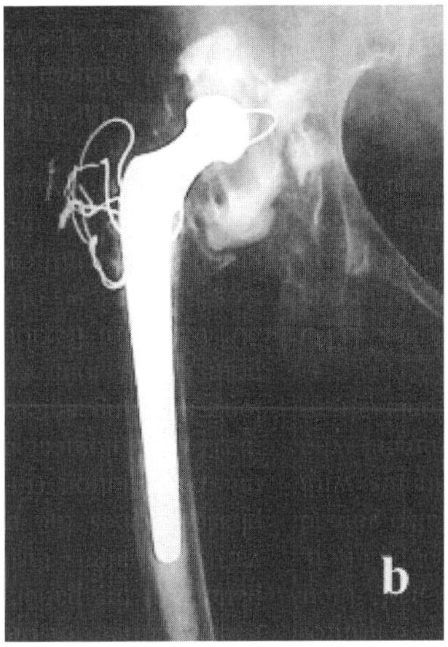

Fig. 9a

Figure 9a – Radiograph showing implantation of the prosthesis at the level of the true acetabulum five years after operation. Figure 9b – Radiograph showing the cup placed at the position of the false acetabulum. It became loose four years after the initial implantation.

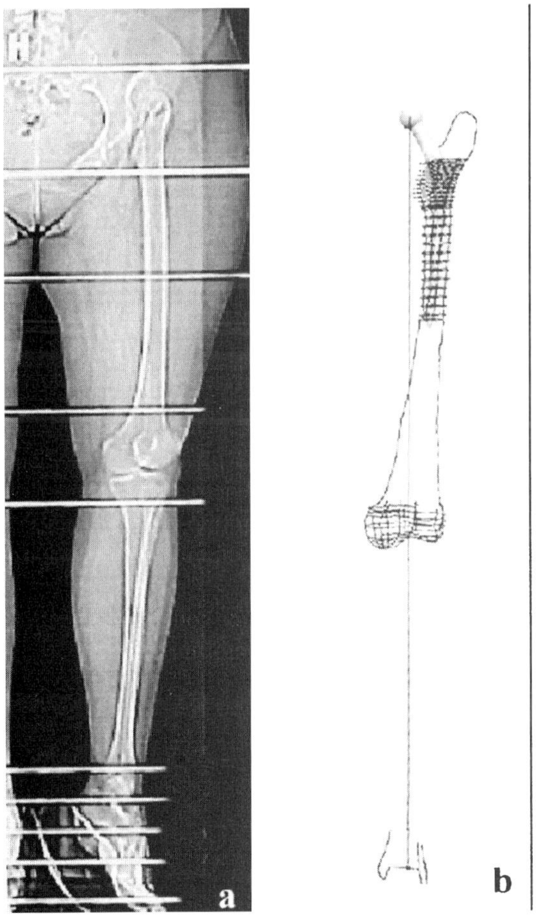

Fig. 10

Figure 10a – Topogram of the left leg with fixed external rotation. Figure 10b – The same leg after computer-assisted mathematical correction and simulated implantation of the prosthesis (with permission of TST Ltd, Ioannina, Greece).

It is not uncommon to find differences in the lengths of the bones between the healthy and the dislocated limb. In only one-third of patients are both lower limbs the same length; often the dislocated leg is longer. This is especially important when the hip is restored to the normal centre of rotation after implantation of the arthroplasty because if the skeleton of the limb is longer a shortening osteotomy of the femur will be required (Fig. 6).

Measurement of the dimensions of the true acetabulum should be made. There is usually increased anteversion, and a small anterior diameter. The anterior wall is thin, hypoplastic, shallow and displaced anteriorly within the pelvis (Fig. 7). There is always some osseous 'reservoir' in the posterior aspect of the acetabulum where a relatively adequate space can be created for the implantation of the cup. The technique of 3D image reconstruction may be used (Fig. 8).

During the preoperative planning the correct positioning of the prosthesis in the true acetabulum is assessed.[10,11] In a series of 284 dislocated hips we have been able to place the arthroplasty in the position of the true acetabulum. In addition to the improved biomechanical function of the joint in this position[9,12] it is thought that the survival of the arthroplasty is increased (Fig. 9).

After the initial measurements, the CT data are loaded onto a Risc 6000 computer for further study and processed using CATIA (a computer-assisted designing/engineering/manufacturing IBM program) and Adobe Photoshop programs. Each sagittal section is related to the X and Y axes and each slice to a specific Z axis. It is thus possible to place the images derived from each slice in space and images with specific dimensions and geometry which occupy a specific position are stored in the computer.[9] A three-dimensional mathematical model can then be created to study the skeleton of the lower limb and to incorporate all

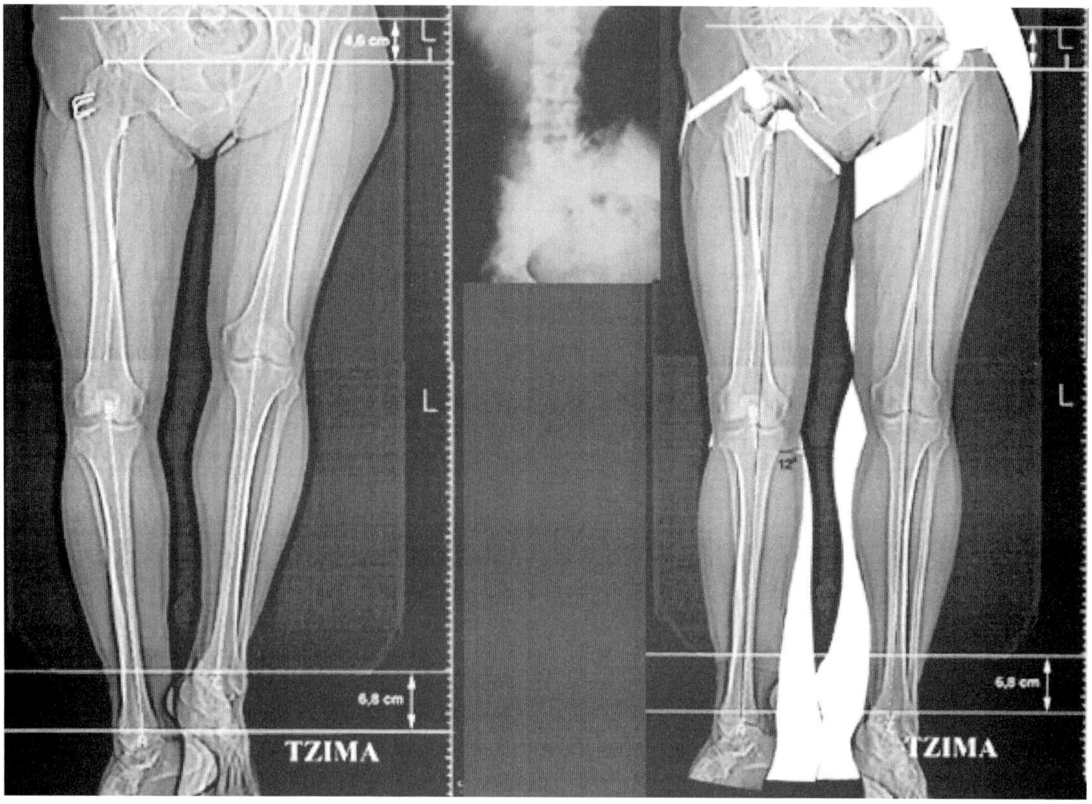

Fig. 11

Figure 11a – Topogram of the fused right hip and dislocated left. Figure 11b – Because the spine was fixed but in a balanced position calculation of the tilted position of the pelvis was accepted. After correction the length of the legs is equal.

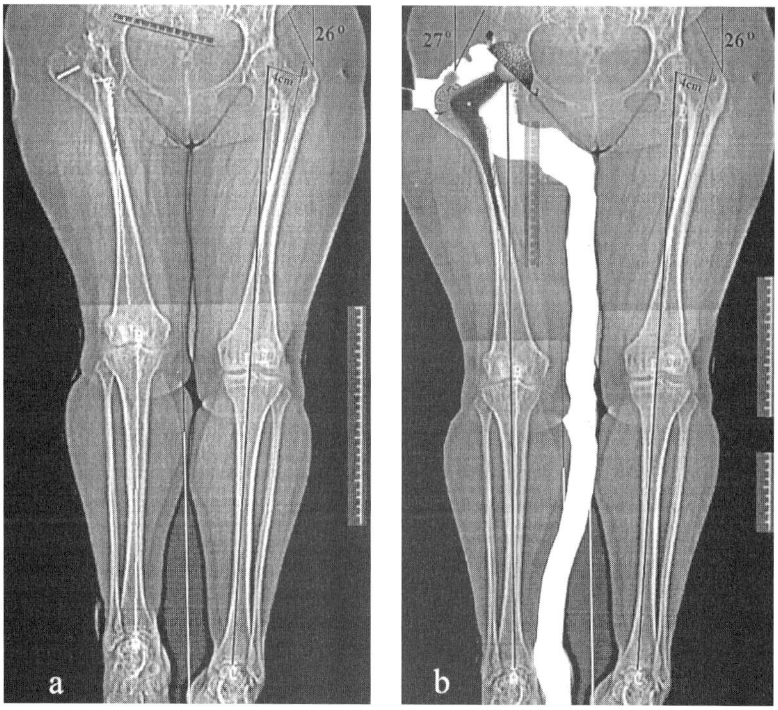

Fig. 12a Fig. 12b

Figure 12a – Topogram of the initial situation of the skeleton of a patient with an osteotomised dislocated right hip, a valgus knee and a dysplastic left hip. Figure 12b – Restoration of the leg length, the position of the abductor muscles and the functional axis of the knee by simulated implantation of a customised prosthesis.

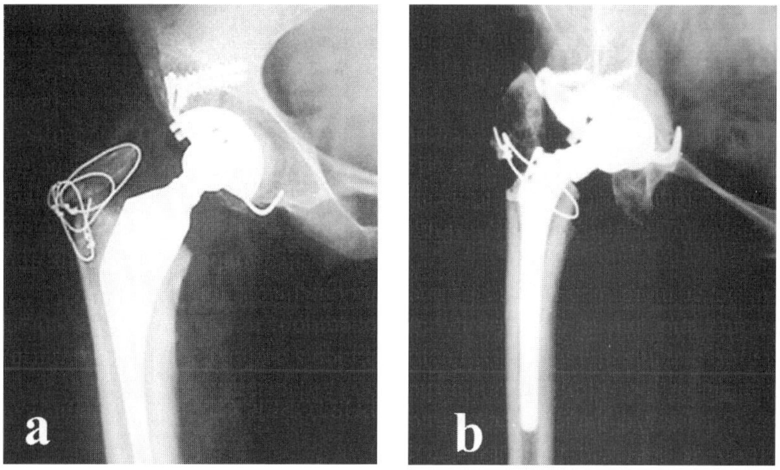

Fig. 13a Fig. 13b

Radiographs showing pseudarthrosis of the greater trochanter.

the surgically designed requirements. In this way the operation to be performed on the patient is simulated on the computer.

The first step is to correct the rotational deformity of the limb (Fig. 10) and this is achieved by positioning the entire model on the computer in such a way that the true frontal plane of the femoral condyles is parallel to the frontal plane of the body. The position of the lesser trochanter is then determined with respect to the ischial ramus at the same place as the healthy opposite site or at the middle point of the ramus. The equality of the limb length is again checked on the computer. If there are minor differences, they can be corrected by making a lower osteotomy of the neck of the femur, by retaining more of the neck, or by using a femoral prosthesis with a longer neck. Significant lengthening of the neck is not advisable because of the stress that will be exerted on the muscles surrounding the hip which may hold the hip in abduction or increase the risk of ectopic ossification.

In order not to cause any disturbance in the area where the arthroplasty will be placed, the osteotomy is performed more distally than the prosthesis and the femur is shortened as much as is required for both limbs to be of equal length (Fig. 11).

If there is also axial deviation of the knee, most commonly in valgus, this may be corrected at the same time by changing the size of the excised piece of bone, which is in the shape of an irregular trapezium, while controlling the alignment of the knee. It is easy to calculate the necessary angles of the osteotomies as well as the length of the portion of bone to be excised on the computer.

The next step is the verification of the position of gluteus medius. After correct aligning of the femur in relation to the pelvis, gluteus medius should gain insertion into the greater trochanter at an angle of 17° to 30° of abduction in relation to the perpendicular. This angle depends on the position of the greater trochanter. An outward shift of the trochanter increases the angle and an inward shift decreases it. Thus, changing the offset of the arthroplasty may be accomplished although there remain some limitations. If the other hip is normal, it is preferable to follow its offset (Fig. 12). The centre of rotation of the hip, the knee and the centre of the ankle should be on the same axis. If the knee is in a significant valgus position then a corrective osteotomy should be performed, otherwise the choice of the offset should not influence the above-mentioned relationship.

Finally, the resistance of the femoral stem against the high bending stresses of the increased offset when a customised arthroplasty with a thin stem is used should be determined. Here, computer-assisted engineering of the resistance of the prosthesis is necessary, or in certain situations the production of a trial prosthesis which is subsequently subjected to mechanical stress to determine the limit of its fatigue before the decision about implantation is made. This, however, is seldom needed.

If it is not possible to restore the direction of gluteus medius by the above method, osteotomy of the greater trochanter and its fixation in a new position which satisfies the functional requirements are required. This procedure is controversial. Some authors suggest that it is a necessary step in performing an arthroplasty in CDH. We use a posterolateral approach to the hip and have never needed to perform an osteotomy of the greater trochanter for reasons of exposure only. We do not, however, consider that osteotomy causes a delay in rehabilitation as a result of delayed union, since the area of bone contact is small in these difficult joints. However, a pseudarthrosis or delayed union may occur which leads to insufficiency of the abductor muscles and limping (Fig. 13).

The next important step is the selection of the type of arthroplasty to be performed. CDH has different requirements as regards the selection of materials in comparison with degenerative arthritis. The bone which will contain the

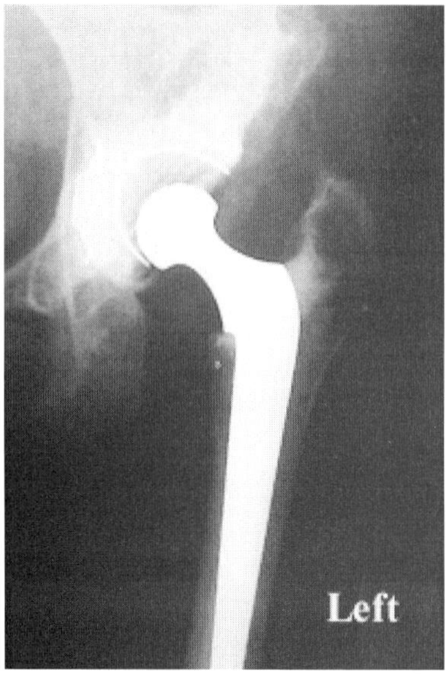

Fig. 14a

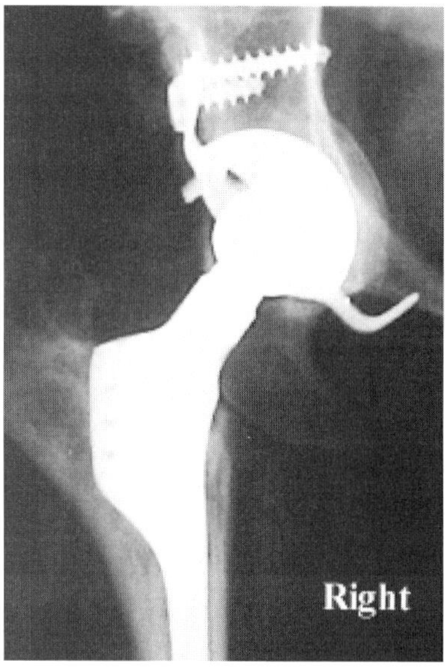

Fig. 14b

Figure 14a – Radiograph showing excellent stability of an offset bore Charnley cup nine years after implantation. Figure 14b – Radiograph of another patient operated on with a special cementless customised (Symbios SA, Yverdon, Switzerland) offset bore cup one year after implantation.

prosthesis may be atrophic because of the lack of loading and this should be taken into consideration when deciding whether a cemented or cementless prosthesis should be used.

As regards the acetabulum, a cup is selected which is expected to give good initial stability and guarantee long-term function. Screw-in cups usually give good stability and in our series of patients did not cause early problems.[13,14] In the long term, however, they are prone to loosening and migration and thus are not recommended. It is very difficult for press-fit cups to acquire sound initial stability in dislocated hips, despite their good long-term results in degenerative joint disease, and there may be early mechanical failure and loosening. In our series they accounted for most of the early failures that led to revision.

We suggest the use of special cups which have a hook for anchorage on the obturator foramen at the level of the tubercle and the potential for screw fixation into healthy ilium. Similarly, good results are achieved with cemented cups after appropriate modelling of the acetabulum by a technique described by Hartofilakidis et al,[1] the so-called cotyloplasty (Fig. 14).

Because of the small dimensions of the true acetabulum prostheses of appropriate size are required. In order to have a layer of polyethylene more than 6 mm thick around the cephalic area of the prosthesis, inserts of diameter 22.2 mm are used and if needed the polyethylene of the cup should have offset modelling so that there is a layer of adequate thickness in the area which bears most load. These offset-bore Charnley cups give exceptionally good results.

Selection of the stem is not easy because of the irregular geometry of the medullary canal of the femur and the requirements described above to restore the functional relations of the joint.

The selection which satisfies the basic requirements is made from a large arthroplasty library in the computer.[16] A comparison is then made between the size and the form of the initially selected arthroplasties and those of the femoral canal with the aim of achieving a good central fit. A trial implantation of the selected prosthesis follows with a simulation process on the computer and finally that which fulfils the criteria of the best implantation is chosen. If the patient is over 65 years of age, or the femur has considerable atrophy, a cemented prosthesis is used.

In this way, the size, the design of the stem and the position of implantation are preselected by computer. If none of the usual prostheses fulfils the criteria for satisfactory implantation, a customised prosthesis is made, based on the computer requirements. In a series of 92 hips in which selection was made according to this computerised technique, there was complete agreement between the findings of the preoperative study and those during surgery (Fig. 15).

PERFORMING THE ARTHROPLASTY

All patients have prophylactic antibiotics and anticoagulants and after operation are given indomethacin to prevent ectopic ossification.

During the operation the patient is placed in a lateral position. We use a posterolateral approach without osteotomy of the greater trochanter unless it was predesigned in the study. The external rotators of the hip are divided and

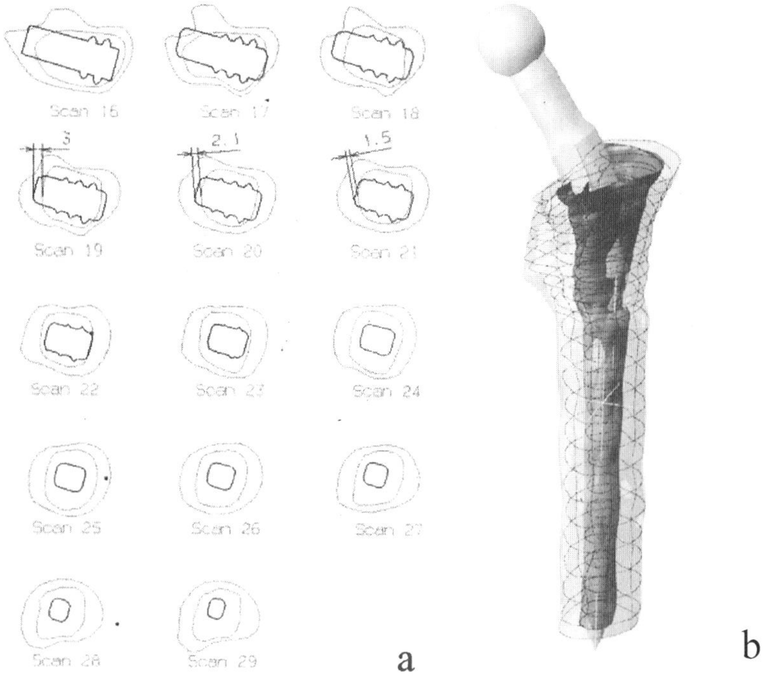

Fig. 15

The simulated implantation of a) a Spotorno femoral stem and b) a Wagner stem (with permission of TST Ltd, Ioannina, Greece).

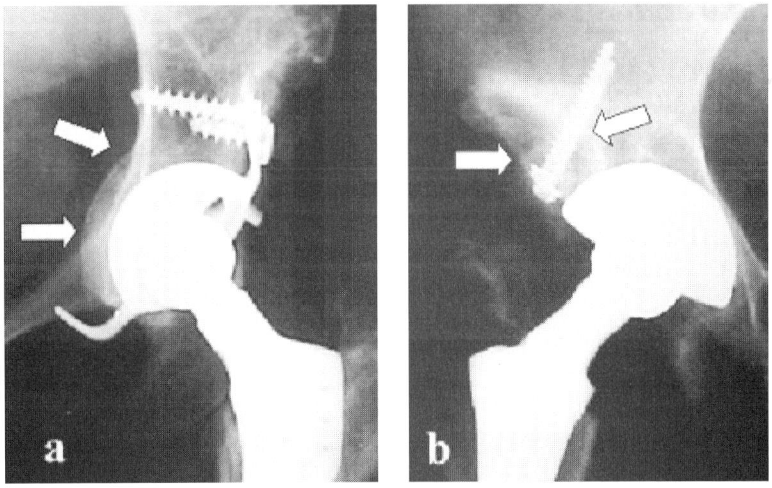

Fig. 16

Radiographs showing a) incorporation of morsellised bone grafts six months after operation and b) good consolidation of a combination of morsellised and spongiosa bone grafts three years later.

held with sutures. Initially, the posterior and then the superior, anterior and inferior parts of the capsule are transected and excised. Osteotomy of the femoral neck is then performed with removal of any osteophytes from the false acetabulum.

Following the direction of the joint capsule the true acetabulum is traced and freed from soft tissue until its entire perimeter is visible. The obturator foramen is identified and the posterior wall is prepared. This is the area where space for the modelling of the true acetabulum will be provided. The extensive preparation of the soft tissues which surround the joint is very important in order to allow reduction of the prosthesis without exerting stress and to prevent damage to the sciatic and femoral nerves.

It should be borne in mind that the nerves surrounding the hip in the dislocated joint have an abnormal course and are rather lax which may explain why no nerve injuries have been described in the reconstruction of neglected CDH.

After identification of the area of the true acetabulum, it is modelled using a Lexer chisel. In shallow acetabula, which are a common finding, the depth is increased by penetrating the medial wall and reconstructing it with a morsellised bone graft from the excised femoral head. This graft cannot be considered as an element of initial stabilisation but over a period of about four months, it is incorporated and forms strong bone within the pelvis. It therefore participates in the resulting stabilisation and may be a source of bone stock.[15]

Often, in a lower dislocation, a hollow space is found in part of the roof of the acetabulum. This is preserved and filled with morsellised bone graft. Similarly, these grafts cannot function as support and have been known to fail,[16] and thus should be avoided (Fig. 16).

After the final modelling of the acetabulum, the cup is placed accurately with relative ease in the predesigned position.

The next step is the placement of the femoral stem which should be achieved easily and successfully with little potential for error.

If a shortening osteotomy is to be performed, contrary to the advice of other authors[12,17] we prefer to place it distal to the femoral stem, as mentioned above. Initially, the proximal part of the osteotomy is undertaken which frees the proximal portion of the femur and the prosthesis. The arthroplasty may then be reduced relatively easily since there is no tension from the muscles which insert around the knee; the limb is not lengthened at this phase. Traction to the limits of muscle tension is then performed so that the amount of bone to be excised can be established and the leg-lengths checked. If these parameters are valid a distal osteotomy is then undertaken which can be oblique if knee correction is deemed necessary.

Fixation of the osteotomy is achieved by a LC-DCP titanium plates with 8 to 10 holes. Adequate space should be available for the placement of the screws distal to the stem. In a small number of patients it is impossible to stretch the muscle mass fully and thus it is necessary to excise a larger length, but never more than 6 mm of bone (Fig. 17).

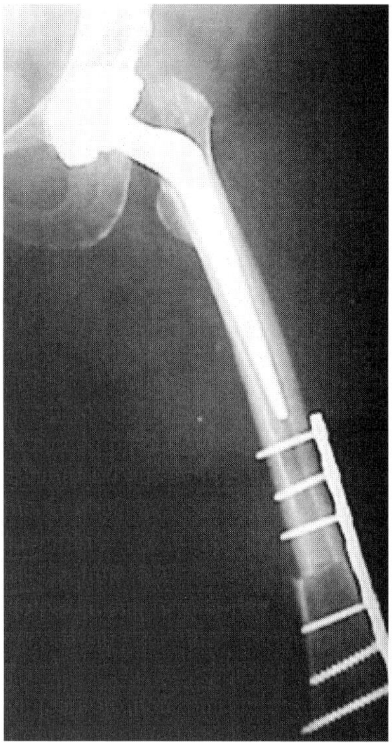

Fig. 17

Radiograph showing a shortening femoral osteotomy distal to the femoral stem in a patient operated on for a dislocated left hip.

It may be possible to achieve full equality of length if the soft tissues were freed from the femur, but this would mean exerting high tension on the nerves with the risk of development of neurological complications. We do not attempt this in our patients.

If osteotomy of the greater trochanter has been performed, it is then placed in the predetermined position. The surface of the bone at this site should be prepared and in some cases a graft may be needed. Stabilisation of the trochanter is not easy because of its small size of the bone and it is often brittle. We use wires and especially strong delayed absorption sutures.

Because of the small size of the bone it has been occasionally necessary to create special holes in the customised stems through which sutures can be passed for stabilisation of the greater trochanter. Complications such as pseudarthrosis, incomplete union and absorption of the greater trochanter may occur. More often ectopic ossification is observed.

POSTOPERATIVE REHABILITATION

Patients are given antibiotics during the first 24 hours after operation, low-molecular-weight heparin for 21 days and indomethacin for 15 days.

Assisted mobilisation begins immediately after operation with a regime of physiotherapy. The use of regular analgesics is necessary during the first 48 hours after operation and thereafter depending on the patient's condition.

Patients are usually mobilised on the second day on crutches with partial weight-bearing. They usually leave hospital five days later and follow a mild regime of physiotherapy. Radiological examination is performed at 1.5, 3, 4.5 and 6 months after operation and then once a year.

Walking with one crutch is usually allowed 1.5 months after operation and completely free walking at three months depending on the progress of union of the greater trochanter and the osteotomy of the femur, if these have been performed.

REFERENCES

1. **Hartofilakidis G, Stamos K, Ioannidis T.** Low-friction arthroplasty for old untreated congenital dislocation of the hip. *J Bone Joint Surg [Br]* 1988;70-B:182-9.

2. **Bobyn JD, Tanzer M, Brooks CE.** Noncemented total hip arthroplasty in the young patients: considerations for optimizing long-term implant survival. *Instr Course Lec* 1994;43:299-313.

3. **Chandler HP, Reineck FT, Wixson RL, McCarthy JC.** Total hip replacement in patients younger than thirty years old. *J Bone Joint Surg [Am]* 1981;63-A:1426-34.

4. **D'Antonio JA.** Preoperative templating and choosing the implant for primary THA in the young patient. *Instr Course Lect* 1994;43:339-46.

5. **Dorr LD, Takei GK, Conaty JP.** Total hip arthroplasty in patients less than forty-five years old. *J Bone Joint Surg [Am]* 1983;65-A:474-9.

6. **Argenson J-N, Aubaniac J-M.** Preoperative planning of total hip reconstruction for congenital dislocation of the hip using custom cementless implants. *S Orthop J* 1994;3:11-8.

7. **Dias JJ, Johnson GV, Finlay DBL, Stoyle TF.** Preoperative evaluation for uncemented hip arthroplasty: the role of computerised tomography. *J Bone Joint Surg [Br]* 1989;71-B:43-6.

8. **Husmann O, Rubin PJ, Leyvraz PF, de Roguin B, Argenson JN.** Three-dimensional morphology of the proximal femur. *J Arthroplasty* 1997;12:444-50.

9. **Xenakis ThA, Gelalis ID, Koukoubis ThD, et al.** Neglected congenital dislocation of the hip: role of computed tomography and computer-aided design for total hip arthroplasty. *J Arthroplasty* 1996;11:893-8.

10. **Pagnano MW, Hanssen AD, Lewallen DG, Shaughnessy WJ.** The effect of superior placement of the acetabular component on the rate of loosening after total hip arthroplasty. *J Bone Joint Surg [Am]* 1996;78-A:1004-14.

11. **Vasu R, Carter DR, Harris WH.** Stress distributions in the acetabular region. I. Before and after total joint replacement. *J Biomech* 1982;15-3:155-64.

12. **Paavilainen T, Hoikka V, Solonen KA.** Cementless total replacement for severely dysplastic or dislocated hips. *J Bone Joint Surg [Br]* 1990;72-B:205-11.

13. **Duparc J, Massin P.** Total hip prosthesis with screw rings: results over 2 years of 198 consecutive prostheses. *Rev Chir Orthop* 1991;77:221-34.

14. **Snorrason F, Karrholm J.** Primary migration of fully threated acetabular prostheses: a roentgen stereophotogrammetric analysis. *J Bone Joint Surg [Br]* 1990;72-B:647-52.

15. **Xenakis Th, Koukoubis T, Hantes K, Varytimidis S, Soucacos PN.** Bone grafting in total hip arthroplasty for insufficient acetabulum. *Acta Orthop Scand* 1997;275:33-7.

16. **Mulroy RD, Harris WH.** Failure of acetabular autogenous grafts in total hip arthroplasty. *J Bone Joint Surg [Am]* 1990;72-A:1536-40.

17. **Reikeraas O, Lereim P, Gabor I, Gunderson R, Bjerkreim I.** Femoral shortening in total arthroplasty for completely dislocated hips: 3-7 year results in 25 cases. *Acta Orthop Scand* 1996;67:33-6.

HIGH TIBIAL OSTEOTOMY

CONDITIONS, INDICATIONS, TECHNIQUES, PROBLEMS, RESULTS

WERNER MÜLLER

From the Kantonsspital, Bruderholz, Basel, Switzerland

Osteotomy is an old and well-established orthopaedic technique. Fixation in a plaster cast, however, sometimes for long periods, results in loss of range of movement (ROM) and atrophy of the muscles. This was a limiting factor in the indications for treatment of unicompartmental osteoarthritis by a varus or valgus osteotomy.

After World War II and with the introduction of antibiotics there has been further development of all types of high tibial osteotomy (HTO). In 1958 Jackson,[1] in 1961 Jackson and Waugh[2] and then later Coventry[3,4] published reports of new techniques of osteotomy around the knee with the introduction of sophisticated technical equipment. Since then we have become more critical in the evaluation of the safest, the best and the most economic procedure considering the rates of complication, the time off work, and the overall long-term results.

Younger patients with post-traumatic deformity including ligamentous laxity of the knee, and older patients with unicompartmental or asymmetrical osteoarthritis with a different level of demand must be judged separately. There is also a difference between populations of different parts in the world in terms of levels of demand, compliance and acceptance.

HTO may be a difficult procedure with an unpredictable outcome and many orthopaedic surgeons have instead preferred to do unicompartmental (UKA) or total knee arthroplasty (TKA). Since both UKA and TKA also have their problems, especially in an active and younger population, there has now been a trend back to HTO. It has also gained in importance since there are many young patients with ligamentous instability and pathological malalignment who require an osteotomy to regain dynamic functional alignment of their limb.

Nevertheless, in spite of new tools and techniques, HTO is still a demanding procedure with a long learning curve. Failure will occur if the indications, including consideration of the ligamentous conditions and instabilities, are not well recognised, and when the operative experience and treatment of complications are inadequate.

INDICATIONS

There are six main indications.

1) Correction of a congenital deformity.
2) Correction of a deformity after conditions such as rickets and Paget's disease.
3) Correction of a deformity after growth disturbance (Blount's disease or trauma to the growth plate).
4) Correction of post-traumatic deformity.
5) Correction of load balance in ligamentous instability.
6) Correction of alignment in unicompartmental osteoarthritis.

THE SEVEN PRINCIPLES FOR PERFORMING AN HTO

1) Measurement of the static and dynamic angles (preoperative, perioperative and postoperative).
2) The morphotype must be considered: varus, internal rotation; valgus, external rotation; and genu flexum, hyperextension.
3) Ligamentous instability.
4) Choice of the angle of correction.
5) Choice of the appropriate technique.
6) Maintenance of the angle of correction achieved peroperatively.
7) Avoidance of later loss of correction.

Measurement of the static and dynamic angles. The gait pattern of the patient must be assessed. Is there additional varus or valgus thrust during the stance and acceleration phases? Does the patient walk with the knee or leg in internal rotation (in-toeing) or external rotation (out-toeing)? Radiological examination is then carried out using long standing anteroposterior radiographs in extension of both knees, long standing posteroanterior radiographs in 30° to 45° of flexion (the Schuss views of the French, the Rosenberg views of the English), varus-valgus stress radiographs for identification or differentiation of bone defects or ligamentous instability, and occasionally whole-leg standing radiographs of both limbs simultaneously while weight-bearing.

Respecting the morphotype. Limited mobility of the hip, especially rotation, may influence the gait pattern and the dynamic load. The varus knee with internal rotation requires more valgus correction than with the normal position of the foot, and the valgus knee with external rotation more varus correction than with the normal position of the foot.

Ligamentous instability. Instability of the lateral collateral ligament with insufficiency of the lateral structures needs an increase in valgus correction of 2° to 3° for the varus knee and, similarly, more varus correction in the valgus knee with medial ligament instability.

If there is anterior instability, the HTO should be performed without an increase in the slope angle of the tibial plateau. Sometimes lowering of the plateau is beneficial. In the case of posterior instability the slope of the plateau has to be slightly raised by anterior elevation, but it should be remembered that elevation of the slope more than 10° can cause a chronic insufficiency of the anterior cruciate ligament.[5,6]

Choice of the angle of correction. This is probably the most critical part of HTO and is very difficult. Measurements of the angle, the dynamic conditions and the general clinical data, including the height of the patient and his leg length, are very important. Small patients with short femora need a greater degree of correction than those with long femora. Since the femur grows only 30% to 35% at the level of the head and neck and 65% to 70% in the distal growth plate, the neck length is relatively shorter in tall people with long femora and is relatively longer in short femora. The femorotibial angle is therefore 9° in short, 7° in medium and 5° in tall subjects (Fig. 1). There are also population variations, especially in Asia, where many people have short internally-rotated varus legs.

This may be the reason why in the literature the recommended degrees of correction-overcorrection vary enormously, e.g., 12° to 16° of valgus, minimally 8° of valgus, >7° or <3° to <6°.

Choice of appropriate technique. There is no easy method of operation without risk of later complications. Some techniques are easier to perform, but it is essential that at the end of the procedure the angle of correction corresponds to that calculated to give the best long-term results.

The same concerns apply to maintenance of the achieved angle and the avoidance of later loss of correction. The new fixation systems and computer-assisted procedures will not totally remove these problems but help to improve the primary control of the alignment.

Maintenance of the peroperative angle of correction. The relatively soft proximal tibia must be stable on its medial and lateral columns. The opposite pillar must be stabilised by internal fixation systems and sometimes external fixation is required.[7]

Stability of the anterior pillar is ensured since all HTOs are carried out above the tibial tuberosity where the cancellous bone is very dense and consolidates quickly. The thickest cortical bone of the proximal tibia is on the posterior aspect. There is usually a safe buttressing contact in closing-wedge HTOs, but the opening-wedge technique creates an unstable situation in the posterior aspect of the osteotomy. Fortunately, the muscle belly of popliteus with its fibrous reinforcements lies posteriorly just above the area of the osteotomy, thus protecting the popliteal vessels and nerve bundles which are close to the site. The tension of these structures adds stability by ligamentotaxis in the open-wedge technique and usually helps to avoid bleeding into the popliteal fossa.

Avoidance of later loss of correction. The bone structure of the proximal tibia is very delicate. Aglietti et al[8] described loss of correction during the healing phase in 10% of

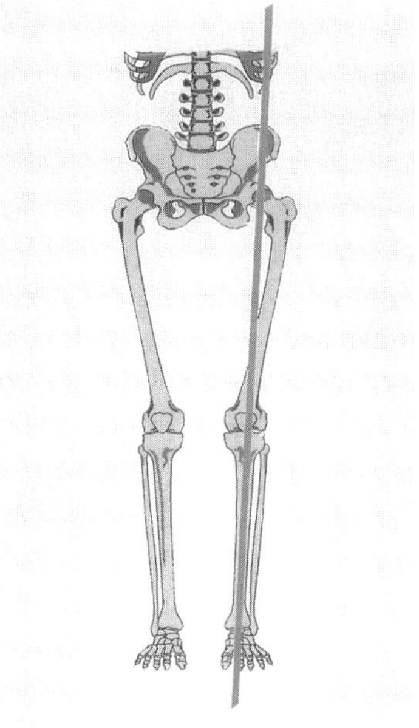

Fig. 1a

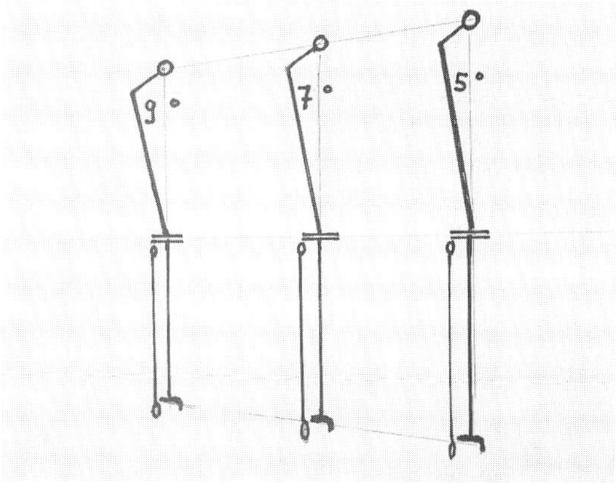

Fig. 1b

Figure 1a – Diagram of the hip-knee-ankle mechanical axis (Mikulicz axis for normal alignment). Figure 1b – The femorotibial angle is formed by the two anatomical axes of femur and tibia. With a normal mechanical Mikulicz axis it is different in short (9°), medium (7°) and tall (5°) subjects.

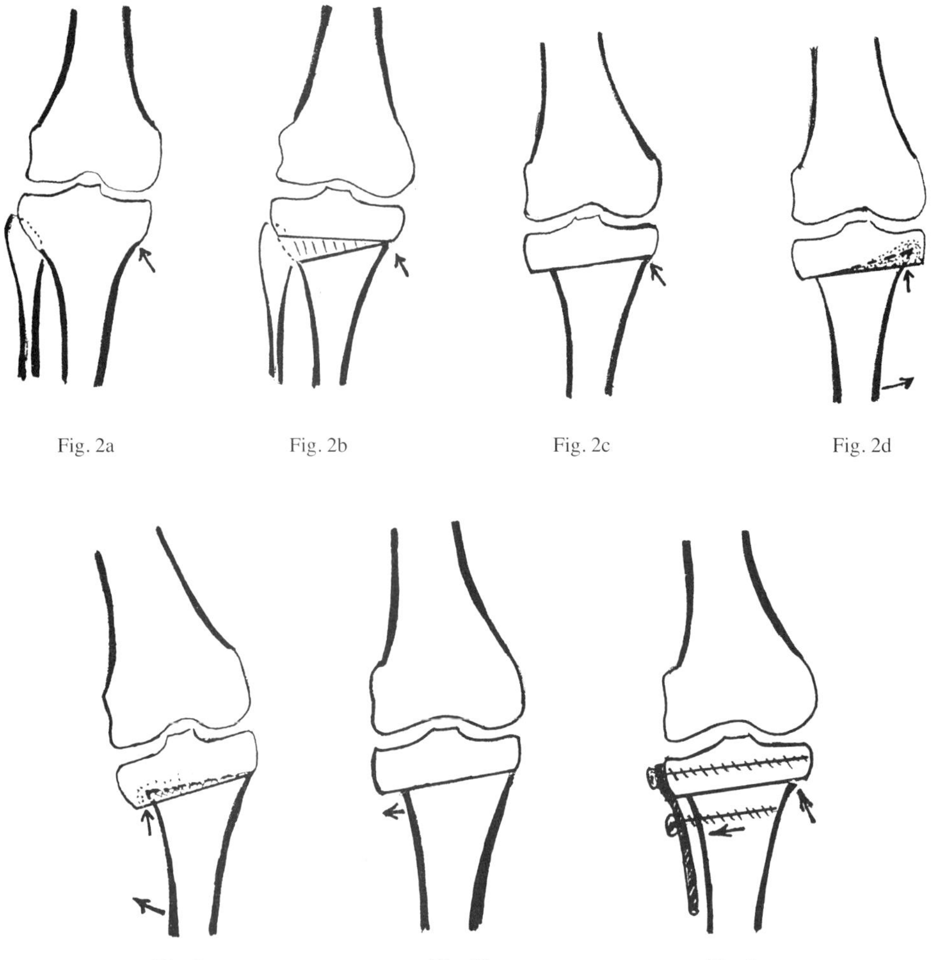

Fig. 2a Fig. 2b Fig. 2c Fig. 2d

Fig. 2e Fig. 2f Fig. 2g

Diagrams of the distribution of and relation between the hard cortical bone (thicker lines) and the soft cancellous bone (thinner lines) in the upper tibia, showing: a) and b) the hard cortical bone ending just under the area of the HTO which is at risk for postoperative loss of correction; c) a transverse HTO with a critical step; d) the medial distal cortical spur sinking into the proximal cancellous fragment leading to recurrence of varus after valgus HTO; e) the lateral distal cortical fragment sinking into the proximal softer cancellous fragment leading to additional excessive valgus deformation after valgus HTO; and f) and g) complications during internal fixation in which the screw distal to the line of the osteotomy pulls the distal fragment laterally and destabilises the osteotomy with possible revarisation d) or excessive valgus deformation.

cases of HTO. The circumferential cortical part is mechanically resistant as long as the entire area is undamaged. The cancellous bone inside is relatively soft, however, and shows a tendency to collapse if there is no additional peripheral support from a congruent cortical shell or fixation material.

The proximal tibia is shaped almost like the end of a trumpet. The thin cortex is reinforced by tension-band layers of collagenous tissues such as the medial collateral ligament, pes anserinus, the fan of the insertion of semimembranosus poteromedially, the iliotibial tract system on Gerdy's tubercle, the aponeurosis of tibialis anterior as well as extensor digitorum communis, and posterolaterally the tendinuous part of popliteus. The handling of these soft tissues in the surgical approach for an HTO and the placement of the internal fixation are important. This peripheral network of collagenous tissues must be respected and preserved as much as possible to help to avoid collapse of the bone.

If an osteotomy ends or cracks just where the cortical layer becomes thicker and stiffer, about 3 to 5 cm distal to the medial joint line, the softer proximal cancellous bone sinks down over the harder and stiffer cortical spur, resulting in later loss of correction which may lead to failure (Fig. 2). To avoid this serious complication, which can happen with all lateral closing-wedge techniques, it is best to leave the medial corticocancellous part intact. If it breaks through, strict postoperative control is necessary. When collapse occurs, an additional medial buttressing fixation must be undertaken.

In the last 35 years we have performed more than 2000 osteotomies around the knee. I shall therefore describe our experience including the difficulties and complications of the operation.

TYPES OF HIGH TIBIAL ANGULAR CORRECTION OSTEOTOMY

These are as follows:

1) Frontal plane: varus and valgus osteotomies.
2) Sagittal plane: antecurvatum, elevation, flexion osteotomy; recurvatum, lowering, extension osteotomy.
3) All planes: reconstruction osteotomy after traumatic disorders.

For all of these it is mandatory that the balance of passive and dynamic forces be restored by considering the axial alignment, the ligamentous stability and the muscular control under dynamic load of the limb. For a successful valgus HTO the lateral compartment with its cartilage layers must be in good condition as must the medial compartment for a varus HTO.

CONTRAINDICATIONS

These include rheumatoid arthritis, more than 10° of extension deficit, less than 100° of flexion, soft atrophic bone, correction angles exceeding 15° to 20°, and elderly patients with difficulty mobilising the limb after operation.

THE IMPORTANT AXES AND ANGLES FOR HTO

The important axes. Table I gives the details according to the criteria of Brown and Amendola.[9]

The important angles about the knee and limb alignment. These angles are formed by the different axes. The transverse axis of the knee is the tangential line to the distal femoral condyles. The mechanical axes of either the femur or of the tibia are not perpendicular to the transverse axis of the knee.

Frontal plane. The lateral distal femoral angle (LDFA) is given by the femoral mechanical axis and the transverse axis. The medial proximal tibial angle (MPTA) lies between the tibial mechanical axis and the transverse axis of the knee. The joint line convergence angle (JLCA) is formed by the tangential line of the femoral condyles (the transverse axis of the knee) and the tangential line of the tibial plateau. These two lines are not parallel. The JLCA converges on the medial side of the joint line because the cartilage layers in the lateral compartment of the knee, comprising the lateral meniscus and the articular cartilage over the dome-shaped lateral tibial plateau, are thicker than those on the medial side with the more concave plateau of the tibia. The lateral distal tibial angle (LDTA) is formed by the tibial mechanical axis and the transverse axis of the ankle, a line tangential to the dome of the talus.

There is considerable anatomical variation in these angles:[9] LDFA, 85.9° to 91.4°, ϕ~87° to 88°; MPTA, 82.6° to 89.2°, ϕ~87°; JLCA, 0.4° to 3.0°, ϕ~1.7° to 1.9°; LDTA, 83.8° to 91.8°, ϕ~88° to 89°.

Sagittal plane. The PTSA (posterior tibial slope angle) is formed by a line perpendicular to the longitudinal axis of the tibia in the lateral view and a line parallel to the joint surface of the medial tibial plateau, with a variation of 6° to 13°, ϕ~10°.

Angles of correction and indications. Any excessive overcorrection should be avoided because it leads to progressive valgus degeneration of more than 186°.[10] Undercorrection (less than 183°) in cases of osteoarthritis leads to a recurrence of varus OA (Fig. 3).

In an arthroscopic control study Fujisawa, Masuhara and Shiomi[11] showed that insufficient lateralisation of the mechanical axis led to further deterioration in the medial compartment and that a shift of weight-bearing into the medial one-third of the lateral compartment (30%) was clearly associated with reduction in degenerative ulceration of the articular cartilage, with some restructuring of the cartilage layers.

Noyes et al[12] reported that a shift of the mechanical axis into the lateral compartment to the point of 62% of the total width of the tibial joint surface (0° from the medial edge to 100% at the lateral edge) was the best position for the corrected mechanical axis of the width of the tibial joint line (Fig. 4). The value of 30% of the lateral compartment of Fujisawa et al[11] is measured from the spine in the centre

Table I. The important axes for high tibial osteotomy according to the criteria of Brown and Amendola[9]

	Axis	Description
Femur	Anatomical	From the centre of the knee through the middle of the shaft at the junction of the middle and distal thirds
	Mechanical	From the centre of the knee to the centre of the hip
Tibia	Anatomical axis Mechanical axis	Identical in the shaft from centre of the knee to the centre of the ankle (midpoint of the talus)
	The weight-bearing line (mechanical axis of the lower limb)	From the centre of the hip to the centre of the ankle
	The total transverse line through the knee (joint line is given as 100%)	100%: starting 0% on the medial side ending 100% at the lateral side

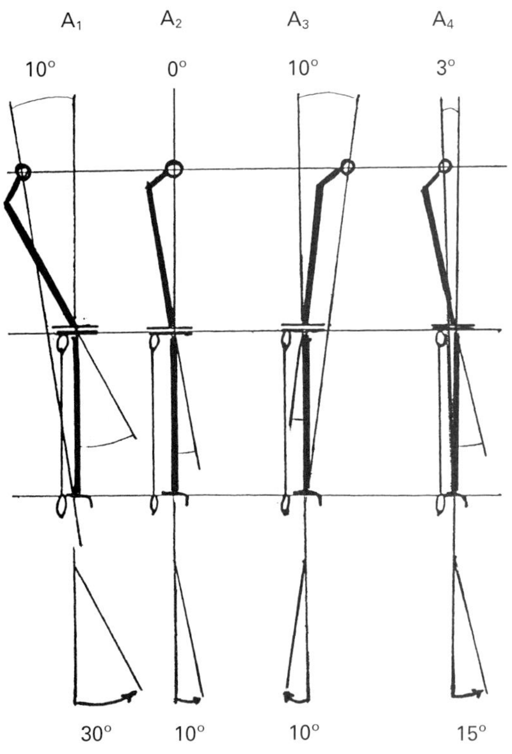

Fig. 3a

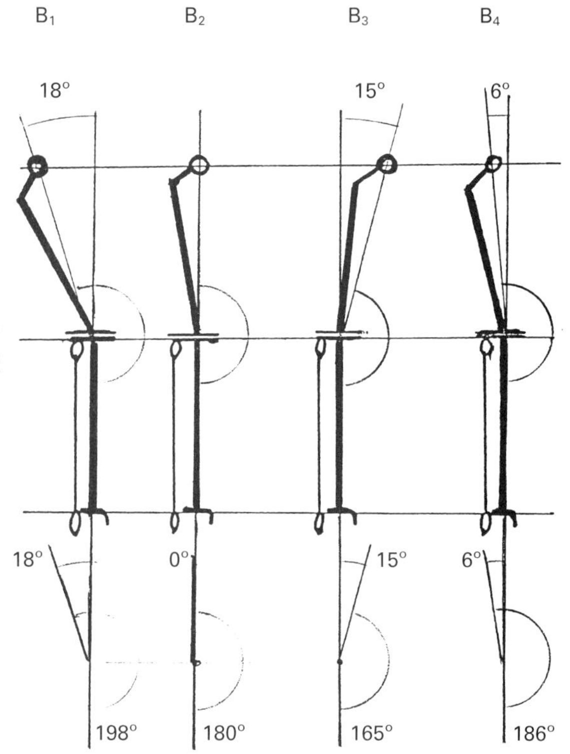

Fig. 3b

Diagrams showing the axes and angles: A1/B1 valgus knee; A2/B2 normal knee; A3/B3 varus knee; and A4/B4 62% corrected knee. Figure 3a – The weight-bearing line equals the mechanical axis of the limb, the tibial anatomical axis. Above, the angle between the weight-bearing line and the tibial anatomical axis and below the angle between the femoral and tibial anatomical axis. Figure 3b – The angle between the mechanical axis of the femur and the anatomical axis of the tibia is the hip-knee-ankle angle.

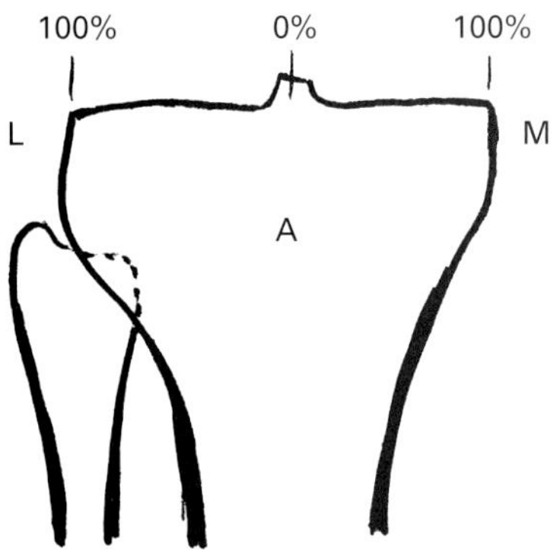

Fig. 4a

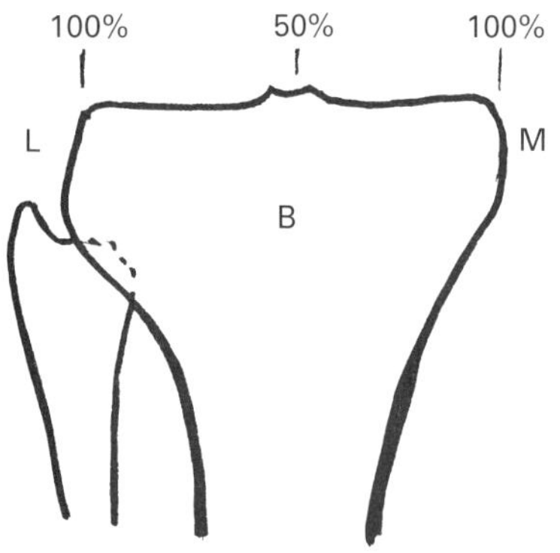

Fig. 4b

Diagrams showing the definition of the width of the tibial plateau (%) according to a) Fujisawa et al[11] and b) Noyes et al.[12].

(0%) to the medial or lateral edge (100%) and corresponds relatively closely to the 62% of Noyes et al[12] whose measurement begins on the medial edge (0%) and goes to the lateral edge (100%) (Fig. 4). In our hands this amount of correction is adequate when the extent of degenerative change is grade II to grade III according to Ahlbäck[13], or in cases of instability of the lateral ligament. It seems to be too much for the post-traumatic deformity or insufficiency of the anterior cruciate ligament (ACL) without osteoarthritis. However, the existing degree of internal or external-rotation should be borne in mind.

Angles of correction for six different types of disorder. Table II gives the angles of correction which have been beneficial and lead to good long-term results. With the ACL-insufficient knee, an anatomical reconstruction of the ACL often corrects by itself up to 5° of valgus. Overcorrection should therefore be avoided in a combined procedure of ACL reconstruction with valgus HTO.

Table II. Correction angles for the six different types of disorder

Group	Description	Correction angle	Overcorrection (degrees)
A	Post-traumatic deformation	Normal correction	1 to 2
B	ACL insufficiency, no osteoarthritis	ACL rec + normal correction	1 to 2
C	PCL-, PCL- + lat. insufficiency		2 to 4 to 5
D	Cartilage damage, repair		3 to 5
E	Unicompartmental osteoarthritis I and II*		3 to 5
F	Unicompartment osteoarthritis grade III* (IV)†		4 to 6

* according to Ahlbäck[13]
† exceptionally

RISKS, ADVANTAGES AND DISADVANTAGES OF THE VARIOUS TECHNIQUES OF HTO

Fibular osteotomy (FOT). Because the peroneal nerve and its distribution lie close to the fibula there is an inherent risk of nerve damage during manipulation and dividing of the fibula.

Thirty years ago, because of the observed paralysis of extensor hallucis longus, we performed FOT at all levels from 10 cm above the malleolar syndesmosis up to the proximal third of the fibula. There was no real safe area, not even in the zone later described by Kirgis and Albrecht[14] at 40 to 68 mm below the neck. Therefore we used two specially designed spoon-shaped Hohmann elevators, placed circularly around the bone to protect the soft tissues when the fibula was divided, but even then this did not always protect the branches supplying extensor hallucis. There was also, but now very rarely, a temporary neurapraxia of this branch possibly due to compression by the elevators themselves. Another reason for moving the level of FOT proximally was the development of a painful pseudarthrosis which required secondary treatment by decortication of the Judet type.

With previous techniques of HTO which did not allow patients to bear weight for 6 to 12 weeks the fibula always consolidated in time. With our technique of elastic HTO,[12] described later, there was earlier consolidation which allowed weight-bearing at four weeks after operation in 80% of cases. In this short time the fibula may not be consolidated and sometimes pseudarthrosis may develop. Apart from rare minor neurological disturbances with rapid recovery, in 1992 I had a case with a more serious lesion induced by a drill bit when the soleus muscle did not cover, as is normal, the posterior aspect of the head and the neck of the fibula with the proximal extension of its muscle belly. Thus the nerve was lying unprotected immediately behind the bone. In this case the traumatised perineurium was closed with a fine suture and there was fortunately considerable improvement in function within two years. Only dysaesthesia of the toes and a weakness of the small peripheral muscles on the dorsal aspect of the foot remained. Since then we have performed FOT at the level of the fibular neck after identification of the peroneal nerve.

The passage of the nerve lateral to the neck of the fibula is normally not protected by muscle. We therefore identify the nerve and protect it while the FOT is performed (see Fig. 12). Over the last eight years in 200 FOTs we have had no damage and the overall incidence of risk factors for significant nerve damage is under 1 in 1000 and for minor changes under 5 in 1000 in our very large series.

For HTOs with a small correction of the valgus angle in knees with ligamentous instability in younger people, in whom a lateral closing-wedge technique of less than 5° has been used, a FOT may not be necessary because the fibula is able to glide against the tibia.

In most cases the fibular head lies under the roof of the lateral tibial plateau and cannot glide proximally (Fig. 5). FOT is therefore necessary, even for a few degrees of correction. Lateral malleolar pain may occur later if this is not respected and the fibula is too long.

Resection of the proximal tibiofibular joint or of the head of the fibula loosens the lateral antivarus tension band system (LCL with biceps, ITT, ITB and popliteus). A few degrees (~2° to 3°) more valgus correction are then needed in order to compensate for that loss. This may be the reason why some early exponents of HTO advocated valgus overcorrection by as much as 8°.

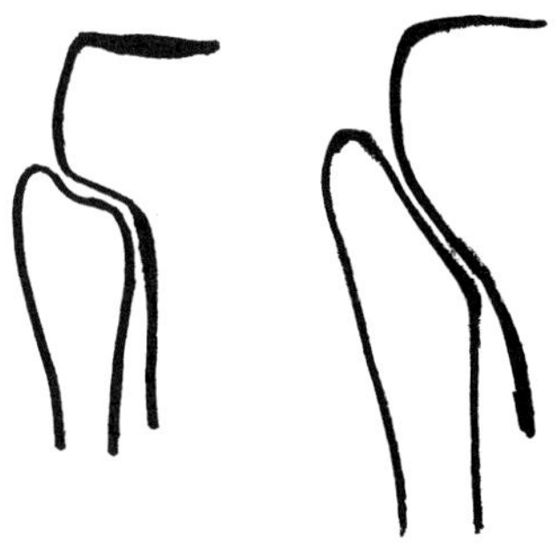

Fig. 5

Diagram showing the relation of the fibula to the upper tibia: a) no gliding (often better visible on a lateral radiograph); and b) some gliding possible.

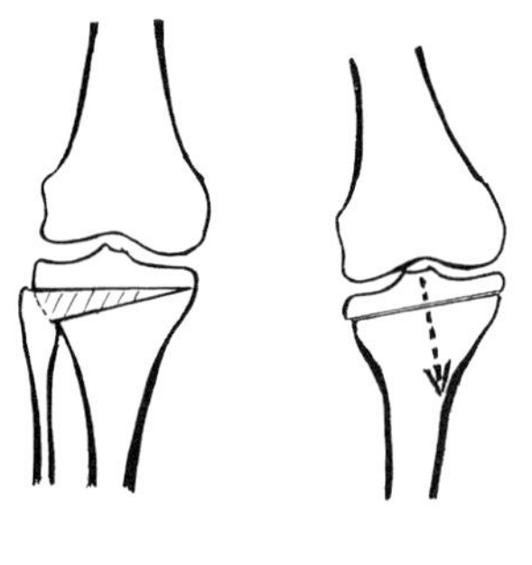

Fig. 6a

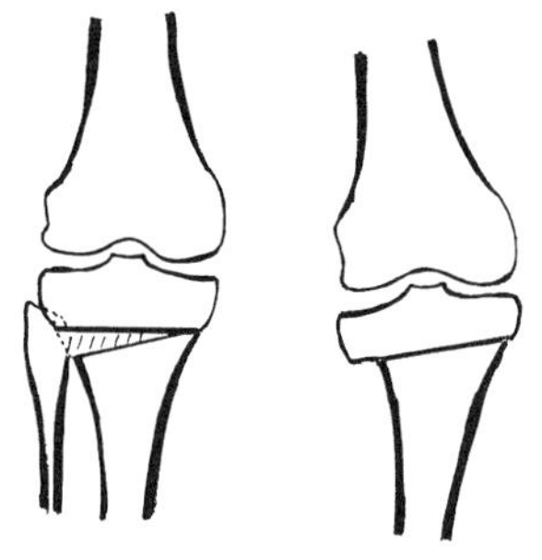

Fig. 6b

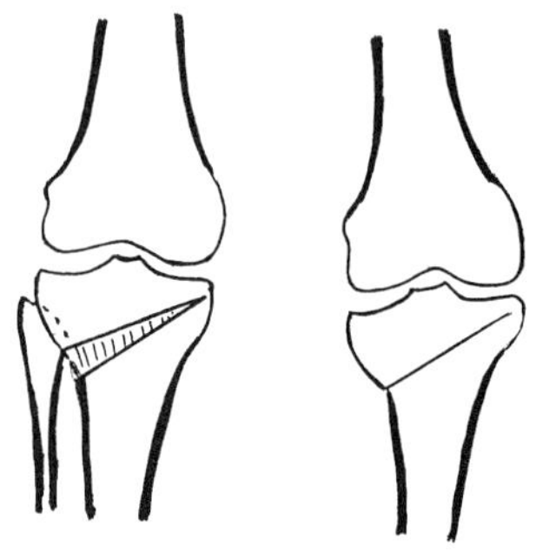

Fig. 6c

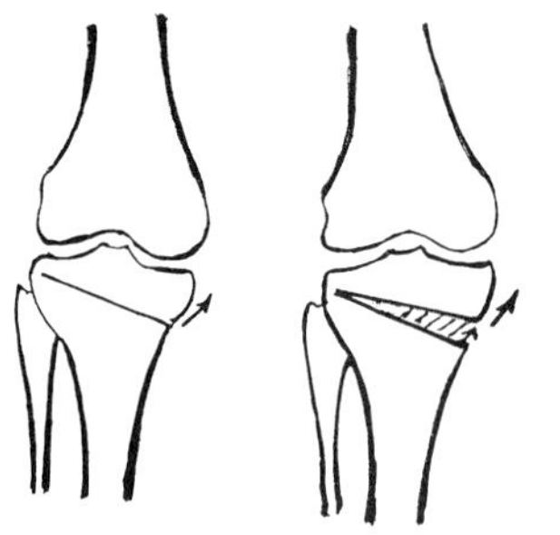

Fig. 6d

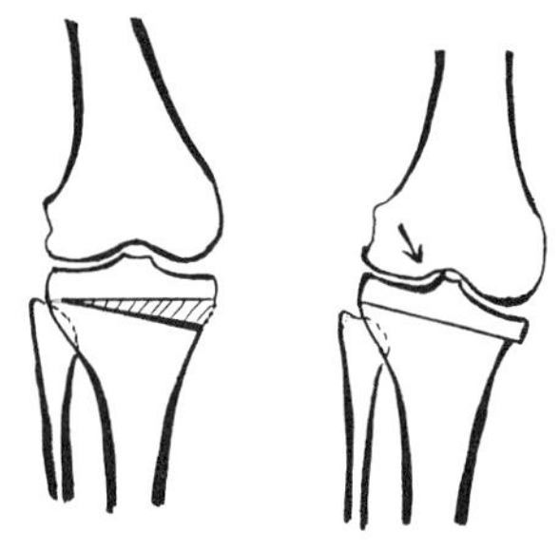

Fig. 6e

Diagrams showing that the deformation of the proximal tibia is different depending on the level of the cut and on its obliquity. Figure 6a – A very proximal valgus closing wedge with marked deformation, a possible problem with later TKA. Figure 6b – A transverse valgus closing wedge above the tibial tuberosity creating a step on the lateral side with less deformation. Figure 6c – A lateral oblique closing wedge which creates no step; the deformation is less than in (b). Figure 6d – A medial valgus opening wedge which lifts the medial plateau up with less deformation. Figure 6e – A medial varus closing wedge which creates a tilt of the plateau with shear forces.

Proximal lateral transverse closing-wedge HTO. This may also weaken the dynamic antivarus system and therefore more overcorrection may be necessary. In the most proximal area of the tibia, where the circumference is the longest, the contact surface of the osteotomy is the largest possible and leads to rapid consolidation if the blood supply is good, and the fixation, usually with Blount-clamps, is secure. Great care is required not to harm the joint surface by penetration. Stuart[15] gave a good description of the safe technique for this HTO. If a large wedge is removed postoperative deformation of the proximal tibia is significant (Fig. 6a) and may be a problem for later TKA with straight stems.

Transverse high lateral closing-wedge osteotomy above the tibial tuberosity. The main risk here lays in the medial part of the osteotomy which ends just above the beginning of the hard and stiff distal cortical fragment (Fig. 6b). Another disadvantage is the postoperative new configuration of the proximal tibia with a step on the lateral cortical wall. Because of this step the distal fragment is sometimes pulled laterally moving the hard cortical spur of the distal medial fragment laterally under the soft cancellous bone of the proximal fragment (Fig. 2f). The postoperative deformity of the proximal tibia is less significant than with the previous osteotomy.

HTO with the Charnley external fixator system. In 1964, the Orthopaedic University Clinic in Basel used this technique with the aim of fixing the osteotomy peroperatively in the appropriate angle of correction. Problems with the pins in elderly osteoarthritic patients resulted in the method being abandoned in favour of internal fixation with the new AO L-plate implants, which allow much earlier discharge from hospital.

The dome-shaped HTO. This technique was one of the earlier attempts at obtaining the angle of correction peroperatively as with the Charnley external fixation technique, the elastic closing HTO or with the opening-wedge HTO (Fig. 7a).

There is a considerable learning process, however, and during the consolidation period the angle achieved at operation was not always maintained. The osteotomy goes through the medial and the lateral cortical pillars thereby destabilising them. Internal fixation from one side does not satisfactorily control the fragments. Therefore Naumann, Köhler and Stephan[16] and Naumann and Stephan[17] used external fixators in a series of 428 patients. The incidence of damage to the deep branch of the peroneal nerve was 9.3% for temporary paralysis and 3.5% for persistent paralysis.[14] Depending on the method of fixation the incidence was 9.8% with an external fixator, 1% with Blount clamps and 2.3%

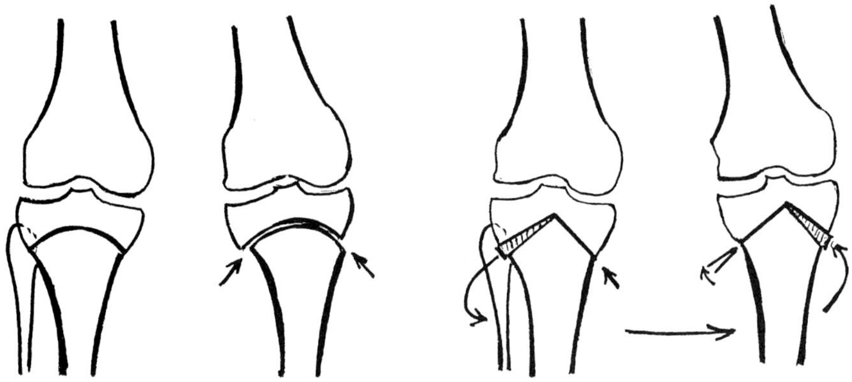

Fig. 7a Fig. 7b

Diagrams showing both so-called 'Pendel-osteotomies' with a) a dome osteotomy and b) a lateromedial double-wedge osteotomy which destabilises the medial and the lateral supporting pillar making it difficult for internal fixation to maintain the achieved angle (often external fixators were necessary).[14,16]

with fixation in a plaster cast. Additional fixation in a plaster cast and immobilisation are not desirable in osteoarthritic knees with damaged cartilage. For these knees any further loss of movement because of immobilisation is detrimental.

The V-shaped 'Pendel-HTO'. The same problems occurred with the V-shaped HTO. This points proximally above the tuberosity of the tibia and takes a smaller wedge out on the lateral side thus filling the opening gap on the medial side to realign the knee into valgus. Safe fixation and the avoidance of bony collapse are the problems with this method (Fig. 7b).

The oblique lateral closing-wedge valgus HTO. This technique of wedge excision from distally upwards to the proximal medial cancellous part of the tibia combines several advantages without avoiding all risks (Fig. 6c). The soft medial bone remains in place and there is a very large surface contact of the osteotomy. Both sides of the wedge are of equal length, so that there is no remaining lateral cortical step. There is no significant deformity after the correction which could create a later problem if TKA has to be performed, and there is the opportunity for internal fixation with thinner and lighter plates and screws.

The complication of all oblique HTOs is the creation of a rotational deformity, which may be more than 10° to 15° when the opening or closing occurs asymmetrically, or when the cut of the osteotomy is not perpendicular to the long axis of the tibia.

Technical aids. For the above HTOs there are many systems for cutting out precisely angled wedges and for introducing different internal fixation devices. Maintaining the angle of correction can be achieved with a fixed angled blade-plate which guarantees the angle and fixation. Nevertheless the preoperative calculation can still be a problem and requires some arbitrary judgement. The angle of bowing of these plates may be large in order to withstand the forces and obtaining soft tissue cover may be a problem. There are also less voluminous but less constraining plates. Experience is needed to place these so that the planned angle of correction is obtained with appropriate stability. None of these devices guarantees the avoidance of failure.

The lateral elastic valgus HTO and the operative technique. This was developed at the Kantonsspital Bruderholz/Basel by Müller, Kentsch and Schäfer.[18] The main principle is to preserve the continuity of the metaphyseal bone of the tibia but to allow its deformation with up to 10° to 15° of axial correction (Fig. 8).

Approach. A straight lateral incision is used starting beside the patella and continuing between the tibial tuberosity and Gerdy's tubercle for about 10 cm distal to the joint line. The aponeurosis of the anterior compartment must be incised to reach the lateral aspect of the tibia. The iliotibial band must be reflected posteriorly with the aponeurosis. Transverse incision of the iliotibial tract is avoided in order not to weaken the active lateral antivarus tension band-system. The approach to the fibula is by the same incision.

Technique. We do not resect a predetermined wedge over the width of the head of the tibia but remove an appropriate trapezoidal piece of bone and leave a significant bony bridge on the medial side (Fig. 9). The resection runs from the lateral side distally in an oblique direction to a point situated 1.5 cm from the joint surface, 1.5 cm from the medial cortex and 1.5 cm from the medial distal tibial cortex. This oblique direction of the HTO gives alignment from cortex to cortex without a step. The remaining bridge of bone is still thick and strong enough to withstand valgus deformation without breaking through when the piece of trapezoid bone has been removed. The required individual angle of correction should be determined from the preoperative long standing radiographs. After deformation the new angle is checked during operation by radiography with a metal rod placed from the centre of the hip to the centre of the tibiotalar joint. This axis should cross the knee at the centre through the spines (50% of the width of the tibial plateau) (Fig. 4) for a normal correction (5°, 7°, 9°), and for overcorrection, laterally from the intercondylar spine at about 60% to 65% of the width of the plateau from the medial side, corresponding to a point situated at about one-quarter to one-third lateral to the spine in the lateral compartment (Fig. 10). Fixation is achieved by using an ASIF L-plate and compression device. Enough time has to

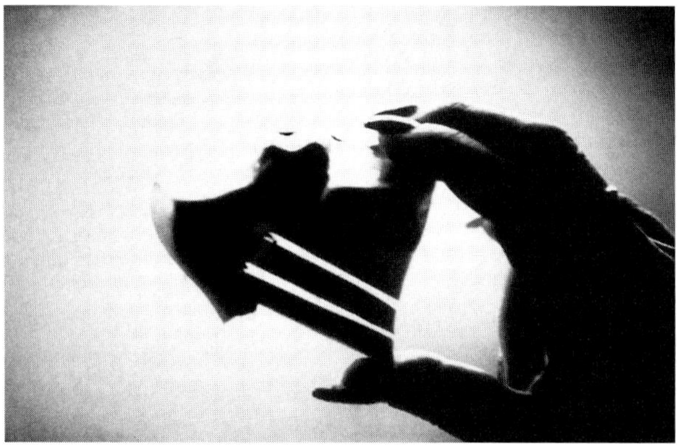

Fig. 8a

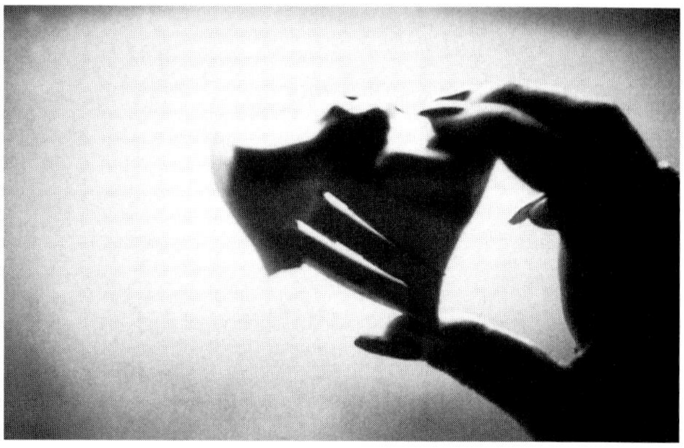

Fig. 8a

Photographs showing the elastic valgus HTO a) before deformation and b) after deformation (here with two resected slots).

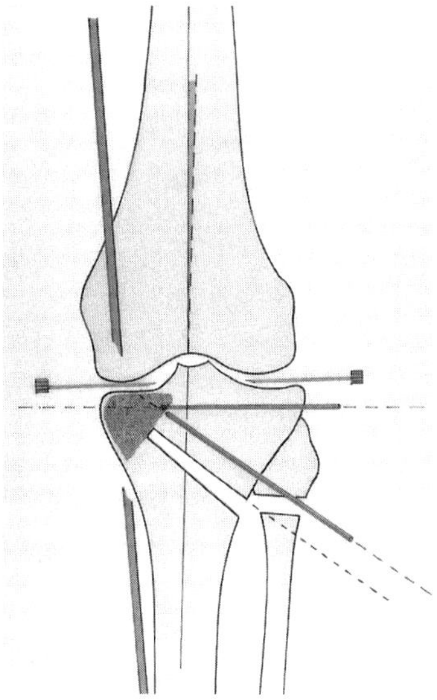

Fig. 9a

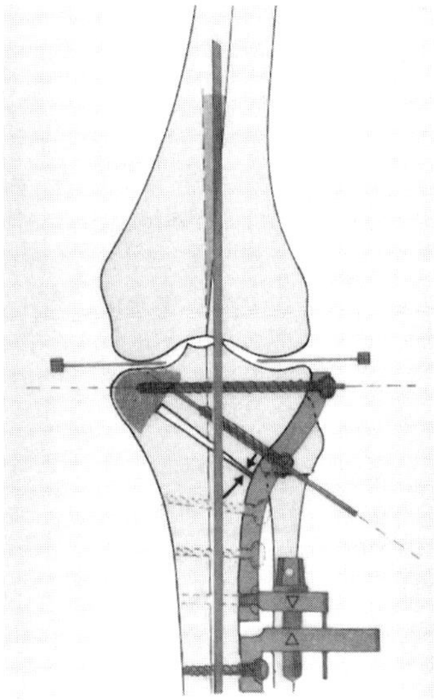

Fig. 9b

Photographs of the elastic valgus HTO showing a) the trapezoid bone resection and medial deformation area and b) compression with the mechanical axis centred after the elastic deformation.

be given to deform the bone up to the necessary correction angle without it breaking. If the correction does not progress steadily and easily or comes to a halt the gap must be cleared, and probably more bone should be removed.

The medial closing-wedge varus HTO. This type of HTO has been used for correction of the valgus knee. Since the approach and the osteotomy were easier on the tibial than on the femoral side this procedure was in favour for some time. A varus HTO of the tibia is contrary to the basic principles for a successful osteotomy around the knee. At the end of the realignment of the limb the joint line of the knee should remain more or less parallel to the ground. The shear forces on the cartilage during normal stance should be minimal for a good long-lasting result. Therefore sometimes a sequential double osteotomy of the distal femur and proximal tibia should be performed to obtain correct alignment and a horizontal joint line. Biomechanically, a significant varus HTO is not a correct procedure since the plateau becomes tilted into an oblique position. Because of the resulting shear slide of the lateral femoral condyle towards the intercondylar tibial spine, the main weight-bearing is in the lateral compartment.[19] The osteoarthritis is not stabilised and progresses further (Fig. 6e).

The lateral varus opening-wedge HTO. This HTO was also used for tightening the lateral ligament system, but biomechanically it was not successful. It may have helped in cases of minor instability in a knee with a minor valgus deformity. Now it is no longer used.

The medial valgus opening-wedge HTO. This oblique HTO is of value in a varus knee with instability of the medial ligament. It allows the angle of correction to be determined peroperatively (Fig. 6d).

The main disadvantages are breakthrough of the opposite cortex which causes an unstable situation and difficulty in

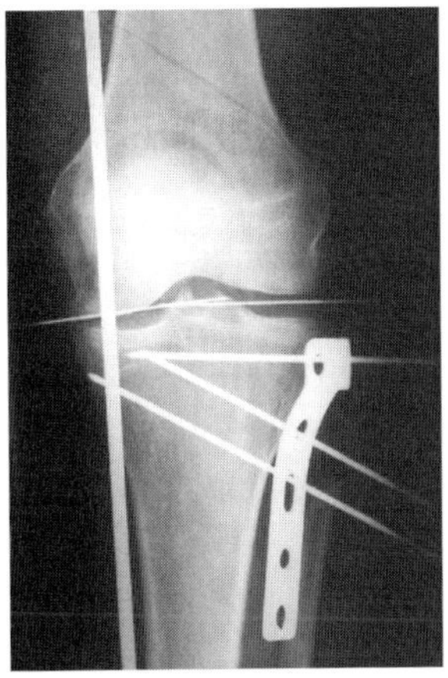

Fig. 10a

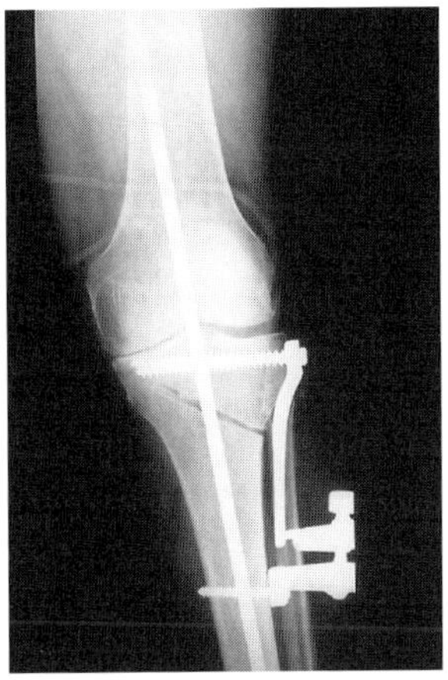

Fig. 10b

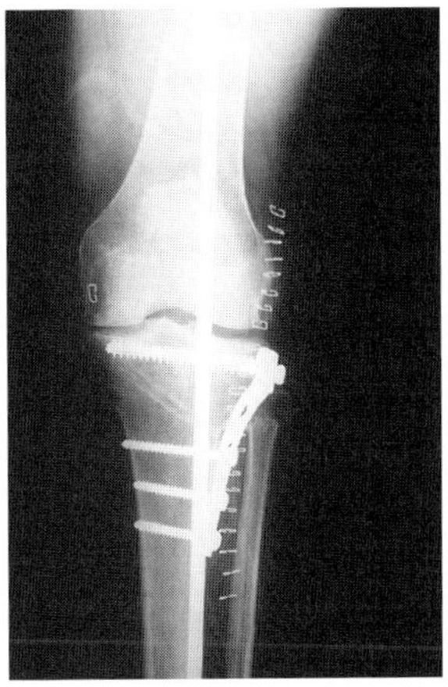

Fig. 10c

Radiographs showing the elastic valgus HTO a) peroperatively with guide pins, b) the attained normal correction and c) overcorrection of ± 2°.

maintaining the calculated angle of correction. Asymmetrical opening can produce a significant rotational deformity, sometimes of more than 15° of malrotation and also a genu flexum if the HTO opens more in front than in the back. This complication occurs quite often. In the back where there is hard cortex and important musculotendinous insertions such as semimembranosus, obtaining the correct degree of opening is not easy and may require considerable soft-tissue release. The medial ligament system may also have to be released.

In 2000 Fowler, Tan and Brown[20] described the technique for the opening-wedge HTO using the new Puddu plate[21] (Fig. 11). They report optimistically about this procedure but warn of destabilising the opposite cortical hinge. Their postoperative management is to place the operated leg in a padded hinge brace for six weeks with partial weight-bearing and crutches, followed by another six weeks of "full protected weight-bearing. Usually union is complete by 12 weeks. If the lateral cortex is violated, a more conservative approach to the weight-bearing schedule is recommended."

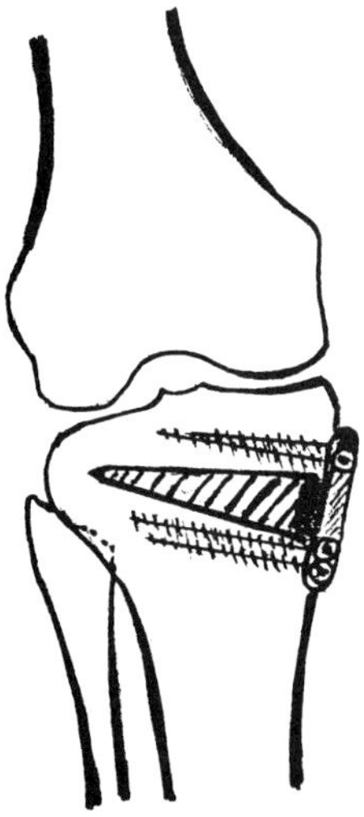

Fig. 11

Diagram of the medial opening-wedge HTO with the Puddu plate system.

Recently, De Simoni, Stäubli and Appenzeller[22] demonstrated a new fixation system for use with an opening-wedge HTO, which is similar to the new LISS (Less Invasive Stabilising System) of the AO IF-techniques. A multicentre study with this implant is currently in progress.

Finally, mention must be made of the possibility of a continuously opening medial wedge using the Heidelberg External Fixator System (HEFS) by callus distraction. The external fixation has to be worn for six weeks and the patients have to be carefully selected because of the daily self-administered distraction. The advantages are the choice of the best angle of correction and of fast consolidation by callus distraction.

EFFECT OF HTO ON PATELLOFEMORAL OSTEOARTHRITIS

In all cases of grade-II, grade-III and even grade-IV osteoarthritis with marked preoperative patellofemoral osteoarthritis there is a significant improvement in the latter with almost full relief from pain after closing-wedge valgus HTO. The preoperative lateralisation of the patella is reduced. We suggest that as a result of the valgus correction, the antivarus dynamic tension-band forces are decreased. The closing-wedge technique also lengthens the lateral part of the patellar tendon and reduces its tension. It remains to be seen whether opening-wedge valgus HTO which increases the patellofemoral pressure by relatively shortening the patellar tendon will also improve the symptoms of patellofemoral osteoarthritis (Fig. 12).

The general advantages and disadvantages of both techniques are given in Table III.

LENGTHENING OR SHORTENING OF THE TIBIA AFTER HTO

Changing a varus into a valgus knee does not alter the length markedly. In order to calculate the objective difference in

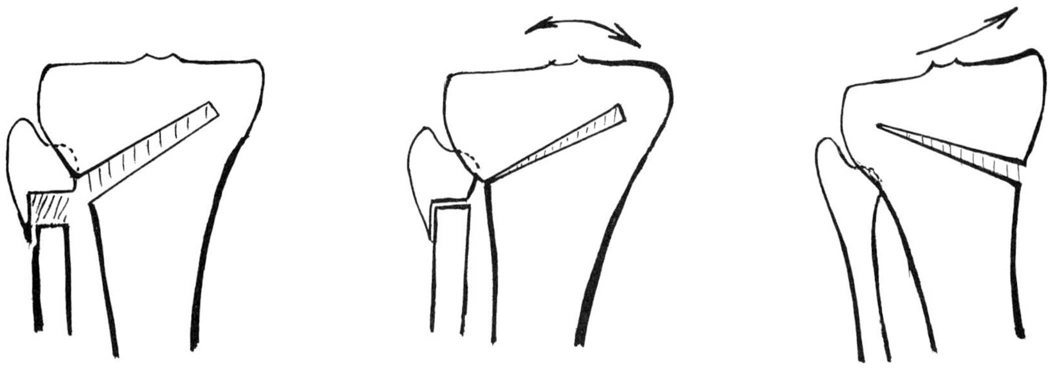

Fig. 12a Fig. 12b Fig. 12c

Diagrams showing the different deformations of the tibial plateau in the closing and opening-wedge techniques. Figure 12a – The bone cuts for elastic VHTO and proximal FOT. Figure 12b – After valgus deformation with a bent medial tibial plateau. Figure 12c – After a medial opening wedge for VHTO with elevation and bending up of the medial tibial plateau: (b) and (c) can be observed on postoperative radiographs after open or elastic closing-wedge procedures.

Table III. General advantages and disadvantages of opening- and closed-wedge HTOs

	Advantages	Disadvantages
Opening wedge	No FOT, less risk for the peroneal nerve Less exposure necessary Correction angle peroperatively and after	Limited in opening Limited in correction angle Higher compression in the medial compartment Fixation less stable Longer protection time and non-weight-bearing
	Technically less demanding	Risk of creating genu flexum malrotation Medial skin incision (saphenous nerve) Patellofemoral osteoarthritis
Closing wedge	Larger correction angle possible Better control of the medial compartment with early full movement and stable fixation	FOT Higher risk for the peroneal nerve Greater soft-tissue exposure Elastic closing technically more demanding Compartment syndrome (rare)
	Less risk of malrotation or of genu flexum Lateral skin incision, less nerves involved Patellofemoral osteoarthritis improved	

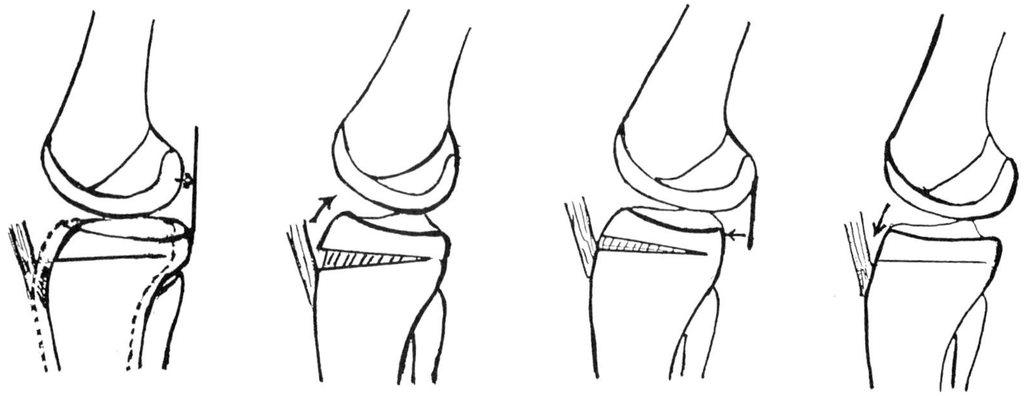

Fig. 13a Fig. 13b Fig. 13c Fig. 13d

Diagrams of sagittal HTO showing a) and b) the elevation of the tibial slope for genu recurvatum or instability of the PCL or PCL-posterolateral instability and c) and d) deflection for chronic anterior subluxation in instability of the ACL.

length, the angle and size of the wedge must be considered in the centre of the tibia where the mechanical axis passes. This is equally true for a closing or an opening wedge. With a wedge height of 9 mm at the periphery, the lengthening or shortening in the central mechanical axis of the tibia is only 4 to 5 mm. For the total length of the limb this is not a problem, but relative shortening of the patellar tendon of 5 mm in opening-wedge HTO may be significant.

HTO IN THE SAGITTAL PLANE

Dejour et al[5] and Neyret et al[6] reported that deformity after growth disturbance, genu recurvatum and chronic instability of the ACL or PCL are the main indications for restoring the angle of slope of the tibia or for changing it (Fig. 13). Instability of the ACL requires a reduction of the slope, that of the PCL an anterior elevation for the biomechanical balance of the forces. Sometimes a combination of valgus and varus HTO is necessary.

GENERAL REMARKS CONCERNING THE SURGICAL APPROACHES

The medial side of the knee is copiously supplied by sensory nerves from the expansion of the saphenous nerve. All incisions divide some of these branches leaving numbness and paraesthesia which often prohibits kneeling. Release of the medial collateral ligament is often necessary.

The lateral side contains much less important sensory nerve branches. The denervated area after any lateral incision is smaller and the anterior part of the knee especially retains its intact sensitivity, but the development of a compartment syndrome is possible.

RESULTS OF HTO IN THE LITERATURE

Results for varus HTO. Coventry[4] reported optimistically on 45 knees operated between 1960 and 1979. After correction the medial tilt of the plateau was less than 10°. He stated that the tibial spine was load-bearing on its lateral slope towards the lateral compartment, especially in the presence of a pre-existing varus tilt. Shoji and Insall[23] reported 49 knees in 45 patients which had had varus HTO. After a follow-up of 31 months only 53% of patients had relief of pain; 14% had partial relief and 33% had none. They did not recommend varus HTO. Chambat et al[24] and Dejour et al[5] supported the procedure if the required correction did not exceed 10°. Their favoured alternative was a varus osteotomy of the distal femur.

Results for valgus HTO. Jenny, Jenny and Morscher[25] reported the short- and long-term results of 783 transverse closing-wedge HTOs. Of these, 587 (75%) were very satisfactory or satisfactory, 130 (15%) showed no marked improvement and in 66 (10%) there was increased pain a few months after operation. In the further evaluation of their results they found that the group of satisfied and very satisfied patients increased after more than ten years. Those with no marked improvement remained more or less constant over ten years and then deteriorated. The group of the dissatisfied patients deteriorated almost immediately after the HTO and continued to do so. Fifteen (2%) required reosteotomy and 8.7% of the dissatisfied group required TKA, in 19 within two years.

Odenbring et al[26] and Odenbring[27] reported 314 patients who had had HTO with a follow-up of 10 to 14 years. Of these, 52 had TKA, 10 had a further HTO, 54 of 170 had revision of undercorrected HTO, and 8 of 144 had revision of normal or overcorrected HTO.

Yasuda et al[28] described satisfactory results in 85% of 50 HTOs after six years and in 62% after ten years. All of these series show that the results are not easily comparable. Depending on the indication and on the angle of correction they may be good and satisfying in the long term while the unsatisfactory group tended to deteriorate soon after the operation.

Within the last five decades HTOs have been carried out for very different indications, and in different populations. Yasuda et al[28] have had experience of a population which is small in stature and with knees in internal rotation. These would have required overcorrection which in northern Europe would have resulted in progressive valgus deformity.[10]

ELASTIC VALGUS HTO

Before the success of TKA, HTO was used mainly for elderly patients with marked stage-III or stage-IV osteoarthritis who required some overcorrection. Cosmetically, it was not so important how the overcorrections appeared, but now this is no longer the case. In our country some patients still want a HTO instead of a TKA because they like to maintain walking and are worried that a TKA would not withstand such demands over a long period of time without wear and loosening. They trust the good results of HTO. In addition, younger patients with, for example, post-traumatic instability, represent a new group of indications. They have greater demands in terms of the cosmetic appearance etc.

We have therefore developed a technique termed the 'elastic HTO'. With this method we can choose peroperatively the correct angle by marking the mechanical axis with a rod on the radiographs. In especially difficult cases we also compared the required axis with the axis of the opposite leg and thus achieved a cosmetically acceptable result and a biomechanically correct alignment in this younger population.

We have evaluated a series of 100 elastic valgus HTOs operated on between 1989 and 1990 with a minimal follow-up of 36 up to 48 months.[18] This series contained all the indications including normal correction, slight overcorrection in ligamentous instability, a grade-I and grade-II osteoarthritis and marked grade III to, exceptionally, grade IV.

The angle of correction was between 4° and 18°. The mean valgus correction for a preoperative varus of 7.1° was 8.9°. The mean postoperative femorotibial anatomical angle was 187°. Overall, 26% of patients were very satisfied, 52% satisfied, 18% partially satisfied and 8% not satisfied.

Nowadays, the indication for some patients in this series would have been for a primary TKA, because the results of TKA are more reliable since systems with meniscal bearings give much better results even with a higher demand.

In the series complications included loss of correction in three patients, in two of whom this was minor but the third required operative correction with medial buttressing. There were two cases of transient lesions of the peroneal nerve and none of deep-vein thrombosis. In addition, in the last 18 years we have observed three cases of infection, one of a compartment syndrome, and one of aneurysm of the anterior tibial artery.

REFERENCES

1. **Jackson JP.** Osteotomy for osteoarthritis of the knee. *J Bone Joint Surg [Br]* 1958;40-B:826.
2. **Jackson JP, Waugh W.** Tibial osteotomy for osteoarthritis of the knee. *J Bone Joint Surg [Br]* 1961;43-B:746-51.
3. **Coventry MB.** Osteotomy of the upper portion of the tibia for degenerative arthritis of the knee: a preliminary report. *Clin Orthop* 1989;248:4-8.
4. **Coventry MB.** Proximal tibial varus osteotomy for osteoarthritis of the lateral compartment of the knee. *J Bone Joint Surg [Am]* 1987;69:32-8.
5. **Dejour D, et al.** Tibial antirecurvatum osteotomies. *Oper Techn Sports Med* 2000;8:67-70.
6. **Neyret Ph, et al.** Tibial deflexion osteotomy. *Oper Techn Sports Med* 2000;8:1:61-6.
7. **Catagni MA, et al.** The role of external fixation in antivarus tibial osteotomy. *Oper Techn Sports Med* 2000;8:1:39-43.
8. **Aglietti P, Buzzi R, Gaudenzi A, Sangregorio P, Scrobe F.** Accuracy in high tibial osteotomy in varus gonarthrosis. *Arch Putti Chir Organi Mov* 1989;37:271-82.
9. **Brown GA, Amendola A.** Radiographic evaluation and preoperative planning for high tibial osteotomies. *Oper Techn Sports Med* 2000;8:1:2-19.
10. **Hernigou P, Medevielle D, Debeyre J, Goutallier D.** Proximal tibial osteotomy for osteoarthritis with varus deformity: a ten to thirteen-year follow-up study. *J Bone Joint Surg [Am]* 1987;69:332-54.
11. **Fujisawa V, Masuhara K, Shiomi S.** The effect of high tibial osteotomy on osteoarthritis of the knee: an arthroscopic study on 54 knee joints. *Orthop Clin North Am* 1979;10:585-608.
12. **Noyes FR, Schipplein OD, Andriacchi TP, Saddemi SR, Weise M.** The anterior cruciate ligament-deficient knee with varus alignment: an analysis of gait adaptations and dynamic joint loadings. *Am J Sports Med* 1992;20:707-16.
13. **Ahlbäck S.** Osteoarthritis of the knee: a radiographic investigation. *Acta Radiol* 1968;277:7-72.
14. **Kirgis A, Albrecht MS.** Palsy of the deep peroneal nerve after proximal tibial osteotomy: an anatomical study. *J Bone Joint Surg [Am]* 1992;74-A:1180-5.
15. **Stuart MJ.** Tibial antivarus closing wedge osteotomy. *Oper Techn Sports Med* 2000;8:1:27-31.
16. **Naumann I, Köhler G, Stephan E.** Komplikationen bei Tibiakopfosteotomien in Abhängigkeit von der Fixierung. *Orthop Praxis* 1987;23:466-71.
17. **Naumann I, Stephan E.** Ergebnisse von 221 Tibiakop-Pendelosteotomien. *Orthop Praxis* 1984;20:914-6.
18. **Müller W, Kentsch A, Schäfer N.** The elastic high tibia valgus osteotomy in the varus deformity. *Oper Techn Sports Med* 2000;8:1:19-26.
19. **Goutallier D, Hernigou P, Lenoble E.** Treatment of lax arthrotic genu valgum using Debeyre's unicondylar osteotomy: a radioclinical study of 55 knees operated on more than 5 years ago. *Rev Chir Orthop Reparatrice Appar Mot* 1988;74:753-63.
20. **Fowler PJ, Tan JL, Brown G.** Medial opening wedge high tibial osteotomy: how I do it. *Oper Techn Sports Med* 2000;8:1:32-8.
21. **Puddu G, Franco V.** Femoral antivalgus opening wedge osteotomy. *Oper Techn Sports Med.* 2000;8:1:56-60.
22. **De Simoni C, Stäubli A, Appenzeller A.** Neue Fixationstechnik für mediale open-wedge osteotomien der proximalen Tibia. Abstr SGO Congress (Schweizerische Gesellschaft für Orthopädie 7-9 Sept Davos. In: *Schweiz Med Wochenschrift* 2000;119:130.
23. **Shoji H, Insall J.** High tibial osteotomy for osteoarthritis of the knee with valgus deformity. *J Bone Joint Surg [Am]* 1973;55-A:963-73.
24. **Chambat P, et al.** Varus tibial osteotomy. *Oper Techn Sports Med* 2000;8:1:44-7.
25. **Jenny K, Jenny H, Morscher E.** Indications, surgical technique and results of transcondylar tibia osteotomy in gonarthrosis: experiences based on a follow-up study of 783 tibia osteotomies. *Orthopade* 1985;14:161-71.
26. **Odenbring S, et al.** Revision after OT for gonarthrosis: a 10-19 years follow-up of 314 cases. *Acta Orthop Scand* 1990;61:128-30.
27. **Odenbring S.** *Osteotomy for medial gonarthrosis.* Lund: Ortonova AB Sweden, 1991.
28. **Yasuda K, et al.** A ten- to 15-year follow-up observation of high tibial osteotomy in medial compartment osteoarthrosis. *Clin Orthop* 1992;282:186-95.

REVISION SURGERY IN FAILED TOTAL KNEE ARTHROPLASTY

D. HUTEN

From Bichat Hospital, Paris, France

Revision of total knee arthroplasty (TKA) is becoming a more common procedure because of the increasing number of TKAs performed each year and the decreasing age of the patients undergoing surgery. Nevertheless, revision of a TKA remains much less common than that of a total hip arthroplasty.

Many complications of TKA may require a revision procedure. These include aseptic loosening, osteolysis, stiffness, laxity, patellar complications, periprosthetic fracture, mechanical failure, rupture of the extensor mechanism and unexplained pain.

Each complication may require a specific procedure such as arthrolysis, secondary patellar resurfacing, or exchange of a part or the whole prosthesis. Infection and postoperative skin necrosis which often coexist, lead to other specific problems and will not be discussed here. We participated in a symposium of the French Society of Orthopaedic Surgery (SOFCOT) in 2000, dedicated to revision of TKA and will now report its conclusions.[1]

The first step is to identify the complication. It is often easy to recognise aseptic loosening or patellar dislocation but it can be difficult to identify flexion instability,[2] patellar clunk syndrome, or dissociation of a tibial component.[3] In these difficult cases, specialised investigations such as imaging or arthroscopy are required.

The second step is to understand the mechanism of failure. Long-term wear of tibial polyethylene, a poor prosthetic design or malalignment can explain loosening. It is often more difficult to identify the reason for tilt or dislocation of the patella (malposition of a femoral or tibial component, contraction of the lateral retinaculum of the patella), laxity (ligament insufficiency, malalignment, wear of tibial polyethylene), or stiffness (difficult rehabilitation, reflex sympathetic dystrophy, component malposition).

The revision must correct the cause of the complication. Thus, there are many aspects to revision, ranging from the exchange of a tibial implant, arthrolysis or secondary patellar resurfacing to the exchange of the whole prosthesis. A revision procedure is not limited to prosthetic exchange although this is the most common operation. Prosthetic exchange may be required for different complications such as loosening, osteolysis, stiffness, laxity or fracture.

EVALUATION OF FAILED TOTAL KNEE ARTHROPLASTY

A complete evaluation is needed, including the aetiology, previous procedures (osteotomy, ligament reconstruction, unicompartmental arthroplasty), length of follow-up, type of implant, immediate postoperative course (pain, stiffness, history of infection), onset of the symptoms (immediately after the initial procedure or delayed), pain (location, mechanical or inflammatory), effusion, chronic instability, crepitus and the medical background of the patient (age, medical history, particularly cardiovascular).

During the physical examination, the alignment of the knee, the quality of the skin and scar(s), effusion, range of movement, anteroposterior (AP), varus and valgus stress laxity, and localised pain on palpation or during patellar mobilisation should be recorded.

Standard radiographs (AP, lateral, patellar skyline view) will provide the following data: 1) the type of prosthesis, sacrificing or retaining the posterior cruciate ligament (PCL), cemented or not, with or without patellar resurfacing); 2) the individual placement and size of the component; 3) joint line and patellar height; 4) patellar alignment; 5) fixation of components (radiolucent lines, migration); and 6) patellar and tibial polyethylene wear.

Signs of periprosthetic osteolysis or of infection (periosteal reaction) should be noted. A full-length standing AP radiograph will determine accurately the position of the components.

Infection must be eliminated. Febrile episodes, long periods of postoperative antibiotic therapy, evidence of inflammation on inspection of the knee, osteolysis and an elevated level of C-reactive protein should be recorded. If suspicion of infection prevails, aspiration is required and a cell count, measurement of glucose levels and culture of organisms should be carried out.

Other investigations may be required. Stress radiographs are helpful in evaluating laxity or to identify loosening without migration of components. CT may be used to measure the angle between the transverse axis of the femoral component and the transepicondylar line, the femoral neck axis compared with the other side, and between the

AP mid-axes of the tibial component and the tibial tubercle. Bone scans may be helpful when loosening or infection is suspected but the sensitivity and specificity are poor.

The requirements for these tests are based on the type of complication and the proposed revision procedure.

ASEPTIC LOOSENING AND OSTEOLYSIS

Aseptic loosening is the major indication for revision which consists of exchanging a part of or the whole prosthesis. The technical requirements are identical to those of a primary TKA although they are more difficult to meet. They are as follows:

1) There must be a normally aligned knee in the coronal and sagittal planes.
2) The distal femoral and tibial cuts in the coronal plane must be perpendicular to the mechanical axis of the lower limb (or parallel to the ground, during one-leg standing i.e., with a 3° varus cut).
3) The joint line and patella must be located at a normal height.
4) There must be satisfactory and balanced tension of capsuloligamentous structures in flexion and extension. It must be remembered that the tibial cut contributes to ligament tension during extension and in 90° flexion, while the distal femoral cut contributes only in extension and the posterior femoral cut only in 90° flexion.
5) The range of movement should be identical to the maximum predicted range for the implant, without impingement, usually 0° to 120°.
6) The patella must track normally with balanced tension of the patellar retinacula.

The amount of epiphyseal bone loss and the condition of the collateral ligaments must be considered during preoperative planning. The degree of bone loss, however, can best be assessed during surgery. There are different classifications of bone loss after removal of the components.[4,5] That of the SOFCOT symposium[6] is based on the condition of the bone stock after the bone cuts. It applies to both tibial and femoral condyles and includes three parameters, namely, the level of bone cuts, the symmetry or asymmetry of the tibial and distal femoral cuts, and loss of bone, i.e., absent, cavitary or segmental.

For the patella, we have considered three 'possibilities': 1) no or minimal loss of bone allowing a satisfactory reimplantation of a new component; 2) loss of bone making reimplantation uncertain; and 3) loss of bone preventing reimplantation.

It is more difficult to identify the condition of the collateral ligaments before and even during the procedure. Before the revision, examination must be made for previous ligament injuries, either traumatic or surgical, or a history of significant deformity with stretching of ligaments on the convex side and contraction on the concave side. Laxity or a subluxation of the prosthesis must be noted. Standing and stress radiographs are helpful. Pseudolaxity, however, is created by component wear (Fig. 4) or migration, and should not be confused with true ligamentous deficiency.

Technical errors at the initial operation need to be identified on the radiographs of the affected knee. Comparison with the contralateral knee is necessary to identify the size of the components, the height of the patella and the joint line.

Thus, preoperative planning can allow the selection of a revision system with augments, stems, standard and constrained tibial plateaux and will assess the need for bone allografts. The exchange of a single component is sometimes possible, provided that a replacement is still available.

The incision is determined by the previous surgery and must avoid creating extensive flaps which may lead to skin necrosis and infection. A previous midline or medial parapatellar incision is preferred. A lateral incision should only be used when close to the joint and may require an associated osteotomy of the tibial tubercle. If multiple longitudinal scars are present, the most lateral is the safest. A plastic surgical intervention should be considered in cases of poor previous wound healing or multiple incisions.

Exposure may be critical, especially if the knee is stiff. Avulsion of the patellar tendon is difficult to treat and has a poor prognosis. Removal of one or both components, when possible, relaxes soft tissues and often avoids a relieving incision in the quadriceps[7] or an osteotomy of the tibial tubercle.[8] This osteotomy, when necessary, must detach a long fragment and be separated from the tibial cut by a bridge of bone. It allows a good exposure but may lead to secondary displacement or nonunion. We prefer the relieving incision in the quadriceps because it is easy to repair and does not weaken the quadriceps. The V-Y quadriceps turndown[7] devascularises the patella and weakens the quadriceps.

Removal of loose components is easy. Conversely, removal of adequately fixed components, especially when they are uncemented, is difficult. Polyethylene tibial and patellar components may be transected by an oscillating saw and the peg(s) removed. Use of an oscillating or a Gigli saw for the cement-bone interface is of value for metal components, although metal pegs may limit this. Several osteotomes can be inserted on top of one another to separate the metal components from bone. Lever-arm manoeuvres are dangerous. Direct impaction onto the components is less dangerous but may remove cancellous bone with the components.

Hypertrophic synovial membrane and granulomatous tissue should be removed very carefully.

The first step is the tibial cut. It should be perpendicular to the axis of the tibia in both the coronal and sagittal planes (or with a 3° posterior slope). Either intra- or extramedullary instrumentation may be used. An overly

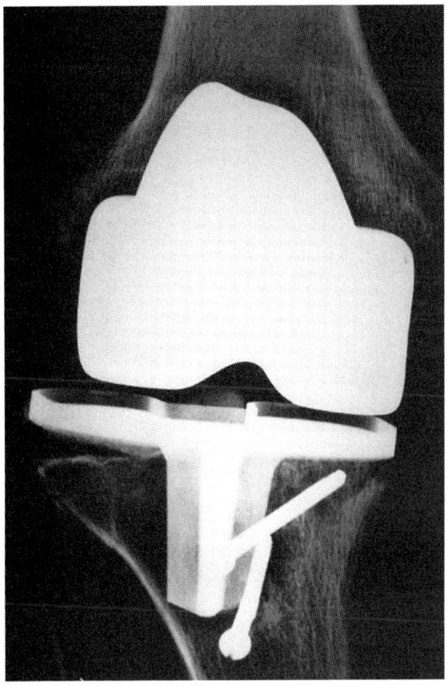

Fig. 1a

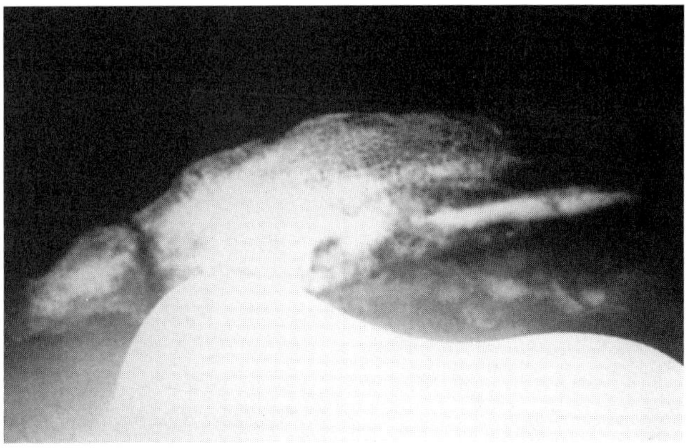

Fig. 1b

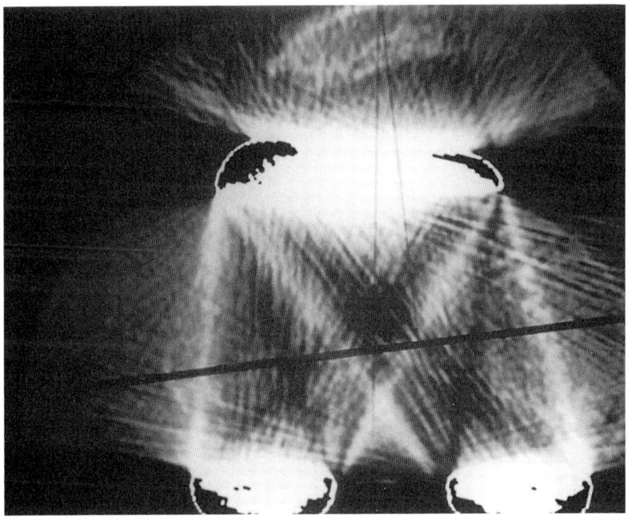

Fig. 1c

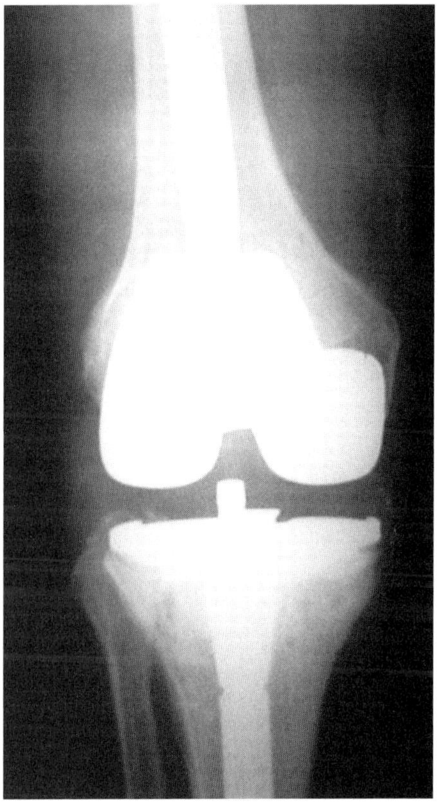

Fig. 1d

Figure 1a – Radiograph showing aseptic tibial loosening with varus migration and osteolysis of the medial tibial plateau. Figure 1b – Radiograph showing lateral subluxation of the patella with associated fracture and loosening of the component. Figure 1c – CT shows internal rotation of the femoral component of 7°. Figure 1d – Radiograph showing a Wallaby III revision TKA, with bone grafting of the medial tibial plateau and uncemented stems.

distal cut eliminates all bone defects but decreases the width of the cut surface which will support the tibial component. An overly proximal cut retains large bone defects and weak bone which is unable to support the component. An intramedullary stem is often required and many ancillary systems are based on intramedullary press-fit stems. They are stable but may lead to malposition of the components if the axis of the stem differs from the anatomical axis of the tibia.

The trial tibial baseplate and the trial tibial plateau should restore the appropriate height of the joint line. This can be measured on the preoperative radiographs, taking the opposite knee as a reference. The distance can be checked during the procedure, taking the head of the fibula or the tibial tubercle as a landmark.

On the femoral side, the distal cut should be perpendicular to the mechanical axis of the femur. The angle between the anatomical and mechanical axis must be considered, and the intramedullary instrumentation should allow a 3, 5 or 7° valgus cut, according to this angle. If a stem is used, different stems with these different valgus angles are needed. The most frequent errors are to undersize the femoral component, to position it too proximally and to use a thick tibial component to obtain tension of the soft tissues. When selecting the femoral size, that of the previous femoral component must be considered. The contralateral radiograph is more useful. The femoral component should stabilise the knee in flexion with the selected tibial plateau, without medial or lateral overhang. The proximodistal position of the femoral component should stabilise the knee in extension with this same tibial plateau. If the soft tissues are normal, the height of the joint line is normal. If they are lax, an adequate femoral reconstruction does not provide stability. A thicker tibial component will result in an excessively proximal joint line and a patella baja. More distal positioning of the femoral component and a larger femoral component should be considered if possible.

With 90° flexion, the rotation of the femoral component and the stability in flexion should be determined. Rotational landmarks are identified. The guidelines vary according to the different authors. In revision surgery, the posterior aspect of the femoral condyles and the Whiteside line are not available. The epicondylar axis may be used and is considered by many authors as the best landmark[9-13] but it is sometimes difficult to identify both epicondyles, especially the medial one. When the femoral component has not migrated, preoperative CT will measure the angle between the transverse axis of the component and the epicondylar line (Fig. 1). This procedure helps to rotate the new femoral component appropriately. This landmark leads to slight external rotation of the femoral component and also to external rotation of the tibial component which has to be congruent with the femoral component in extension. It moves the trochlear groove laterally, thus improving patellar tracking. It also increases the tension of the lateral soft tissues, and decreases this on the medial side.

Stability in flexion is checked with the tibial plateau and the femoral trial component. If the flexion gap is asymmetrical, the contracted soft tissues should be released. In cases of flexion instability, the height of the joint line i.e., the thickness of the tibial plateau, and the anteroposterior size, frequently underestimated, of the femoral component should be checked (Fig. 2). Flexion instability may also be due to stretching of the soft tissues. Once a femoral size has been selected, the amount of posterior femoral bone loss can be estimated.

With the knee in extension, the proximodistal position of the femoral component stabilising the knee with the tibial plateau, without fixed flexion or recurvatum, should be determined. If the extension gap is asymmetrical, the contracted soft tissues must be released. Most often there is distal femoral loss of bone and the femoral component has to be more distal on one or both sides of the knee. This step is facilitated by ancillary systems which can align a trial femoral component along a centromedullary stem. More rarely, a fixed flexion deformity may require a more proximal femoral component and a distal resection is needed. Distal femoral resection which is too great, however, makes the collateral ligaments loose and leads to mid-flexion instability. It is better to perform a posterior release.

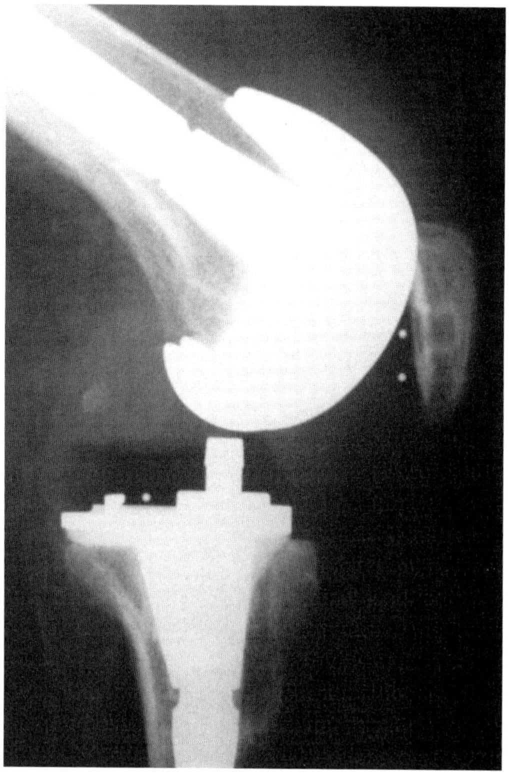

Fig. 2

Radiograph showing dislocation of a revision prosthesis. The selected femoral component is too small and does not restore the anteroposterior size of the femur before arthroplasty (flexion instability).

Once both the flexion and extension gaps are determined, the femoral chamfer and the intercondylar region are prepared. A trial is performed with the femoral component and a posterostabilised tibial plateau. The rotation of the tibial component is then determined. The middle of the tibial plateau must be opposite the mid-third of the tibial tubercle. The tibial post should also be fully congruent with the femoral box in extension. Patellar tracking is most satisfactory in this position. In case of patellar subluxation, a lateral retinacular release is needed.

Cavitary defects may be filled with cement if moderate, but a morsellised and impacted bone graft is preferable. It is much more difficult to reconstruct segmentary defects. Cement, with or without screws, cannot be pressurised and has no mechanical efficiency. Quadrangular femoral augments and triangular or quadrangular tibial augments are reliable and easy to use. Ancillary systems allow bone cuts according to their shape and size. In some revision systems thicker femoral components are also available and allow reconstruction of larger defects. When the augments are too small, as in segmentary defects over 8 or 10 mm, structural and, more rarely, massive bone grafts are needed.[5] Bony fragments with collateral ligament origins should be reattached.

Centromedullary stems are needed in the case of large segmentary defects or weak bone. Uncemented large press-fit stems are usually preferred,[14] but are difficult to use for the following reasons. The femur is curved and long stems impinge against the anterior cortex. This impingement may prevent their use or may be painful.[15] The angle between the anatomical and mechanical axes of the femur varies. For this reason, stems with different valgus angles are needed (3, 5, 7°). The tibial or the femoral shaft may sometimes present a distal valgus or varus curve. In these cases a stem in the proximal tibia or the distal femur leads to valgus or varus of the tibial or femoral component and may impinge against the cortex. The anatomical axis of the tibial shaft is often not aligned with the middle of the epiphysis.[16] A stem may impinge against the tibial cortex. Moreover, the tibial component may overhang unless a smaller component is used. For this reason, offset stems may be needed. In many ancillary systems, positioning of the components is based on centromedullary stems: misalignment of a stem leads to component malposition. If the stems are introduced through the trial components, they can impinge on the cortex. It is easier to use cemented stems. They are thinner and do not impinge, but they are difficult to remove in the case of infection or loosening.

In most of the total knee revision systems, standard posterostabilised and constrained posterostabilised tibial plateaux are available. Constrained plateaux limit varus/valgus and rotation. They enhance knee stability but increase the risk of loosening and require the use of stems for this reason. All the trials are done with an unconstrained standard tibial plateau. If the joint is stable in extension and flexion, no further constraint is required. In other cases, a coronal, rotational femoral, or tibial malalignment, or an overly proximal joint line must be ruled out and the use of a constrained plateau considered. It can control isolated instability in flexion but is unable to control instability in extension, especially if medial. Instability in extension is due to deficient medial or lateral tissues which must be recognised preoperatively or as early as possible during the procedure. If necessary, a rotating hinge prosthesis must be used to resolve this problem.

An unresurfaced patella may or may not be resurfaced if the trochlear design is adequate,[17] but in our experience relief of pain is better when the patella has been resurfaced.[1] A well-fixed and intact patellar prosthesis is retained if it can be coupled with the revision femoral component. In other cases, the available bone stock will determine if the component should be removed and changed. It is better to revise a well-fixed metal-backed patellar component, but it is difficult to remove it and the patella may even be fractured. The clinical relevance of the condition of the patella at the end of the procedure is controversial.[18,19] We prefer to resurface the patella whenever possible.

The functional results of prosthesis exchange are satisfying but long-term results are uncertain, and the survival rate at eight years was only 83% in the series of Hass et al.[14]

OTHER REVISIONS

Stiffness. Preoperative stiffness, post-traumatic osteoarthritis, multiple previous operations, neuromuscular disorders, difficult rehabilitation, and reflex sympathetic dystrophy (RSD) promote stiffness. It may also be due to technical errors such as malposition, oversized components, or increased patellar thickness. While not proven, stiffness is more probable with prostheses which retain the PCL or both cruciate ligaments. If the range of movement does not improve in spite of adequate rehabilitation a manipulation is indicated before four or at most eight weeks. For this reason, patients have to be seen at four weeks after the initial procedure. Late manipulations may give satisfying results,[20] but there is a risk of femoral or tibial fracture and rupture of the extensor mechanism.

Arthrolysis may be indicated when malalignment has been ruled out. In surgical arthrolysis, all intra-articular adhesions in the suprapatellar pouch, and the medial and lateral gutters can be released. A lateral retinacular release is often needed. A PCL which is too tight can be partially detached from its femoral or tibial origin.[21] The improvement in the arc of movement is assessed after each step. Removal of a modular tibial plateau facilitates the exposure and allows release of the posterior capsule in the case of a flexion deformity. A patella that is too thick can be thinned. A modular tibial plateau that is too thick can be changed.

Arthroscopic arthrolysis is less invasive but also less efficient. A flexion deformity cannot be treated. It requires greater experience. There is a risk of scratching the components and of postoperative bleeding. In the absence of a significant flexion deformity it may be indicated with more recently occurring stiffness. In difficult cases it can be converted into an open procedure.

Prosthesis exchange may be necessary in cases of malpositioned or oversized components. It can also be carried out after a failed arthrolysis. The exposure is difficult and may require a quadriceps release or osteotomy of the tibial tubercle. Removal of well-fixed components can be difficult and create loss of bone which will need reconstruction. The technical errors of the initial operation must be identified and corrected to achieve satisfactory kinematics. Sacrifice of a previously retained PCL facilitates the procedure and the postoperative rehabilitation.

The range of movement achieved by the weight of the leg is noted at the end of the procedure. A long and intensive postoperative rehabilitation is required. Nevertheless, some movement will be lost during the postoperative course.[1] The most important risk is recurrent or

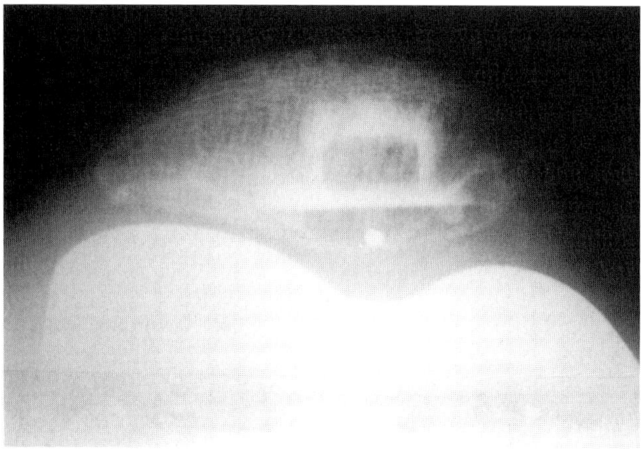
Fig. 3a

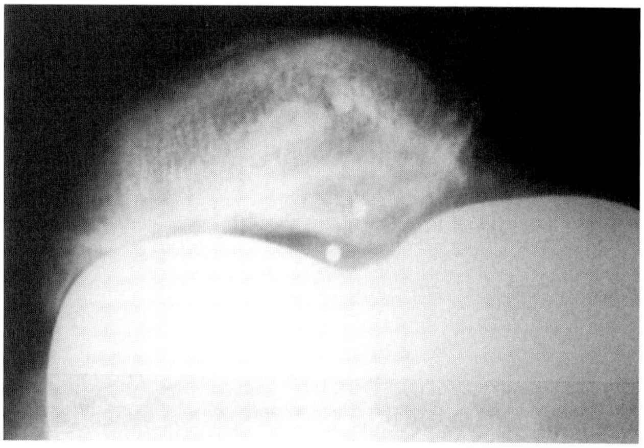
Fig. 3b

Radiographs showing a) the inlay patellar component and b) six years later with asymptomatic migration, fracture of the cement and lateral tilting and impingement of the patella.

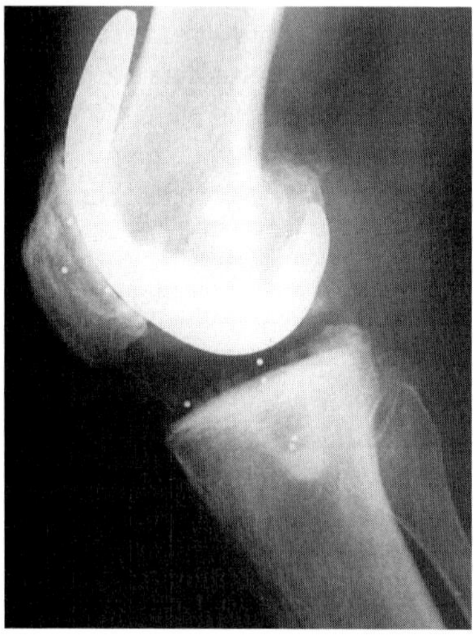
Fig. 4a

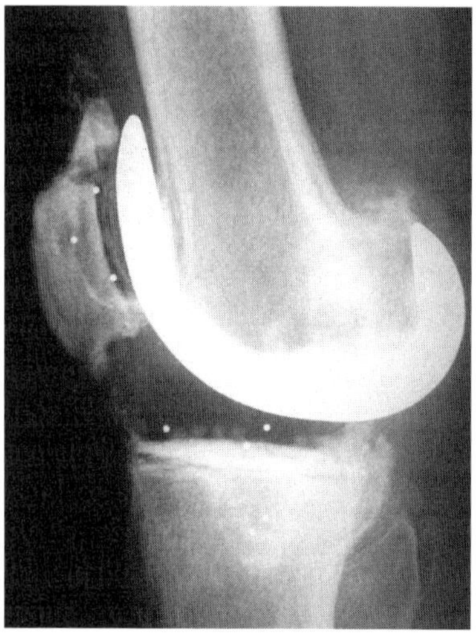
Fig. 4b

Radiographs showing a) a Freeman prosthesis and b) 13 years later with anterior tibial subluxation due to posterior wear of the polyethylene. There is a painful fracture of the proximal pole of the patella.

even increased stiffness and, for this reason, the decision as to whether to revise a stiff TKA is difficult. The improvement in the range of movement is more important when more limited before the procedure. This should be judged according to the degree of stiffness and an associated flexion deformity. In the presence of slight malposition, it is difficult to decide between arthrolysis and exchange.

Laxity. This may be revealed by different symptoms. Posterostabilised total knees may dislocate, most often in the first postoperative months. Chronic instability with pain, swelling, giving-way and a feeling of insecurity, can be observed with both PCL-sacrificing and PCL-retaining prostheses. It can occur both early, in the case of malalignment or ligament deficiency, or late and may then be attributed to wear of the tibial polyethylene causing progressive subluxation. Instability in flexion may only be revealed by pain and chronic swelling and, even then, is difficult to diagnose.[2]

Dislocation of posterostabilised prostheses (Fig. 2) occurs most often in full flexion in patients having an excellent postoperative range of flexion.[22] In obese patients, this complication is associated with impingement between the hypertrophic soft tissues of the thigh and the calf. Dislocation may be isolated or associated with chronic instability. Once the dislocation has been reduced, either under anaesthesia or not, coronal and anteroposterior stability must be assessed in extension and especially in flexion. An initial dislocation with a patient having a good functional result and a well-aligned prosthesis does not require a revision. Conversely, in recurrent dislocations or associated chronic instability, a revision must be considered. If there is balanced extension and flexion laxity but no malposition, a thicker tibial component can stabilise the knee. In some total knee systems, a plateau with a higher post (thicker or of the same thickness) can be used, but it is more constraining and the risk of loosening is increased. In other cases, prosthetic exchange is indicated.

Chronic instability is due to technical errors, associated ligament deficiency, or polyethylene wear (see Fig. 4). Exchange of the plateau is rarely indicated, but in some PCL-retaining prosthesis systems, ultracongruent plateaux are available and may heal a posterior laxity due to rupture of the PCL. In most cases, prosthetic exchange is the only option.

For prosthetic exchange, the condition of the collateral ligaments must be noted. If they are intact, correction of the technical errors of the initial procedure due to malaligned or undersized components and a standard posterostabilised plateau are adequate. A constrained posterostabilised plateau may be required if isolated flexion instability persists. In cases of extension instability due to a severe (especially medial) deficiency of the collateral ligament, a rotating hinge prosthesis should be considered.

Patellar complications. There are many patellar complications: pain, instability, necrosis, fracture, clunk syndrome, wear and loosening. In metal-backed patellar components, no longer used today, wear of the polyethylene may lead to rupture or disassociation.[23] Metal-on-metal contact releases metal particles thus inducing osteolysis and loosening which requires revision.

When facing patellar complications, the first step is to look for femoral or tibial malposition. A CT scan is needed. Excessive femorotibial valgus, internal femoral (Fig. 1) or tibial rotation, femoral or tibial medialisation, oversizing of the femoral component or a protruding trochlea due to flexion or anterior translation of the femoral component favour lateral patellar instability. It may be revealed by pain, swelling, recurrent or permanent dislocation, and a feeling of instability. Radiographs will demonstrate patellar malalignment (tilting, subluxation, dislocation), and, in some cases, wear of the lateral aspect of the patella (Fig. 3). The best treatment is correction of the femorotibial malalignment but it requires exchange of one or both components. In moderate malpositioning, especially if tibial, a transfer of the tibial tubercle can be considered but there is a risk of secondary displacement and nonunion. The alternative is a soft-tissue method such as Insall's proximal realignment procedure.

When the patellar complication cannot be explained by femorotibial malposition, the origin of the symptoms in the patellofemoral compartment must be sought. An unresurfaced patella may be painful, especially if the trochlear design is maladapted.[17] After secondary resurfacing, pain is frequently but not always relieved. Persisting pain after secondary resurfacing probably does not arise from the patella. An oblique patellar cut leads sometimes to painful bone-on-metal contact as well as an excessive tension of the lateral retinaculum if the lateral facet was insufficiently resected. Exchange or removal of the patellar component is indicated. Lateralisation of the patellar component and thickness of the patella greater than 4 mm[24] also favour patellar instability and should be corrected.

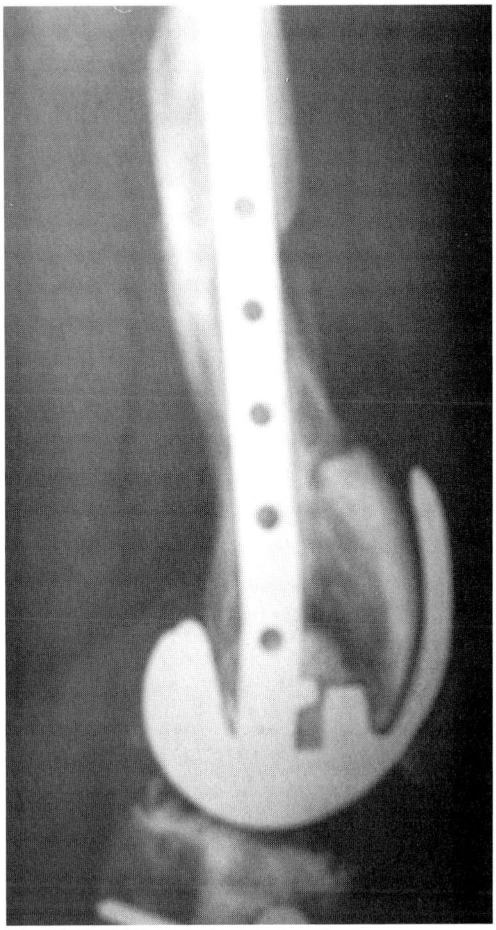

Fig. 5

Radiograph showing recurvatum malunion of the distal femur six years after locked retrograde intramedullary nailing. There is associated asymptomatic loosening of the femoral component, but the patient is free from pain.

Patellar fractures (Figs 1, 3 and 4) may be asymptomatic and revealed by routine radiographs. Different types have been described (marginal, transverse and shear fractures) and may compromise the fixation of the component and the continuity of the extensor mechanism.[25] Fractures without loosening or discontinuity of the extensor mechanism are treated conservatively.[25,26] In other cases, active extension lag and/or pain require a revision. Internal fixation and prosthetic reimplantation are rarely possible. Isolated removal of the loose component may be indicated or a partial or total patellectomy with reconstruction of the extensor mechanism. Pain is relieved but the quadriceps is weakened.[26] In asymptomatic fractures with associated loosening and release of particles, a revision has to be considered. With fractures, results of revisions are poor if an associated femorotibial malposition is not treated.

The clunk syndrome is a complication of posterostabilised total knees. It is due to a fibrous nodule at the superior pole of the patella locked in the intercondylar notch as the knee is brought from the flexed position to extension. The nodule suddenly pops out proximally and the patient experiences a clunking sensation. It requires surgical or arthroscopic removal of the nodule.[27] A superior overhang of the patella, a sharp anterior notch in the femoral component or a patella baja could result in irritation, leading to the formation of fibrous tissue and explain recurrence after excision of the nodule.

Isolated patellar loosening may be asymptomatic (Fig. 3) or painful which may then require exchange or removal of the loose component if bone stock is inadequate. A three-peg implant may be useful when revising a one-peg component, and vice versa. Component reimplantation combined with bone grafting[28] is an uncertain procedure.

When a patellar component is removed, the remnants of the patella may be spongialised to allow remodelling against the trochlea. A shell-shaped patella may be filled with morsellised bone graft maintained by a synovial flap. In revisions for patellar complications, the treatment of any associated femorotibial malposition such as varus or anterior tilt of the tibial component should be considered, especially if radiolucent lines or wear are present.

Femoral and tibial fractures. These are rare.[29,30] Osteoporosis due to ageing or steroid treatment predisposes to this complication. The role of anterior femoral notching is significant. The fracture may be at the level of or away from the component and isolated or associated with malposition, loosening or wear.

In isolated fractures, conservative treatment is possible with undisplaced and stable injuries. Otherwise, internal fixation is required. Plating decreases the blood supply to bone fragments. It is not stable in osteoporotic patients, and thus may lead to nonunion. Blade-plates and screw-plates with large epiphyseal screws improve the stability and for this reason are preferred to conventional plates.[1] Locked anterograde or retrograde femoral nailing is a less invasive treatment. A limited exposure may be necessary. Infection and rates of nonunion are decreased but malunion is more frequent and will make revision difficult. Retrograde nailing is not possible in PCL-sacrificing prostheses and with components which have a narrow intercondylar notch. This procedure often leads to recurvatum angulation because the entry point of the nail is too posterior (Fig. 5). Rush nails ascending from the area of both epicondyles have been recommended[31] but we have no personal experience of this.

In fractures associated with malpositioning, loosening or wear, exchange of the prosthesis should be considered, but this is a much more demanding procedure. Fixation of the fracture has to be combined with the prosthetic exchange, thus rendering positioning of the component and soft-tissue balancing more difficult. Reconstruction of the associated bone loss is necessary. Segmental or massive bone grafts or a large prosthesis may be required. Elderly patients are often ill-prepared for such a procedure as their general condition may be poor. In these cases internal fixation may be preferred. Once the fracture has healed, clinical and radiological symptoms may require exchange of the prosthesis.

Mechanical failure. There are many types of mechanical failure because of modularity, poor prosthetic design and materials and technical errors such as disassociation of the tibial plateau, fracture of the tibial tray, accelerated wear of the tibial plateau, and rupture of the tibial post. Frequently, symptoms such as pain, effusion and laxity are present and associated osteolysis due to wear particles may occur. The diagnosis may be difficult in cases of undisplaced fracture of the tibial tray or disassociation without any displacement of the tibial plateau.[3]

Revision is needed to exchange the deficient component. Scratching or burnishing of the retained metal components should be sought. These need to be changed since they may release wear particles and accelerate polyethylene wear, leading to osteolysis and loosening.

Rupture of the extensor mechanism. This is a rare but severe complication. The most common causes are manipulation under anaesthesia, severe eversion of the patella and impingement of the patellar tendon against the tibial plateau of mobile-bearing total knees. It may also occur after extensive dissection of the patellar tendon with lateral retinacular release and excision of the fat pad, and secondary to stiff knees, revision surgery, rheumatoid arthritis, and trauma.

Rupture of the patellar tendon is the most frequent and is difficult to treat. Recent and peroperative ruptures can be sutured. A patellotibial cerclage is needed. Tendon augmentation using the tendon of semitendinosus or gracilis may be helpful. Longstanding ruptures require a difficult and uncertain reconstruction using these tendons. Results of allografts of the extensor mechanism seem to be disappointing. Nonunion of the tibial tubercle is also difficult to treat, especially with displacement.

Unexplained pain. A painful prosthesis without any radiological abnormality is a difficult problem[32] and may be caused by referred pain from the spine or the hip, periarticular disorders including neuromas, pes anserinus tendinitis and patellar tendon tendinitis, or impingement of the popliteus tendon or hamstring tendons against the components. Some complications such as low-grade infection, flexion instability, slight loosening, and micromobility of an uncemented component are difficult to diagnose. An overhang of an oversized or poorly centred component, intra-articular fibrous bands, a PCL which is too tight, wear of polyethylene and a patella baja with contact between the anterior surface of the tibial component and the inferior border of the patella, are possible explanations. An arthroscopy may be useful.

The results of such revisions are uncertain and patients have to be informed that the rate of failure is high. During the revision, the soft tissues and components are inspected. Attempts to mobilise the components can sometimes identify or verify the origin of the pain. In our experience, it can be more frequently identified when there has been a pain-free interval after the initial procedure.[1] When it cannot be determined, a decision is difficult.

CONCLUSIONS

There are many reasons to revise a total knee prosthesis and, for each, different procedures may be required. The first step is to identify the nature of the complication and determine its cause in order to select the appropriate treatment. Exchange of the prosthesis is not the only procedure but it is the most frequent and can be indicated for different complications. The technical errors have to be identified and then treated. The most important difficulties are bone loss and occasional associated ligamentous deficiencies. In the most severe cases, a rotating hinged prosthesis may be needed and therefore must be available.

REFERENCES

1. **Symposium of the SOFCOT 2000.** Revision total knee arthroplasty. *Rev Chir Orthop Reparatrice Appar Mot* 2000:in press.
2. **Pagnano MW, Hanssen AD, Lewallen DG, Stuart MJ.** Flexion instability after primary posterior cruciate retaining total knee arthroplasty. *Clin Orthop* 1998;356:339-46.
3. **Davis PF, Bocell JR, Tullos HS.** Dissociation of the tibial component in total knee replacements. *Clin Orthop* 1991;272:199-205.
4. **Engh GA.** Bone defect classification. In: Engh GA, Rorabeck CH, eds. *Revision total knee arthroplasty.* Baltimore: Williams and Wilkins, 1997:63-120.
5. **Ghazavi MT, Stockley I, Yee G, Davis A, Gross A.** Reconstruction of massive bone defects with allograft in revision total knee arthroplasty. *J Bone Joint Surg [Am]* 1997;79-A:17-25.
6. **Burdin Ph.** Classification des pertes de substance osseuse. In: Symposium sur les reprises de prothèse totale du genou. *Rev Chir Orthop Reparatrice Appar Mot* 2000;in press.
7. **Garvin KL, Scuderi G, Insall JN.** Evolution of the quadriceps snip. *Clin Orthop* 1995;321:131-7.
8. **Whiteside LA.** Exposure in difficult total knee arthroplasty using tibial tubercle osteotomy. *Clin Orthop* 1995;321:32-5.
9. **Berger RA, Rubash HE, Seel MJ, Thompson WH, Crossett LS.** Determining the rotational alignment of the femoral component in total knee arthroplasty. *Clin Orthop* 1992;286:40-7.
10. **Churchill DL, Incavo SJ, Johnson CC, Beynnon BD.** The transepicondylar axis approximates the optimal flexion axis of the knee. *Clin Orthop* 1998;356:111-8.
11. **Mantas JP, Bloebaum RD, Skedros JG, Hofmann AA.** Implications of reference axes used for rotational alignment of the femoral component in primary and revision knee arthroplasty. *J Arthroplasty* 1992;7:531-5.
12. **Olcott CW, Scott RD.** Femoral component rotation during total knee arthroplasty. *Clin Orthop* 1999;367:39-42.
13. **Poilvache P, Insall JN, Scuderi GR, Font-Rodriguez DE.** Rotational landmarks and sizing of the distal femur in total knee arthroplasty. *Clin Orthop* 1996;331:35-46.
14. **Haas SB, Insall JN, Montgomery W III, Windsor RE.** Revision total knee arthroplasty with use of modular components with stems inserted without cement. *J Bone Joint Surg [Am]* 1995;77-A:1700-7.
15. **Barrack RL, Rorabeck C, Burt M, Sawhney J.** Pain at the end of the stem after revision total knee arthroplasty. *Clin Orthop* 1999;367:216-25.
16. **Hicks CA, Noble Ph, Tullos H.** The anatomy of the tibial intramedullary canal. *Clin Orthop* 1995;321:111-6.
17. **Whiteside LA.** Selective ligament release in total knee arthroplasty of the knee in valgus. *Clin Orthop* 1999;367:130-40.
18. **Barrack RL, Matzkin E, Ingraham R, Engh GA, Rorabeck C.** Revision knee arthroplasty with patella replacement versus bony shell. *Clin Orthop* 1998;356:139-43.
19. **Pagnano MW, Scuderi GR, Insall JN.** Patellar component resection in revision and reimplantation total knee arthroplasty. *Clin Orthop* 1998;356:134-8.
20. **Esler CAN, Lock K, Harper WM, Gregg PJ.** Manipulation of total knee replacements: is the flexion gain retained? *J Bone Joint Surg [Br]* 1999;81-B:27-9.
21. **Ritter MA, Faris PM, Keating EM.** Posterior cruciate ligament balancing during total knee arthroplasty. *J Arthroplasty* 1988;3:323-6.
22. **Fehring TK, Valadie Al.** Knee instability after total knee arthroplasty. *Clin Orthop* 1994;299:162.
23. **Rosenberg AG, Andriacchi TP, Barden R, Galante JO.** Patellar component failure in cementless total knee arthroplasty. *Clin Orthop* 1988;236:106-14.
24. **Star MJ, Haufman KR, Irby SE, Colwell CW.** The effects of patellar thickness on patellofemoral forces after resurfacing. *Clin Orthop* 1996;322:279-84.
25. **Goldberg V, Figgie HE III, Inglis AE, et al.** Patellar fracture type and prognosis in condylar total knee arthroplasty. *Clin Orthop* 1988;236:115-22.
26. **Hozack WJ, Goll SR, Lotke PA, Rothman RH, Booth RE.** The treatment of patellar fractures after total knee arthroplasty. *Clin Orthop* 1988;236:123-7.
27. **Lucas TS, Deluca PF, Nazarian DG, Bartolozzi AR, Booth RE.** Arthroscopic treatment of patellar clunk. *Clin Orthop* 1999;367:226-9.
28. **Tabutin J.** Osseous reconstruction of the patella with screwed autologous graft in the course of repeat prosthesis of the knee. *Rev Chir Orthop Reparatrice Appar Mot* 1998;84:363-7.
29. **Engh GA, Amneen DJ.** Periprosthetic fractures adjacent to total knee implants: treatment and clinical results. *J Bone Joint Surg [Am]* 1997;79-A:1100-13.
30. **Felix NA, Stuart MJ, Hanssen AD.** Periprosthetic fractures of the tibia associated with total knee arthroplasty. *Clin Orthop* 1997;345:113-24.
31. **Ritter MA, Keating EM, Faris PM, Meding JB.** Rush rod fixation of supracondylar fractures above total knee arthroplasties. *J Arthroplasty* 1995;10:213-6.
32. **Mont MA, Serna FK, Krackow KA, Hungerford DS.** Exploration of radiographically normal total knee: replacement for unexplained pain. *Clin Orthop* 1996;331:216-20.

ANTERIOR KNEE PAIN

ANDREW M. JACKSON

From London, England

Troublesome anterior knee pain is a common problem in active adolescents and young adults and the complex of symptoms is well known.[1,2] The pain is worse when the patellofemoral joint is under load as when descending stairs, squatting and jumping. Symptoms are eased at rest, especially if the knee is held straight. The 'cinema' symptom in which pain is produced by prolonged sitting with the knee in the flexed position is often present. Crepitus is a sign of variable significance. The symptoms tend to be worse with overuse and often limit sporting activities.

Sometimes a definite diagnosis, such as Osgood-Schlatter disease, can be made quickly and logical advice and treatment given. On other occasions, however, the symptoms can be severe and disabling and yet no obvious cause for pain is found. At times there may be a credibility gap between the subjective and the objective and this can be equally frustrating for the patient as well as the surgeon. If a proper diagnosis cannot be made then treatment must be empirical. Referred pain from the hip must always be excluded and it should not be forgotten that Osgood-Schlatter disease and slipped upper femoral epiphysis occur in the same age group and could conceivably coexist.

From a clinical viewpoint it is convenient to consider the causes of anterior knee pain under the headings of 'Distinct' and 'Obscure' (Table I). The first group consists mainly of focal lesions which can be clinically and radiologically defined and for which local treatment can be applied and outcomes predicted. The second includes dynamic problems, such as maltracking and the excessive lateral pressure syndrome, as well as idiopathic chondromalacia and psychogenic pain.

The frequency of anterior knee pain is related to the very considerable compression and sheer forces which are transmitted through the patellofemoral joint. One important function of the patella is to displace the patellar tendon away from the centre of rotation of the knee and so increase its moment arm. The contact point between the patella and the trochlear groove is a fulcrum and on the patellar side of the articulation an area of contact sweeps up from the inferior to the superior pole as the knee flexes from full extension to 90° of flexion.[3] Static experiments show that at 60° of knee flexion over twice the body-weight is transmitted through the patellofemoral joint, while dynamic studies in serious weight-lifters suggest a patellar tendon tension of 17.5 times the body-weight when pushed to the extreme.[4,5] It is therefore not surprising that the patello-

Table I. Causes of anterior knee pain

Distinct	Obscure
Overuse Osgood-Schlatter, Sinding-Larsen-Johansson, jumper's knee, quadriceps tendinitis, bipartite patella, stress fracture	Idiopathic knee pain
Trauma-related lesions Osteochondritis dissecans, bone bruising, post-traumatic degenerative change	Chondromalacia
Syndromes and dysplasias	Maltracking, subluxation/tilt
Tumours Dorsal defect of patella, giant-cell tumour, osteosarcoma, etc	Excessive lateral pressure syndrome
Miscellaneous Plicae, bursae, patellar tendon ossification, posterior cruciate ligament rupture	Reflex sympathetic dystrophy
Iatrogenic Hauser procedure, infrapatellar contracture syndrome, neuroma	Psychogenic

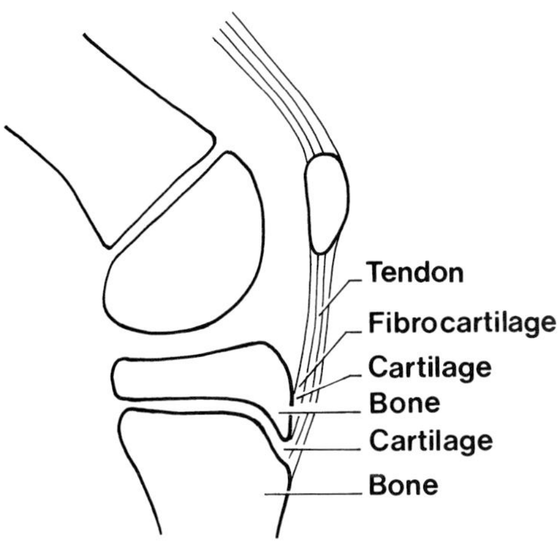

Fig. 1

Diagram showing the tenuous anchorage of the patellar tendon in the immature skeleton (reproduced with permission of Harcourt Publishers Ltd).

femoral joint has the thickest articular cartilage of any joint in the body and that peripatellar failure of the extensor mechanism is such a common problem. Acute failure is of course, manifest as 'fracture' or 'rupture' while subacute and chronic failure give rise to anterior knee pain. The origin of the pain is a subject of debate since articular cartilage is devoid of nerve endings. Cartilage also has very limited powers of repair and regeneration once fibrillation and ulceration have occurred.

Overuse and repeated minor trauma commonly play a part in the production of anterior knee pain, especially when sufficient time is not allowed for the resolution of subliminal damage. Paradoxically, underuse can also be incriminated as a cause of damage to the articular surface, for example the chondromalacia which is seen on the medial or odd facet of the patella. This small area does not come into contact with the femur until the knee flexes past 130° and therefore in most patients is a very underused part of the articular surface. Osteoporosis of the patella often accompanies anterior knee pain although it is difficult to know if it is a cause or effect. It reduces the stiffness of the patella and causes thinning of the subchondral bone plate, thus decreasing the ability of the patella to cope with the huge forces already referred to.

DISTINCT CAUSES OF ANTERIOR KNEE PAIN

Overuse

Juvenile traction osteochondritis. Osgood-Schlatter disease is commonly seen in boys aged between 12 and 14 years and less often in girls and at a slightly younger age. The diagnosis is easy if the patient points to the tibial tubercle and a prominence is already obvious. Kneeling is painful. The condition occurs at a time when increasing demands are made on a still immature skeleton. The adult patellar tendon is firmly anchored to bone by Sharpey's fibres, but in the growing child the anchorage is more tenuous (Fig. 1).[6] Repeated microavulsion injuries accompanied by half-hearted fibro-osseous repair results in prominence of the tubercle. Its fragmented appearance on radiography is due to partial separation of chondro-osseous fragments. Very rarely, infection or trauma may masquerade as Osgood-Schlatter disease and plain radiography should be a routine procedure, especially in the unilateral case.

Treatment is conservative in the first instance, reducing activity to a level at which symptoms become manageable. Short-term immobilisation in a cast is very rarely necessary and bilateral casting is a definite mistake since it will result in a very disabled child. The natural history is for the symptoms to disappear within one to two years, leaving the bony prominence as a permanent marker of the event. If symptoms remain troublesome into the late teens, radiographs will probably show an ossicle in the substance of the tendon adjacent to the tubercle. Removal of the ossicle and sometimes an associated bursa will be curative and most patients are asymptomatic in adult life.[7]

Sinding-Larsen-Johansson disease occurs in the same age group, but the point tenderness and pathology are located at the lower pole of the patella. The lateral radiograph of the patella may be normal or show some speckled calcification in the patellar tendon adjacent to the lower pole. Treatment is along the same lines as for Osgood-Schlatter disease. Usually the area of speckled calcification heals leaving the familiar elongated lower pole of the patella which is so often seen in footballers. Occasionally, a troublesome ossicle persists and requires excision. Very rarely, traction osteochondritis similar to Sinding-Larsen-Johansson disease may be seen at the proximal pole of the patella.[8] The differential diagnosis of abnormal calcification at the lower pole of the patella lies between Sinding-Larsen-Johansson disease, bipartite patella, stress fracture and impending sleeve fracture.

Jumper's knee. This is the name given to tendinitis at the tendon-bone interface at the lower pole of the patella after skeletal maturity. Again the problem is overuse and jumping is not the only cause. Focal tenderness at the lower pole of the patella is the key physical sign and this can often be eliminated if the patient is asked to do a straight-leg raising test and to hold the leg a few inches off the couch. This shows that the tender area can be protected by the tensed superficial fibres of the patellar tendon and that the problem lies at a deeper level.

Conservative treatment demands a period of rest, perhaps combined with pain-relieving physiotherapy which includes ultrasound, deep friction, isometric exercises and hamstring stretches. Oral anti-inflammatory agents can be helpful but local injections of steroids are contraindicated in case of rupture of the tendon. If conservative treatment fails and ultrasound or MRI shows abnormalities in the substance of the tendon surgical exploration may be indicated in that small group of patients who are professional

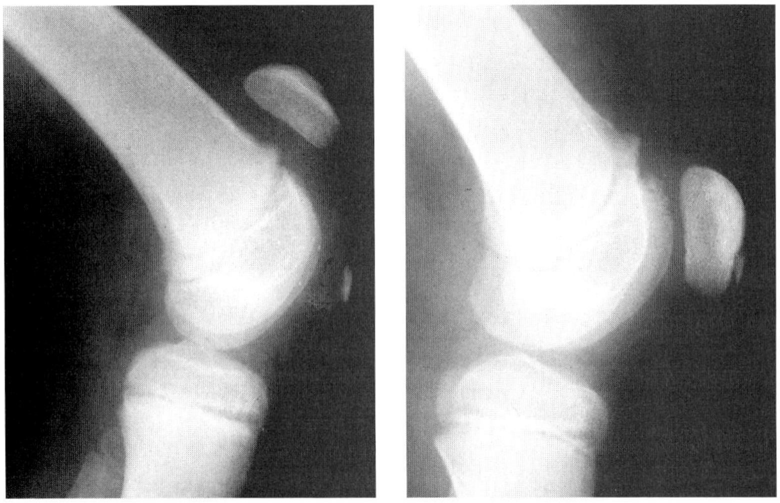

Fig. 2a Fig. 2b

Radiographs of a 12-year-old boy showing a) a widely displaced sleeve fracture and b) the opposite knee with the characteristic bipartite lower pole. Separation occurs through the line of the synchondrosis. If pain is associated with such a picture there must be concern about impending separation (reproduced with permission of Harcourt Publishers Ltd).

Fig. 3

Radiograph of an adult footballer with acute-on-chronic anterior knee pain. The right patella is tracking better perhaps because the stress fracture has acted as an autolateral release.

athletes and who refuse to give up sporting activities which exacerbate the condition.

A variety of different procedures has been recommended, but not surprisingly the concept of inflicting surgical trauma on a degenerative tendon in order to stimulate healing does not always work. The simplest operation is to split the tendon at the site of maximal tenderness and, if a granuloma is found, to scrape it away with a curette. If the deeper half of the tendon is involved it can be stripped off the lower pole of the patella and some authors have advocated drilling of the distal pole in order to bring in a new blood supply.[9] The knee should be protected in a splint for four weeks before beginning a rehabilitation programme. For recalcitrant cases in top athletes, Blazina et al[10] claim success with resection of the lower pole of the patella and reattachment of the tendon. More recently, it has been proposed that the cause of the problem is impingement of the deeper fibres of the patellar tendon against the lower pole of the patella in flexion rather than traction. Accordingly, arthroscopic trimming of the lower pole of the patella has its advocates.[11] This procedure not only brings in new blood supply but also exposes the deep fibres of the patellar tendon at its origin to synovial fluid, which may be beneficial.

Bipartite patella. Bipartite patella is common in childhood. It is often bilateral and usually regarded as a variation of normal ossification. The two centres may proceed to fusion in the second decade. Very rarely, in response to overuse or acute injury, the synchondrosis separating the two centres may become painful and the site of local tenderness. There are three sites at which bipartite patella is found and each has an important soft-tissue attachment:

1) The distal pole of the patella with attachment of the patellar tendon.

2) The lateral margin of the patella with attachment of the lateral retinaculum.

3) The superolateral corner, the insertion of vastus lateralis. This is the commonest site for symptoms.

It is conceivable that in some patients the type-1 lesion may represent the endstage of Sinding-Larsen-Johansson syndrome. In others, there is no doubt about the bipartite nature of the lower pole of the patella and in this context the sleeve fracture of the patella is a fascinating entity.[12] Perhaps patients with a bipartite lower pole with its characteristic appearance are at high risk of sustaining a fracture (Fig. 2). Certainly, if such a patient presents with pain and tenderness at the lower pole, this should be viewed as indicating separation, and activities should be curtailed. The fracture, when it occurs, is along the line of the synchondrosis; the avulsed distal pole is largely cartilaginous. It is always much larger than the radiographs suggest and must be reattached.

The type-2 lesion, if not bipartite, may be caused by direct injury or by a stress phenomenon related to a tight lateral retinaculum and maltracking of the patella. A mobile lateral marginal stress fracture of the patella with the synovial fluid gap at the site of the injury may perhaps represent an autolateral release of a tight retinaculum (Fig. 3).

The type-3 lesion is the commonest cause of symptoms which occasionally are severe enough to merit surgery. The simplest and most effective procedure is excision of the superolateral fragment. If the excision is performed through an incision in line with the fibres of vastus lateralis and by peeling back the insertion of this muscle to the patella rehabilitation can be rapid. Alternatively, Ogata[13] has shown that simple detachment of vastus lateralis from the fragment can often remove the stress and allow the fragment to heal spontaneously.

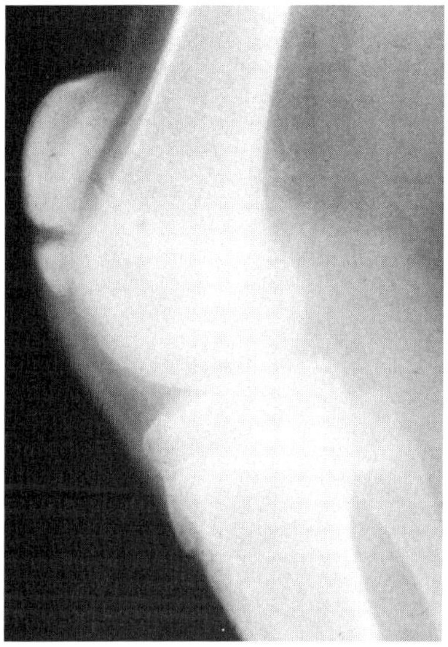

Fig. 4

Radiograph of the knee of a teenage spastic diplegic with deteriorating crouch gait. There is a combination of stress fracture/separation of the lower pole of the patella, Osgood-Schlatter disease and patella alta (reproduced with permission of Harcourt Publishers Ltd).

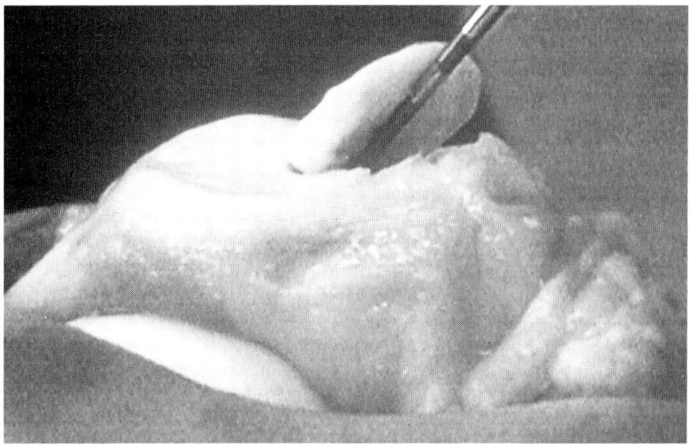

Fig. 5

A large osteochondritis dissecans lesion of the patella. Fixation failed and patellectomy was eventually required (reproduced with permission of Harcourt Publishers Ltd).

Stress fracture of the patella. This was first described in the English literature by Devas.[14] The transverse stress fracture is the most common form and is seen in athletes as well as in patients with cerebral palsy who overload the patella by walking with a crouch gait.[15] It is a mistake to assume that deteriorating gait in a spastic who is entering the teenage years is due simply to an increase in weight combined with a decrease in motivation. The problem, not always obvious, may be the result of a stress fracture and avulsion of the lower pole of the patella (Fig. 4). In these cases management must include release of the hamstrings and correction of the flexed knee deformity. The distinction between a stress fracture and a bipartite patella remains difficult. It is said that the line of a stress fracture passes vertically through the patella while that of a synchondrosis of a bipartite patella runs more obliquely. Histologically, the presence of callus is proof of a genuine stress lesion, and excessive mobility of a fragment with sclerotic margins and a synovial gap would suggest established nonunion of a fracture.

Trauma-related lesions

Osteochondritis dissecans of the patella. This is a rare cause of anterior knee pain in the young athlete. Repeated microtrauma and particularly sheer stress to the articular surface are thought to be the cause.[16] Sometimes the lesion is associated with maltracking of the patella. In addition to pain there may be obvious crepitus when the knee extends against load, and perhaps a moderate effusion. Pain inhibition may cause giving-way. If the lesion is small a painful arc may be found as the point of patellar contact with the femur passes over the lesion.

Plain radiographs, including the 30° skyline view, will usually confirm the diagnosis although, if in doubt, more detailed images may be obtained by CT or MRI which will show whether separation has occurred. On the plain film subchondral sclerosis usually indicates loosening of the fragment within the crater. The best way to stage the lesion is at arthroscopy when the surgeon must distinguish between the following conditions:

1) An intact lesion with no break in the articular cartilage which on probing reveals no movement of underlying bone.
2) A separated lesion in which there is no break in the articular cartilage but the probe shows that beneath this intact layer the bone has separated.
3) A trapdoor lesion in which the articular cartilage is breached for part of the circumference of the lesion. The fragment of osteochondritis dissecans is partially detached from the articular surface.
4) A totally detached lesion (= loose body).

Conservative treatment with rest is appropriate for intact lesions which will usually show no sclerosis, and in patients presenting under the age of 13 or 14 years when healing is the rule. There is a good case for attempting to stabilise separated lesions, and biodegradable polylactic acid pins may be of value. Lesions which are partially or

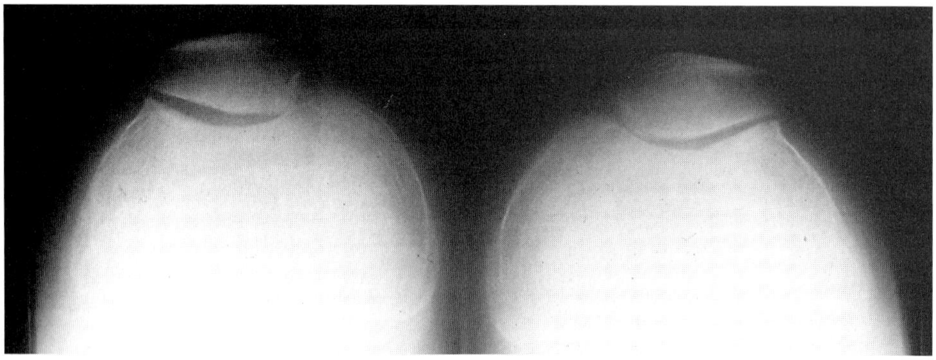

Fig. 6

Radiograph showing premature osteoarthritis in the dysmorphic knee of a patient born with Stickler's syndrome.

completely separated from the articular surface have been treated by excision leaving vertical edges to the crater, curettage and drilling, with the aim of healing the defect with fibrocartilage. With smaller lesions of the patella, good or excellent results have been recorded with follow-up as long as 15 or 19 years, but the larger craters still remain a problem[17,18] (Fig. 5). Autologous implantation of cartilage may offer hope when previously patellectomy was the final solution.

Bone bruising. When seen on MRI of a post-traumatic knee bone bruising is most often a minor feature of a more complex picture and of variable significance. It may result from direct trauma or from indirect forces which have produced patellar subluxation or dislocation. In such a case anterior knee pain may persist for three or four months as part of the post-traumatic symptoms. Very occasionally, a full-thickness fragment of overlying articular cartilage may be shed into the joint a month or two after the injury and this will be accompanied by a sudden deterioration in symptoms and an effusion in the knee.

Post-fracture. Successful treatment of patellar fractures demands accurate reduction of the fracture, adequate fixation and restoration of a nearly normal joint surface. The state of the articular cartilage is often worse than plain radiographs suggest and the gliding surface must always be inspected by the operating surgeon. There is a tendency to try to preserve the patella at all costs, but if a reasonable joint surface cannot be reconstructed patellectomy is preferable to the months of fruitless rehabilitation which follow a poor operation.

Syndromes and dysplasias. Dysplasia of the patella and condylar surfaces can lead to incongruity and premature degenerative change as well as maltracking and a liability to patellar dislocation. Anterior knee pain due to incongruity is seen in Stickler's syndrome (arthro-ophthalmoplegia) (Fig. 6). When patellar dislocation occurs in childhood there is often a positive family history, and associated dysplasia may be associated with a neuromuscular problem or a syndrome (for example nail-patella, Down's syndrome or the Marfan syndrome).

Tumours. Primary, metastatic and even metabolic brown tumours have all been reported within the patella (Fig. 7). The usual presentation is non-specific anterior knee pain but, occasionally, a lytic lesion is the site of a pathological fracture. It should not be forgotten that osteomyelitis of the patella can resemble a bone tumour. The dorsal defect of the patella is an oddity and presents as a lytic lesion at the superolateral aspect of the patella in the same region as in a type-3 bipartite patella. It may or may not be symptomatic and the surface of the joint is not involved. Very occasionally, such a lesion is so large that it may require curettage and grafting. Very rarely, soft-tissue tumours may occur within the fat pat and synovial tumours such as pigmented villonodular synovitis can cause anterior knee pain, clicking and catching.

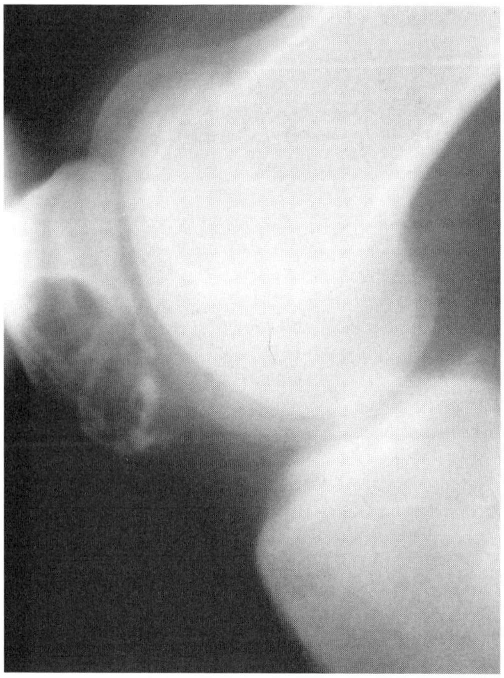

Fig. 7

Radiograph showing chondroblastoma of the patella.

Miscellaneous

Plicae. These are found at four sites within the knee. They are infolded shelves or partitions of synovial lining and contain a core of fibrous tissue. They are inconstant, vary in size and can be regarded as normal anatomical variants; only rarely do they cause symptoms.

The medial plica in particular has become a much overrated focus of attention and many innocent plicae have been removed for no reason. If there is local tenderness at the correct site, a synovial snap between 30° and 60° of flexion, a fibrotic plica and an adjacent erosion on the condyle then the diagnosis should be considered to be correct. Surgery in such cases will be rewarding.[19] To incriminate the plica in the absence of these symptoms and signs is a result of ignorance. The complete suprapatellar plica which separates the suprapatellar pouch from the joint proper may occasionally be a cause of symptoms. On occasion, MRI has shown an effusion in the upper compartment which does not communicate with the joint below. The infrapatellar plica or ligamentum mucosum sometimes forms a complete curtain between the two halves of the knee. Apart from obstructing the arthroscopist, this pilca has little clinical relevance nor does the somewhat thicker lateral pilca, which is encountered as the arthroscopist manoeuvres down the lateral gutter.

Hoffer's syndrome. There is no doubt that some patients have an outsized infrapatellar fat pad which bulges out on either side of the patellar tendon when the knee is extended. Arthroscopically when viewed from above, it may seem to protrude more than normal into the distended knee. There may be areas of fibrosis and inflammation in the fat pad suggesting that it has been trapped or pinched from time to time, but there is uncertainty as to whether it has ever been truly pathological.

Bursae. These are common and well recognised and should be treated conservatively in the first instance avoiding irritation to the front of the knee. They may contain blood or synovial fluid. The prepatellar bursa is responsible for housemaid's knee and the infrapatellar bursa for the clergyman's variety. There is a third bursa between the patellar tendon and the upper tibia which is not easily seen and symptoms from this area may be confused with those of Hoffer's disease.

Rupture of the posterior cruciate ligament. Chronic deficiency of the posterior cruciate ligament is associated with patellofemoral arthritis presumably because the posterior displacement of the tibia increases the resultant force on the patellofemoral joint.

Ossification of the patellar tendon. This may be related to injury and can be a cause of continuing minor disability (Fig. 8). Matsumoto et al[20] reported two cases and it seems that over the years as the ossification matures, pain, stiffness and disability will increase. In their series resection of the calcified tendon and reconstruction with a Leeds-Keio ligament was recommended.

Iatrogenic

Some adverse effects may follow operations such as the Hauser procedure for recurrent dislocation of the patella, in which the tibial tubercle is transferred medially and distally. While the distal displacement should never be more than is necessary to correct patella alta, the more harmful component of this operation is the medial shift. This inevitably recesses the insertion of the patellar tendon posteriorly and runs directly contrary to the Maquet principle. An increased incidence of late-onset osteoarthritis has been attributed to this procedure.[21]

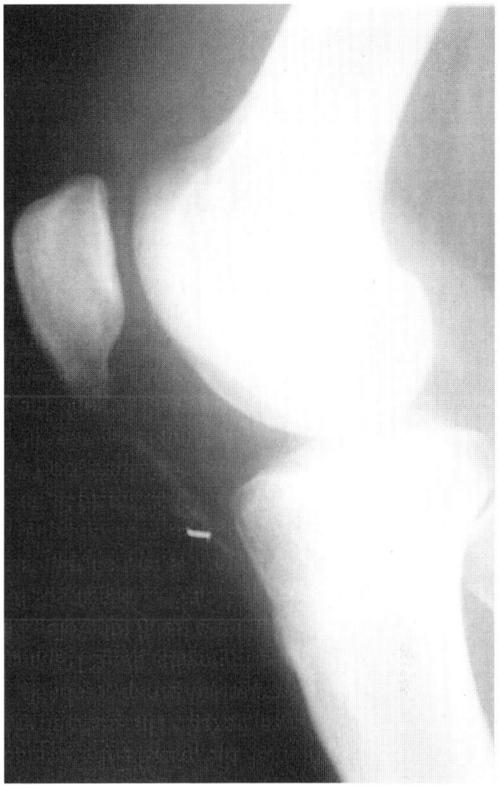

Fig. 8

Radiograph showing ossification of the patellar tendon associated with anterior knee pain in a 20-year-old woman.

The infrapatellar contracture syndrome. This form of patella infera may follow injury or surgery and is made worse by prolonged immobilisation. The knee is stiff and painful with restricted patellar mobility and swelling is obvious around the patellar tendon and the fat pad. Early recognition and treatment by vigorous physiotherapy and with anti-inflammatory drugs are important, but if the condition becomes established surgery is best delayed until the inflammatory phase dies down. This may take two or three months. The surgery involves extensive medial and lateral retinacular releases with the division of intra-articular adhesions and excision of the fibrous tissue which has replaced the fat pad. Sometimes it is necessary to slide the tibial tubercle proximally to re-establish the correct patellar height.[22] Patella infera may follow epiphyseal leg lengthening (Fig. 9).

Post-traumatic neuroma. Neuromas may complicate scars in front of the knee just as at other sites. In particular, care

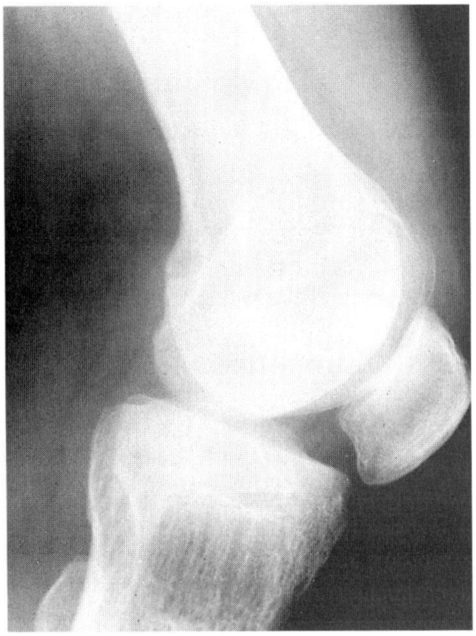

Fig. 9

Radiograph showing iatrogenic patella infera after epiphyseal lengthening of the tibia.

must be taken not to damage the saphenous nerve when harvesting the hamstring tendons.

OBSCURE CAUSES OF ANTERIOR KNEE PAIN

How should one approach patients in whom the diagnosis is not obvious? The problem can be studied clinically, by imaging and at arthroscopy and it is helpful to try to place patients into one of the categories suggested in Table I.

Idiopathic knee pain. It must be acknowledged that in some patients the precise cause of pain will never be established. These are often young patients with high expectations and who place great demands on their knees. Clearly, overuse is part of the problem. On the other hand inert and overweight patients can present with similar symptoms.

Fairbank et al[23] found that clinical examination was of little help in assessing patients with idiopathic knee pain. Joint mobility, the 'Q' angle, genu valgum and anteversion of the femoral neck were not found more commonly in patients with anterior knee pain than in a control group. Tight hamstrings and the "hamstrung knee" as described by Hughston[24], however, do seem to be a real entities which will respond to physiotherapy and stretching. These patients need to be reassured as to the benign nature of their pain. Protection from overuse, a review of sports and training activities, stretches when necessary and a programme of isometric and inner-image exercises on the quadriceps are beneficial. Patellar mobilisation with the aim of stretching the lateral retinaculum, which arises largely from the iliotibial band, is also helpful. Knee braces and supports should be avoided.

A reasonable outcome can be expected after six months of conservative treatment. Kannus et al[25] reported a seven-year follow-up of patients with chronic patellofemoral pain syndrome; 75% of their patients had recovered by six months and the results were little changed when seen at seven years. Interestingly, one of their subgroups was treated with intra-articular glycosaminoglycan polysulphate with no beneficial effect. Leslie and Bentley[26] showed that nearly 60% of their patients with anterior knee pain and a normal articular surface at arthroscopy were asymptomatic at one year. It is therefore clear that conservative treatment for six months will solve most problems, but a small hard core of patients will remain a therapeutic challenge.

In this recalcitrant group MRI or arthroscopy will probably show some degree of chondromalacia. It is wise to check again that there is no subtle element of maltracking which is contributing to this. In the absence of maltracking the choice of surgical treatment lies between chondral shaving, curettage and drilling, resurfacing the articular surface and, ultimately, patellectomy. A reasonable outcome from patellectomy was reported by Bentley[27] who found good or excellent results in 77% of 60 patellectomies performed for severe chondromalacia at a mean follow-up of seven years.

Chondromalacia. The term describes a pathological lesion of articular cartilage which, when mild, may be reversible but when severe can lead ultimately to osteoarthritis. Chondromalacia patellae may be idiopathic or secondary to maltracking, but since it is most often seen on the medial facet of the patella and osteoarthritis on the lateral facet, it can be concluded that the one does not necessarily lead to the other.[28] As with osteoarthritis the symptoms do not always reflect the macroscopic appearance. Standard radiographs are often normal when the malacic changes are relatively advanced, hence the importance of MRI and arthroscopy. When inspecting the articular surfaces of the patella it is important to try to distinguish between pathological abnormality and chondral changes that are part of the normal ageing process. A fine hairy appearance of the articular cartilage, in the absence of softening or fissuring, is most likely to be due to age-related wear on the surface. Ultimately, this may lead to osteoarthritis but in its early stages it is probably asymptomatic.[29]

True chondromalacia has a separate clinical appearance. The four stages as defined by Outerbridge[29] can be modified to suit the arthroscopist:

Grade 1. Closed disease:

(a) At first sight the surface looks normal, but the probe reveals a soft spongy feel or pitting oedema. The surface is intact and the softening probably reversible.

(b) A blister or raised portion of the articular surface is seen but examination with a probe shows this to be boggy. The surface is still intact.

Grade 2. Open disease. The probe will now reveal fissures which may or may not be obvious at first sight.

Grade 3. Severe exuberant fibrillation or 'crabmeat' appearance.

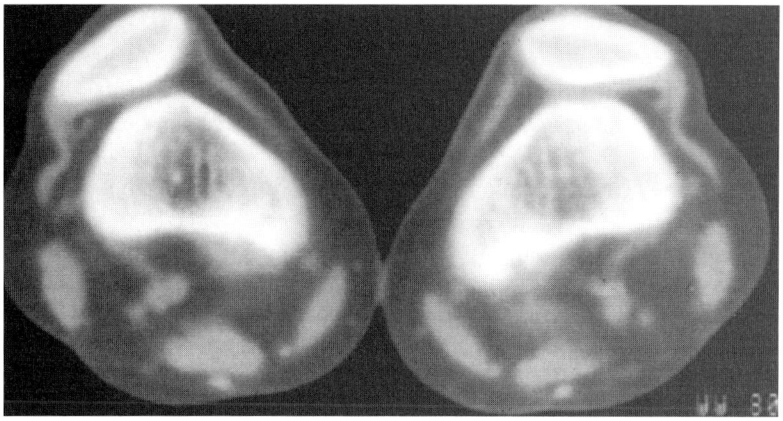

Fig. 10

Lateral subluxation of the patella in extension. The lateral retinaculum is lax and plays no part in causing the subluxation.

Grade 4. The fibrillation is full thickness and the erosive changes extend down to bone which may be exposed. This is in effect osteoarthritis. The size of the lesion also needs to be recorded.

There is conflicting evidence as to the true pathological nature of chondromalacia. Goodfellow, Hungerford and Woods[30] described primary changes in the deep and intermediate layers of the articular cartilage and referred to the process as 'basal degeneration'. This seems to fit well with the appearance at arthroscopy in grade-1 disease. Bentley,[31] however, has biopsied malacic areas on the medial facet and provided evidence of surface fibrillation and loss of superficial matrix. He believes that this marks the commencement of chondromalacic change.

How does chondromalacia develop? Cartilage can be regarded as a compressed matrix. The type-II collagen fibres tightly bind together the proteoglycans which carry a very high negative charge and are strongly hydrophilic. If the collagen breaks down the unconstrained proteoglycans will inevitably draw more water into the hydrated matrix causing boggy swelling.[32] Fissuring is the next step in this destructive process, followed by fragmentation and ulceration.

Maltracking of the patella. This may lead to excess overload with sheer forces being applied to the articular cartilage in some areas while underloading may occur in others. Both hyperpression and hypopression may be detrimental to nutrition of the cartilage.[33] The more extreme cases of maltracking will predispose to recurrent dislocation of the patella and this can be particularly damaging to the patellofemoral joint. The traditional tangential skyline views provide static images from which it is difficult to understand fully the dynamics of patellar tracking. Subtle disorders may be overlooked and it has been shown that as the normal knee moves from 90° flexion to full extension the patella shifts and tilts medially with respect to the tibial tubercle, with a slight clockwise rotation of the patella on the right and anticlockwise on the left.[34] These movements may not be clinically detectable but may be relevant. Some obvious signs such as the 'Q' angle, valgus deformity, recurvatum, triple deformity and patella alta may all be factors in producing maltracking, but when it comes to treatment it is the pattern of maltracking which matters most. This requires definition before recommending corrective surgery. It is most important to distinguish between lateral subluxation in extension and in flexion.

Lateral subluxation in extension is best demonstrated by clinical examination. The patient, sitting on the edge of the couch, extends the knee against gravity and as the patella disengages from a position of bony stability in the trochlear groove it kicks laterally. This physical sign is usually seen as the knee extends from 20° flexion up to full extension and may be associated with pain and crepitus. This pattern of maltracking is commonly associated with recurrent dislocation of the patella during childhood and adolescence but less degrees of maltracking can cause pain and a feeling of instability. Since the problem occurs in the last 20° of extension, inner range exercises of the quadriceps that are freely prescribed for anterior knee pain are not appropriate for this group of patients. The principal cause of this problem is malalignment of the quadriceps which produces a bowstring effect between its mean point of origin and its insertion on to the tibial tubercle. The lateral retinaculum is not tight and surgical correction must include some type of distal realignment (Fig. 10). Most patients in this group whose symptoms are limited to pain and feelings of instability will respond to physiotherapy.[35,36]

By contrast, maltracking in flexion is difficult to see clinically but can be radiologically defined on skyline radiographs taken between 20° and 45° of flexion. A standard technique is most important and the view of Merchant et al[37,38] is probably the most popular. In this method the knee is at 45° and the x-ray beam angled towards the foot. Fulkerson and Shea[39] have emphasised the importance of tilt and subluxation and have described three pathological patterns (Fig. 11). Tilt is produced by the posterior pull of the lateral retinaculum and can be recognised by drawing the line of Laurin et al[40] which connects the tips of the medial and lateral femoral condyles as a reference line. The congruence angle is a method of measuring subluxation.

CT is used to study tilt/subluxation. Overlapping of images is avoided and reference points can be more precise. The knee can be studied as it approaches full extension and

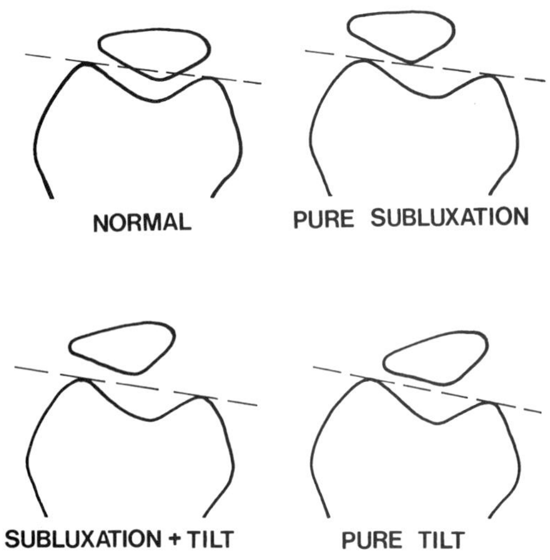

Fig. 11

Diagram showing the concept of tilt, subluxation and combined subluxation and tilt as different entities (reproduced with permission of Harcourt Publishers Ltd).

the sophisticated scans described by Kawakubo, Fujikawa and Matsumoto[41] have allowed the study of patellofemoral contact in the moving knee. These showed that in patients with recurrent dislocation of the patella the contact area moved laterally as the knee flexed. The contact area was smaller than in a normal controlled group, probably resulting in overloading. By superimposing the CT scans taken through the femoral sulcus and the tibial tubercle, the tibial tubercle/femoral sulcus distance can be measured. If this is greater than 20 mm it is pathological and an indication for medial transfer of the tibial tubercle.

Arthroscopic assessment of patellar tracking is undertaken through an anterolateral or superolateral portal. Incremental patellar tracking can be studied at various angles between 0° and 90°. At 45° flexion and beyond the patella should be centred and congruent in the trochlear groove even although the knee is distended.[42] The arthroscopist can also observe overhang of the lateral facet.

Excessive lateral pressure syndrome. Ficat and Hungerford[43] first recognised a situation in which there was no subluxation or maltracking but, nevertheless, a tight retinaculum placed the lateral patellar facet under increased load. Occasionally, the patella tilts without subluxation. This is most commonly seen when there is a predominantly "one facet patella". The subchondral bone under the lateral facet is sclerotic while the medial third of the patella is osteoporotic. The skyline view may show lateral beaking or a marginal fracture which is taken as evidence of excessive traction on the lateral margin of the patella. At operation softening or fissuring of the articular cartilage of the lateral facet will probably be found and this is an indication for lateral release. As the joint becomes progressively more arthritic with loss of joint space, secondary subluxation and tilt will occur (Fig. 12).

Stiff painful knee/reflex sympathetic dystrophy. A typical patient in this group suffers from intractable knee pain of considerable duration and is severely disabled often walking with crutches. Time will have been lost from school or work and the patient is anxious and depressed. Often, such a patient is best admitted to hospital for 'the team' approach (Fig. 13). The knee must be fully investigated so that unlikely lesions such as osteoid osteoma are excluded. The usual concern is that there may be an element of reflex sympathetic dystrophy; lately renamed "complex regional pain syndrome".[44] The patients whom we are considering are type 1 rather than type 2 which is the group associated with peripheral nerve injury.

The challenge in this group is early diagnosis and successful treatment. The diagnosis itself is not difficult once it has been considered. The patient presents with severe intractable pain which is out of proportion to the original injury. Occasionally, it may follow an operation, particularly when there has been difficulty with the immediate postoperative rehabilitation and mobilisation. In the leg the knee is commonly involved but, of course, the entire limb can be affected. Autonomic dysfunction is manifest by cyanosis or mottling, most easily seen when the patient is standing and there may be a noticeable temperature difference between the affected area and the opposite side. In late

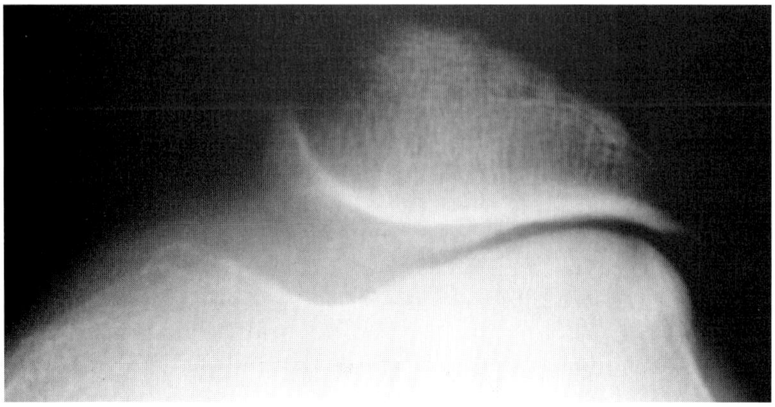

Fig. 12

Radiograph showing beaking of the lateral margin of the patella, sclerosis of the lateral facet and osteoporosis of the medial patella. They suggest that the subluxation and tilt in this patient may be the result of loss of joint space and that the causative factor here is excessive lateral pressure syndrome.

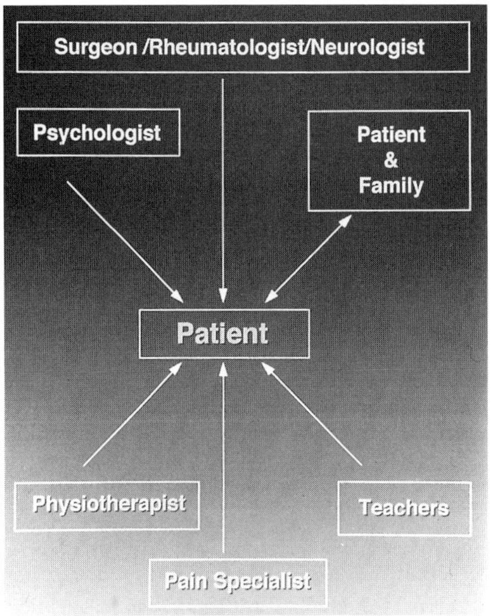

Fig. 13

Diagram showing those involved in the team approach.

cases there are trophic changes involving the skin as well as wasting of the quadriceps and stiffness of the joint. The inability to function and chronic pain feed the depression.

The dysfunction leads to radiological osteoporosis which may become apparent within a month of onset of symptoms. The periarticular medullary bone may have a moth-eaten appearance (Fig. 14).

A three-phase technetium bone scan can be helpful in diagnosis but less so in the younger patient.[45] The most useful diagnostic test is a trial of sympathetic block and the simplest of these is the phentolamine test. Al Duri and Aichroth,[46] in their excellent review of this difficult subject, agree with the consensus view to divide reflex sympathetic dystrophy into three stages as follows:

Stage I. 0 to 3 months; pain and hypersensitivity are dominant features.

Stage II. 3 to 6 months; diffuse radiating pain, stiffness, swelling, osteoporosis. Colour changes may appear.

Stage III. Over 6 months; the pain may begin to recede leaving osteoporosis, atrophy and stiffness.

Stiffness may be due to arthrofibrosis. Infrapatellar fibrosis may drag the patella downwards and in severe long-standing cases there may be irreversible chondral damage. The first line of treatment includes intensive physiotherapy with a prolonged blockade, for example, epidurally with an indwelling catheter. This problem is far from solved. If there is not an autonomic-mediated component to the pain the problem is likely to be psychogenic and should perhaps be regarded as a sort of orthopaedic version of 'anorexia' and equally mysterious.

The possibility of focal dystonia should not be forgotten.

TREATMENT OF OBSCURE KNEE PAIN

Surgery should not be performed in the absence of a demonstrable abnormality. When operation is indicated, the choice lies between the correction of maltracking if this has been demonstrated, a local procedure to repair or improve the articular surface or a biomechanical manoeuvre to reduce load on the patellofemoral joint. A combination of approaches may be appropriate. In some instances a trial of a minor operation such as lateral release may be worth pursuing before proceeding with a longer procedure, especially if the chondral changes are mild. When damage to the articular cartilage is severe and irreversible, patellectomy is the last resort.

Surgery for maltracking. Lateral subluxation of the patella in extension, if causing sufficient pain and crepitus, is an indication for distal realignment of the tubercle with or without proximal medial advancement of the patellofemoral ligament and the lower oblique fibres of vastus medialis. Lateral release alone will achieve nothing since the lateral retinaculum is not tight.[47]

Pure subluxation in flexion is usually associated with mild chondral damage and the symptoms are pain and

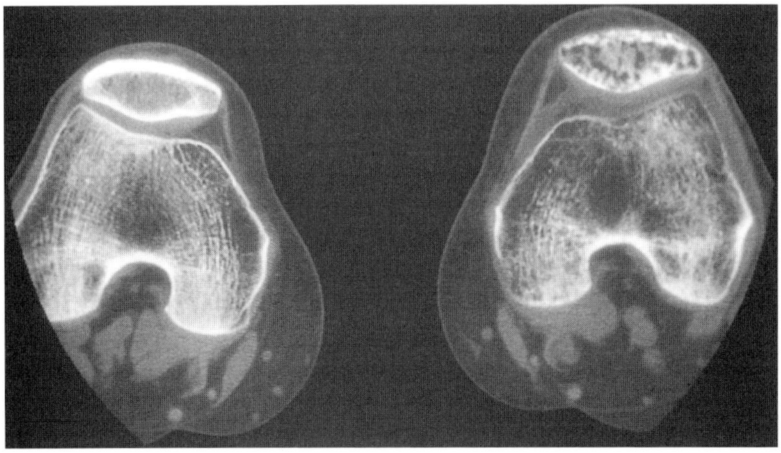

Fig. 14

The typical mottled appearance and osteoporosis seen in stage-II reflex sympathetic dystrophy.

instability. A simple lateral release often suffices but if this fails or if chondral damage is severe distal realignment in the form of an Elmslie-Trillat procedure or Fulkerson anteromedial transfer may be undertaken.[48] With combined subluxation and tilt the lateral facet is overloaded, the chondral damage is likely to be more severe, and the threshold for performing a distal realignment is lower. Pure tilt is probably the most sinister maltracking problem. This is stable maltracking and it leads to excessive lateral pressure syndrome, retinacular pain and rapid progression to osteoarthritis. In some of these patients the wear process can be relatively asymptomatic so that osteoarthritis of the lateral facet is severe at the time of presentation.

Open lateral release is best performed through an incision of 1 to 2 cm with the knee flexed so that the retinaculum is under tension at the moment of division. The release extends from the lower fibres of vastus lateralis down as far as the joint line. The superior lateral geniculate artery is secured and the wound infiltrated with local anaesthetic and adrenaline to diminish bleeding. Closed lateral release has become unpopular because of the high incidence of postoperative haemarthrosis, swelling and stiffness. This may have changed with the advent of newer electrosurgical instruments which vaporise rather than burn the tissue and which can be used in saline. The standard method is to place the arthroscope in the anteromedial portal and to use the cutting electrode in the anterolateral portal. The fibres of vastus lateralis must not be divided from the superolateral margin of the patella in case of producing iatrogenic medial subluxation. As the retinaculum is divided extravisated irrigation fluid will be seen subcutaneously in the line of the cut. If patellar shaving is contemplated it is best to divide the retinaculum first since this improves access to the articular surface of the patella.

Chondral surgery. Attempts to improve or repair the articular surface of the patella are most appropriate when the area of damage is limited and the chondromalacia is idiopathic and not related to subluxation/tilt. Patellar shaving was first popularised by Wiles et al[47] who described an open procedure which has since been revisited by arthroscopists. It has not been found to be a rewarding procedure. Nevertheless, when there is severe fibrillation with effusion and small fragments of articular cartilage in the joint, it does seem reasonable to try to tidy up the articular surface. By reducing the amount of debris in the joint and the release of proteolytic enzymes, synovitis may be minimised and the onset of osteoarthritis delayed.[49]

Excision of circumscribed malacic areas of chondromalacia and drilling of subchondral bone have met with some success. The defect will fill with repair fibrocartilage. This is viable but does not withstand huge loads and sheer forces because it lacks the properties of hyaline cartilage. In order to reinforce this fibrocartilage carbon fibre pads have been used at some centres with moderate success in the short term. Pongor et al[50] have reported pain relief in 67% of patients at three years and Muckle and Minns[49] describe the formation of a smooth low-friction surface with the abolition of crepitus in 70% of patients. However, Meister, Cobb and Bentley[51] subsequently reported disappointing results in 27 patients in whom there was a poor outcome in 48% and which resulted in patellectomy in 30%.

Osteochondral grafting in the form of mosaicplasty can be moderately successful for defects on the femoral condyles. It has not been helpful on the patellar surface. It is still early days for the technique of autologous chondrocyte implantation which may improve as different scaffolds are developed to carry the chondrocytes.

Biomechanical surgery. Maquet[52] described how anterior displacement of the tibial tubercle reduces the forces acting across the patellofemoral joint. His initial operation was used in the treatment of osteoarthritis but its application soon spread to the management of anterior knee pain. It was thought that the larger the advancement the better the result and advancement of 2 to 3 cm was recommended as routine. There was a high cosmetic price to pay for improving the mechanics since the resulting knees were ugly, and stretching of the skin over the tibial tubercle led to problems of skin necrosis and infection. Ferguson et al[53] subsequently pointed out that a large advancement of the tubercle reduced the vector force across the patellofemoral joint but also the area of contract stress between the patella and condyles because of rocking of the patella. A compromise had to be struck and advancement of 1.5 cm was recommended. Extreme advancement is no longer recommended, but elements of the principle of Maquet are incorporated into the Fulkerson anteromedial realignment as well as the Elmslie-Trillat procedure which invariably leaves a slightly elevated tubercle.

Various tangential and sagittal patellar osteotomies have been described, but none of these operations has been received with much enthusiasm.

Ablative surgery. Patellectomy is indicated when the articular surface of the patella is severely damaged over a wide area and the rest of the knee looks normal. The repair of the quadriceps mechanism should be such as to allow rapid postoperative rehabilitation protected by a hinged knee brace. After patellectomy patients can expect little problem in day-to-day living but sporting activities will likely be curtailed. Even with vigorous rehabilitation some wasting of the quadriceps will remain and various authors have estimated that extensor power will never be better than 70% of normal. There is likely to be some loss of flexion and instability may become a problem if high demands are placed on the joint. The results are worse in the knee which has had multiple previous operations. The complications include rupture or persistent subluxation of the quadriceps mechanism and pain after the procedure. The Maquet procedure may be helpful in treating the latter problem.

The simplest method is enucleation of the patella through a minimal incision, otherwise known as the 'snatch patellectomy', but it may not be the best. Gunal et al[54] maintain that by advancing the oblique fibres of vastus medialis over the longitudinal repair they can overcome the problem of weakness of the quadriceps after patellectomy. Alternatively, if repair of the defect of the quadriceps seems tenuous it can be reinforced by turning down half the thickness of the rectus tendon which, incidentally, gives a better cosmetic result. When patellectomy is to be performed for an unstable patella the method of West and Soto-Hall[55] which combines realignment of the quadriceps with patellectomy can still be recommended.

THE GENUPATH

No discussion of anterior knee pain is complete without alerting the reader to the existence of the genupath. The entire life and being of these unusual individuals centre around their knee symptoms which become chronic and are blamed for failure both at work and in their private lives.

With consummate skill and patience they can manipulate a succession of orthopaedic surgeons to perform a series of procedures, each one more drastic than the last. In some, self-mutilation may be suspected and in most, litigation is used at some stage to bankroll the lifestyle. The disruptive chain of events invariably commences as 'anterior knee pain of unknown cause' in adolescence and this progresses in stages which include patellectomy, knee replacement, arthrodesis and even above-knee amputation in just ten to 15 years. Orthopaedic surgeons must be on their guard since these patients will be deliberately misleading and they need psychiatric help, not surgery. With the exception of diagnostic arthroscopy, it is wise to make a rule never to operate on the basis of subjective symptoms alone and to adhere to it.

REFERENCES

1. **Insall J.** Patellar pain. *J Bone Joint Surg [Am]* 1982;64-A:147-52.
2. **Dowd GSE, Bentley G.** *Anterior knee pain in knee surgery: current practice.* London: Martin Dunitz, 1992:724-35.
3. **Goodfellow J, Hungerford DS, Zindell M.** Patello-femoral joint mechanics and pathology. I: Functional anatomy of the patello-femoral joint. *J Bone Joint Surg [Br]* 1976;58-B:287-90.
4. **Perry J, Antonelli D, Ford W.** Analysis of knee-joint forces during flexed-knee stance. *J Bone Joint Surg [Am]* 1975;57-A:961-7.
5. **Zernicke RF, Garhammer J, Jobe FW.** Human patellar-tendon rupture: a kinetic analysis. *J Bone Joint Surg [Am]* 1977;59-A:179-83.
6. **Ogden JA.** *Skeletal injury in the child.* 2nd Ed. Philadelphia: WB Saunders Company, 1990:791.
7. **Krause BL, Williams JP, Catterall A.** Natural history of Osgood Schlatter disease. *J Pediatr Orthop* 1989;9:216-8.
8. **Batten J, Menelaus MB.** Fragmentation of the proximal pole of the patella. *J Bone Joint Surg [Br]* 1985;67-B:249-51.
9. **Smillie IS.** *Injuries of the knee joint.* 4th Ed. Edinburgh: E & S Livingstone Ltd, 1962.
10. **Blazina ME, Kerlan RK, Jobe FW, Carter VS, Carlson GJ.** Jumper's knee. *Orthop Clin North Am* 1973;4:665-78.
11. **Johnson DP.** Arthroscopic surgery for patellar tendinitis. *J Bone Joint Surg [Br]* 1996;78-B;Suppl II, 144.
12. **Houghton GR, Ackroyd CE.** Sleeve fracture of the patella in children, a report of three cases. *J Bone Joint Surg [Br]* 1979;61-B:165-8.
13. **Ogata K.** Painful bipartite patella: a new approach to operative treatment. *J Bone Joint Surg [Br]* 1994;76-A:573-8.
14. **Devas MB.** Stress fractures of the patella. *J Bone Joint Surg [Br]* 1960;42-B:71-4.
15. **Lloyd Roberts GC, Jackson AM, Albert JS.** Avulsion of the distal pole of the patella in cerebral palsy: a cause of deteriorating gait. *J Bone Joint Surg [Br]* 1985;67-B:252-4.
16. **Marandola MS, Prietto CA.** Arthroscopic Herbert screw fixation of patella osteochondritis dissecans. *Arthroscopy* 1993;9:214-6.
17. **Desai SS, Patel MR, Michelli LJ, Silver JW, Lidge RT.** Osteochondritis dissecans of the patella. *J Bone Joint Surg [Br]* 1987;69-B:320-5.
18. **Schwarz C, Blazina ME, Sisto DJ, Hirsh LC.** The results of operative treatment of osteochondritis dissecans of the patella. *Am J Sports Med* 1988;16:522-9.
19. **Johnson DP, Eastwood DM, Witherow PJ.** Symptomatic synovial plicae of the knee. *J Bone Joint Surg [Am]* 1993;75-A:1485-95.
20. **Matsumoto H, Kawakabo M, Otani T, Fujikawa K.** Extensive post-traumatic ossification of the patella tendon. *J Bone Joint Surg [Br]* 1999;81-B:34-6.
21. **Hampson WGJ, Hill P.** Late results of transfer of the tibial tubercle for recurrent dislocation of the patella. *J Bone Joint Surg [Br]* 1975;57-B:209-13.
22. **Paulos LE, Pinkowski JL.** Patella infera. In: Fox JM, Del Pizzo W, eds. *The patellofemoral joint.* New York: McGraw-Hill Inc, 1993.
23. **Fairbank JCT, Pynsent PB, van Poortvliet JA, Phillips H.** Mechanical factors in the incidence of knee pain in adolescents and young adults. *J Bone Joint Surg [Br]* 1984;66-B:685-93.
24. **Hughston JC.** Extensor mechanism examination. In: Fox JM, Del Pizzo W, eds. *The patellofemoral joint.* New York: McGraw-Hill Inc, 1993.
25. **Kannus P, Matri A, Paakkala T, Jarvimen M.** An outcome study of chronic patellofemoral pain syndrome. *J Bone Joint Surg [Am]* 1999;81-A:355-63.
26. **Leslie IJ, Bentley G.** Arthroscopy in the diagnosis of chondromalacia patellae. *Ann Rheum Dis* 1978;37:540-7.
27. **Bentley G.** The surgical treatment of chondromalacia patellae. *J Bone Joint Surg [Br]* 1978;60-B:74-81.
28. **Bentley G.** Is chondromalacia patellae a precursor of osteoarthritis of the knee? *J Bone Joint Surg [Br]* 1988;70-B:334.
29. **Outerbridge RE.** The aetiology of chondromalacia patellae. *J Bone Joint Surg [Br]* 1961;43-B:752-7.
30. **Goodfellow J, Hungerford DS, Woods C.** Patello-femoral joint mechanics and pathology. 2. Chondromalacia patellae. *J Bone Joint Surg [Br]* 1976;58-B:291-9.
31. **Bentley G.** Articular cartilage changes in chondromalacia patellae. *J Bone Joint Surg [Br]* 1985;67-B:769-74.
32. **Newman AP.** Articular cartilage repair. *Am J Sports Med* 1998;26:309-24.
33. **Ficat RP, Hungerford DS.** *Disorders of the patello-femoral joint.* Paris: Masson, 1977.
34. **Reider B, Marshall JL, Ring B.** Patellar tracking. *Clin Orthop* 1981;157:143-8.
35. **Dandy DJ.** Recurrent subluxation of the patella on extension of the knee. *J Bone Joint Surg [Br]* 1971;53-B:483-7.
36. **Jackson AM.** Recurrent dislocation of the patella. *J Bone Joint Surg [Br]* 1992;74-B:2-4.
37. **Merchant AC, Mercer RL, Jacobsen RH, Cool CR.** Roentgenographic analysis of patellofemoral congruence. *J Bone Joint Surg [Am]* 1974;56-A:1391-6.
38. **Carson WG, James SL, Larson RL, Singer KM, Winternitz WW.** Patellofemoral disorders: physical and radiographic evaluation. Part II: radiographic examination. *Clin Orthop* 1984;185:178-86.
39. **Fulkerson JP, Shea KP.** Disorders of patellofemoral alignment. *J Bone Joint Surg [Am]* 1990;72-A:1424-9.
40. **Laurin CA, Lévesque HP, Dussault R, Labelle H, Peides PJ.** The abnormal lateral patellofemoral angle: a diagnostic roentgenographic sign of recurrent patellar subluxation. *J Bone Joint Surg [Am]* 1978;60-A:55-60.
41. **Kawakubo M, Fujikawa K, Matsumoto H.** Evaluation of patellofemoral joint congruency using three-dimensional computed tomography. *Knee* 1999;6:165-70.

42. **Johnson L.** Arthroscopic evaluation of the patellofemoral articulation. In: Fox JM, Del Pizzo W, eds. *The patellofemoral joint.* New York: McGraw-Hill Inc, 1993:335-50.

43. **Ficat RP, Hungerford DS.** Disorders of the patellofemoral joint. Paris: Masson 1997:123-48.

44. **Lindenfeld TN, Bach BR Jr, Wojtys EM.** Reflex sympathetic dystrophy and pain dysfunction in the lower extremity. *J Bone Joint Surg [Am]* 1996;78-A:1936-44.

45. **Wilder RT, Berde CB, Woloham M, et al.** Reflex sympathetic dystrophy in children: clinical characteristics and follow-up of seventy patients. *J Bone Joint Surg [Am]* 1992;74-A:910-9.

46. **Al Duri Z, Aichroth PM.** Reflex sympathetic dystrophy of the knee. *Knee surgery: current practice.* London: Martin Dunitz, 1992;742-52.

47. **Wiles P, Andrews PS, Bremner RA.** Chondromalacia of the patella: a study of the late results of excision of the articular cartilage. *J Bone Joint Surg [Br]* 1960;42-B:65-70.

48. **Chrisman OD.** The role of articular cartilage in patellofemoral pain. *Orthop Clin North Am* 1986;17:231-4.

49. **Muckle DS, Minns RJ.** Biological response to woven carbon fibre pads in the knee: a clinical and experimental study. *J Bone Joint Surg [Br]* 1990;72-B:60-2.

50. **Pongor P, Betts J, Muckle DS, Bentley G.** Surface replacement of the knee with woven carbon. *J Bone Joint Surg [Br]* 1991;73-B:Suppl I:89.

51. **Meister K, Cobb A, Bentley G.** Treatment of painful articular cartilage defects of the patella by carbon fibre implants. *J Bone Joint Surg [Br]* 1998;80-B:964-70.

52. **Maquet P.** Advancement of the tibial tuberosity. *Clin Orthop* 1976; 115:225-30.

53. **Ferguson AB Jr, Brown TD, Fu FH, Rotkowski R.** Relief of patellofemoral contact stress by anterior displacement of the tibial tubercle. *J Bone Joint Surg [Am]* 1979;61-A:159-66.

54. **Gunal I, Taymaz A, Kose N, Göktürk E, Seker S.** Patellectomy with vastus medialis obliquus advancement for comminuted patellar fractures: a prospective randomised trial. *J Bone Joint Surg [Br]* 1997;79-B:13-6.

55. **West FE, Soto-Hall R.** Recurrent dislocation of the patella in the adult: end results of patellectomy and quadricepsplasty. *J Bone Joint Surg [Am]* 1958;40-A:386-94.

COMPLICATIONS OF KNEE ARTHROSCOPY

ROBIN ALLUM

From Wexham Park Hospital, Slough, England

Although arthroscopy of the knee is a minimally invasive procedure with less risk than endoscopy of the visceral cavities complications can and do occur. The operation is performed in very large numbers worldwide and although the percentage of patients experiencing problems is relatively small the total number is not insignificant. Complications are more likely to occur with more complex procedures such as meniscal repair, synovectomy and intra-articular reconstruction of both the anterior (ACL) and posterior (PCL) cruciate ligaments.

DeLee[1] reported a retrospective review of 118 590 arthroscopies carried out by the Arthroscopy Association of North America (AANA). There were 930 complications (0.8%). It was felt that this probably underestimated the total number of problems since it was a retrospective review based on surgeons' memories. In 1986 Small[2] carried out a further retrospective review of 395 566 arthroscopies. There was an overall complication rate of 0.56%. The percentage was higher in the more complex procedures, 2.4% in meniscal repair and 1.8% in reconstruction of the ACL. In a further prospective study in 1998[3] reviewing 10 262 procedures he found an overall complication rate of 1.68%. The most common complications in this study were haemarthrosis (60.1%), infection (12.1%), thromboembolic disease (6.9%), anaesthetic complications (6.4%), instrument failure (2.9%), reflex sympathetic dystrophy (RSD) (2.3%), ligament injury (1.2%) and fracture or neurological injury (0.6% each). Sherman et al[4] retrospectively reviewed 2640 arthroscopies performed by four surgeons. Overall, there were 216 complications (8.2%) of which 126 were designated as major and 97 as minor. The major complications were infection, haemarthrosis, adhesions, effusions, cardiovascular and neurological problems, RSD and instrument breakage, and the minor were difficulties with wound healing and ecchymoses. A number of predisposing factors were recognised. There was a higher incidence of neurological complications and RSD in patients with an industrial injury. As would be expected the lowest complication rate occurred with diagnostic arthroscopy. A higher overall complication rate occurred with partial medial meniscectomy and the incidence of haemarthrosis was highest in this procedure. Instrument breakage occurred most frequently during partial lateral meniscectomy. The largest number of problems with wound healing occurred after abrasion arthroplasty and lateral release was the commonest cause of adhesions. Slightly surprisingly, the complication rate was unrelated to the experience of the surgeon. The gender of the patient and the use of a tourniquet also had no influence. The length of time of inflation of the tourniquet did appear to be significant, with a higher risk in those patients who had a tourniquet time of 60 minutes or longer. Patients over 50 years old also were more subject to problems.

OPERATIVE COMPLICATIONS

Leg holder. Leg holders or posts are commonly used to aid exposure, particularly of the posterior horn of the medial meniscus. As in any surgical procedure in the anaesthetised patient there is the potential for damage by the injudicious application of force and it is possible to rupture the medial collateral ligament by the use of excessive valgus stress to open up the medial compartment. Injury to the lateral ligament due to varus stress is much less likely. Small[2] reported 160 knee ligament injuries, 143 of which involved a leg holder. These were reported in 0.04% of all cases of arthroscopy in the AANA.[1] Treatment is normally conservative by functional bracing with initial restriction of extension. Care needs to be taken in the application of a valgus force (Fig. 1), particularly when trying to view the posterior horn of the medial meniscus in a tight medial compartment in a middle-aged or elderly patient in whom the soft tissues are likely to be less flexible.

Tourniquet. A temporary paresis may occur after prolonged inflation of the tourniquet. It is important that regular checks are made on the accuracy of tourniquet pressures and it should be deflated after a maximum of two hours.

In the series of Sherman et al[4] the rate of complications was directly related to age and tourniquet time. Patients less than 50 years old with a tourniquet time of less than 40 minutes were in the low-risk group with a predicted complication rate of 6.7%. Patients over the age of 50 with a tourniquet time of less than 40 minutes or under the age of

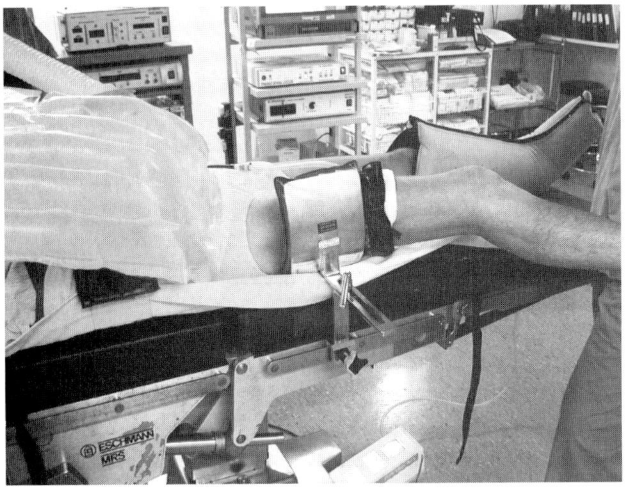

Fig. 1

Photograph showing that care should be taken when using a valgus force to open up the medial compartment with a leg holder.

50 with a tourniquet time of between 40 and 59 minutes were categorised as of average risk with a predicted complication rate of 10.1%. Those older than 50 years with a tourniquet time of between 40 and 49 minutes were classed as a moderate risk with a predicted complication rate of 16.4%. The high-risk patients were those who had a tourniquet time of greater than 60 minutes, regardless of age, when the predicted complication rate was 28.6%. Regarding major complications, patients under the age of 30 years with a tourniquet time of less than 40 minutes were in the low-risk group with a predicted complication rate of 3.2%. Patients over the age of 30 with a tourniquet time of less than 40 minutes or under the age of 30 with a tourniquet time between 40 and 59 minutes were in the average-risk group with a predicted complication rate of 5.2%. Patients over the age of 30 with a tourniquet time of between 40 and 59 minutes were in the moderate-risk group with a predicted complication rate of 8.1% and in the high-risk group the tourniquet time was greater than 60 minutes regardless of age with a predicted complication rate of 14.3%.

Compartment syndrome. There have been isolated reports of a compartment syndrome occurring during arthroscopic surgery.[5,6] For this to occur there must be a defect in the capsule. Increased irrigation pressure or blockage of the drainage will increase the risk. Noyes and Spievack[7] demonstrated in a cadaver study that fluid can extravasate into the thigh from a rupture of the suprapatellar pouch and into the calf from a rupture of the semimembranosus bursa. Peek and Haynes[5] showed in an animal model that the elevated compartment pressure in the calf returned to normal after 15 minutes, but in the presence of a fascial defect the pressure remained elevated for eight hours leading to muscle necrosis. In the cases reported by Peek and Haynes[5] and Fruensgaard and Holm[6] fasciotomies were carried out.

It is important to perform a preliminary examination under anaesthesia in the patient with an acute injury. If there is a significant disruption of a collateral ligament the risks of arthroscopy may outweigh any possible benefits. If a decision is made to proceed, care needs to be taken with infusion of the irrigation fluid and the thigh and calf need to be checked at regular intervals to ensure that no leakage is occurring.

Intra-articular damage. Any intra-articular structure can be damaged in an invasive procedure. It is important not to use a sharp trocar to introduce the arthroscope into the knee. A portal of adequate size should be made so that a blunt obturator can be used (Fig. 2). The anterior horns of the menisci are vulnerable when the incisions for the anteromedial and anterolateral portals are being made and it is wise to cut upwards with the knife away from the meniscus rather than downwards. Apart from the first portal the knife blade should be observed from within the joint (Fig. 3). Damage to the articular cartilage is not uncommon, but decreases with experience. It is essential that the placement of the portal is correct to allow easy passage of instruments within the joint. Operating instruments should

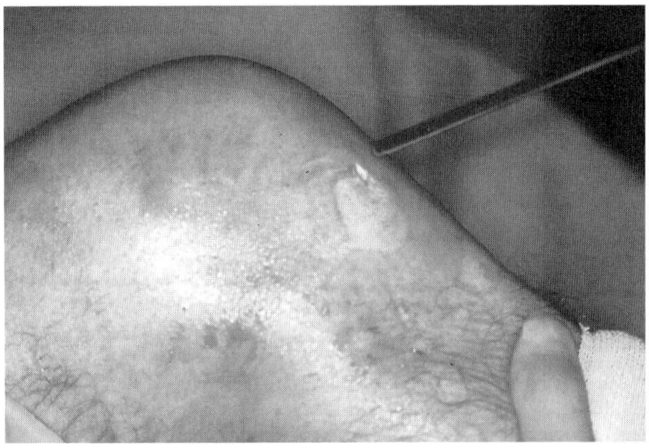

Fig. 2

Photograph showing the use of a blunt obturator to introduce the arthroscope into the knee.

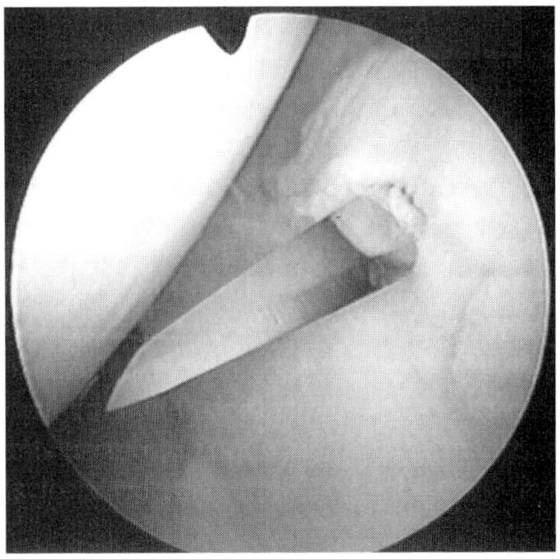

Fig. 3

The knife blade being observed from within the joint.

not be used unless they can be clearly seen and tissue should never be cut blindly, but always under direct vision. Great care needs to be taken with power instruments since they can do much damage very quickly, particularly to soft tissue. The inflow of fluid must be sufficient to maintain a clear operating field because power shavers remove relatively large quantities of fluid from the knee by suction.

It is important to limit meniscal resection to areas which are clearly unstable. The meniscus is the shock-absorber of the knee and overenthusiastic removal of meniscal tissue will lead to increased mechanical stress on the articular cartilage with a greater risk of post-traumatic osteoarthritis. The surgeon should always try to preserve a rim of meniscal tissue so that the hoop stress function can at least be partly maintained.

The cruciate ligaments can be vulnerable during meniscal excision when an intercondylar attachment is being removed.

Instrument breakage. This problem is less frequent than in the early days of arthroscopic surgery since the design of instruments has been improved and they have become more robust. It does, however, still occur. When this happens, if the broken fragment is visible the flow through the knee should be stopped by switching off both the irrigation and the outflow. A grasping instrument such as a pituitary rongeur needs to be passed carefully and gently across the joint to remove the fragment. If the fragment is not visible, irrigation may wash it into the field of vision. The use of an image intensifier may be necessary to localise it. It may be prudent to leave the fragment if it is small and inaccessible since removal may cause more harm than good. Magnetised instruments are available and may help in a difficult situation.

Neurological injury. Rodeo, Forster and Weiland[8] reported four mechanisms by which neurological damage can occur during arthroscopy. These are: 1) direct trauma; 2) pressure secondary to a compartment syndrome occurring as a result of extravasation of fluid; 3) tourniquet damage; and 4) dysfunction due to the ill-understood condition of RSD.

Injury to a nerve is rare. In Small's initial series[2] there were 229 nerve injuries in 375 069 knee arthroscopies, an incidence of 0.06%. The saphenous nerve was the most commonly involved (42%). The peroneal nerve was damaged in 5%, the femoral nerve in 3% and the sciatic nerve in 3%. In the remaining 47% the details of the involved nerve were not specified. In a further study by Small[3] there was only one instance of nerve damage in 8791 knee arthroscopies (0.01%). This was an injury to the saphenous nerve which occurred during a repair of the medial meniscus. In DeLee's study[1] there were 63 neurological complications in 118 590 arthroscopies, an incidence of 0.05% of which 25 involved the peroneal nerve, 23 the saphenous nerve, seven the femoral nerve, four the tibial nerve and four the sciatic nerve. On the medial side of the knee the saphenous nerve is potentially vulnerable posteromedially. It can be damaged by a posteromedial portal or during repair of the medial meniscus. The nerve lies deep to sartorius and is protected to a certain extent when the knee is flexed. The safe area for a posteromedial portal or incisions for medial meniscal repair lie between the posterior edge of the medial collateral ligament and the anterior margin of the tendon of pes anserinus. If there is any doubt, the nerve can be exposed directly or may be visualised by transillumination. During meniscal repair, as long as the needles exit anterior to the pes anserinus tendon, the nerve should be safeguarded. The anatomy of the saphenous nerve is variable making it very difficult to avoid injury completely during repair of the medial meniscus. Austin and Sherman,[9] in a review of the complications of this procedure, felt that saphenous neuropathies are an unavoidable and acceptable complication of this procedure.

Injury to a superficial nerve is not uncommon. The infragenicular branch of the saphenous nerve (IGBSN) runs a variable course and at times damage by anterior portals may be unavoidable. Injury to the IGBSN has been reported after knee arthroscopy.[4,10] In the study of Sherman et al[4] there was an incidence of 22.2% of sensory change in the distribution of the IGBSN after standard portals had been utilised. Although 'safe zones' have been advocated, the wide variability in the course of the nerve precludes the absolute avoidance of damage.[11,12] Mochida and Kikuchi[13] recommended that arthroscopic portals should be positioned close to both the patella and the patellar tendon if injury to the IGBSN is to be avoided.

On the lateral side the common peroneal nerve is vulnerable and the effects of injury to this structure are significant. Again damage is most likely to occur during meniscal repair. There has been one report of injury to the common peroneal nerve during lateral meniscectomy,[14] but in all other cases injury has occurred during meniscal suture.[14] Proximally, above the level of the knee, the nerve lies medial to the biceps tendon, between the biceps and the lateral head of gastrocnemius (Fig. 4). At the level of the joint it passes posterior to the biceps to wind around the neck of the fibula. Flexion of the knee will allow the nerve to drop back posteriorly making it less vulnerable. The safe

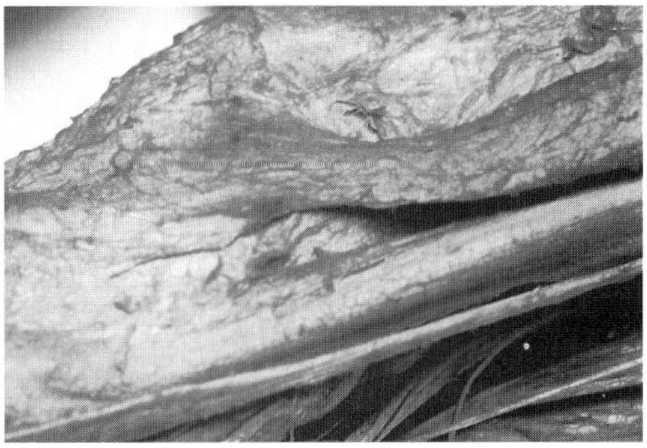

Fig. 4

Photograph showing the lateral popliteal nerve medial to biceps.

area is between the posterior edge of the iliotibial band and the biceps, preferably deep to the lateral head of gastrocnemius. To aid identification of the correct site for placement of a portal or an incision for meniscal repair, the joint can be transilluminated from within or a needle can be passed into the posterolateral joint and its position checked with the arthroscope. The interval between the iliotibial band and the biceps is developed. To confirm the position a probe can be passed across the joint from the anteromedial portal to tent the posterolateral capsule from within. The lateral head of gastrocnemius can be identified and its lateral border freed by blunt dissection. During in-to-out meniscal suture, the needles must be passed out of the joint under direct vision and as long as they are anterior to the biceps and lateral to the lateral head of gastrocnemius the peroneal nerve will be safeguarded. Use of the contralateral portal allows a relative anterior and lateral deviation of the repair needle further safeguarding the nerve, and this is also true posteromedially. Occasionally, formation of a neuroma can be troublesome and it is possible that a relatively minor nerve injury can lead to RSD.

Vascular injury. Jackson[15] reported the occurrence of injury to the popliteal artery leading to amputation. In the AANA review[1] there were six cases of penetrating injury of the popliteal artery. Four of these patients required amputation. There were 12 vascular injuries in Small's 1986 report,[2] but no vascular complications were listed in his later study.[3] Beck, Robison and Hallett[16] described a case of a pseudoaneurysm of the popliteal artery after arthroscopy and in 1987 Jeffries et al[17] presented two cases of injury to the popliteal artery occurring during arthroscopic lateral meniscectomy using power tools. Both lesions required repair. The popliteal neurovascular bundle is in close proximity to the posterior capsule of the knee and is clearly potentially vulnerable. It is important that the tip of any surgical instrument must be seen clearly at the back of the knee. Particular care needs to be taken with power tools and it is imperative that the operative field is clear at all times with adequate irrigation. If a vascular injury is suspected because of either excessive bleeding at the site of operation or compromise of the distal circulation, it is imperative that an urgent vascular opinion is sought followed by prompt arteriography and appropriate surgery when indicated. Any delay may result in the need for amputation. Fasciotomy may also have to be considered after any period of ischaemia. Vascular injury is more likely to occur during meniscal repair and the precautions outlined previously must be followed to safeguard the popliteal artery, particularly during repair of the lateral meniscus.

The superior lateral geniculate artery is vulnerable during a procedure for lateral release. The risk of bleeding can be minimised by the use of electrocautery. It is wise to infiltrate the incision with Marcaine and adrenaline and to use a drain for 24 hours. There is also the possibility of damage to this vessel during synovectomy.

The saphenous vein may be damaged when using a posteromedial portal or during repair of a medial meniscus and the same precautions need to be taken as outlined in the previous section on neurological injury.

Diagnostic errors. Arthroscopy is an invasive procedure and it is not a substitute for other methods of diagnosis. It is vital that a careful evaluation of the patient is carried out by standard clinical means with a history, examination and appropriate investigations. Often the history alone will provide the diagnosis. A careful systematic examination is essential. Plain radiographs should always be taken. MRI is a very effective non-invasive method of diagnosis and rarely should the arthroscope now be used solely for this purpose. Its function is predominantly to enable appropriate intra-articular surgery to be carried out after a definitive diagnosis has been made. Joyce and Mankin[18] described 12 cases in which significant diagnostic errors were made because of inadequate preoperative evaluation. Six patients had a significant neoplastic lesion visible on plain radiographs.

During the procedure itself the inexperienced surgeon may have problems with visualisation because of poor technique. It is important that adequate supervision is given in the early stages of the learning curve so that the important technical aspects of the operation are addressed. These include placement of the portals, positioning of the knee, triangulation and adequate irrigation.

POSTOPERATIVE COMPLICATIONS

Pain. Control of pain after operation is of the utmost importance. It is rarely a problem after diagnostic or simple operative arthroscopy but may occur after more complex procedures such as meniscal repair, synovectomy or intra-articular reconstruction of ligaments. There are a number of options for the management of pain. Opiates and other potent analgesics can be given as an intermittent fixed dose, into the epidural space, or as an intra-articular injection.[19] Local anaesthetic can also be given by the intra-articular route.[20] Non steroidal anti-inflammatory drugs (NSAIDs) are effective orally, by injection or rectally. Physical measures such as cold therapy have also been used with variable success.[21-27] All these methods have disadvantages and none is ideal. As well as the important factor of the comfort of the patient the level of pain experienced on coming round from the anaesthetic in the recovery room may well determine progress in the early stages after operation. A minimal level of pain has a very positive effect on the morale of the patient which may help the early programme of rehabilitation, particularly in the recovery of movement. Severe pain will impede this.

Haemarthrosis. The incidence of this complication is approximately 1%.[28] It is more common after lateral release because of damage to the superior lateral geniculate artery, and an incidence of between 5% and 42% has been reported after this procedure.[29] If a painful tense haem-

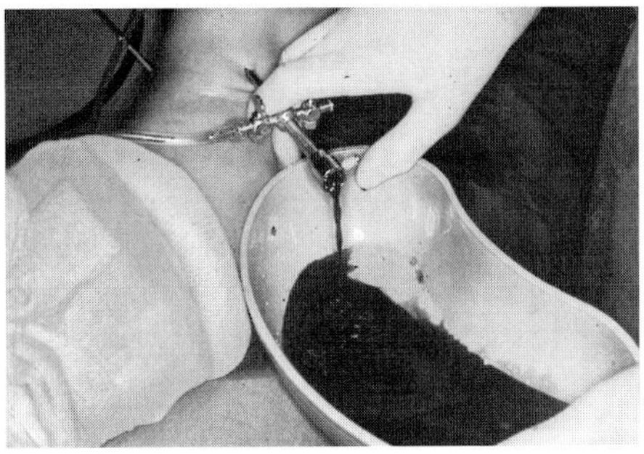

Fig. 5

Photograph showing the washing out of a haemarthrosis.

arthrosis develops the knee should be washed out arthroscopically (Fig. 5), local anaesthetic with adrenaline infiltrated into the joint and a pressure bandage applied. Consideration should be given to introducing a suction drain for 24 hours.

Thromboembolism. The risk of thromboembolic disease after arthroscopy is clearly low since the procedure is relatively short and mobilisation is quick. The incidence in the AANA study[1] was 0.1% and in Small's studies,[2,3] 0.17% and 0.13%, respectively. In the AANA study[1] 23% of patients with a deep-vein thrombosis (DVT) developed a pulmonary embolism (PE) and there were four deaths. The figures for DVT were probably an underestimate as the reviews were based on clinical symptoms. The overall reported incidence of DVT after arthroscopy of the knee ranges from 0% to 7.3% and PE from 0% to 0.32%.[30] In a study using venography[31] the incidence of DVT was 4.2%. There are a number of factors which are associated with an increased risk of thromboembolism. Patients over the age of 40 years are more likely to develop postoperative thrombosis. A prolonged operating or tourniquet time is also a risk factor but there is no definite evidence that the tourniquet itself increases the risk. When there is a previous history of thrombosis or embolism the risk of thromboembolic complications increases significantly. Kakkar et al[32] reported an incidence of DVT of 100% in a group of patients with a history of previous PE. There is no indication for routine thromboprophylaxis in arthroscopic surgery, but the operating and tourniquet times should be kept to a minimum and postoperative mobilisation should be as rapid as possible. Some form of prophylaxis should be considered for patients in the risk groups mentioned above particularly those with a previous thromboembolism.

Infection. Infection after arthroscopy is uncommon. The knee is the largest synovial cavity in the body and septic arthritis is therefore a very serious complication. DeLee[1] reported an incidence of 0.08%, Sherman et al[4] 0.1%, D'Angelo and Ogilvie-Harris,[33] 0.23% and Armstrong, Bolding and Joseph,[34] 0.42%. Diagnosis is not always straightforward. In classical septic arthritis there is acute pain, swelling, warmth and erythema accompanied by the systemic signs of fever and malaise together with a leucocytosis, with a raised ESR and level of C-reactive protein (CRP). *Staphylococcus aureus* is the most common infecting organism under these circumstances. The presentation, however, can be more insidious with a subacute onset of pain, swelling, mild fever and minimal or no leucocytosis, which may be associated with a coagulase-negative staphylococcus. Under these circumstances a Gram stain of the synovial fluid may be negative and a culture is required to confirm the diagnosis. Infection is more common among patients with longer operating times, an increased number of procedures during surgery, prior procedures and in those having chondroplasty or soft-tissue debridement.[34] A number of authors have also reported an increased incidence of septic arthritis after the administration of intra-articular corticosteroids at the time of arthroscopy. There is almost certainly impairment of local and systemic immune defence mechanisms.[34,35] Prophylactic antibiotics are not routinely used for arthroscopic surgery apart from more complex procedures such as reconstruction of the ACL. D'Angelo and Ogilvie-Harris,[33] however, have suggested that there may be a case for their use from the point of view of cost-benefit. Certainly, the treatment of septic arthritis of the knee is expensive. The patients in the series of D'Angelo and Ogilvie-Harris[33] were in hospital for a mean of 20 days, but this length of stay may not always be necessary. There is no definite consensus in the literature regarding the management of established septic arthritis after arthroscopy. There is general agreement that intravenous antibiotics are indicated initially based on the sensitivities from the synovial Gram stain or culture. The duration of treatment recommended varies from a few days to six weeks. It would seem wise to continue with intravenous antibiotics until the patient is clearly responding and the systemic signs resolving. Any pus or infected synovial fluid in the knee should be removed. Simple aspiration under local anaesthesia can be carried out, but this is likely to be a painful procedure and it is very difficult to remove all the fluid and the fibrin and other debris related to the infective process. Adequate removal of all infected material can only be achieved by an arthroscopic washout using copious lavage with several litres of fluid. After this a drain may be inserted for 24 to 36 hours. An irrigation-suction system can be set up but these are difficult to manage and there is no definite evidence that there is any advantage over lavage itself. This may have to be repeated after 48 to 72 hours. The joint should be rested initially but as soon as the infection is under control a graduated programme of rehabilitation needs to be instituted concentrating on the return of movement. Continuous passive motion (CPM) may be useful in the early stages of recovery.

Armstrong et al[34] made the following recommendations concerning infection.

1) Local injection of intra-articular corticosteroid should not be given at the time of arthroscopy.

2) If a patient develops persistent pain and swelling after arthroscopy culture of the synovial fluid is required. The

absence of erythema, fever, leucocytosis or obvious infection in the synovial fluid does not exclude infection.
3) Coagulase-negative staphylococci may cause a postoperative septic arthritis and a positive culture therefore may indicate infection rather than contamination.
4) The appropriate treatment of established septic arthritis is arthroscopic lavage.
5) Intravenous antibiotics for two weeks is sufficient if the condition is diagnosed and treated promptly.
6) An irrigation-suction system is not necessary.

Effusion and synovitis. An effusion is not uncommon after arthroscopy but rarely causes a problem. The reported incidence varies between 0% and 15%.[36] It may persist after arthroscopic surgery particularly for degenerative joint disease. The knee will remain painful, irritable and swollen because of postoperative synovitis. This can be a difficult and recalcitrant condition. Treatment is essentially conservative with rest, ice, compression and elevation together with NSAIDs and physiotherapy. If symptoms continue further investigation may be indicated. A full blood count, ESR and CRP should be undertaken to exclude infection, and also plain radiography. An isotope bone scan can be useful to determine the extent of the inflammatory response. MRI may be necessary to exclude a continuing mechanical problem. A further arthroscopic procedure with a washout should be considered if the joint does not respond to conservative measures, but there is no guarantee that this will lead to resolution of the symptoms of a postoperative inflammatory synovitis.

Synovial fistula. In DeLee's survey[1] there were 30 cases of synovial fistula, 70% of which responded to immobilisation in a cast. Details of treatment in the remaining 30% were not given. Proffer, Drez and Daus[37] retrospectively reviewed 976 arthroscopies over a period of three years. Six patients developed synovial fistulae; all were men with a mean age of 35.8 years. The fistulae developed between three and ten days after surgery with a mean of six days. Significant degenerative changes were present in at least one compartment in five cases. The portals involved were the posteromedial in three, superomedial in two and posterolateral in one. All cultures were sterile. Treatment was by immobilisation in extension together with prophylactic administration of oral cephalosporins. The fistulae closed after a mean of nine days (7 to 14). No patient required surgery and there were no recurrences. The combination of degenerative joint disease and posterior portals was felt to increase the risk but the numbers were not of statistical significance. The authors concluded that simple immobilisation in extension until the fistula closed, using a commercially available knee immobiliser was all that was required. Since no positive cultures were obtained prophylactic antibiotics were not necessary.

Complex regional pain syndrome 1. The International Association for the Study of Pain[38] has renamed RSD as complex regional pain syndrome 1 (CRPS 1). The purpose of the change in nomenclature is to introduce a descriptive diagnosis as opposed to one based on the questionable assumptions that the syndrome is always reflex in nature, mediated through the sympathetic nervous system with a consistently displayed dystrophy. The new definition expresses the complexity and variety of clinical presentations of the condition and the regional distribution of the characteristics presented where pain is considered to be a constant feature. CRPS 1 of the knee displays many symptoms and signs that are characterised by a disproportionate amount of pain, loss of function and a number of features which appear at first sight to be difficult to evaluate. Some are so random, bizarre and unconfined to dermatomes that it is tempting to regard the patient as mentally disturbed. Most, however, are sufficiently constant to demand further questioning and investigation.

CRPS 1 can occur after any type of injury to the knee including arthroscopic surgery. In making a diagnosis when the patient presents with a painful knee after an arthroscopic procedure it is essential to carry out appropriate investigations first to exclude a mechanical or inflammatory disorder. When these have been eliminated those features which would support a diagnosis of CRPS 1 should be sought. Does the patient suffer from Raynaud's disease or migraine? Women appear to be at a considerably greater risk of developing CRPS 1 than men. The syndrome may occur at any age and may be seen both in children and in the elderly, with the peak incidence between the third and fourth decades. The patellofemoral joint seems to be particularly vulnerable and most series in the literature report a relatively high incidence of problems associated with patellofemoral injury, disease or surgery. Injury to cutaneous nerves may also precipitate an exaggerated autonomic response and the saphenous nerve and its branches appear to be particularly vulnerable.[39,40] Katz and Hungerford[39] described 36 patients with CRPS 1, 69% of whom were female. Their mean age was 39.6 years (13 to 70). Of these 64% had had either an injury or an operation involving the patellofemoral joint, 41% had had previous surgery and 47% trauma to the front of the knee. The average number of operations before diagnosis was 1.2 and in 17% there was evidence of nerve injury. The mean delay in diagnosis was 29 months (3 weeks to 11 years). One patient had been submitted to an arthroscopy, three manipulations, another arthroscopy, an arthrotomy and patellar realignment, a PCL reconstruction and a further manipulation followed by a total knee replacement without resolution of symptoms! In a review of 19 patients Ogilvie-Harris and Roscoe[40] described 13 women and six men with a mean age of 40 years (15 to 49). Sixteen had sustained injuries and three had undergone surgery, two meniscectomies and one Maquet procedure. Poehling, Pollock and Koman[41] found that all 35 patients with CRPS 1 had evidence of damage to the infrapatellar branch of the saphenous nerve, either by trauma or surgery. Their mean age was 42 years (19 to 80) and 73% were women. Cooper, DeLee and Ramamurthy[42] reviewed the results of epidural anaesthesia in CRPS 1 in

14 patients in a younger age group with a mean age of 29 years (21 to 39); there were eight women and six men, of whom 11 had had surgery to the patella. Fulkerson and Hungerford[43] also highlighted the vulnerability of the patellofemoral joint because of the superficial subcutaneous position of the patella. In their experience the most common type of trauma is a direct blow to the patella, such as occurs in a dashboard injury or a fall onto the front of the knee. Indirect injuries such as twisting injuries or patellar dislocation are considered to be less likely to lead to CRPS 1.

In a large series of 60 patients from the Hospital for Special Surgery, New York, O'Brien et al[44] reported a similar age distribution with a mean age of 37.5 years (15 to 70). Of the 60 patients, 41 were women. Two-thirds had had previous knee surgery and 13 of the remaining 20 patients had pain arising from the patellofemoral joint.

The only certainties about this syndrome are its unpredictability and variability. The spectrum of severity ranges from mild transient symptoms to a severe disabling long-term problem. Pain is the main symptom and typically is out of proportion to that expected after injury or operation. Night pain may be particularly troublesome. Anatomically, the pain does not specifically follow the distribution of a single peripheral sensory nerve.[45] The knee will be diffusely tender and hyperaesthetic and there may be trigger points which can cause excruciating pain. The other clinical features of this syndrome relate to vasomotor instability. The initial response is one of vasodilatation and the skin becomes pink, warm and dry. Changes in sweating are termed sudomotor changes. The combination of swelling and inactivity due to the constant pain leads to stiffness. The clinical picture then changes and after a variable period of time vasoconstriction occurs. The knee becomes blue and cold and the skin shiny or contracted. Hair growth and on occasions ipsilateral nail growth are affected. Later, the knee becomes atrophic with thinning of the skin and loss of subcutaneous fat. Pigmentation changes may also occur, leading to dark or pale patches of melanin redistribution.

Most authors have described three phases in the vasomotor changes in CRPS 1 as follows.

Phase 1. The early vasomotor response of swelling and vasodilatation when the knee is hot pink and dry. This usually occurs within three months of the precipitating episode.

Phase 2. The dystrophic phase with predominant vasoconstriction, continuing oedema and cold thin skin together with increasing stiffness, developing between three and 12 months after the onset.

Phase 3. The atrophic phase with increasing atrophy of skin, muscle and soft tissue with fibrosis and contracture. Diffuse bony changes also occur. These later changes may be irreversible and cause a permanent disability. This phase occurs at a variable time but usually after at least 12 months.

The diagnosis depends very much on awareness of the condition and it should be considered in any patient who has persistent pain after arthroscopic surgery which is out of proportion to the normal postoperative discomfort. Radiological changes normally appear between two and eight weeks after the onset of symptoms. The essential change is one of demineralisation. The osteoporosis is commonly patchy with a band-like distribution predominantly affecting the subchondral bone, epiphysis and metaphyseal region (Fig. 6). Both cortical and cancellous bone is involved. The changes are different from the generalised ground-glass appearance of disuse atrophy. The joint space remains normal and there is no evidence of an inflammatory arthropathy such as erosions. Soft-tissue swelling may also be visible. The severity of the radiological changes is very variable as is the clinical syndrome and in a small proportion of patients the radiographs may be normal. The osteoporosis resolves after clinical recovery but some of the radiological changes may be irreversible. Bone scanning is a useful investigation and is certainly sensitive although not specific. Typically, the ^{99}Tc scan will show increased uptake in the early stages of the disease (Fig. 7). The bone

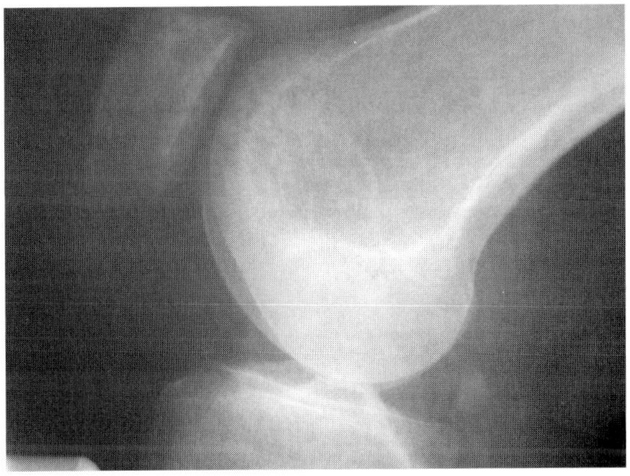

Fig. 6

Lateral radiograph of CRPS 1, showing patchy osteoporosis with a band-like distribution predominantly affecting the subchondral bone, epiphysis and metaphyseal region.

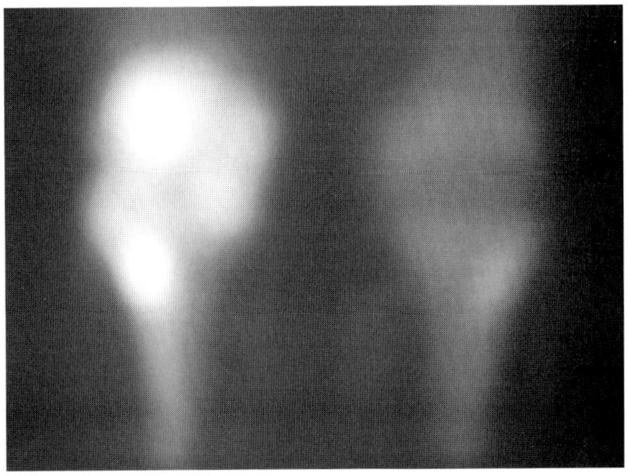

Fig. 7

Bone scan in CRPS 1 showing marked increased activity.

scan is abnormal before the radiological changes appear. There is increased uptake in the whole area affected by the disease. Both the blood-pool phase and the delayed image show increased activity. The changes may be widespread with increased activity in the other joints of the affected limb, and the whole limb itself may be involved and also changes in the contralateral limb may be seen. The exception to this is in children, in whom the bone scan may not change. Later, the scan returns to normal. Ogilvie-Harris and Roscoe[40] reported that all patients who presented early had positive scans, whereas in the group presenting later, only six of eight scans were positive. In the large series described by O'Brien[44] all 19 patients who had bone scans demonstrated some asymmetry of uptake, and two with good results from treatment had repeat scans which showed decreased activity. Bone scanning is therefore a reliable indicator of CRPS 1 and, if the bone scan is normal in an adult, particularly in the early stages, the diagnosis must be doubtful. Other investigations such as MRI and CT do not provide useful information.

Other causes of unresolved pain are infection, inflammatory joint disease and circulatory disturbances including DVT. The patient with CRPS 1 will be well with no systemic signs and the appropriate haematological investigations including full blood count, ESR, CRP, rheumatoid factor, uric acid and serum biochemistry will be normal. The radiological signs will be confined to the bone and the joint space will be normal or at least unchanged from previous radiographs. A venogram is advisable if DVT is clinically suspected.

The main objective of treatment is to alleviate pain as a prelude to rehabilitation.[46] The mainstays of treatment are the use of analgesics including NSAIDs, neurotransmitter blockers, physiotherapy and regional blocks. The transcutaneous nerve stimulator is also thought to be effective. The management of this condition is difficult and a prolonged treatment and rehabilitation programme is almost invariably required. The services of a pain clinic are invaluable particularly with respect to sympathetic blockade. Progress can be painfully slow and much patience is required on the part of the patient, surgeon and physiotherapist. The recovery period is measured in years rather than months or weeks.

Infrapatellar contracture syndrome. Paulos et al[47] and Paulos, Wnorowski and Greenwald[48] have described a group of patients with a combination of both significant loss of movement and reduced patellar mobility after operation or trauma. It most commonly occurs after reconstruction of the ACL but may arise after less complex arthroscopic procedures. In the original series[47] there were 28 patients, in 26 of whom the condition developed after operation and in two after minor trauma to the anterior aspect of the knee. There were 19 ACL reconstructions, two PCL reconstructions, two arthroscopic meniscectomies, one arthroscopic lateral retinacular release, one diagnostic arthroscopy and one each of proximal and distal patellar realignment. All patients had a significant lack of extension ranging from 7° to 35° of fixed flexion. Knee flexion ranged from 60° to 139°. Common symptoms were stiffness, pain, swelling after activity, crepitation, weakness and giving-way. Physical signs included an antalgic or flexed knee gait, quadriceps atrophy and patellofemoral crepitation with a shelf sign at the distal attachment of the patellar tendon because of induration around the tendon. There was significant loss of patellar mobility. The patellar tendon was short with obvious patella infera in 16% of cases. Radiographs showed disuse osteoporosis in the patellofemoral joint in most cases. Patella infera was usually associated with narrowing of the joint space and the formation of osteophytes.

The management is very difficult. Paulos et al[48] described three stages of this syndrome. In stage I, the prodromal stage, there is diffuse oedema and a painful range of movement together with restricted patellar mobility. Patients fail to gain the expected range of movement after operation. Stage II, or the active stage, follows with restriction of movement, atrophy of the quadriceps and patellofemoral crepitus. At this stage vigorous physiotherapy or manipulation will only aggravate the problem. In stage III, there is patella infera and evidence clinically and radiologically of patellofemoral osteoarthritis. The key to the diagnosis clinically is reduced patellar mobility. A zero or negative passive patellar tilt or superior or inferior glide of less than 2 cm confirms the diagnosis. It is then important to determine whether the problem is predominantly suprapatellar or infra- and peripatellar. Suprapetallar entrapment with adhesions in the suprapatellar pouch usually responds to arthroscopic debridement and manipulation. If the pathology is infra- and peripatellar then all vigorous rehabilitation should cease. The patient is placed on a gentle exercise programme with NSAIDs. If these measures do not resolve the problem open surgery is indicated, with intra- and extra-articular removal of adhesions, release of the patellar tendon and a lateral retinacular release. If patella infera of 8 mm or more is present, osteotomy of the tibial tubercle may be advisable, moving the tubercle proximally and anteriorly. The postoperative regime consists of CPM with a graduated range of movement, with splintage in extension if necessary. A further arthroscopic procedure may be required. Paulos et al[48] reported that after this regime the desired range of movement was achieved in most patients, but residual symptoms, patellofemoral dysfunction and activity-related pain and swelling were considerable.

ARTHROSCOPIC RECONSTRUCTION OF THE ANTERIOR CRUCIATE LIGAMENT

Reconstruction of the ACL is now commonly performed arthroscopically and it is therefore appropriate to consider the specific complications of this procedure. They may be operative or postoperative.

Operative complications

These can be related to the three stages in the operation: graft harvest, graft placement and graft fixation.

Graft harvest. The extensor mechanism is a vulnerable structure. It is possible to violate the patellar tendon when making the preliminary arthroscopy portals. The medial or lateral border may be damaged, making it difficult to use the middle third if a bone-patellar-tendon-bone (B-P-T-B) graft is being harvested. Since the patella can be fractured when taking the bone block, care must be taken not to lever too hard on the block until it has been cut completely. It is likely that some degree of microscopic damage will occur to the articular cartilage and subchondral bone by the vibrations from the power saw, however carefully it is used.

Harvest of the hamstring tendons is more demanding technically and it is not difficult to divide the tendons with inadequate length for reconstruction. Care should be taken to release all the peritendinous adhesions before passing the tendon stripper. If this does not pass freely, it should be removed and the tendon released by further dissection.

Graft placement. It is of prime importance to replace the ACL anatomically so that its function can be reproduced as closely as possible.

If the tibial tunnel is positioned too far forward, extension will be limited.[49-51] The reference points for the intra-articular opening of the tibial tunnel are the PCL, the anterior horn of the lateral meniscus and the stump of the ACL. The tip of the guide-wire should emerge posterior to the posterior edge of the anterior horn of the lateral meniscus, which is 5 to 7 mm anterior to the anterior attachment of the PCL. The hole should be drilled through the posterior part of the stump of the ACL, if still visible. If the drill hole is anterior to this point impingement may occur on the roof of the intercondylar notch causing limitation of extension. Commercially-produced drill guides are available for this step. Care must be taken to ensure that the tip of the drill guide is placed sufficiently posteriorly (Fig. 8). Commonly, the guide is designed so that the guide-wire hits the 'axilla' of the intra-articular portion rather than the tip and this may produce a tunnel which is too anterior.

Extension may also be limited by a build-up of scar tissue at the front of the intercondylar notch, the so-called 'cyclops' lesion[52] (Fig. 9). The stump of the ACL should be removed from the tibia and the 'trapdoor' formed by drilling the tunnel should be shaved away.

The most common fault is to place the femoral tunnel too anteriorly.[49] When this occurs flexion will be limited and/or the graft will stretch.[53] The architecture of the intercondylar notch may well be altered by osteophytes and scar tissue which has formed in response to instability. It is essential to identify the back of the intercondylar notch accurately. The so-called 'resident's ridge' approximately 1 cm in front of the posterior edge of the intercondylar notch may cause confusion to the inexperienced. This is a ridge of bone which initially appears to represent the back of the intercondylar notch but on probing it becomes clear that there is more bone posteriorly. Defining the anatomy is easier with modern arthroscopic equipment and certainly there are advantages over conventional open surgery as regards visualisation. If the notch is narrowed, an arthroscopic osteotome can be used to open up the front of the intercondylar area. The posterior part of the fat pad can be removed with a shaver, so that the arthrosope can be backed up for a clearer view of the intercondylar notch. Using a combination of hand instruments, soft-tissue shavers and bony burrs the lateral wall of the intercondylar notch is cleared until a probe can be passed clearly over the back. As in all arthroscopic surgery observation must be reinforced by palpation and there is no substitute for feeling the probe pass out over the back of the notch which is completely different from the probe passing over the 'resident's ridge'. A bridge of bone of 1 to 2 mm only should be left at the posterior edge of the femoral tunnel (Fig. 10) and commercially-available drill guides can be used for this important step. The tunnel is drilled at the 11 o'clock position for the

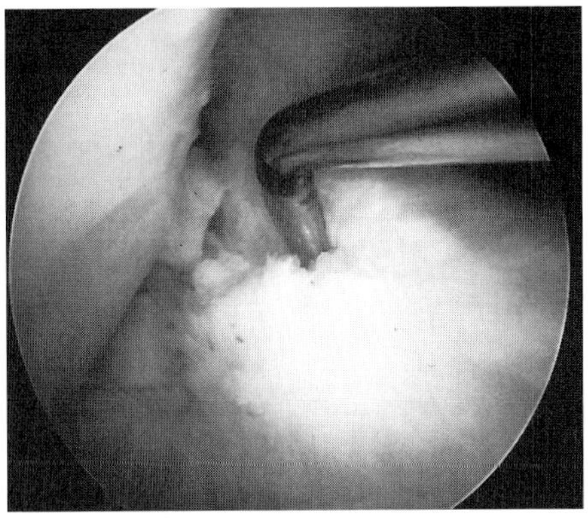

Fig. 8

Tibial tunnel drill guide in the posterior part of the ACL stump.

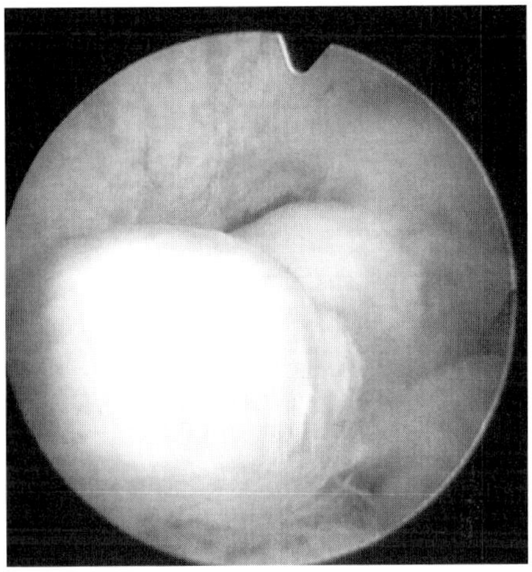

Fig. 9

The 'cyclops' lesion.

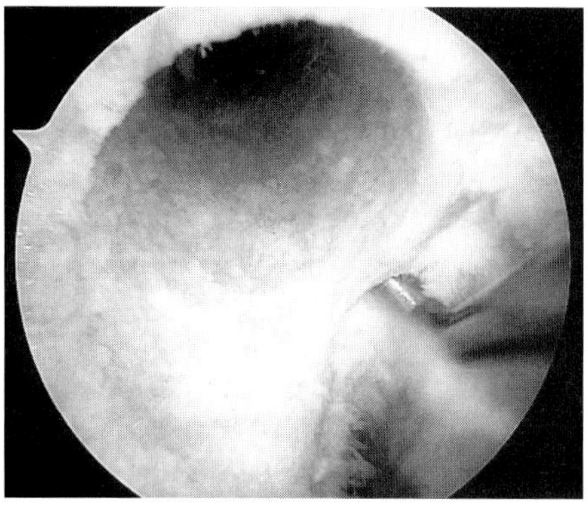

Fig. 10

Femoral tunnel with a 1 to 2 mm bridge of bone posteriorly.

right knee and at 1 o'clock for the left. Failure to visualise adequately the posterior aspect of the intercondylar notch may result in too anterior a position of the femoral tunnel. This will restrict flexion and/or lead to stretching and rupture of the graft.

Graft fixation. Interference screws can be dangerous if used incorrectly. When a B-P-T-B graft is employed it will not always follow the track between the bone block and the wall of the tunnel, and fixation may be inadequate if divergence occurs. Guide-wires are commercially available but they are easily bent. It is important to insert the screw at the correct angle. The knee must be flexed to at least 90° and drilling the femoral tunnel through the medial portal rather than through the tibial tunnel will facilitate this step. The graft must be taut when the screw is inserted to reduce the risk of damage as a result of the screw catching on the soft tissue. The bone block in the femoral tunnel should be inserted with the cancellous surface uppermost and the screw superiorly so that the screw threads are well away from the soft-tissue part of the graft.

The fixation of hamstring grafts is more challenging. Soft tissue has to be fixed to bone rather than bone-to-bone. EndoButton, screw-washer, belt-buckle staples, ligament anchors, and interference screws all appear to be satisfactory. At least 2 cm of graft is required in the bone tunnels for adequate fixaton.

Postoperative complications

The donor site

Anterior knee pain. Anterior knee pain after B-P-T-B reconstruction of the ACL is well documented.[54-60] The use of hamstring tendons for the graft is generally thought to reduce the incidence of anterior knee pain. There have, however, been conflicting reports in the literature.[61-65] In anatomical terms, the pain can arise from the skin, the prepatellar tissues, the patellar tendon or its sheath, the patella itself, and in the case of hamstring tendons the tissues adjacent to the insertion of the pes anserinus.

Pain and discomfort on kneeling are very common and this may be troublesome in those patients whose job involves kneeling. A neuroma of the infrapatellar branch of the saphenous nerve may cause considerable symptoms. Patellar tendinitis has been reported in patients after harvest of the patellar tendon. Most cases settle with time. The patellofemoral joint is a very vulnerable structure and chondromalacia can be a problem as a consequence of the injury, the surgery, or the postoperative immobility.

Chondromalacia may be inevitable in some patients after a serious injury to the knee. Harvest of the patellar tendon must damage the patella, no matter how careful and gentle the surgery, and there must be a disturbance of patellofemoral biomechanics. It has been suggested that careful attention to a vigorous and aggressive rehabilitation regime will reduce the incidence of postoperative patellofemoral problems[66] and it is important to achieve and maintain full extension for the well-being of the patellofemoral joint.

Fracture of the patella and rupture of the patellar tendon. After any major operation on the knee there is inevitably a degree of limitation of movement no matter how successful the surgery and rehabilitation. The extensor mechanism is therefore vulnerable if the knee is injured. Increased forces will be transmitted across the patella and its tendon because of the lack of mobility of the joint. Also, there will be a defect in the anterior aspect of the patella after harvest of the graft which will take some months to fill in. This will act as a stress riser and a fracture may occur at the junction between the defect and the normal bone.

Femoral fracture. Cases have been reported of fracture of the distal femur in relation to the stress risers at the bone tunnel or the site of fixation.

Muscle weakness. Some degree of muscle weakness is inevitable after such a major surgical procedure, but it can be a long-term problem.

Rupture of the graft. The graft may fail because of either a new injury or a technical error in insertion, usually poor tunnel placement or inadequate notchplasty leading to impingement.

Limitation of movement. Any loss of movement after injury or surgery will lead to considerable disability. Patients requiring reconstruction of the ACL are usually involved in considerable athletic activity and will therefore need maximum mobility of their knees. Even if the knee is perfectly stable postoperatively a patient with severe limitation of movement may well not be able to return to his or her sport. Loss of extension causes particular problems during sport and in normal gait and function. Knee flexion of less than 125° interferes with activities such as sitting, squatting, stair-climbing and running. Loss of movement, particularly extension, leads to an increased incidence of patellofemoral problems with anterior knee pain and painful patellofemoral crepitus. Rehabilitation is obviously slower and return to physical activity both at work and on the sports field will be delayed. The gait pattern never returns to normal and muscle function recovers slowly and incompletely.

A loss of extension of between 50° and 10°, and flexion

to only 125° or 130° has been reported.[53,58,67-69] The incidence of stiffness therefore varies, depending on the definition, but problems with loss of movement have been reported in up to 24% of cases.[54] Sachs et al[54] carried out a survey of 50 prominent knee surgeons who had published in the field of reconstruction of the ACL. From the 40 who replied, flexion contracture was the most common complication after ligament surgery. It is associated with a high level of patient dissatisfaction and is very frustrating for the patient, surgeon and physiotherapist. Treatment is difficult, requiring hard work on the part of the patient and progress is usually slow. Shelbourne, Patel and Martini[70] have devised a classification of arthrofibrosis based on a review of 72 patients. There are four types as follows.

Type 1. Extension loss of <10° with normal flexion.

Type 2. Extension loss of >10° with normal flexion.

Type 3. Extension loss of >10°, with loss of >25° of flexion and a tight patella.

Type 4. Extension loss of >10°, with loss of 30° of flexion or more, and patella infera with marked patellar tightness.

A number of risk factors have been suggested.

Age. The older patient will recover more slowly from reconstructive surgery because of age-related changes in connective tissue. There is, however, no conclusive evidence that the results of reconstruction of the ACL in this age group are any worse than in the younger patient.[71]

Early surgery. This is open to debate. As with many controversial subjects a search through the literature will produce more than one opinion. Several papers suggest that there is a strong link between early surgery and postoperative limitation of movement[69,72-74] and a number support the opposite view.[75-77] It would seem wise to wait for the inflammatory reaction in the knee to settle after injury so that the knee is 'quiet'. Certainly, to operate on a knee that has considerable restriction of movement, particularly extension, would be unwise.

Concomitant injury. The more widespread the injury to the knee, the more likely it is that there will be complications such as stiffness.

Additional surgery. Similarly, additional operations such as meniscal repair (Fig. 11) or other operations on the ligament will increase the risk of limitation of movement. Meniscal injury commonly accompanies rupture of the ACL and may lead to a dilemma in management, as it is wise to let the knee settle down before undertaking a major reconstructive procedure, but it may be felt that meniscal surgery should not be delayed. There is no evidence that delaying meniscal surgery has a harmful effect and the results of repair are probably not prejudiced by delay. Indeed, a proportion of acute peripheral meniscal tears occurring at the time of injury to the ACL may have the capacity to heal spontaneously. The haemarthrosis and inflammatory response to the acute injury create an ideal environment for healing. An aggressive attitude towards meniscal repair at an early stage may result in unnecessary procedures being carried out, and it has been noted that some acute peripheral tears have healed when the arthroscopy is repeated at the time of reconstruction of the ACL. Fitzgibbons and Shelbourne[78] have shown that certain types of lateral meniscal tear can be left alone at the time of reconstruction of the ACL without causing later symptoms. These are avulsion tears of the posterior horn, vertical tears posterior to the popliteus tendon and stable longitudinal tears usually of one surface only. This may partly explain the success of meniscal repair at the time of reconstruction of the ACL. Stabilising the knee may reduce the stress on the meniscus and the tear then either heals or remains mechanically stable. The only situation in which early surgery must be seriously considered occurs when the knee is locked due to a displaced bucket-handle meniscal tear. The mechanical block needs to be dealt with before a fixed flexion deformity develops. Shelbourne and Johnson[79] have recommended a two-stage procedure with a partial meniscectomy or meniscal repair followed by reconstruction of the ACL when the knee has recovered from the initial surgery. This is said to have several advantages including the more aggressive use of repair, the prevention of problems in regaining movement, a second look to judge the success of the meniscal repair and time for the patient to prepare for the reconstruction physically, mentally and socially. Certainly, a major surgical reconstruction carried out in a locked knee carries a considerable risk of limitation of movement. Care should be taken when carrying out an in-to-out meniscal repair not to tie the sutures with the knee flexed, particularly on the medial side, since this will cause restriction of extension due to tethering of the capsule.

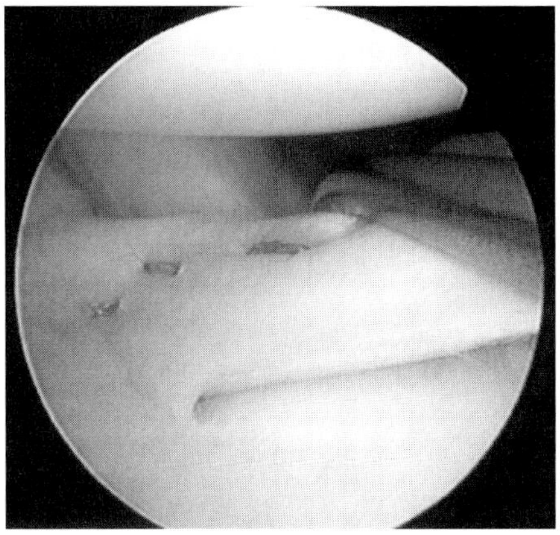

Fig. 11

Meniscal repair. Any other surgery will increase the risk of limitation of motion after ACL reconstruction.

Injuries to the medial collateral ligament (MCL) may occur in association with rupture of the ACL. In recent years, the approach to this injury has become more conservative. There appears to be no advantage in surgical repair of the MCL in association with rupture of the ACL.[80,81] Certainly, there is a risk with open surgery to the MCL and the posteromedial capsule that postoperative

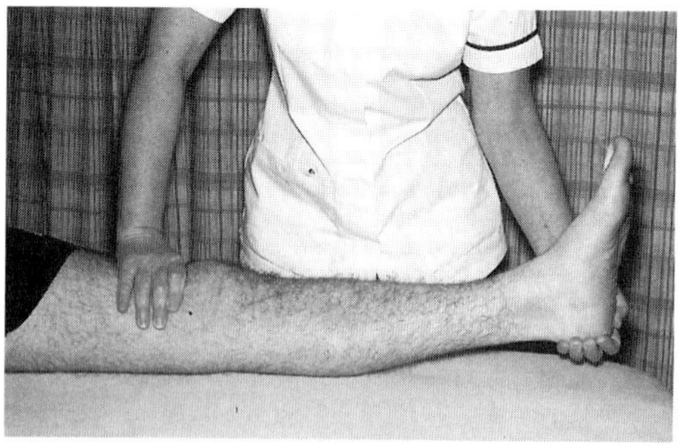

Fig. 12

It is important that the patient undergoes an adequate and appropriate rehabilitation programme for the return of full movement and function, particularly extension.

scarring may lead to difficulty in regaining a full range of movement, particularly extension.

There are few reports in the literature regarding combined ACL and PCL injuries and ACL and lateral complex injuries. After operation recurrent instability is more likely to be a problem than limitation of movement and the advantages of early repair may outweigh the risks of limitation of movement.

Inadequate rehabilitation. An adequate and appropriate rehabilitation programme is essential for the return of full movement and function, particularly extension (Fig. 12). This has been emphasised by several authors, notably Shelbourne and Nitz.[82] The correct surgical technique and adequate fixation of the graft should allow early aggressive restoration of movement, particularly extension.

The management of rehabilitation is not easy and requires a great deal of care and patience. Progress is almost invariably slow. If the patient fails to regain movement satisfactorily in the early postoperative phase despite adequate conservative measures, a decision will have to be made regarding more active intervention. The timing is difficult. If an invasive procedure is carried out when the knee is still inflamed from the surgery the problem may be aggravated. If there is undue delay, an established contracture may occur which will be difficult to correct. With modern techniques of accelerated rehabilitation manipulation under anaesthetic (MUA) and arthroscopy are indicated between six and 12 weeks after operation if there is fixed flexion of 10° or more.[82,83]

Ideally, the patient should achieve 120° of flexion by six weeks after surgery and failure to achieve this target or to progress satisfactorily indicates that further measures may be necessary. Each patient must be individually assessed and several factors may have to be taken into consideration in deciding on management. It may be better to rest the knee and stop active rehabilitation for a short period to allow the joint to settle, particularly if the patient has been working the knee very vigorously. If the knee is tender, swollen and inflamed, excessive manipulation or physiotherapy may make matters worse.

If arthroscopy is felt to be necessary, adhesions are removed with a combination of hand instruments and power shavers. The position and state of the graft are checked and the knee is put through as full a range of movement as possible to check that there is no impingement, particularly in extension. Watanabe and Howell[84] have described the typical radiological, MRI and arthroscopic appearances of impingement. Notchplasty is carried out if indicated. A gentle MUA is also carried out. If there are significant technical errors partial or total resection of the graft with or without revision will have to be considered.

The postoperative management must be closely supervised. Pain should be minimised with an aggressive approach to return of movement with both active and passive exercises. A bivalved cast or extension board may be used if fixed flexion is a problem and CPM may help to maintain improvement in the range of movement. Shelbourne et al[70] described the management of the 72 patients with established arthrofibrosis who formed the basis for the classification system described previously. Arthroscopy was carried out at a mean of 12.5 months after reconstruction of the ACL. Patients with type-1 arthrofibrosis had an arthroscopic resection of scar tissue from the front of the intercondylar notch, including the cyclops lesion if present, so that full extension was possible without impingement. This was followed by appropriate postoperative physiotherapy. In the type-2 patients, extrasynovial scar tissue anterior to the proximal tibia required excision as well as a full clearance of the anterior part of the intercondylar notch. An extension cast was applied for 24 hours, followed by extension exercises and prone hanging with further casting on a daily basis for two or three days if full extension could not be achieved. Patients in the type-3 group required resection of scar tissue from between the fat pad and the patellar tendon, into the fat pad and proximally as far as the insertion of vastus medialis obliquus and vastus lateralis. If the ACL graft was too anterior the anterior fibres were resected and a notchplasty was performed. A similar procedure was carried out in the type-4 patients with a more extensive scar resection medial and lateral to the patella. An MUA was carried out in all type-3 and type-4 patients followed by serial casting usually for three to four days, with physiotherapy and a bivalved cast at night. Once full extension was achieved and maintained, flexion exercises were introduced. Using this regime at a mean follow-up of 35 months, type-1 patients gained a mean of 7° of extension, type-2 patients 14° of extension, type-3 patients 13° of extension and 28° of flexion and type-4 18° of extension and 27° of flexion. No patients in any group developed problems with symptomatic instability or on objective testing despite partial resection of the graft in ten and complete resection in four. In the type-4 patients, the mean length of the patellar tendon increased from 42 mm preoperatively to 45 mm postoperatively.

To summarise the management of this difficult condition:

1) Prevention is better than cure.
2) Operation should be performed when the knee is 'quiet' with no significant restriction of movement.
3) The tunnels must be in the right place.

There must be adequate postoperative analgesia with correct rehabilitation, concentrating on immediate return of full extension.

CONCLUSIONS

No invasive procedure will be entirely free from risk and arthroscopy of the knee is no exception. Patients should be made aware of this fact. Complications are relatively rare but can have serious and significant consequences when they occur. Not all are unavoidable and it is important to exercise due care in all phases of the surgical process, including preoperative assessment, the surgery itself and aftercare.

REFERENCES

1. **DeLee JC.** Chairman, Committee on Complications of Arthroscopy Association of North America. Complications of arthroscopy and arthroscopic surgery: results of a national survey. *J Arthroscopic Rel Surg* 1985;1:214-20.
2. **Small NC.** Complications in arthroscopy: the knee and other joints, Committee on Complications of the Arthroscopy Association of North America. *Arthroscopy* 1986;2:253-8.
3. **Small NC.** Complications in arthroscopic surgery performed by experienced arthroscopists. *Arthroscopy* 1988;4:215-21.
4. **Sherman OH, Fox JM, Snyder SJ, et al.** Arthroscopy - "No Problem Surgery": an analysis of complications in two thousand six hundred and forty cases. *J Bone Joint Surg [Am]* 1986;68-A:256-65.
5. **Peek RD, Haynes DW.** Compartment syndrome as a complication of arthroscopy: a case report and a study of interstitial pressures. *Am J Sports Med* 1984;12:464-8.
6. **Fruensgaard S, Holm A.** Compartment syndrome complicating arthroscopic surgery: brief report. *J Bone Joint Surg [Br]* 1988;70-B:146-7.
7. **Noyes FR, Spievack ES.** Extraarticular fluid dissection in tissues during arthroscopy: a report of clinical cases and a study of intra-articular and thigh pressures in cadavers. *Am J Sports Med* 1982;20:346-51.
8. **Rodeo SA, Forster RA, Weiland AJ.** Current concepts review: neurological complications due to arthroscopy. *J Bone Joint Surg [Am]* 1993;75-A:917-26.
9. **Austin KS, Sherman OH.** Complications of arthroscopic meniscal repair. *Am J Sports Med* 1993;21:864-8.
10. **Carson RW.** Arthroscopic meniscectomy. *Orthop Clin North Am* 1979;10:619-27.
11. **Ebraheim NA, Mekhail AO.** The infrapatellar branch of the saphenous nerve: an anatomic study. *J Orthop Trauma* 1997;11:195-9.
12. **Pagnani MJ, Warner JJP, O'Brien SJ, Warren RF.** Anatomic considerations in harvesting the semitendinosus and gracilis tendons and a technique of harvest. *Am J Sports Med* 1993;21:565-71.
13. **Mochida H, Kikuchi S.** Injury to the infrapatellar branch of the saphenous nerve in arthroscopic knee surgery. *Clin Orthop* 1995;320:88-94.
14. **Rodeo SA, Sobel M, Weiland AJ.** Deep peroneal-nerve injury as a result of arthroscopic meniscectomy: a case report and review of the literature. *J Bone Joint Surg [Am]* 1993;75-A:1221-4.
15. **Jackson RW.** Current concepts review: arthroscopic surgery. *J Bone Joint Surg [Am]* 1983;65-A:416-20.
16. **Beck DE, Robison JG, Hallett JW Jr.** Popliteal artery pseudoaneurysm following arthroscopy. *J Trauma* 1986;26:87-9.
17. **Jeffries JT, Gainor BJ, Allen WC, Cikrit D.** Injury to the popliteal artery as a complication of arthroscopic surgery: a report of two cases. *J Bone Joint Surg [Am]* 1987;69-A:784-5.
18. **Joyce MJ, Mankin HJ.** Caveat arthroscopy: extra-articular lesions of bone stimulating intra-articular pathology of the knee. *J Bone Joint Surg [Am]* 1983;65-A:289-92.
19. **Joshi GP, McCarroll SM, Cooney CM, et al.** Intra-articular morphine for pain relief after knee arthroscopy. *J Bone Joint Surg [Br]* 1992;74-B:749-51.
20. **Chirwa SS, MacLeod BA, Day B.** Intraarticular bupivacaine (marcaine) after arthroscopic meniscectomy: a randomized double-blind controlled study. *Arthroscopy* 1989;5:33-5.
21. **Cohn BT, Draeger DP, Jackson DW.** The effects of cold therapy in the postoperative management of pain in patients undergoing anterior cruciate ligament reconstruction. *Am J Sports Med* 1989;17:344-9.
22. **Schroder D, Passler HH.** Combination of cold and compression after knee surgery: a prospective, randomised study. *Knee Surg Sports Traumatol Arthrosc* 1994;2:158-65.
23. **Barber FA, McGuire DA, Click S.** Continuous-flow cold therapy for outpatient anterior cruciate ligament reconstruction. *Arthroscopy* 1998;14:130-5.
24. **Paessler HH, Shelbourne KD.** *Biological, biomechanical and clinical approaches to the follow-up treatment of ligament surgery in the knee.* In: Sports exercise and injury Pearson Professional Ltd, 1995;1:83-95.
25. **Daniel DM, Stone ML, Arendt RN.** The effect of cold therapy on pain, swelling and range of motion after anterior cruciate ligament reconstructive surgery. *Arthroscopy* 1994;10:530-3.
26. **Edwards DJ, Rimmer M, Keene GCR.** The use of cold therapy in the postoperative management of patients undergoing arthroscopic anterior cruciate ligament reconstruction. *Am J Sports Med* 1996;24:193-5.
27. **Konrath GA, Lock T, Goitz HT, Scheidler J.** The use of cold therapy after anterior cruciate ligament reconstruction: a prospective, randomised study and literature review. *Am J Sports Med* 1996;24:629-33.
28. **Dandy DJ, O'Carroll PF.** Arthroscopic surgery of the knee. *Br Med J* 1982;285:1256-8.
29. **McGinty JB.** Complications of arthroscopy and arthroscopic surgery. In: McGinty JB, Caspari RB, Jackson RW, eds. *Operative arthroscopy.* Philadelphia: Lippincott-Raven, 1996:71-81.
30. **Poulsen KA, Borris LC, Lassen MR.** Thromboembolic complications after arthroscopy of the knee. *Arthroscopy* 1993;9:570-3.
31. **Stringer MD, Steadman CA, Hedges AR, et al.** Deep vein thrombosis after elective knee surgery: an incidence study in 312 patients. *J Bone Joint Surg [Br]* 1989;71-B:492-7.
32. **Kakkar VV, Howe CT, Nicolaides AN, Renney JTG, Clarke MB.** Deep vein thrombosis of the leg: is there a "high risk" group? *Am J Surg* 1970;120:527-30.
33. **D'Angelo GL, Ogilvie-Harris DJ.** Septic arthritis following arthroscopy, with cost/benefit analysis of antibiotic prophylaxis. *Arthroscopy* 1988;4:10-4.
34. **Armstrong RW, Bolding F, Joseph R.** Septic arthritis following arthroscopy: clinical syndromes and analysis of risk factors. *Arthroscopy* 1992;8:213-23.
35. **Gosal HS, Jackson AM, Bickerstaff DR.** Intra-articular steroids after arthroscopy for osteoarthritis of the knee. *J Bone Joint Surg [Br]* 1999;81-B:952-4.
36. **Dandy DJ.** Complications and technical problems. In: Dandy DJ, ed. *Arthroscopic management of the knee.* 2nd ed. Edinburgh: Churchill Livingstone, 1987:64-71.
37. **Proffer DS, Drez D Jr, Daus GP.** Synovial fistula of the knee: a complication of arthroscopy. *Arthroscopy* 1991;7:98-100.
38. **Merskey H, Bogduk N, eds.** *Classification of chronic pain: descriptions of chronic pain syndromes and definition of pain terms.* Seattle: IASP Press, 1994.
39. **Katz MM, Hungerford DS.** Reflex sympathetic dystrophy affecting the knee. *J Bone Joint Surg [Br]* 1987;69-B:797-803.
40. **Ogilvie-Harris DJ, Roscoe M.** Reflex sympathetic dystrophy of the knee. *J Bone Joint Surg [Br]* 1987;69-B:804-6.
41. **Poehling GG, Pollock FE Jr, Koman LA.** Reflex sympathetic dystrophy of the knee after sensory nerve injury. *Arthroscopy* 1988;4:31-5.
42. **Cooper DE, DeLee JC, Ramamurthy S.** Reflex sympathetic dystrophy of the knee: treatment using continuous epidural anesthesia. *J Bone Joint Surg [Am]* 1989;71-A:365-9.

43. **Fulkerson JP, Hungerford DS, eds.** *Disorders of the patellofemoral joint.* 2nd ed. Baltimore: Williams and Wilkins, 1990:247-64.

44. **O'Brien SJ, Ngeow J, Gibney MA, Warren RF, Fealy S.** Reflex sympathetic dystrophy of the knee: causes, diagnosis and treatment. *Am J Sports Med* 1995;23:655-9.

45. **Lindenfield TN, Bach BR, Wotjys EM.** Reflex sympathetic dystrophy and pain dysfunction in the lower extremity: an Instructional Course Lecture: the American Academy of Orthopaedic Surgeons, 1996;78:1936-44.

46. **Stanton-Hicks M, Baron R, Boas R, et al.** Complex regional pain syndromes: guidelines for therapy. *Clin J Pain* 1998;14:155-66.

47. **Paulos LE, Rosenberg TD, Drawbert J, et al.** Infrapatellar contracture syndrome: an unrecognised cause of knee stiffness with patella entrapment and patella infera. *Am J Sports Med* 1987;l5:331-41.

48. **Paulos LE, Wnorowski DC, Greenwald AE.** Infrapatellar contracture syndrome: diagnosis, treatment and long-term follow-up. *Am J Sports Med* 1994;22:440-9.

49. **Fu FH, Bennett CH, Ma CB, Menetrey J, Lattermann C.** Current trends in anterior cruciate ligament reconstruction. Part II. Operative procedures and clinical correlations. *Am J Sports Med* 2000;28:124-30.

50. **Howell SM, Clark JA, Farley TE.** A rationale for predicting anterior cruciate graft impingement by the intercondylar roof: a magnetic resonance imaging study. *Am J Sports Med* 1991;19:276-82.

51. **Howell SM, Barad SJ.** Knee extension and its relationship to the slope of the intercondylar roof: implications for positioning the tibial tunnel in anterior cruciate ligament reconstructions. *Am J Sports Med* 1995;23:288-94.

52. **Jackson DW, Schaefer RK.** Cyclops syndrome: loss of extension following intra-articular anterior cruciate ligament reconstruction. *Arthroscopy* 1990;6:171-8.

53. **Mueller W.** *The knee: form, function and ligament reconstruction.* New York: Springer Verlag, 1983;8-75.

54. **Sachs RA, Daniel DM, Stone ML, Garfein RF.** Patellofemoral problems after anterior cruciate ligament reconstruction. *Am J Sports Med* 1989;17:760-5.

55. **O'Brien SJ, Warren RF, Pavlov H, Panariello R, Wickiewicz T.** Reconstruction of the chronically insufficient anterior cruciate ligament with the central third of the patellar ligament. *J Bone Joint Surg [Am]* 1991;73-A:278-86.

56. **Rosenberg TD, Franklin JL, Baldwin GN, Nelson KA.** Extensor mechanism function after patellar tendon graft harvest for anterior cruciate ligament reconstruction. *Am J Sports Med* 1992;20:519-26.

57. **Aglietti P, Buzzi R, D'Andria S, Zaccherotti G.** Arthroscopic anterior cruciate ligament reconstruction with patellar tendon. *Arthroscopy* 1992;8:510-6.

58. **Wojtys EM.** The ACL deficient knee. *American Academy of orthopaedic Surgeons Monograph* 1994:90.

59. **Bach BR Jr, Tradonsky S, Bojchuk J, et al.** Arthroscopically assisted anterior cruciate reconstruction using patellar tendon autograft: five- to nine-year follow-up evaluation. *Am J Sports Med* 1998;26:20-9.

60. **Burwell JMR, Davies AJ, Allum RL.** Anterior knee symptoms after reconstruction of the anterior cruciate ligament using patellar tendon as a graft. *The Knee* 1998;5:245-8.

61. **Marder RA, Raskind JR, Carroll M.** Prospective evaluation of arthroscopically assisted anterior cruciate ligament reconstruction: patellar tendon versus semitendinosus and gracilis tendons. *Am J Sports Med* 1991;19:478-84.

62. **Otero AL, Hutcheson L.** A comparison of the doubled semitendinosus/gracilis and central third of the patellar tendon autografts in arthroscopic anterior cruciate ligament reconstruction. *J Arthroscopy* 1993;9:143-8.

63. **Sgaglione NA, Del Pizzo W, Fox JM, Friedman MJ.** Arthroscopically assisted anterior cruciate ligament reconstruction with the pes anserine tendons: comparison of results in acute and chronic ligament deficiency. *Am J Sports Med* 1993;21:249-56.

64. **Aglietti P, Buzzi R, Zaccherotti G, De Biase P.** Patellar tendon versus doubled semitendinosus and gracilis tendons for anterior cruciate ligament reconstruction. *Am J Sports Med* 1994;22:211-8.

65. **Karlson JA, Steiner ME, Brown CH, Johnston J.** Anterior cruciate ligament reconstruction using gracilis and semitendinosus tendons: comparison of through-the-condyle and over-the-top graft placements. *Am J Sports Med* 1994;22:659-66.

66. **Shelbourne KD, Trumper RV.** Preventing anterior knee pain after anterior cruciate ligament reconstruction. *Am J Sports Med* 1997;25:41-7.

67. **Graf B, Uhr F.** Complications of intra-articular anterior cruciate reconstruction. *Clin Sports Med* 1988;7:835-48.

68. **Fu FH, Irrgang JJ, Harner CCD.** Loss of motion following anterior cruciate ligament reconstruction. In: Jackson DW, ed. *The anterior cruciate ligament, current and future concepts.* New York, NY: Raven Press, 1993:373-80.

69. **Harner CD, Irrgang JJ, Paul J, Dearwater S, Fu FH.** Loss of motion after anterior cruciate ligament reconstruction. *Am J Sports Med* 1992;20:499-506.

70. **Shelbourne KD, Patel DV, Martini DJ.** Classification and management of arthrofibrosis of the knee after anterior cruciate ligament reconstruction. *Am J Sports Med* 1996;24:857-62.

71. **Heier KA, Mack DR, Moseley JB, Paine R, Bocell JR.** An analysis of anterior cruciate ligament reconstruction in middle-aged athletes. *Am J Sports Med* 1997;25:527-32.

72. **Mohtadi NGH, Webster-Bogaert S, Fowler PJ.** Limitation of motion following anterior cruciate ligament reconstruction: a case-control study. *Am J Sports Med* 1991;19:620-5.

73. **Shelbourne KD, Wilckens JH, Mollabashy A, DeCarlo M.** Arthrofibrosis in acute anterior cruciate ligament reconstruction: the effect of timing of reconstruction and rehabilitation. *Am J Sports Med* 1991;19:332-6.

74. **Shelbourne KD, Foulk DA.** Timing of surgery in acute anterior cruciate ligament tears on the return of quadriceps muscle strength after reconstruction using an autogenous patellar tendon graft. *Am J Sports Med* 1995;23:686-9.

75. **Majors RA, Woodfin B.** Achieving full range of motion after anterior cruciate ligament reconstruction. *Am J Sports Med* 1996;24:350-5.

76.**Marcacci M, Zaffagnini S, Iacono F, Neri MP, Petitto A.** Early versus late reconstruction for anterior cruciate ligament rupture: results after five years of follow-up. *Am J Sports Med* 1995;23:690-3.

77. **O'Neill D.** Arthroscopically assisted reconstruction of the anterior cruciate ligament: a prospective randomized analysis of three techniques. *J Bone Joint Surg [Am]* 1996;78-A:803-13.

78. **Fitzgibbons RE, Shelbourne KD.** 'Aggressive' nontreatment of lateral meniscal tears seen during anterior cruciate ligament reconstruction. *Am J Sports Med* 1995;23:156-9.

79. **Shelbourne KD, Johnson GE.** Locked bucket-handle meniscal tears in knees with chronic anterior cruciate ligament deficiency. *Am J Sports Med* 1993;21:779-82.

80. **Hillard-Sembell D, Daniel DM, Stone ML, Dobson BE, Fithian DC.** Combined injuries of the anterior cruciate and medial collateral ligaments of the knee: effect of treatment on stability and function of the joint. *J Bone Joint Surg [Am]* 1996;78-A:169-76.

81. **Shelbourne KD, Porter DA.** Anterior cruciate ligament-medial collateral ligament injury: non-operative management of medial collateral ligament tears with anterior cruciate ligament reconstruction: a preliminary report. *Am J Sports Med* 1992;20:283-6.

82. **Shelbourne KD, Nitz P.** Accelerated rehabilitation after anterior cruciate ligament reconstruction. *Am J Sports Med* 1990;18:292-9.

83. **Brown HR, Indelicato PA.** Complications of anterior cruciate ligament reconstruction. *Oper Tech Orthop* 1992;2:125-35.

84. **Watanabe BM, Howell SM.** Arthroscopic findings associated with roof impingement of an anterior cruciate ligament graft. *Am J Sports Med* 1995;23:616-25.

STATIC METATARSALGIA

MICHAEL M. STEPHENS

From the Mater Misericordiae Hospital, Cappagh Orthopaedic Hospital, The Children's Hospital and Central Remedial Clinic, Dublin, Ireland

Static metatarsalgia is a term used to describe pain in the forefoot which is of mechanical rather than of inflammatory origin[1] (e.g., systemic arthropathies). It is located distal to the tarsometatarsal joints and is usually found in the region of the metatarsal heads. In adults it is a common reason for referral and presentation to foot clinics. The disorders which cause this symptom are anatomical and biomechanical in origin, and, rarely, can arise from congenital or acquired abnormalities of the structure and architecture of the foot. They have the effect of changing the biomechanics of the foot so that there is abnormal distribution of weight on the sole, causing pain.

NORMAL ANATOMY

The normal alignment of the metatarsal heads is in a curve (Fig. 1A) as described by Lelièvre.[2] On a weight-bearing dorsal plantar radiograph the centre of the first metatarsal head is at the same level as the second and the lateral three metatarsal heads are progressively more proximal, giving this curve. On contact with the ground the five metatarsal heads are equidistant from the weight-bearing surface. The so-called 'distal transverse metatarsal arch' is only present in the non-weight-bearing foot and therefore is functionally irrelevant. The first metatarsal is inclined or pitched at an angle of 20° to the weight-bearing surface, which gradually lessens to 5° for the fifth metatarsal. The five metatarsals are connected by four intermetatarsal ligaments in each web space which allows all five to act as a flexible unit. The pitch of the metatarsals means that there is a medial and lateral arch. The former is made up of the calcaneus, talus, navicular, medial cuneiform and first metatarsal, while the latter comprises the calcaneus, cuboid and fifth metatarsal. This implies that there is a functional midfoot transverse arch at the level of the tarsometatarsal joints. Unlike the rest of the foot, the bony configuration of this area gives stability through the shape, particularly of the cuneiforms which form a 'gothic arch', i.e., they are wedge-shaped, being thicker dorsally and more narrow at their plantar surface.

In general, the plantar capsules and ligaments are thicker and therefore stronger than their dorsal neighbours since they are on the tension-band side of the pedal skeletal structure. At the metatarsophalangeal (MTP) joints, these stabilising soft tissues are further reinforced by the fibrocartilaginous volar or plantar plates. These not only prevent dorsal dislocation of the proximal phalanx but also act as a functional weight-bearing organ, particularly from late mid-stance to toe-off. The plantar fascia gives further support to this longitudinal arch[3] by its insertion into the calcaneus posteriorly and, among others, the plantar plates distally.

The musculotendinous units can be divided into extrinsic, i.e., those arising proximal to the foot, and intrinsic, those arising within the foot. The tibialis posterior supports the medial longitudinal arch by its insertion into the navicular and also the whole transverse arch of the midfoot through its insertion into the bases of the metatarsals. Peroneus longus and brevis are its antagonists, the former

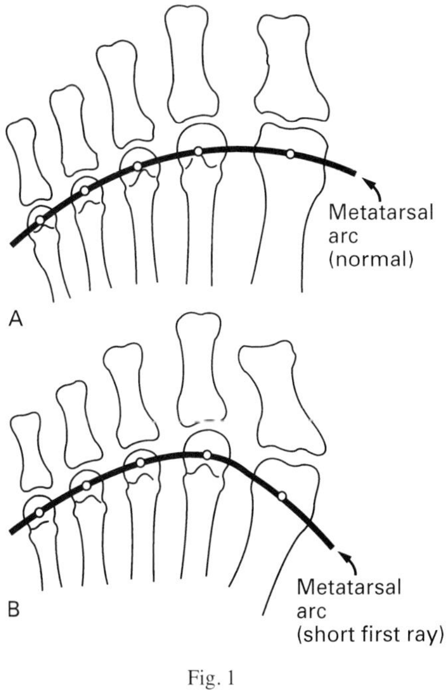

Fig. 1

Diagram showing the alignment of weight-bearing of the metatarsal heads, in the case of A) a normal foot and B) a short first metatarsal.

plantar flexing the first metatarsal and thus giving further support to the medial longitudinal arch. Peroneus brevis, through its insertion to the base of the fifth metatarsal, works to balance the distal and lateral extensions of tibialis posterior. Flexor hallucis longus further supports the medial longitudinal arch late in the cycle, near toe-off. Flexor digitorum longus has a similar function but only to a minor degree, but the tendinous interconnection between flexor digitorum longus and flexor hallucis ensures that the metatarsal heads and toes act in unison.[4] The intrinsic muscles, acting primarily through the extensor hood, give further stability to the MTP joints to prevent hyperextension and subluxation.

NORMAL BIOMECHANICS

Normal function of the forefoot relies on the five metatarsals acting in unison, linked proximally by the tarsometatarsal joints and distally by the intermetatarsal ligaments. This has developed because of the bipedal gait of man, the foot being no longer a prehensile organ. The stability of the forefoot is maintained by the skeletal structure, particularly at the tarsometatarsal joints, the dynamic stabilisers (musculotendinous groups) and the static stabilisers (ligaments). During the stance phase on heel strike, the forefoot is relatively flexible, but as body-weight is transmitted to the forefoot later in the stance phase nearer toe-off, it becomes more rigid for the propulsive stage of gait. In mid-stance, the mobility of the forefoot is in a state between fully flexible and relatively rigid. This change in forefoot biomechanics between heel strike and toe-off occurs predominately through the musculotendinous unit but also through the static stabilisers of the plantar fascia, the volar plates and the skeletal configuration of the angles obtained by the MTP break (Fig. 2). At heel strike, the paying out of the hamstring muscles allows the knee to straighten. Tibialis anterior maintains ankle dorsiflexion, which then slowly pays out to allow the foot-flat stage of gait. Tendo Achillis contracts to stabilise the hindfoot in the flat-foot stage and this then pays out to allow some dorsiflexion before heel-off. From heel-strike to toe-off there is a progressive decrease in ankle dorsiflexion to a plantar flexed position at toe-off.[5] As the foot moves from heel- to toe-off there is increasing contracture of tibialis posterior which supinates the subtalar joint and forefoot, the former by its attachment to the tuberosity of the navicular and the latter by its attachments distally to the plantar aspect of the bases of the metatarsals.[6] For forefoot stability its antagonist, peroneus longus, contracts to balance its contraction. Nearer to toe-off, flexor hallucis longus gives further stability to the first ray for the final effort of propulsion. There is a minor contribution from flexor digitorum longus and the intrinsics. Flexor hallucis and flexor digitorum longus, however, act in unison because of the tendinous connections between these tendons on the plantar aspect distal to the tarsometatarsal joints.[4] This means that in most people, flexor hallucis aids flexion of the second toe and less frequently the other lesser toes.

As these musculotendinous units convert the foot from a flexible shock-absorbing organ at heel-strike to a rigid organ for push-off, the skeleton of the foot is also changing in its orientation. On heel-strike the subtalar joint is in relative valgus, in mid-stance it is in the mid-position and at toe-off it is in varus. Because of the changing axes of rotation of the talonavicular and calcaneocuboid joint, Chopart's joint becomes more rigid the further the hindfoot supinates or inverts.[7] This gives skeletal stability to the midfoot to allow the maximum transmission of forces through the musculotendinous units at toe-off.

The MTP break (Fig. 2) is the line which connects the first to the second metatarsal heads which are normally at right angles to the line of progression of the foot. The line joining the second to the fifth metatarsal head is an oblique axis. This means that as the foot moves from the start of

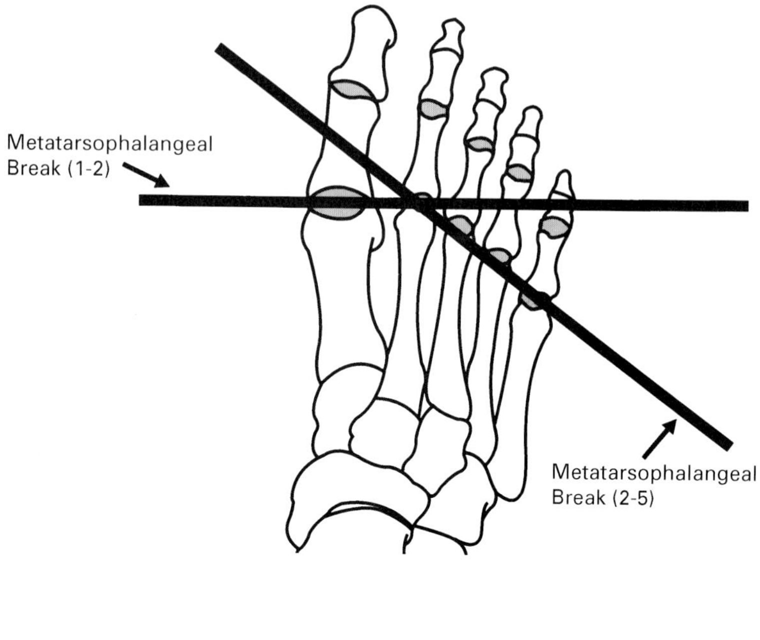

Fig. 2

Diagram showing that the MTP break line (2-5) functions immediately after heel rise, while the break (1-2) acts at the end of heel-rise towards toe-off.

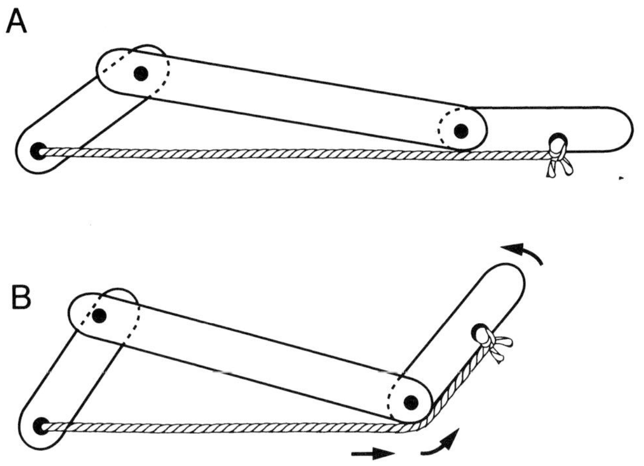

Fig 3

Diagram showing the windlass effect. The fixed length of the plantar fascia is represented as a string acting upon the skeletal structure, which is represented as two lever arms. Figure 3A – Foot flat in mid-stance. Figure 3B – As the toes dorsiflex on heel-rise the distal lever arm forces the proximal lever arm to plantar flex (first ray).

heel-rise to the beginning of toe-off the forefoot, and indirectly the hindfoot, is forced to supinate along this oblique axis between the second and fifth metatarsal heads. Just before toe-off the axis between the first and second metatarsal heads comes into play allowing the correct plane for dorsiflexion of the first ray at toe-off.

The plantar fascia, which is a static ligamentous structure with a fixed length between the base of the proximal phalanges to its insertion into the calcaneus (Fig. 3), has to act as a 'windlass' late in the stance phase. This means that as the toes extend after heel-rise, this windlass effect forces relative plantar flexion of the first ray at the midfoot, increasing the medial longitudinal arch and stabilising the forefoot.[3]

It is clear that this fine balance and interaction between the musculotendinous units, the static stabilisers and the skeleton of the foot are mandatory for normal bipedal gait. Any disturbance of these functions can lead to abnormal forefoot loading and/or an increased time of forefoot loading in the gait cycle, which can ultimately result in pain or the symptoms of metatarsalgia.

EXTRINSIC ABNORMALITIES (TABLE I)

Flexion contractures of the hip and tight musculotendinous units of the hamstrings will limit extension of the knee. This results in more anterior movement of the body-weight so the flat-foot stage and forefoot loading in stance occur earlier. A tight tendo Achillis will have the same effect, loading the forefoot earlier in the gait cycle and for a longer time. In the unlikely event of only one of these groups being tight, the others can compensate; for example, with tight hamstrings, tendo Achillis will have to stretch more to allow further dorsiflexion. More frequently, however, both hamstrings and the triceps suri are tight. With this combination, minor degrees of tightness will produce loading of the forefoot earlier in the gait cycle and, therefore, overuse. Discrepancy of leg length will increase loading of the forefoot by the relative equinus position of the foot to compensate on the short-leg side. On the long side, a compensatory mechanism of persistent valgus will lead to a persistent pronated position of the hindfoot and delayed locking of the mid-tarsal joints in mid-stance. Genu varum is compensated by continual pronation in the subtalar joint to allow the forefoot to be plantigrade. Similarly, at heel-rise, the pronated hindfoot is preventing the normal physiological locking of the midfoot and therefore lessening stability of the midfoot and forefoot. Genu valgum is accommodated by the foot with subtalar supination so that it no longer acts as a good shock absorber on heel-strike, and there is a tendency for increased loading of the first ray in mid-stance, which is the opposite to the tendency for lateral forefoot loading with genu varum.

HINDFOOT MALALIGNMENT (TABLE II)

The subtalar joint acts as an 'Archimedes screw'. When the heel is in valgus, the subtalar joint is pronated. As the foot moves into the later stages of stance the heel moves into varus. The joint then becomes supinated. For this to occur the calcaneus internally rotates and moves slightly forwards so that it lies more underneath the talus. When the heel is valgus the axes of rotation of the calcaneocuboid and talonavicular joint are relatively parallel. This means they can act as a unit and therefore the midfoot joint of Chopart is relatively flexible, allowing the foot to act as a shock-absorber after heel-strike. As the calcaneus moves underneath the talus into a varus position late in the stance phase, these axes of rotation become oblique and lock the midfoot, making the foot relatively rigid. Hypothetically, in mid-stance, when the foot is giving body support, the subtalar joint should be in the mid-position, between valgus and varus, pronation and supination and flexible and rigid. If there is abnormal alignment of the talus with regard to the calcaneus this balance is upset. To assess the position of the subtalar joint in mid-stance the talonavicular joint is neut-

Table I. Extrinsic abnormalities

Hip flexion contractures
Tight hamstring muscles
Tight tendo Achillis (triceps suri)
Discrepancy in leg length
Genu varum
Genu valgum

Table II. Hindfoot malalignment

Weight-bearing heel varus
Weight-bearing heel valgus
Subtalar joint varus (talonavicular joint neutral)
Subtalar joint valgus (talonavicular joint neutral)
Dysfunction of tibialis posterior
Overactivity of peroneus longus

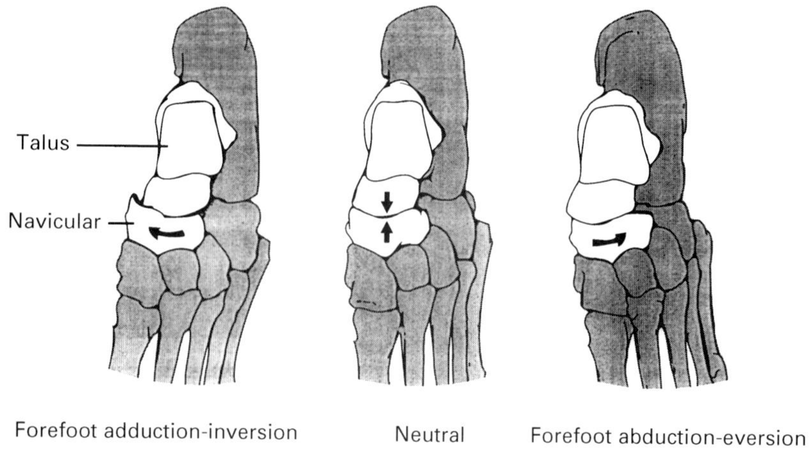

Fig. 4

Diagram showing the relationship of the talonavicular joint. When the forefoot is inverted, adducted and supinated (varus), the navicular moves medially in relation to the talar head. When the forefoot is abducted, everted and pronated (valgus), the navicular moves laterally on the talar head.

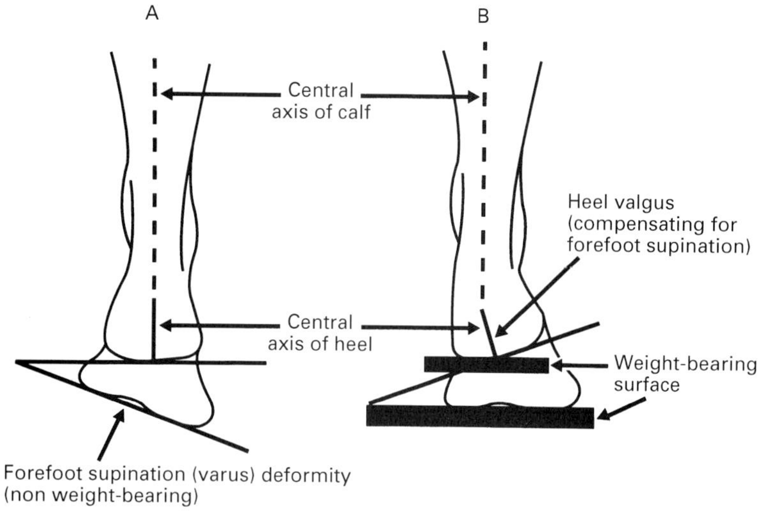

Fig. 5

Diagram showing a forefoot varus deformity. Figure 5A – When the talonavicular joint is in the neutral position the forefoot is in a supinated or varus position. Figure 5B – When this foot bears weight the heel has to drift into valgus to compensate for the forefoot supination or varus.

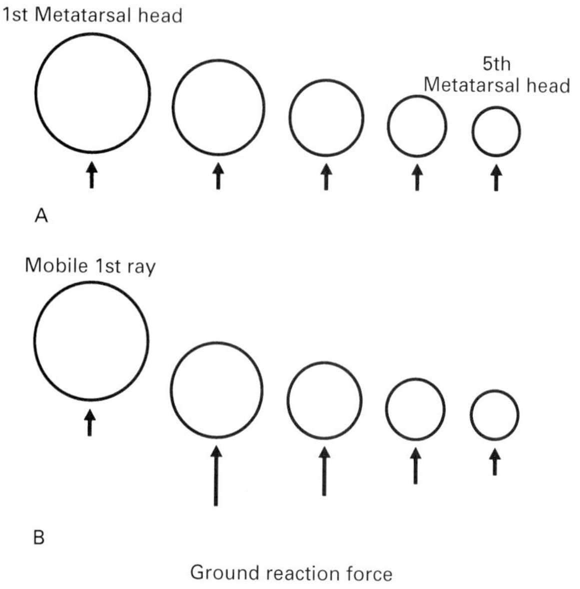

Fig. 6

Diagram to show loading of the metatarsal head. Figure 6A – The ground resection force should be equally distributed over all five metatarsal heads in the normal foot with no distal transverse metatarsal arch on weight-bearing. Figure 6B – A mobile first ray in a foot which pronates, or is in valgus in the mid-stance, causes increased load on the immobile second metatarsal head as the first ray dorsiflexes.

ral, i.e., the navicular is perfectly placed on the end of the head of the talus and it is not moving laterally, as when the heel is in valgus, or medially as when the heel is in varus (Fig. 4). In mid-stance with a neutral talonavicular joint the heel should be neutral underneath the tibia and the forefoot is also neutral, i.e., not supinated or pronated. If the subtalar joint is not aligned properly the calcaneus and forefoot are not in this normal relationship in mid-stance.[8] For example, when the talonavicular joint is neutral and the forefoot is supinated or in varus, the heel in mid-stance has to be proportionally more in valgus to allow the forefoot to be plantigrade. This is seen classically in pes planus. The opposite occurs when the talonavicular joint is neutral, the forefoot is in valgus or pronated and the heel has to move into varus to allow the forefoot to become plantigrade (Fig. 5). In pes planus, Chopart's joint is relatively unlocked and therefore as the foot moves forward to heel-rise the normal midfoot locking is not complete. Tibialis posterior has to act excessively because the navicular is still relatively lateral. Similarly, the plantar fascia is stretched because of the relative pes planus. This excessive valgus forces the first ray to elevate, increasing the load on the second metatarsal which is stiff at its tarsometatarsal joint because

Table III. Forefoot disorders

Abnormalities of the metatarsal head alignment-arcade
Short metatarsal
Mobile first ray
Hallux valgus/metatarsus primavarus
Bunionette deformity/fifth metatarsal valgus
Morton's neuroma
Hammer/claw toes
Sesamoid abnormalities
Stress fracture
Freiberg disease

it is wedged between the medial and lateral cuneiforms. It therefore has to carry more weight which can lead to synovitis in the second MTP joint or a stress fracture (Fig. 6). This will have a direct effect on the forefoot disorders of static metatarsalgia. When the varus foot is examined it means that this foot is relatively stiff which is easily observed in clinical practice. This will make the forefoot excessively loaded and give a higher risk of stress fractures, particularly on the lateral border of the foot.

FOREFOOT DISORDERS (TABLE III)

As seen in the previous sections, extrinsic abnormalities and hindfoot malalignment can influence the forefoot directly, leading to overuse/overload and static metatarsalgia. There are other local disorders. Metatarsal length, particularly the relative lengths of the first and second metatarsals, may alter forefoot loading. Ideally, the heads of the first and second metatarsal are the same length sharing weight-bearing towards toe-off. If the first metatarsal is short the second metatarsal will be loaded excessively, leading to stress fractures and synovitis of the second MTP joint. If it is longer, there is increased pressure on the head of the first metatarsal and its sesamoids (Fig. 1B), but the second MTP joints are more commonly affected since the first tarsometatarsal joint is more mobile, i.e., if the heel is still in valgus late in the stance phase at heel-rise peroneus longus may not have contracted enough to support the first ray. This means that as heel-rise progresses and weight is transferred more distally, it is transferred more to the second and even the third MTP joint as the first metatarsal moves dorsally.

There is a normal arcade running proximally from the second metatarsal to the fifth, and if there are abnormalities in the length of the metatarsal, i.e., if this line is broken by one being too short or too long, it will affect the weight-bearing of the metatarsals. This is because those which are weight-bearing will have to carry more load and therefore are at greater risk of developing syndromes of overuse such as stress fractures, synovitis and excessive clawing of the toes. These deformities of the lesser metatarsals are rare but can be seen on occasions after childhood fractures which affect the growth plate, or in congenital hypoplasia or hyperplasia.

As a hallux valgus increases so does the intermetatarsal angle, as does pronation of the first metatarsal in relation to the rest of the foot.[9] Thus the hallux valgus escapes from the pull of the adductor hallucis allowing the metatarsal to move further into abduction and the phalanx more into adduction, with the flexors and extensors also acting as adductors. As this happens the first ray migrates dorsally, further increasing loading on the second MTP joint. This results in the relatively common calluses seen underneath the second MTP joint in association with hallux valgus. There is usually associated splaying of the foot and this will include a relative valgus of the fifth metatarsal leading to a bunionette deformity. Again the fifth tarsometatarsal joint is relatively mobile and therefore weight will be transferred to the fourth and third MTP joints. Synovitis of these MTP joints causes stretching of the capsule and therefore laxity, with stretching of the volar plate. At the same time the intrinsics are stretched allowing an intrinsic minus deformity. As the intrinsics lose power, the long flexors and extensors attempt to accommodate for this, leading to a progressive claw-toe deformity. Ultimately attrition rupture occurs at the volar plate, leading to subluxation and dislocation of the MTP joint,[10] and the intrinsic muscles become extensors of the MTP joint, as they move dorsal to the axis of rotation of the joint.

Morton's neuroma is a particular disorder which is predominately found within the third web space because the common digital nerve to the third space has an interconnection or communicans branch to the second common digital nerve. This makes it relatively immobile and it becomes stretched over the intermetatarsal ligament, made worse if the toes are clawed. In pes planus, since the fourth metatarsal is more mobile than the third, there are increased sheer forces on the common digital nerve.[11] Fibrosis of the nerve ultimately leads to formation of a 'neuroma' and the symptoms of a Mulder's click.[12]

Sesamoiditis is most commonly seen in the relatively rigid foot. The hindfoot is in varus when weight-bearing and when the talonavicular joint is neutral the forefoot is in valgus. A plantar flexed first ray further increases the load on the first MTP joint and its sesamoids. Sesamoiditis can also occur in the presence of hallux valgus because as the first metatarsal deviates medially the sesamoids move relatively laterally, and the tibial sesamoid comes to lie on the crest of the plantar surface of the first metatarsal head. In this position it becomes more prominent, particularly if the first tarsometatarsal joint is relatively stiff.

Freiberg's disease or osteochondritis of the second metatarsal head occurs and presents in the skeletally immature patient. It is probably related to all the above causes of excessive loading of the second ray and repetitive trauma, i.e., hindfoot valgus, supinated forefoot, a mobile first ray and a long second ray.[13]

MANAGEMENT

A treatment programme cannot be instigated until the cause of the metatarsalgia has been clearly outlined. In my experience it is rarely unifactorial. This is particularly relevant in those patients with a high demand on their feet, for example, athletes. In these cases there are usually several minor abnormalities which act to summate and reduce pain in an overused/overloaded area of the forefoot. The onus therefore is on the clinician to assess the patient with static metatarsalgia, starting in the proximal leg and moving distally, examining muscle groups for tightness as outlined in the section on extrinsic abnormalities. The hindfoot and the forefoot are similarly examined, particularly their relationship to each other and to the subtalar joint. This is normally assessed while the patient is first standing and then prone with the feet over the end of the examination couch, with the talonavicular joint held in neutral. This allows the intimate relationship between the forefoot and the hindfoot through the subtalar joint to be ascertained. Once this is done factors which predispose to abnormal forefoot loading and abnormal biomechanics in the stance phase are demarcated. The final part of the clinical examination is in relation to the precise site of the symptoms. Palpation localises a tender metatarsal head or volar plate. Plantar flexion of this MTP joint tightens the collateral ligaments and therefore increases the joint pressure. If there is inflammation and an effusion in the joint, these will stimulate the primary source of pain. Compression testing between the first and fifth metatarsal, i.e., side-to-side, with pressure on the third web space, may elicit pain indicative of a Morton's neuroma. This is usually a painful click, i.e., a positive Mulder's sign.[12] Pain along the shafts of the metatarsals may indicate a stress fracture, or on the tibial sesamoids, sesamoiditis. A bony overgrowth may be palpated over the dorsal aspect of the second metatarsal head indicating Freiberg's osteonecrosis. The clinical examination will also finally give some indication of the type of foot and the line of the MTP break, particularly in relation to a short first ray and a relatively long second ray. Radiological assessment generally confirms the clinical diagnosis. The anteroposterior weight-bearing radiographs will outline the arcade of the MTP joint in relation to the classic curve of Lelièvre.[2] It is also useful for the assessment of splaying of the foot in relation to the one/two and four/five intermetatarsal angle. This radiograph will also show any abnormality in the development of the lesser metatarsals, i.e., short lesser metatarsals. On the weight-bearing lateral view, metatarsal pitch will indicate the presence of abnormalities such as a plantar flexed first ray, and talonavicular or navicular cuneiform sag associated with a valgus deformity. An oblique radiograph rarely gives more information, except for demonstrating early subluxation of the MTP joints. Technetium bone scanning is useful to confirm a stress fracture and is its primary indication. It is sometimes useful to confirm an inflamed second MTP joint in its early stages when there is doubt clinically. Ultrasound has probably been replaced by MRI for the diagnosis of Morton's neuromas and conditions such as an intermetatarsal ganglion and a synovial cyst.

After this assessment, management can be planned under two headings. First, there must be treatment for the predisposing causes which give increased forefoot loading. For example, tight hamstrings and tendo Achillis must be treated by intensive stretching to decrease forefoot loading. Night splinting is useful in severe cases to treat this extrinsic cause. The position of the foot, with the subtalar joint in a neutral position, may indicate, for example, a forefoot varus or supination deformity, i.e., on weight-bearing this foot tends to be pronated with the heel in valgus. If the forefoot is supported by an orthosis medially, in mid-stance the subtalar joint will be in neutral, preparing the foot to move into the propulsive phase. Secondly, local relief of pain is addressed. The forefoot orthosis may have cushioned cutouts to decrease the loading on a particular metatarsal head. By treating what could be described as indirect forces which cause metatarsalgia, pain is often slowly alleviated, but in intractable cases further treatment may be required temporarily to make the patient more comfortable. Topical and systemic non-steroidal anti-inflammatory drugs and local steroid injections have their place occasionally. Care must be taken when injecting metatarsophalangeal joints as this may cause rupture of the volar plate.

Surgical treatment is only indicated when all conservative means with treatment for the local pain and the predisposing causes have failed. Operations must be biomechanically based, and procedures which were carried out in the past, such as excision of metatarsal heads, should be condemned. The goal for the orthopaedic surgeon is to equalise the weight-bearing across all five metatarsal heads so that the ground reaction forces are distributed over a larger area and thus reduce pressure.

Surgical treatment often depends on the primary aetiology and is generally performed for fixed deformity as flexible deformities are most commonly successfully treated conservatively. Such management can be planned appropriately and may include dorsiflexion osteotomy of the first ray for intractable pain in the first ray, and shortening procedures on the second metatarsal when this is relatively long and there is overload on the MTP joint. The Weil osteotomy is probably most appropriate for this, certainly before there has been dislocation of the joint.[14] In revision cases it may be necessary to realign all the metatarsals to restore the normal arcade of the MTP break. Freiberg's disease in the early stages may be treated by dorsal cheilectomy and drilling, and later a dorsiflexion rotational osteotomy, to move the articular surface from underneath to the end of the metatarsal. Morton's neuroma and neuritis may be treated by either decompression or excision, making sure that the common digital nerve in the third web space is divided as proximally as possible so that any plantar branches are excised, allowing the nerve to retract into the midfoot. The latter procedure is probably more popular now. Metatarsus varus of the first ray may be corrected by some form of derotational plantar flexion translational osteotomy, e.g., a rotational proximal Chevron osteotomy.[15] In this way the first ray is encouraged to become functional again, reducing the load on the second metatarsal. Less commonly, a similar procedure may be required for metatarsus valgus of the fifth ray. Localised, painful and intractable plantar keratosis (IPK) may only gain limited benefit from conservative management, and orthoses will only be helpful after minor surgery has been performed. For example, IPK over the tibial sesamoids is easily treated by excision of the plantar half of the sesamoid through a medial approach, protecting the medial digital nerve to the hallux. Similarly, a plantar condylectomy of the fifth metatarsal is useful for IPK in this area, but patients must be warned that insoles are often required despite this surgery.

CONCLUSIONS

Static metatarsalgia is only a symptom. It behoves a clinician to rule out systemic disorders, for example rheumatoid, psoriasis, colitis and gouty arthritides. Careful clinical examination of the whole lower limb is required to find the predisposing causes and the localised area of pain. Treatment programmes may fail unless all the predisposing factors are addressed. If the pain is treated in isolation there may be temporary relief but it will recur unless the other factors which overload the forefoot are addressed. Surgical treatment is indicated when conservative management has failed and must be based on good biomechanical principles to try to restore the foot to normal function as it moves from heel strike and shock absorption, to mid-stance and body support, to toe-off and propulsion.

REFERENCES

1. **Eulry F.** Static metatarsalgia. *Rev Prat* 1997;47:37-42.
2. **Lelièvre J.** *Patologie du pied.* 5th ed. Paris: Masson, 1971: 526-8.
3. **Stainsby GD.** Pathological anatomy and dynamic effect of the displaced plantar plate and the importance of the integrity of the plantar plate-deep transverse metatarsal ligament tie-bar. *Ann R Coll Surg Engl* 1997;79:58-68.
4. **Sarrafian S.** *Anatomy of the foot and ankle.* 2nd edition. Philadelphia: Lippincott Co, 1989:240-56.
5. **Nordin M, Frankel V.** *Basic biomechanics of the musculo-skeletal system.* 2nd edition. Philadelphia: Lee & Febiger, 1989:115-82.
6. **Sarrafian SK.** *Anatomy of the foot & ankle: descriptive, topographic, functional.* Philadelphia: Lippincott, 1993;239-40.
7. **Elftman H.** The transverse tarsal joint and its control. *Clin Orthop* 1960;16:41-5.
8. **Stephens MM.** The subtalar joint: biomechanical principles of treatment. *Eur Instr Course Lect* 1997;3:51-7.
9. **Eustace S, O'Byrne J, Beausang O, et al.** Hallux valgus, first metatarsal pronation and collapse of the medial longitudinal arch – a radiological correlation. *Skeletal Radiol* 1994;23:191-4.
10. **Yao L, Cracchiolo A, Farahani K, Seeger LL.** Magnetic resonance imaging of plantar plate rupture. *Foot Ankle Int* 1996;17:33-6.
11. **Jarde O.** Morton's metatarsalgia. *Foot Ankle Surg* 1998;4:187-92.
12. **Mulder J.** The causative mechanism in Morton's metatarsalgia. *J Bone Joint Surg [Br]* 1951;33-B:94-55.
13. **Katcherian DA.** Treatment of Freiberg's disease. *Orthop Clin North Am* 1994;25:69-81.
14. **Davies MS, Saxby TS.** Metatarsal neck osteotomy with rigid internal fixation for the treatment of lesser toe metatarsophalangeal joint pathology. *Foot Ankle Int* 1999;20:630-5.
15. **Borton D, Stephens MM.** Basal metatarsal osteotomy for hallux valgus. *J Bone Joint Surg [Br]* 1994;76-B:204-9.

THE RHEUMATOID FOOT AND ANKLE

A. VILADOT JR, F. ALVAREZ AND R. VILADOT

From the Hospital Sant Rafael, Barcelona, Spain

We understand the term 'rheumatoid foot' to mean the pattern of deformities appearing in the foot during the course of generalised chronic inflammatory disease of the musculoskeletal system. Of these, we highlight rheumatoid arthritis, psoriatic arthritis and the spondylarthropathies. Although they affect the structures of the foot in different ways, all cause a very uniform type of pathology.

The most important, in terms both of its frequency and its severity, is rheumatoid arthritis, which is almost invariably manifest in the foot in advanced stages of the disease, and may often present there first. It is one of the few generalised diseases which can affect the entire foot.

From an epidemiological viewpoint, rheumatoid arthritis can appear at any age, although it is predominant between 25 and 55 years. Two-thirds of the cases are in women, although from the age of 60 upwards, this disproportion between men and women tends to even out. It is a disease which is seen in all countries, in all climates and is suffered by all races. Its systemic nature means that not only are the joints affected, but also the tendons, skin, muscles, vessels and nerves.

In the joints, the first changes are seen in the synovial membrane, in the form of an inflammatory reaction, accompanied by a massive cellular proliferation which produces an invasive granulation tissue known as 'pannus'. It comprises activated macrophages and fibroblasts which gradually erode cartilage, bone, tendons and ligaments.

The disease starts with an initial stage of synovitis, with secondary effects on the capsule and ligaments which lose their mechanical properties, allowing easy subluxation or dislocation of the joints. In a more advanced stage, the cartilage is destroyed and the epiphyseal bone is eroded, which finally leads to total functional destruction of the joint. Ankylosis is not often seen.

Injuries to the tendons usually start in the sheath and the synovitis progressively destroys the tendon. The sheath and the tendon become adherent, the bands are destroyed and subluxation occurs. This leads to functional incapacity and dislocation of the joints.

The skin appears thinned and fragile; it can be injured by minimal trauma and ulceration may result which can take weeks to cure. These symptoms may be exacerbated by medical treatment, often with corticosteroids.

Subcutaneous nodules appear after an arteritis and have three characteristic areas: a central area of fibrinoid necrosis, a crown of fibroblasts and a peripheral area infiltrated with lymphatic cells. The nodules are located in prominent areas, and can be easily palpated under the skin. They are clearly defined and are characteristic of the disease (Fig. 1).

In muscle there is involvement of the interstitial connective tissue of arterioles which, in conjunction with reduced activity in those patients, contributes to the muscular atrophy which is characteristic of this disease.

Another manifestation of the systemic effects is vasculitis. It usually affects minor vessels and is seen by the presence of petechiae. The medium or large vessels are rarely affected. In advanced stages, vasculitis hinders cicatrisation of the skin to a major degree, which must be taken into account when surgery is considered.

Neurologically, the perineurium is affected which may give rise to sensory or motor-sensory neuropathies. Entrapment neuropathies can also occur, particularly in the posterior tibial nerve in the tarsal tunnel, or in the intermetatarsal spaces, causing a characteristic Morton's neuroma. It should be noted, however, that these entrapment neuropathies are much more frequent in the wrist than in the foot.

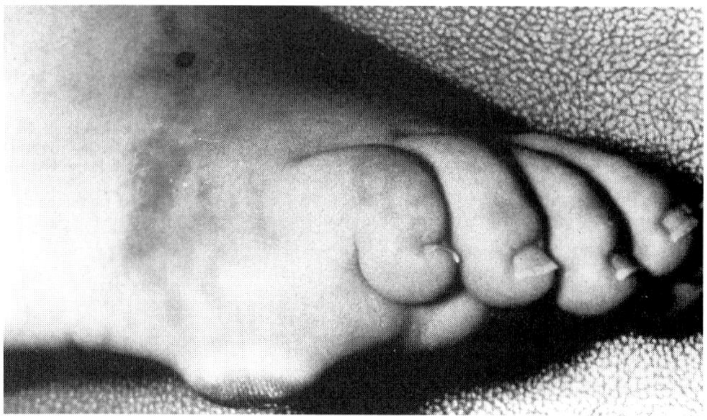

Fig. 1

Photograph of a rheumatoid nodule under the head of the fifth metatarsal.

Treatment of the rheumatoid foot should encompass an overall medicosurgical strategy for the patient, given that in most cases, other areas such as the knees or the hips and the upper limbs are affected. The goal is to relieve the pain and to restore function, in order to enable the patient to walk as independently as possible.

Modern medical treatments which induce remission (methotrexate, sulphasalazine, hydroxychloroquine and cyclosporin) or biological treatment with anti-tumour necrosis factor α, administered early on when the disease is first diagnosed, allow the control of its evolution, thereby reducing the number of joints affected.

In cases in which the whole foot is affected, lesions of the plantar vault should be considered first. Once the normal morphology is restored the deformities of the forefoot should be corrected aligning it with the hindfoot. Lastly, if the ankle is affected, it should be treated.

In view of the complex biomechanics of the foot, we believe that procedures on the tarsus should be based on arthrodesis, with the aim of stabilising the plantar arch. In the ankle and the metatarsophalangeal joints, surgery should maintain mobility since this is fundamental for walking without a limp.

Over recent decades, a large variety of surgical techniques has been described for the treatment of the rheumatoid foot. It is impossible to refer to all of these and we shall therefore set out those which are most frequently used and the criteria for treatment used in our department. We will deal separately with deformities of the hindfoot and midfoot, the forefoot and the ankle.

HINDFOOT AND MIDFOOT

All the joints can be affected by rheumatoid arthritis, but the midtarsal, and in particular the talonavicular joint, is by far the most often damaged.

Before the advent of cortisone, the deformity of the plantar arch seen most commonly was equinovarus. During the acute stages of the disease, the patient would remain bedridden for long periods and the equinus position and the weight of the sheets produced this deformity.

Today, the deformity which is seen most frequently is the valgus flat foot. After involvement of the talonavicular joint, the talus drops down, forwards and inwards, with subluxation of the joint. The midfoot and the forefoot deviate into abduction. Three other factors are involved: 1) the effect of the body-weight; 2) the dysfunction of the tendon of tibialis posterior frequently found in this condition; and 3) dysfunction of the spring ligament, also because of the arthritis.

Involvement of Chopart's joint also affects the subtalar joint, and the calcaneum becomes deviated into valgus. This causes compression between the calcaneum and the lateral malleolus which causes pain and occasionally a stress fracture of the fibula (Fig. 2). The osteoporosis which occurs contributes to this.

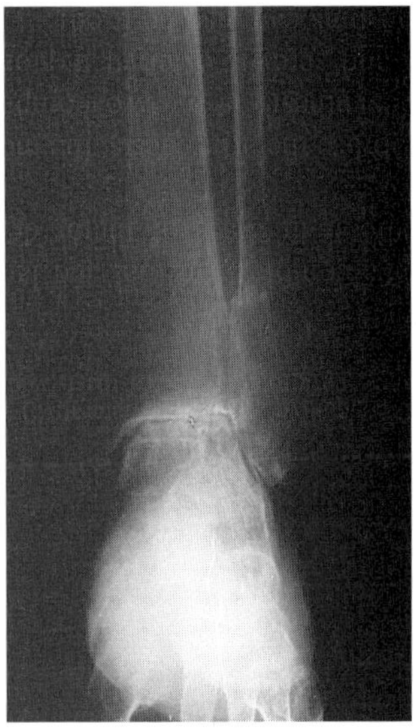

Fig. 2

Radiograph showing a stress fracture of the fibula associated with arthritis of the ankle.

Operative treatment. This is based on arthrodesis which has the double aim of stabilising the foot and eliminating pain.

In cases of isolated involvement of the talonavicular joint, we believe that the arthrodesis should be performed as early as possible so that progressive deformity of the rest of the foot can be prevented (Fig. 3).

In cases of valgus flat-foot deformity, we recommend double arthrodesis using the approach described by Viladot.[1] The technique is performed in the following stages (Fig. 4).

Stage 1. An incision is made on the medial aspect of the foot with release of the tendon of tibialis anterior. Next, a flap based posteriorly is elevated, including the periosteum, the ligaments and the tendon of tibialis posterior. In cases in which a lesion of the latter is suspected, we prolong the incision proximally, behind the medial malleolus, in order to be able to examine it thoroughly and, if possible, repair it.

Stage 2. A lateral skin incision is made and the sinus tarsi and subtalar joint are opened. We resect the articular surfaces and the soft tissues of the sinus tarsi.

Stage 3. A corrective manoeuvre is performed. A blunt instrument is passed between both incisions through the sinus tarsi underneath the neck of the talus and its head is lifted upwards, backwards and outwards. This supinates the hindfoot by positioning the calcaneum under the talus, correcting its valgus position. In order to achieve correction of the medial arch, it may be necessary to perform a wedge resection of this structure.

Stage 4. We insert a cylindrical bone graft into the sinus tarsi, taken with a Cloward instrument from the iliac crest, in order to maintain correction of the valgus and achieve arthrodesis of the subtalar joint.

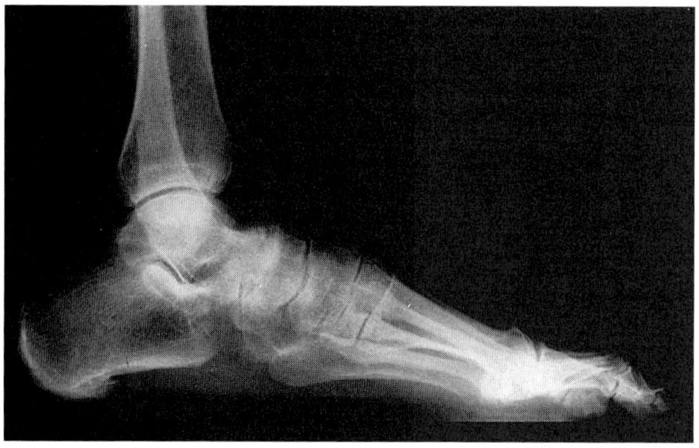

Fig. 3a

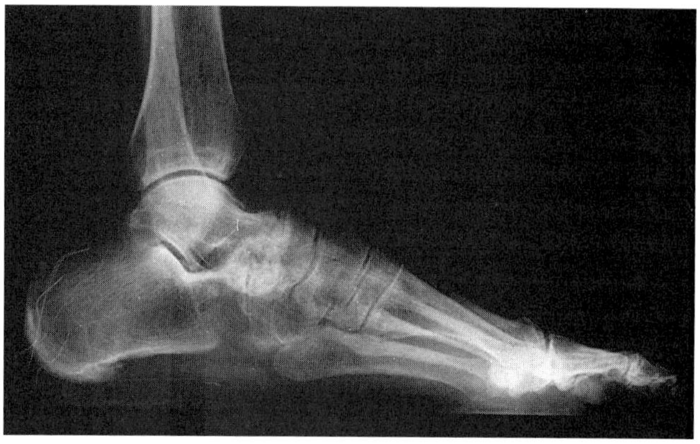

Fig. 3b

Radiographs showing a) isolated arthritis of the talonavicular joint before operation and b) a talonavicular arthrodesis after operation.

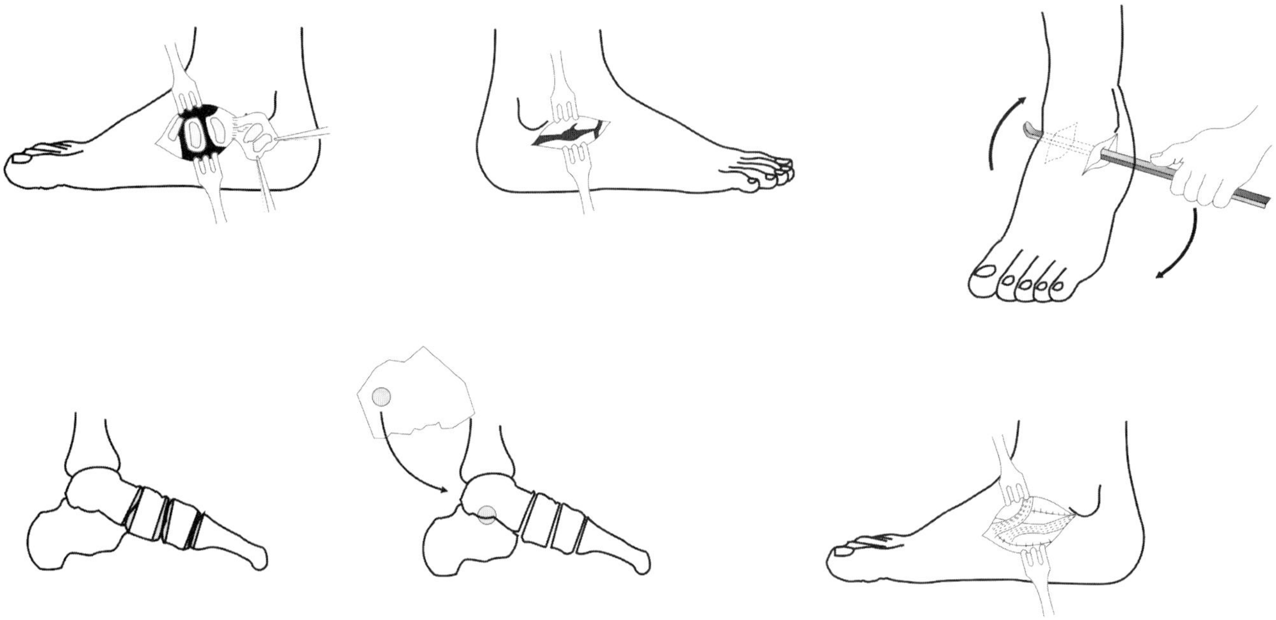

Fig. 4

Diagram showing surgical stages of double arthrodesis from two approaches (see text).

Stage 5. The flap which was elevated in stage 1 is re-attached by tensing the tendon of tibialis posterior and reinforced by the tendon of tibialis anterior.

This technique allows good correction of the deformity and arthrodesis of the affected joints (Fig. 5). It is important to avoid being overambitious in the correction because, if the talus is elevated too much, stress is transferred in the ankle, which has usually lost the elasticity of the tibio-peroneal syndesmosis.

FOREFOOT

In rheumatoid arthritis, the forefoot is affected in a high percentage of cases, usually bilaterally. These are the joints which are most frequently involved and often constitute the first clinical manifestations of the disease, which makes it essential to pay special attention to them because of their value in early diagnosis. The metatarsophalangeal joints of the last four toes and the interphalangeal joint of the first toe are usually involved first.

In the advanced stages, typical deformities appear which Viladot[2] has classified into three types (Fig. 6).

Triangular forefoot. This is the commonest and has the following characteristics. In the first ray hallux-valgus is present with the great toe considerably deviated outwards and the first metatarsal in varus. In the fifth ray, the deformity is symmetrical. The fifth metatarsal is deviated outwards in valgus so that its head is very prominent on the lateral aspect of the foot. The fifth toe goes into varus. In the central rays, the toes may be deformed above or below the great toe. The metatarsophalangeal joints tend to be subluxed dorsally with the metatarsal heads becoming prominent in the plantar aspect of the foot, which causes significant mechanical metatarsalgia.

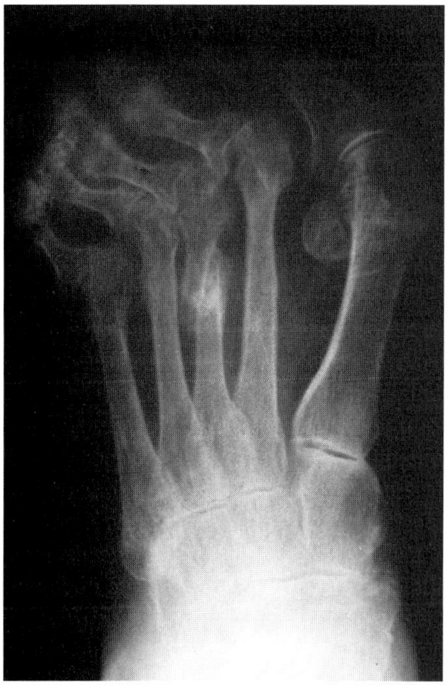

Fig. 5a

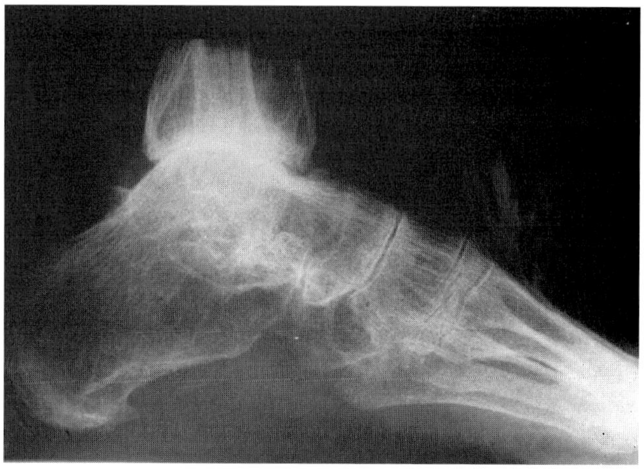

Fig. 5b

AP a) and lateral b) radiographs showing double arthrodesis in a patient affected with flat foot secondary to rheumatoid arthritis. Note the deformities and stress fracture of the forefoot.

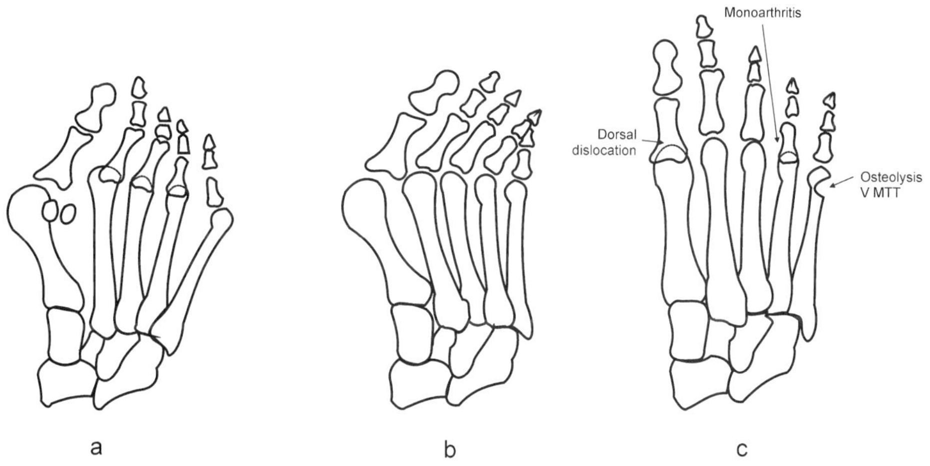

Fig. 6

Diagram showing types of forefoot in rheumatoid arthritis: a) triangular forefoot; b) *coup-de-vent* forefoot; c) atypical forms, monoarticular and polyarticular.

Forefoot in *coup-de-vent péronier*. In this deformity, all the toes are deviated outwards. The deviation is more accentuated in the great toe and decreases towards the lateral side where often the little toe is well aligned.

Atypical form. These are divided into two major groups, monoarticular and total. The former is described by Voutey and Strauss[3] and affects only one metatarsophalangeal joint. In most cases it represents an initial phase of the disease. Galmiche[4] highlights an erosion appearing in the neck of the fifth metatarsal, which is often the first radiological sign of rheumatoid arthritis. However, more severe forms may involve a significant deformity of the entire forefoot. The great toe remains aligned with the metatarsal although it may be subluxed dorsally or be clawed, and the lateral toes suffer totally random deformities.

In a study of 100 rheumatoid forefeet, we found 31% with triangular feet, 34% with *coup-de-vent* appearance, and 35% with the atypical form.[5,6] As regards the last, there were three cases of the monoarticular and 32 of the severe forms. Study of the metatarsal and digital formulae of these forefeet shows that in the triangular forefoot, a long, Egyptian-type great toe was associated with a short first

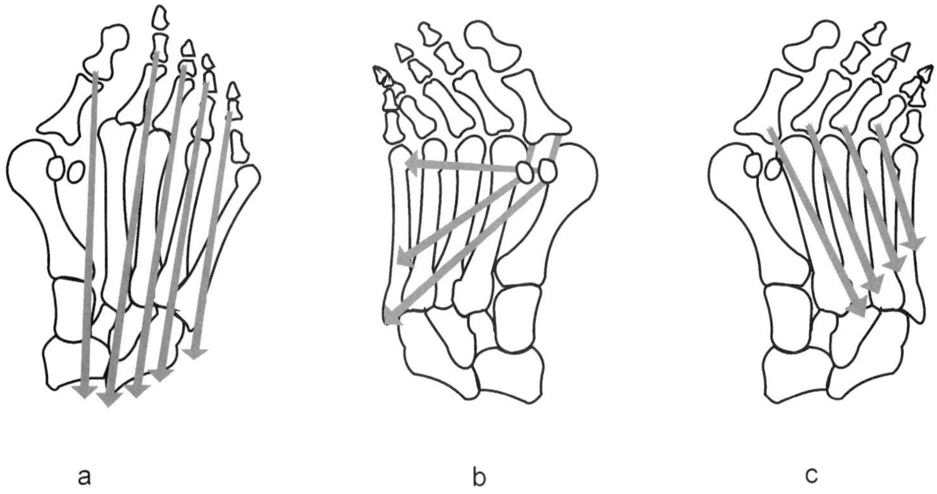

Fig. 7

Diagram showing mechanisms of deformity in the rheumatic forefoot: a) triangular forefoot, action of the long extensor of the toes; b) *coup-de-vent* forefoot, action of the abductor; and c) *coup-de-vent* forefoot, intrinsic contracture.

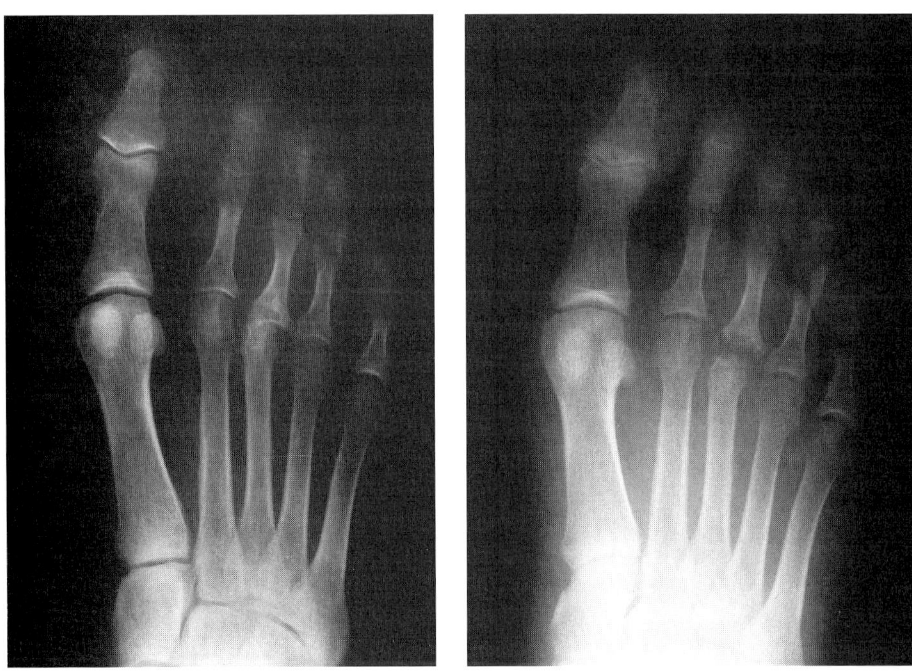

Fig. 8a Fig. 8b

Preoperative a) and postoperative b) radiographs of monoarthritis of the third metatarsophalangeal joint. Note the reduction of the subluxation and remodelling-alignment of the metatarsal head.

metatarsal (index-minus metatarsal formula). In the *coup-de-vent* forefoot, the great toe was also Egyptian, but associated with a powerful first metatarsal, index-plus or index-plus-minus type and in the atypical form, there was no relationship to the metatarsal or digital forms.

From these observations, we can deduce the mechanism of development of the different deformities (Fig. 7). The triangular forefoot is characterised by shortness of the first metatarsal, associated with atrophy of the intrinsic musculature. The metatarsals spread out in a fan-like fashion because of the atrophy of the intrinsic musculature of the first and fifth rays, and of the lumbricals and interossci. This allows predominance of the long flexor and extensor musculature of the first and fifth rays, which fixes the deformity by acting as a bowstring. The atrophy of the short muscles allowing dominance of the long muscles causes dorsal subluxation or dislocation of the middle toes, since the lumbricals and interossei are not powerful enough to keep the toes aligned with the metatarsals. The *coup-de-vent* foot is characterised by the strength of the first metatarsal, which stays in place without deviating into varus. The intrinsic musculature, unlike in the triangular foot, retains its power and keeps the forefoot closed. In this type of foot, the contracture of the short flexor and the abductor of the great toe, because of the rheumatoid disease, deviates the great toe into valgus and this in turn pushes the lateral toes out, giving the typical *coup-de-vent* deformity.

It should be highlighted that feet with a Greek-toe formation deform much less than Egyptian-type feet. We believe that this is explained by the fact that the former are less sensitive to the deforming effects of footwear.

OPERATIVE TREATMENT OF THE FOREFOOT

This has the fundamental aims of relieving pain and correcting deformities to allow the patient to use normal footwear and retain enough mobility to walk without limping.

The efficacy of synovectomies has been much discussed. Brattström[7] and Aho and Halonen[8] state that they give good results. We have had little experience and we believe that they are only indicated in cases of monoarticular involvement. When there is a dislocation of the metatarsophalangeal joint, we combine synovectomy with a remodelling alignment of the head of the metatarsal which allows us to reduce the dislocation (Fig. 8).

The first ray. In the arthritic foot hallux valgus is in most cases accompanied by major destruction of the metatarsophalangeal joint, and therefore, we believe that conservative surgery is not indicated.

There are three options for surgical treatment of the first ray: 1) resection-arthroplasty; 2) arthrodesis; and 3) arthroplasty with an implant.

Resection arthroplasty. We recommend performing the classic procedure of Keller[9] and Brandes[10] with resection of approximately 6 to 7 mm of the base of the first phalanx, which allows the change from an Egyptian digital configuration to the Greek. It is important that the joint remains flexible, preventing stiffness. To this end, if necessary, an associated lengthening of the extensor tendon will be required.

The resection should be associated with correction of the metatarsal varus, which is usually achieved by the capsuloplasty of Lelièvre.[11] In the case of highly accentuated metatarsal varus, an osteotomy may be necessary at the base of the first metatarsal or in the first cuneiform, or in the case of destruction of the cuneometatarsal joint, an arthrodesis.

The advantage of resection arthroplasty is that, because the mobility of the metatarsophalangeal joint is preserved, it allows walking in a more physiological manner. The drawback of the technique is that, because of evolution of the disease, there is a tendency to recurrence of the hallux valgus. This is why authors such as Hasselo et al,[12] McGarvey and Johnson,[13] Mann and Schakel[14] and Cracchiolo, De Stoop and Tilman[15] prefer arthrodesis of this joint.

Arthrodesis. With arthrodesis of the metatarsophalangeal joint, the deformity can be corrected and stabilised. It has the benefit that there is no risk of future recurrence, but the disadvantage is that it allows less physiological walking.

There are several techniques of arthrodesis but, as Mann and Thompson[16] state, creating two parallel flat surfaces encourages intrinsic stability. It is necessary to resect a sufficient amount of bone from the head of the metatarsal and the base of the phalanx so that the ray is not left too long. In this sense, the alignment of the lateral rays should be taken into account.

The final position of the hallux is also important. According to Raunio et al[17] it should be left in 15° of dorsiflexion in relation to the ground and 30° of dorsiflexion in relation to the metatarsal. In the horizontal plane, there should be 20° to 25° of valgus deviation.

Arthroplasty with an implant. Metatarsophalangeal implants constitute for some authors one of the surgical options for the treatment of deformities of the first ray, offering a valid alternative to resection arthroplasty and arthrodesis.

There are numerous techniques and models of implants. The most widely used are hemiarthroplasty with replacement of the articular surface of the proximal phalanx by metal or silicone implants, hemiarthroplasty with replacement of the articular surface of the metatarsal head by metal implants and, lastly, total arthroplasties with a metatarsal metal component and polyethylene in the phalanx. Nowadays the most widely used models in the rheumatoid forefoot are double-stem silicone implants. Since 1985, they have been modified to incorporate press-fit titanium grommets to protect the implant from shearing stresses.

The results obtained with the silicon implant can be considered as good (Cracchiolo et al[18] 84%, Moeckel et al[19] 87%). Most authors agree that the grommets are effective in protecting the implant from shearing stresses and preventing breaking, loosening and the appearance of synovitis due to particles. Some authors[20] have found no significant differ-

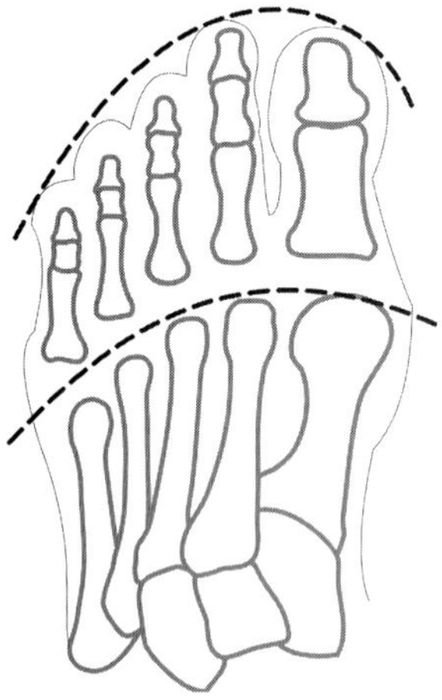

Fig. 9

Diagram showing the ideal forefoot.

ences in comparative series of patients submitted to resection-arthroplasty, arthrodesis and silicone implants. Probably one of the most important differences lies in the treatment options in cases of failure of the implant and of the resection arthroplasty: the conversion into arthrodesis is simpler after a resection arthroplasty.

The lateral rays. Resection arthroplasty of the four lateral rays of the foot is the surgical technique most commonly used for correction of deformities of the rheumatoid forefoot. It has been described with different modifications. Hoffman[21] proposed resection of the heads of the three central metatarsals in severe deformities of the toes. This has the drawback that, since it does not respect the correct metatarsal alignment, the patient develops an overloading of the head of the first and fifth metatarsals in the short term. Fowler[22] proposed plantar resection of the heads of the metatarsals, and of the base of the first phalanx dorsally. Clayton,[23] through a dorsal incision, removed all the metatarsophalangeal joints of the five rays. Kates, Kessel and Kay[24] proposed resection of the five metatarsal heads by a single plantar incision and Lipscomb, Benson and Sones[25] resection of the base of the proximal phalanxes and a plantar condylectomy of the metatarsals.

We recommend performing the metatarsal alignment as described by Lelièvre and Bertrand.[26] This intervention in the arthritic foot has a double aim. First, it restores the normal biomechanics of the forefoot by aiming for the ideal forefoot (Fig. 9), a Greek-type digital formula, with the great toe somewhat shorter than the second, since this is the form least vulnerable to the effects of footwear, and an index plus-minus metatarsal formula. Secondly, synovectomy and resection of diseased tissues are achieved.

The surgical technique is as follows (Fig. 10).

Stage 1. We use a wide transverse plantar incision which, starting in the space between the first and the second metatarsals, runs behind the digitoplantar sulcus towards the outer aspect of the foot. We do not consider it necessary to remove the hyperkeratosed skin, since later, when the increased pressure ceases, the callused areas disappear spontaneously.

Stage 2. We lower a wide flap of skin and subcutaneous tissue which occasionally includes large hygromas. These should be resected. Then a longitudinal incision along the side of the metatarsal head is made, with the aim of separating the flexor tendons and the neurovascular bundle running along its plantar aspect. Upon completion of this stage in all the metatarsals, forced dorsiflexion of the lateral four toes will allow the metatarsal heads to appear, with the tendons and the neurovascular bundle subluxed into the intermetatarsal space.

Stage 3. With a small chisel, we remove the prominences and the condyle from the plantar aspect of the metatarsal head (Du Vries condylectomy operation). Subsequent excision of the head of the metatarsal is then made easier and its true length can be seen more clearly.

Stage 4. Next the distal portion of the metatarsals is removed, taking care to align them correctly. It is necessary to check the correct alignment during the operation using an image intensifier. Once complete, the capsule is sutured, aligning the flexor apparatus beneath the metatarsal.

Stage 5. It is necessary to check if the dorsal dislocations or subluxations of the toes have been corrected. If any of the toes are still dislocated, a dorsal extensor tenotomy and capsulectomy is undertaken.

Stage 6. Next, we make an incision along the medial side of the foot, to expose the metatarsophalangeal joint of the great

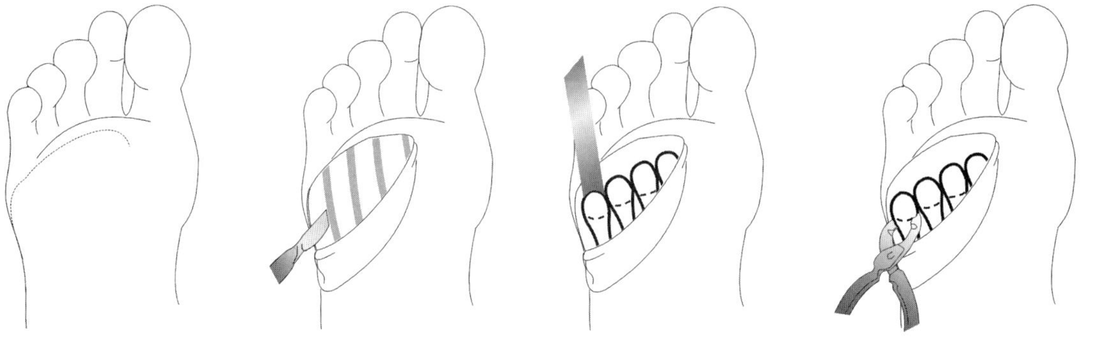

Fig. 10

Diagram showing the surgical stages of metatarsal alignment by the Lelièvre technique (see text).

toe. We perform a resection arthroplasty using the classic Brandes-Keller-Lelièvre techique, ensuring that the great toe is left 1 to 5 mm shorter than the second. If the first metatarsal is longer than the second, we shorten it to obtain an index plus-minus type formula (Fig. 11). We consider that the rheumatoid foot is one of the few situations when this procedure is justified.

Some authors prefer to perform an arthrodesis on the first ray. Vandeputte et al,[27] in a recent publication, made a comparative study between arthrodesis and alignment *versus* arthroplasty and alignment in polyarthritic patients and found no significant differences between the two groups, although the patients were subjectively more satisfied with the resection arthroplasty.

Stage 7. We close the skin of the two incisions and apply a compressive bandage.

Active and passive movements are mandatory from the first day and we allow weight-bearing from the second day.

THE ANKLE

In rheumatoid arthritis, the ankle is affected in 15% to 50% of cases and, in most patients, this is bilateral. Often, the involvement of the ankle is the determining factor in the patient's loss of mobility.

In cases of persistent synovitis when there is no significant radiological involvement, synovectomy may be useful, either open or by an arthroscopic approach. Similarly, there is the option of radioactive synovectomy, although there has been as yet no major experience of this in the ankle.

We usually find that when there is severe radiological involvement in these cases, there are only two options, arthrodesis or arthroplasty with total joint replacement.

Arthrodesis of the ankle. Until now, this has been the most widely used technique. It has the advantage of eliminating pain and, in cases in which the subtalar and Chopart joints are preserved, these compensate for 30% to 40% of the loss of movement of the ankle, thereby allowing fairly normal walking. It should be noted that the flexor-extensor capacity of the subtalar joint is around 25° and the ankle, in the support period of the walking cycle, has a range of movement from 5° dorsiflexion to 20° plantar flexion.

In rheumatoid arthritis, however, arthrodesis of the ankle has several disadvantages. Bilateral involvement may require an arthrodesis of both ankles, which is more incapacitating. Usually, when the ankle is affected, the subtalar and the Chopart joints are already also involved, and the arthrodesis loses its compensatory mechanisms. In such cases, the patient has to use footwear with a rocker-bottom sole. Because of the characteristic vasculitis and treatment with corticosteroids, there is a high incidence of necrosis of the body of the talus, making consolidation of the arthrodesis difficult. The severe osteopenia which also accompanies the disease makes it difficult to use synthetic materials to stabilise the arthrodesis. Both the disease and treatment with corticosteroids cause considerable fragility of the skin, which complicates healing of the wound and facilitates infection.

The most commonly used approaches are the anteromedial, medial to the tendon of anterior tibialis, and the anterolateral, lateral to the tendon of extensor digitorum longus. In either case, the state of the skin may require other approaches, such as posterior, lateral to tendo Achillis

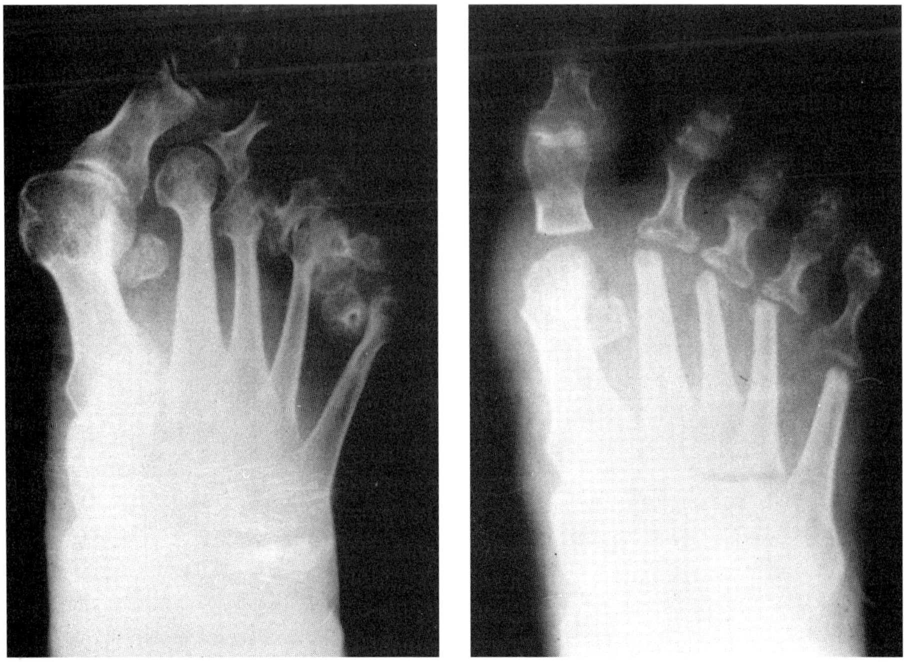

Fig. 11a Fig. 11b

Preoperative a) and postoperative b) radiographs of a rheumatoid forefoot. A Brandes-Keller-Lelièvre operation has been performed on the first ray and a metatarsal alignment on the lateral rays.

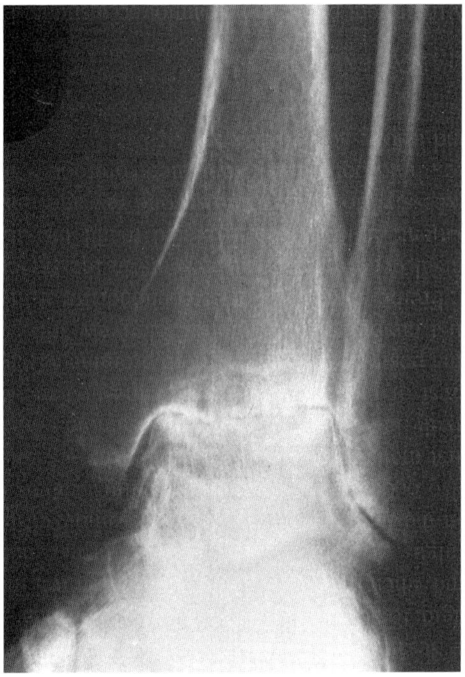

Fig. 12a

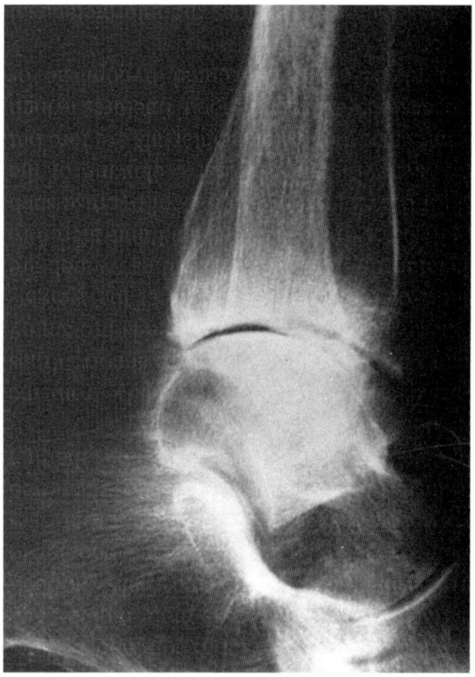

Fig. 12b

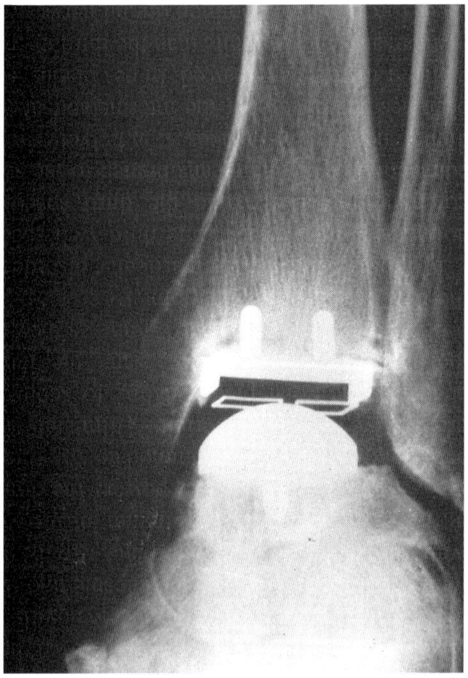

Fig. 12c

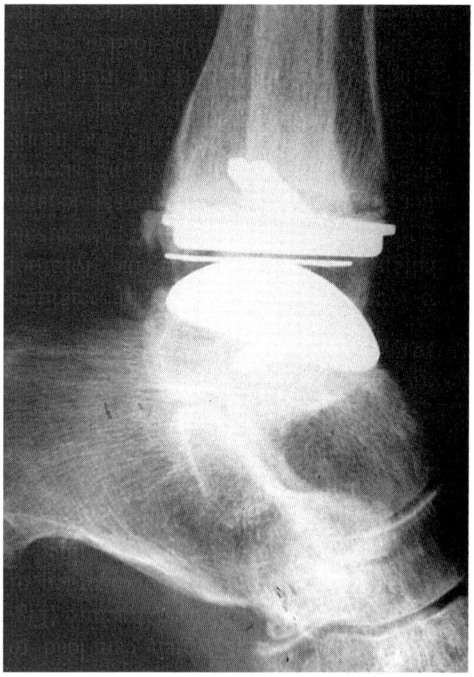

Fig. 12d

Preoperative AP (a) and lateral (b) and postoperative AP (c) and lateral (d) radiographs of a rheumatoid ankle, showing a total ankle prosthesis with three components.

or through it, or a combined medial and lateral technique, through the malleoli in cases of major deformity of the hindfoot.

In order to stabilise the arthrodesis, the most widely used method of osteosynthesis is by two compression screws, although plates and screws, external fixators and percutaneous Steinmann pins can also be used.

In cases in which there is necrosis of the body of the talus, it is advisable to perform a sliding graft from the anterior aspect of the tibia, which is impacted between the neck and the head of the talus. These bones are of better quality and therefore bony consolidation is more likely.

As indicated by King, Watkins and Samuelson,[28] at the end of the operation the ankle should be in a neutral position, without equinus or dorsiflexion, with the heel in about 7° valgus and the foot in 10° of external rotation. In cases in which there is arthrodesis of the tarsus, some authors, such as Cracchiolo et al[15] recommend leaving around 5° of dorsiflexion so that, for instance, standing up from a chair is easier.

Total ankle replacement. In the 1970s, encouraged by positive results obtained with hip and knee implants, the first ankle implants appeared. It is worth highlighting Lord and Marotte,[29] Buchholz, Engelbrecht and Siegel,[30] Freeman et al[31] and Newton.[32] This type of surgery initially appeared to offer several benefits over arthrodesis since in addition to relieving the pain, it preserved articular movement in patients who were already seriously restricted by the polyarticular nature of the disease. This has particular importance in patients with both ankles affected with the consequent transfer of stress to the knees.

Although in the short term the results of the operation appeared promising,[33,34] most authors agree that the results deteriorate at medium- and long-term follow-up.[35-38]

The commonest complications of implants are aseptic loosening, slow healing of the wounds, deep infection and talofibular impingement.

Unconstrained implants, concave-convex in shape allow greater mobility, but present less resistance to wear and deformity, and may have problems of stability.

Constrained implants, cylindrical in shape, have less mobility and greater stability, but they generate major stress at the fixation of the implant to the bone, which leads to loosening.

In an attempt to address these problems three-part implants are currently used. They are inserted with a polyethylene meniscus (Fig. 12), and offer a series of theoretical benefits. They increase the contact surface between the tibial and talar components, thereby enhancing the stability of the implant. The different thicknesses of the polyethylene allow adequate tension of the ligaments, ensuring stability and mobility of the implant. The movement between the different components absorbs the stresses in the attachment of the implant to the bone, and allows mobility of the ankle in different planes.

We believe that the results are improved by using this type of implant. Thus, Buechel, Pappas and Iorio[39] using the LCS implant, achieved a survival rate of 95% at ten years and Kofoed and Sorenson[40] using the STAR implant, 75% at ten years in patients with rheumatoid arthritis. Mandolia,[41] using the RAMSES implant, in its initial stages had good results in 74% of patients at five years.

We believe that patients with rheumatoid arthritis may require ankle replacement for two major reasons. First, bilateral involvement makes arthrodesis of both ankles necessary and this is very incapacitating. Secondly, when there is destruction of the ankle there is usually significant involvement of the subtalar and the Chopart joints, and thus the arthrodesis loses its compensating mechanisms.

In order to be able to perform this type of operation, apart from an acceptable quality of the skin and local blood supply, there must be enough malleolar bone stock to allow the introduction of a stable implant, and no deformities of the plantar arch. If these are present, usually in flat valgus feet, they must be corrected before insertion of a total prosthesis.

In the event of failure of the implant, arthrodesis may be performed.

ORTHOTIC TREATMENT

Conservative orthopaedic treatment is indicated in the initial stages of the disease, when the deformities are incipient and reducible, in those patients in whom surgery is contraindicated for medical reasons, in patients who reject surgical procedures, and lastly as a complement to surgery to prevent recurrent deformity and to provide the patient with greater comfort.

The aim of treatment with an orthosis is to relieve pain and to assist walking. To this end, the areas of increased pressure caused by bony prominences should be relieved using soft leather insoles, cut widely at the dorsal aspect of the foot. The shoe should also be provided with orthotic complements which as far as possible prevent mobilisation of the affected joints during walking.

Frequent use is made of orthopaedic devices for the forefoot and the toes, orthopaedic insoles, standard shoes with modifications and orthopaedic shoes.

Orthopaedic devices for the forefoot and the toes. These may be prefabricated or made-to-measure.

Prefabricated devices. These are very varied and can be bought in chemists and orthopaedic outlets. Some of the most widely used are protective rings and discs, which are applied to treat the pain of dorsal calluses of the middle toes; discs for hard patches on the sole, which are the result of overloading of the central metatarsals; interdigital discs and rings for interdigital hyperkeratoses caused by lateral deviations of the toes causing lesions such as the 'partridge eye', the 'kiss callus', etc; toe spacers made of materials of different consistency; and elastic metatarsal supports when there is excess separation of the metatarsals (splayed feet) and for maintaining correction in the postoperative period after surgery on the forefoot.

Made-to-measure devices. These have similar aims and indications as prefabricated devices. Single-component or dual-component silicones are used in their manufacture. The former are rubbery in consistency and the latter are rigid to a greater or less extent, depending on the amount of catalyst used when the mixture is setting.[42]

It is useful for the surgeon to bear these ortheses in mind since on many occasions they can help to resolve minor, yet troublesome, problems.

Orthopaedic insoles. These have three main aims as follows.

To correct the deformity of the foot. This is only possible in the initial stages of the disease. The developing deformities follow the laws of gravity, and the rheumatoid foot adopts the shape of a flat foot with valgus of the heel. A well-fitted, rigid insole is necessary to prevent the deformity progressing and to maintain correction.[43] Therefore soft insoles are not indicated.[44]

To immobilise painful joints of the hindfoot. Rigid plantar supports are also needed for this.

To redistribute the load. This is done by reducing the pressure on the painful areas. With this aim, special elements are incorporated into the surface of the insole. Depending on the type of discharge, the insoles may therefore have a retrocapital bar, a central pad, a notch under the head of the first or a central metatarsal, or an extension beneath the first or central metatarsals.

Insoles for the rheumatoid foot must have a rigid base since their initial aim is to provide firm support for the longitudinal and transverse arches of the foot. On this rigid base, the necessary elements are incorporated for the protection and support of specific areas.

Insoles must be made to measure. To do this, as a general rule, a negative plaster cast is made and a positive mould is made from this. Modifications are then made for each specific insole.

Computer-based studies of the plantar pressures during walking help to make a correct assessment of the efficacy of the insoles.

The use of orthopaedic insoles is common in rheumatoid patients and helpful in the postoperative period to maintain correction.

Footwear. This is an important aspect in patients with rheumatoid problems in the feet. Footwear has evolved greatly over the last two decades.[45] 'Seamless' shoes are no longer used and have been substituted by shoes in 'plastazote,' a material which, using heat, can be fitted specifically for each foot.[46] A number of manufacturers of sports footwear have designed models for arthritic feet, with good acceptance by patients.

Whenever possible, the patient should use standard footwear, to which the necessary modifications to the heel and the sole can be made.[47] A shock-absorbing element is inserted into the heel and a rocker, of which there are different types, into the sole to limit the mobility of the ankle and the metatarsophalangeal joints, thereby assisting walking.[48]

Orthopaedic or made-to-measure footwear should have three essential qualities. It must be light, well-fitting and as attractive as possible.[49] To achieve lightweight footwear, appropriate materials must be used. The fit must be precise, with sufficient width at the back, to prevent decubitus and ulceration. Lastly, the look is very important, and is the main cause of rejection, particularly by women. Efforts should be made to provide an acceptable shoe and to offer the patient the choice of a different model.

REFERENCES

1. **Viladot A.** Nouvelle technique pour le traitement chirurgical du pie-plat-valgus essentiel. *Cah Chir* 1966;16:8-75.
2. **Viladot R.** Tratamiento quirúrgico de la artritis. *Rev Esp Reum Enf Osteo* 1971;XIV:3:216.
3. **Voutey H, Strauss J.** Synovites subbaigües chroniques des articulations métatarso-phalangiennes. *Podologie* 1973;9:157.
4. **Galmiche FC.** *Thése de médicine.* Paris, 1972.
5. **Viladot A.** *Patologia del antepié.* Barcelona: Ediciones Toray, SA, 1975.
6. **Viladot A Jr, Viladot R.** Biomécanique de l'avant-pied rhumatoide en. In: Claustre J, Simon L, eds. *Le pied en practique rhumatologique: pathologie articulaire.* Paris: Masson, 1983.
7. **Brattström H.** Synovektomien in metatarsophalangealgelenken. *Orthopäde* 1973;2:81.
8. **Aho H, Halonen P.** Synovectomy of MTP joints in rheumatoid arthritis. *Acta Orthop Scand* 1991;61 Suppl 243:1.
9. **Keller WL.** The surgical treatment of bunions and hallux valgus. *N Y Med J* 1904;80:741-2.
10. **Brandes M.** Zur operativen Bahandlung des Hallux valgus. *Zentralbl Chir* 1929;56:2434-40.
11. **Lelièvre J.** *Pathologie du pied.* Paris:Masson et Cie, 1967.
12. **Hasselo LG, Willkens RF, Toomey HE, Karges DE, Hansen ST.** Forefoot surgery in rheumatoid arthritis: subjective assessment of outcomes. *Foot Ankle* 1987;8:148-51.
13. **McGarvey SR, Johnson KA.** Keller arthroplasty in combination with resection arthroplasty of the lesser metatarsophalangeal joints in rheumatoid arthritis. *Foot Ankle* 1988;9:75-80.
14. **Mann RA, Schakel ME 2nd.** Surgical correction of rheumatoid forefoot deformities. *Foot Ankle Int* 1995;16:1-6.
15. **Cracchiolo A, De Stoop N, Tilman K.** The rheumatoid foot and ankle. In: Helal B, Rowley D, Cracchilo A III, Myerson MS, eds. *Surgery of disorders of the foot and ankle.* London: Martin Dunitz, 1996.
16. **Mann RA, Thompson FM.** Arthrodesis of the first metatarso-phalangeal joint for hallux valgus in rheumatoid arthritis. *J Bone Joint Surg [Am]* 1984;66-A:687-92.
17. **Raunio P, Lehtimäki M, Eerola M, Hämäläinen M, Pulkki T.** Resection arthroplasty versus arthrodesis of the first metatarsophalangeal joint for hallux valgus in rheumatoid arthritis. *Rheumatology* 1987;11:173-8.
18. **Cracchiolo A, Weltmer JB Jr, Lian G, Dalseth T, Dorey F.** Letter. Arthroplasty of the first metatarsophalangeal joint with a double-stem silicone implant: results in patients who have degenerative joint disease failure of previous operations, or rheumatoid arthritis. *J Bone Joint Surg [Am]* 1993;75-A:1254-5.
19. **Moeckel BH, Sculco TP, Alexiades MM, et al.** The double-stemmed silicone-rubber implant for rheumatoid arthritis of the first metatarso-phalangeal joint: long-term results. *J Bone Joint Surg [Am]* 1992;74-A:564-70.
20. **Clayton ML, Leidholt JD, Clark W.** Arthroplasty of rheumatoid metatarsophalangeal joints: an outcome study. *Clin Orthop* 1997;340:48-57.
21. **Hoffman P.** An operation for severe grades of contracted or clawed toes. *Am J Orthop Surg* 1911;9:441-9.
22. **Fowler AW.** A method of forefoot reconstruction. *J Bone Joint Surg [Br]* 1959;41-B:507-13.
23. **Clayton ML.** Surgery of the forefoot in rheumatoid arthritis. *Clin Orthop* 1960;16:136-40.
24. **Kates A, Kessel L, Kay A.** Arthroplasty of the forefoot. *J Bone Joint Surg [Br]* 1967;49-B:552-7.
25. **Lipscomb PR, Benson GM, Sones DA.** Resection of proximal phalanges and metatarsal condyles for deformities of the forefoot due to rheumatoid arthritis. *Clin Orthop* 1972;82:24-31.
26. **Lelièvre J, Bertrand M.** La réconstruction de l'avant-pied par l'alignement articulaire. *Podologie* 1963;II:93.
27. **Vandeputte G, Steenwerckx A, Mulier T, Peeraer L, Dereymaeker G.** Forefoot reconstruction in rheumatoid arthritis patients: Keller-Lelièvre-Hoffmann versus arthrodesis MTP1-Hoffman. *Foot Ankle Int* 1999;20:438-43.
28. **King HA, Watkins TB Jr, Samuelson KM.** Analysis of foot position in ankle arthrodesis and its influence on gait. *Foot Ankle* 1980;1:44-9.
29. **Lord G, Marotte JH.** Prothése totale de cheville. *Rev Chir Orthop* 1973;59:239-51.
30. **Buchholz H, Engelbrecht E, Siegel M.** Total ankle endoprosthesis. *St Georg Mod Chirurg* 1973;44:241-4.

31. **Freeman MAR, Kempson GE, Tuke MA, et al.** Total replacement of the ankle with the ICLH prosthesis. *Int Orthop* 1979;2:327-31.

32. **Newton E.** An artificial ankle joint. *Clin Orthop* 1979;142:141-5.

33. **Staufer RM, Segal NM.** Total ankle arthroplasty: four years' experience. *Clin Orthop* 1981;160:217-21.

34. **Viladot A Jr.** La prótesis total de tobillo: aternativa a la artrodesis? *Chir piede* 1986;10:61-5.

35. **Bolton-Maggs BG, Sudrow RA, Freeman MAR.** Total ankle arthroplasty: a long-term review of the London Hospital experience. *J Bone Joint Surg [Br]* 1985;67-B:785-90.

36. **Newton E.** Total ankle arthroplasty: clinical study of fifty cases. *J Bone Joint Surg [Am]* 1982;64-A:104-11.

37. **Kitaoka HB, Patzer GL.** Clinical results of the Mayo total ankle arthroplasty. *J Bone Joint Surg [Am]* 1996;78-A:1658-64.

38. **Viladot A.** Tratamiento dc la artrosis del tobillo mediante endoprótesis. *Rev Ort Traum* 1996;40:389-96.

39. **Buechel FF, Pappas MJ, Iorio LI.** New Jersey low contact stress total ankle replacement: biomechanical rationale and review of 23 cementless cases. *Foot Ankle* 1988;8:279-90.

40. **Kofoed H, Sorensen T.** Ankle arthroplasty for rheumatoid arthritis and osteoarthritis: prospective long-term study of cemented replacements. *J Bone Joint Surg [Br]* 1988;80-B:328-32.

41. **Mandolia G.** Ankle arthroplasty: the RAMSES prosthesis. In: Kofoed H, ed. *Current status of ankle arthroplasty.* Berlin: Springer-Verlag, 1998.

42. **Viladot R, Cohi O, Clavell S.** *Ortesis y prótesis del aparato locomotor. 2.1. Extremidad inferior.* Barcelona:Masson, 1987.

43. **Bowman GD CO, MBAPO.** New concepts in orthotic management of the adult hyperpronated foot: preliminary findings. *J Prosthet Orthot* 1997;9:77-81.

44. **Dennis A, Lavigne A.** *Une nouvelle orthese plantaire antialgique: reunion provinciale de la Société Francaise de Medicine et Chirurgie du Pied.* Niza, 1976.

45. **Dixon A, St J.** Management of the rheumatoid foot (with special reference to footwear and appliances). In: *The advances in orthotics.* Ed. George Murdoch, London:Edward Arnold, 1976:505-11.

46. **Viladot R, Cohi O, Olivella S.** Calzado ortopédico para pacientes poliartríticos. *La técnica ortopédico* 1980;III-3:81-3.

47. **Baungartner R, Stinus L.** *Tratamiento ortésico-protésico del pie.* Barcelona:Masson, 1997.

48. **Baehler A-R.** *Técnica ortopédica: indicaciones. Tomo I. Biomecánica extremidad inferior.* Barcelona:Masson, 1999.

49. **Claustre J, Simon L.** Le chaussage du pied rhumatoide. In: de Claustre J, Simon L, eds. *Le pied en practique rhumatologique Pathologie articulaire.* Monographies de podologie, Paris:Masson, 1983.